OPERATIVE TECHNIQUES IN BREAST, ENDOCRINE, AND ONCOLOGIC SURGERY

OPERATIVE TECHNIQUES IN BREAST, ENDOCRINE, AND ONCOLOGIC SURGERY

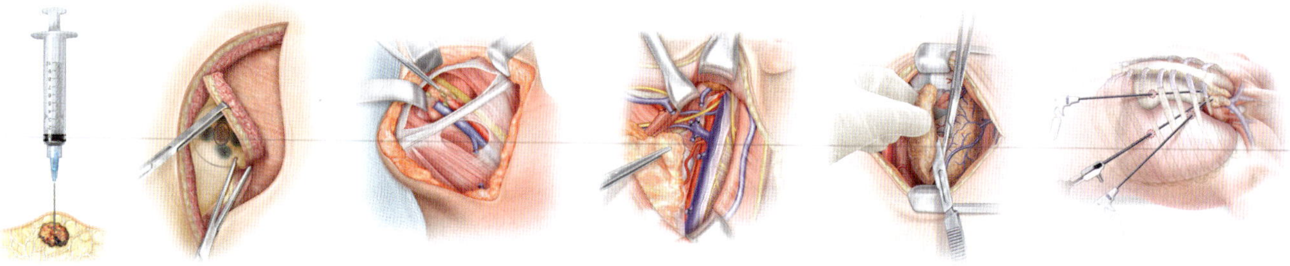

Michael S. Sabel, MD

EDITOR

Chief, Division of Surgical Oncology
Associate Professor of Surgery
University of Michigan Health System
Ann Arbor, Michigan

Michael W. Mulholland, MD, PhD

EDITOR-IN-CHIEF

Professor of Surgery and Chair
Department of Surgery
University of Michigan Medical School
Ann Arbor, Michigan

Illustrations by: BodyScientific International, LLC

Wolters Kluwer

Philadelphia • Baltimore • New York • London
Buenos Aires • Hong Kong • Sydney • Tokyo

Acquisitions Editor: Keith Donnellan
Product Development Editor: Brendan Huffman
Production Project Manager: David Saltzberg
Design Coordinator: Doug Smock
Senior Manufacturing Manager: Beth Welsh
Marketing Manager: Daniel Dressler
Prepress Vendor: Absolute Service, Inc.

9 8 7 6 5 4 3 2 1

Printed in China

Library of Congress Cataloging-in-Publication Data

Operative techniques in breast, endocrine, and oncologic surgery / editor, Michael S. Sabel ; editor-in-chief, Michael W. Mulholland.
p. ; cm.
Includes bibliographical references and index.
ISBN 978-1-4511-9021-2 (alk. paper)
I. Sabel, Michael S., editor. II. Mulholland, Michael W., editor. III. Operative techniques in surgery. Contained in (work):
[DNLM: 1. Breast Neoplasms—surgery. 2. Endocrine Surgical Procedures—methods. 3. Mammaplasty—methods. 4. Melanoma—surgery. WP 870]
RD32
617.9—dc23

2015004607

LWW.com

RRS1503

Dedication

To my wonderful wife, Janeel, and our three beautiful children,
Alex, Madison, and Lauren. Their love and understanding when
family time needed to be compromised is appreciated.
Also to my parents, Steven and Rhoda.
Without their support, none of this would be possible.

—Michael S. Sabel

Contributing Authors

Amy K. Alderman, MD, MPH
Plastic Surgeon
Researcher
Breast Reconstruction
The Swan Center for Plastic Surgery
Alpharetta, Georgia

Benjamin O. Anderson, MD, FACS
Director
Breast Health Clinic
Seattle Cancer Care Alliance
Professor of Surgery and Global Health Medicine
University of Washington
Seattle, Washington

Peter Angelos, MD, PhD
Linda Kohler Anderson Professor of Surgery and Surgical Ethics
Chief
Endocrine Surgery
Associate Director
MacLean Center for Clinical Medical Ethics
The University of Chicago Medicine
Chicago, Illinois

Saïd C. Azoury, MD
Resident
The Johns Hopkins Hospital
Baltimore, Maryland

Jonathan Bank, MD
Department of Surgery
Division of Medicine and Biological Sciences
Section of Plastic and Reconstructive Surgery
The University of Chicago
Chicago, Illinois

Peter D. Beitsch, MD, FACS
Director
Dallas Breast Center
Dallas, Texas

Russell S. Berman, MD
Chief
Division of Surgical Oncology
Program Director
General Surgery
Residency
Associate Professor
Department of Surgery
New York University School of Medicine
New York, New York

Judy C. Boughey, MD
Associate Professor of Surgery
Department of Surgery
Mayo Clinic
Rochester, Minnesota

David L. Brown, MD, FACS
Associate Professor of Surgery
Section of Plastic Surgery
University of Michigan Health System
Ann Arbor, Michigan

Kristine E. Calhoun, MD
Associate Professor
Department of Surgery
University of Washington School of Medicine
Breast Health Clinic, Seattle Cancer Care Alliance
Seattle, Washington

Glenda G. Callender, MD, FACS
Assistant Professor
Department of Surgery
Section of Endocrine Surgery
Director
Endocrine Surgical Oncology Clinical Trials
Yale School of Medicine
New Haven, Connecticut

Anees B. Chagpar, MD, MSc, MPH, MA
Director
The Breast Center—Smilow Cancer Hospital at Yale-New Haven
Associate Professor
Department of Surgery
Yale School of Medicine
New Haven, Connecticut

Amy S. Colwell, MD, FACS
Assistant Professor
Harvard Medical School
Division of Plastic Surgery
Massachusetts General Hospital
Boston, Massachusetts

Amy C. Degnim, MD
Associate Professor of Surgery
Consultant
Division of Subspecialty General Surgery
Department of Surgery
Mayo Clinic
Rochester, Minnesota

Vasu Divi, MD
Assistant Professor
Department of Otolaryngology
Division of Head and Neck Surgery
Stanford University
Stanford, California

Gerard M. Doherty, MD
Surgeon-in-Chief
Boston Medical Center
Utley Professor
Chair
Surgery
Boston University
Boston, Massachusetts

Frank Fang, MD
Department of Surgery
Section of Plastic Surgery
Resident
Section of Plastic Surgery
University of Michigan Health System
Ann Arbor, Michigan

Amy C. Fox, MD
Endocrine Surgeon
Regions Hospital
St. Paul, Minnesota

Douglas L. Fraker, MD, FACS
Jonathan E. Rhoads Professor of Surgical Science
Vice Chairman
Research
Chief
Division of Endocrine and Oncologic Surgery
Department of Surgery
Deputy Director
Clinical Services
Abramson Cancer Center
Penn Medicine: University of Pennsylvania Health System
Philadelphia, Pennsylvania

Paul G. Gauger, MD
Professor
Endocrine Surgeon
A. Alfred Taubman Health Care Center
University of Michigan Health System
Ann Arbor, Michigan

Jeffrey E. Gershenwald, MD
Professor
Department of Surgical Oncology
Division of Surgery
Medical Director
Melanoma and Skin Center
The University of Texas MD Anderson Cancer Center
Houston, Texas

Joseph S. Giglia, MD, FACS
Associate Professor of Surgery
Department of Surgery
Division of Vascular Surgery
University of Cincinnati
Cincinnati, Ohio

Raymon H. Grogan, MD
Assistant Professor
Department of Surgery
Section of General Surgery
Director
Endocrine Surgery Research Program
Pritzker School of Medicine
University of Chicago
Chicago, Illinois

Steven C. Haase, MD
Associate Professor
Department of Surgery
Section of Plastic Surgery
University of Michigan Health System
Ann Arbor, Michigan

Eric G. Halvorson, MD
Assistant Professor of Surgery
Harvard Medical School
Division of Plastic Surgery
Brigham and Women's Hospital
Boston, Massachusetts

Jean-François Henry, MD, FRCS
Professor of Surgery
Consultant
Department of Endocrine Surgery
University-Hospital La Timone
Marseilles, France

Oscar E. Imhof, EKP/ECCP
Clinical Perfusionist
Heartbeat
University Medical Center of Utrecht
Utrecht, The Netherlands

William B. Inabnet, III, MD
The Mount Sinai Hospital
Eugene W. Friedman Professor of Surgery
Chief
Division of Metabolic, Endocrine and Minimally Invasive Surgery
The Mount Sinai Hospital
New York, New York

James W. Jakub, MD
Section Head
Breast and Melanoma Surgery
Division of Gastroenterologic and General Surgery
Department of Surgery
Mayo Clinic
Rochester, Minnesota

Michael G. Johnston, MD
Department of Surgery
Division of Gastrointestinal and Endocrine Surgery
Columbia University College of Physicians and Surgeons
New York, New York

Edwin L. Kaplan, MD
Professor
Department of Surgery
Section of General Surgery
Pritzker School of Medicine
University of Chicago
Chicago, Illinois

Cary S. Kaufman, MD, FACS
Associate Clinical Professor of Surgery
University of Washington
Bellingham Regional Breast Center
Bellingham, Washington

Michael Kim, MD
Fellow in Surgical Oncology
The University of Texas MD Anderson Cancer Center
Houston, Texas

Jeffrey H. Kozlow, MD, MS
Clinical Assistant Professor
Section of Plastic Surgery
University of Michigan Health System
Ann Arbor, Michigan

Bin B.R. Kroon, MD, PhD, FRCS
Emeritus Professor of Surgery
Skin and Melanoma Center
Department of Surgery
The Netherlands Cancer Institute
Amsterdam, The Netherlands

Anita R. Kulkarni, MD
Memorial Sloan Kettering Cancer Center
Section of Plastic Surgery
New York, New York

Anna Kundel, MD
Department of Surgery
Mayo Clinic
Rochester, Minnesota

James A. Lee, MD
Assistant Professor of Clinical Surgery
Department of Surgery
Division of Gastrointestinal and Endocrine Surgery
Chief
Endocrine Surgery
Columbia University College of Physicians and Surgeons
New York, New York

A. Marilyn Leitch, MD
Professor of Surgery
Division of Surgical Oncology
The University of Texas Southwestern Medical Center
Dallas, Texas

Valerie Lemaine, MD, MPH, FRCSC
Assistant Professor of Plastic Surgery
Vice Chair for Research
Department of Surgery
Division of Plastic Surgery
Mayo Clinic
Rochester, Minnesota

Catherine A. Madorin, MD
Department of Surgery
General Surgery
Association of South Bay Surgeons
Torrance, California

Gabriele Materazzi, MD
Department of Surgery
University of Pisa
Pisa, Italy

Christopher R. McHenry, MD
Vice Chairman
Department of Surgery
MetroHealth System
Professor of Surgery
Case Western Reserve University School of Medicine
Cleveland, Ohio

Scott A. McLean, MD, PhD
Assistant Professor
Department of Otolaryngology–Head and Neck Surgery
University of Michigan Health System
Ann Arbor, Michigan

Kelly M. McMasters, MD, PhD
Ben A. Reid, Sr., MD Professor and Chairman
Hiram C. Polk, Jr., MD Department of Surgery
University of Louisville School of Medicine
Louisville, Kentucky

Claire W. Michael, MD
Professor of Pathology
Director
Clinical Research Program and Faculty Career Development
Director
Cytopathology Fellowship
Department of Pathology
Case Western Reserve University
University Hospitals Case Medical Center
Cleveland, Ohio

Paolo Miccoli, MD, FACS
Department of Surgery
University of Pisa
Pisa, Italy

Barbra S. Miller, MD
Staff Physician
Assistant Professor
Department of Surgery
Division of Endocrine Surgery
University of Michigan Health System
Ann Arbor, Michigan

Adeyiza O. Momoh, MD
Department of Surgery
Clinical Assistant Professor of Surgery
Section of Plastic Surgery
University of Michigan Health System
Ann Arbor, Michigan

Maurice Y. Nahabedian, MD, FACS
Department of Plastic Surgery
Georgetown University
Washington, DC

Lisa Newman, MD, MPH, FACS
Director
University of Michigan Breast Care Center
Professor of Surgery
University of Michigan Health System
Ann Arbor, Michigan

Omgo E. Nieweg, MD, PhD
Surgeon
Melanoma Institute Australia
The Poche Centre
North Sydney, Australia

Barnard J. A. Palmer, MD, MEd
Assistant Clinical Professor of Surgery
Department of Surgery
UCSF East Bay Surgery Program
Oakland, California

Judy C. Pang, MD
Assistant Professor
Department of Pathology
University of Michigan Health System
Ann Arbor, Michigan

Julie E. Park, MD
Assistant Professor of Surgery
Director
Breast Reconstruction
Associate Program Director
Department of Surgery
Division of Medicine and Biological Sciences
Section of Plastic and Reconstructive Surgery
University of Chicago
Chicago, Illinois

Ketan M. Patel, MD
Assistant Professor of Surgery
Division of Plastic and Reconstructive Surgery
Keck School of Medicine of USC
Los Angeles, California

Richard A. Prinz, MD
Department of Surgery
Surgery Oncology
NorthShore University Health System
Evanston, Illinois

Andrea L. Pusic, MD, MHS
Department of Surgery
Section of Plastic Surgery
Memorial Sloan Kettering Cancer Center
New York, New York

Emily B. Ridgway, MD
Division of Plastic Surgery
Dartmouth-Hitchcock Medical Center
Lebanon, New Hampshire
Instructor in Surgery
Geisel School of Medicine at Dartmouth
Hanover, New Hampshire

Merrick I. Ross, MD
Charles A. McBride Professor of Surgical Oncology
Chief of the Melanoma Section
Department of Surgical Oncology
The University of Texas MD Anderson Cancer Center
Charles McBride
Houston, Texas

Michael S. Sabel, MD
Chief, Division of Surgical Oncology
Associate Professor of Surgery
University of Michigan Health System
Ann Arbor, Michigan

Amod A. Sarnaik, MD
Assistant Member
Department of Cutaneous Oncology
H. Lee Moffitt Cancer Center and Research Institute
Assistant Professor
Department of Oncologic Sciences
University of South Florida Health Morsani College of Medicine
Tampa, Florida

Brian D. Saunders, MD
Assistant Professor of Surgery and Medicine
Department of Surgery
Penn State Milton S. Hershey Medical Center
Penn State College of Medicine
Hershey, Pennsylvania

Ashok R. Shaha, MD
Attending Surgeon
Jatin P. Shah Chair
Head and Neck Service
Department of Surgery
Memorial Sloan Kettering Cancer Center
New York, New York

Andrew G. Shuman, MD
Surgical Fellow
Head and Neck Service
Department of Surgery
Memorial Sloan Kettering Cancer Center
New York, New York

Rache Simmons, MD
Chief
Breast Surgery
Department of Surgery
Weill Cornell Medical College
New York, New York

Vernon K. Sondak, MD
Chair
Department of Cutaneous Oncology
H. Lee Moffitt Cancer Center and Research Institute
Professor
Departments of Surgery and Oncologic Sciences
University of South Florida Health Morsani College of Medicine
Tampa, Florida

David H. Song, MD, MBA, FACS
Cynthia Chow Professor
Chief
Plastic and Reconstructive Surgery
Vice Chairman
Department of Surgery
Division of Medicine and Biological Sciences
University of Chicago
Chicago, Illinois

Jeffrey J. Sussman, MD, FACS
Professor
Director
Department of Surgery
Division of Surgical Oncology
University of Cincinnati
Cincinnati, Ohio

Geoffrey B. Thompson, MD
Subspecialty General Surgery
Department of Surgery
Mayo Clinic
Rochester, Minnesota

Tiffany A. Torstenson, DO
Breast Surgical Oncology Fellow
Department of Surgery
Mayo Clinic
Rochester, Minnesota

Eleni Tousimis, MD, FACS
Chief
Breast Surgery
President
American Medical Women's Association
MedStar Georgetown University Hospital
Washington, DC

Dale Collins Vidal, MD, MS
Professor of Surgery
Geisel School of Medicine at Dartmouth
Chief
Plastic Surgery
Director
Center for Shared Decision Making
Dartmouth-Hitchcock
Hanover, New Hampshire

Sebastian Winocour, MD, MSc, FRCSC
Resident
Department of Surgery
Division of Plastic Surgery
Mayo Clinic
Rochester, Minnesota

Martha A. Zeiger, MD, FACS, FACE
Professor of Surgery
Department of Surgery
Chief of Oncology, Cellular, and Molecular Medicine
Section of Endocrine Surgery
Johns Hopkins University School of Medicine
Baltimore, Maryland

Series Preface

Operative therapy is complex, technically demanding, and rapidly evolving. Although there are a number of standard textbooks that cover aspects of general, thoracic, vascular, or transplant surgery, *Operative Techniques in Surgery* is unique in offering a comprehensive treatment of contemporary procedures. Open operations, laparoscopic procedures, and newly described robotic approaches are all included. Where alternative or complementary approaches exist, all are provided. The scope and ambition of the project is one of a kind.

The series is organized anatomically in sections covering thoracic surgery, upper gastrointestinal surgery, hepatopancreatico-biliary surgery, and colorectal surgery. Breast surgery, endocrine surgery, and topics related to surgical oncology are included in a separate volume. Modern approaches to vascular surgery and transplantation surgery are also covered in separate volumes.

The series editors are renowned surgeons with expertise in their respective fields. Each is a leader in the discipline of surgery, each recognized for superb surgical judgment and outstanding operative skill. Breast surgery, endocrine procedures, and surgical oncology topics were edited by Dr. Michael Sabel of the University of Michigan. Thoracic and upper gastrointestinal surgery topics were edited by Dr. Mary Hawn of the University of Alabama at Birmingham, with Dr. Steven Hughes of the University of Florida directing the volume on hepato-pancreatico-biliary surgery. Dr. Daniel Albo of Baylor College of Medicine directed the volume dedicated to colorectal surgery. Dr. Ronald Dalman of Stanford University edited topics related to vascular surgery, including both open and endovascular approaches. The discipline of transplantation surgery is represented by Dr. Michael Englesbe of the University of Michigan. In turn, the editors have recruited contributors that are world-renowned; the resulting volumes have a distinctly international flavor.

Surgery is a visual discipline. *Operative Techniques in Surgery* is lavishly illustrated with a compelling combination of line art and intraoperative photography. The illustrated material was all executed by a single source, Body Scientific International, to provide a uniform style emphasizing clarity and strong, clean lines. Intraoperative photographs are taken from the perspective of the operating surgeon so that operations might be visualized as they would be performed. The result is visually striking, often beautiful. The accompanying text is intentionally spare, with a focus on crucial operative details and important aspects of postoperative management.

The series is designed for surgeons at all levels of practice, from surgical residents to advanced practice fellows to surgeons of wide experience. The incredible pace at which surgical technique evolves means that the volumes will offer new insights and novel approaches to all surgeons.

Operative Techniques in Surgery would be possible only at Wolters Kluwer Health, an organization of unique vision, organization, and talent. Brian Brown, executive editor, Keith Donnellan, acquisitions editor, and Brendan Huffman, product development editor, deserve special recognition for vision and perseverance.

Michael W. Mulholland, MD, PhD

Preface

Operative Techniques in Breast, Endocrine, and Oncologic Surgery was created to be a truly unique and comprehensive resource for surgical residents, fellows, and the practicing surgeon. To maximize efficiency, the chapters are presented in outline form, organized to highlight the key components of preoperative assessment and preparation, operative technique, and essential postoperative management. The procedures are broken down step-by-step, with a plethora of images including intraoperative photography and detailed, incomparable artwork. This highly visual format is particularly beneficial when viewed on electronic media devices, a necessary element of any modern textbook.

The authors featured in *Operative Techniques in Breast, Endocrine, and Oncologic Surgery* represent not only some of the preeminent surgeon-educators in breast surgery, oncology, and endocrine surgery but also innovators in the development of novel surgical techniques. Particular attention is devoted to the rapid evolution of the field, including the role of surgery in the context of multidisciplinary care and the incorporation of minimally invasive approaches in oncologic and endocrine surgery.

Special recognition is necessary for the editor-in-chief Dr. Michael W. Mulholland and the editorial and project management staff at Wolters Kluwer Health, including Brendan Huffman and Keith Donnellan. Their vision and encouraging guidance are directly responsible for the completion of what is hopefully an extremely valuable reference for surgeons of all levels.

Michael S. Sabel, MD

Contents

Chapter 1

Fine Needle Aspiration of a Breast Mass

Judy C. Pang Claire W. Michael

DEFINITION

- Fine needle aspiration (FNA) biopsy is a percutaneous procedure that uses a fine gauge needle with or without a syringe to sample fluid from a cyst or extract cells from a solid palpable mass for cytologic analysis.

PATIENT HISTORY AND PHYSICAL FINDINGS

- A focused history should be obtained from the patient including duration of the mass, changes in size, associated pain, or fluctuations of the mass with menstrual cycle. Prior history of trauma or malignancies should also be ascertained. On physical examination, localizing the mass as within the breast parenchyma, lower axilla, or subcutaneous/cutaneous tissue of the chest wall is important. The differential diagnoses may be different. In addition, noting any skin changes such as redness, warmth, or edema is also helpful. Determining the size and quality of the mass as well as depth and relation to other structures is essential for an adequate sample while minimizing complications. There are no absolute contraindications to FNA.

IMAGING AND OTHER DIAGNOSTIC STUDIES

- Mammographic and ultrasound findings can be helpful in arriving at an accurate diagnosis. Knowing whether a lesion is solid or cystic can help select the appropriate needle and syringe. For lesions that are nonpalpable or difficult to palpate, image-guided (i.e., ultrasound) FNA is recommended to ensure proper sampling of the mass.

DIFFERENTIAL DIAGNOSIS

- Benign (i.e., fibroadenoma, cyst)
- Malignant (i.e., carcinoma, lymphoma)
- Atypical (core biopsy or surgical excision required for definitive diagnosis)

NONOPERATIVE MANAGEMENT

- For patients who opt not to undergo a biopsy, short-term follow-up (4 to 6 months) with repeat imaging and clinical examination to document stability or changes is recommended.

SURGICAL MANAGEMENT

- Alternative procedures to FNA biopsy are core needle biopsy and surgical excision of mass.
- For solid masses, FNA biopsy provides cells for cytology, whereas core needle biopsy obtains tissue. In situations where an experienced cytopathologist is not available or tissue architecture is necessary to make a diagnosis (e.g., differentiating between in situ and invasive disease), core needle biopsy is preferred.
- Surgical excision should be reserved for cases where FNA or core needle biopsy was inconclusive. It may be considered for small breast masses where the patient is strongly desirous of excision.

Preoperative Planning

- Prior to the FNA, the location of the palpable mass should be confirmed with the patient. The mass should be examined in the upright and supine position to determine the ideal position for the biopsy.

Positioning

- The patient may be upright or supine depending on the location of the mass. The patient should be positioned to optimize palpation and sampling of the mass.

Approach

- FNA can be performed using (1) a needle, syringe, and syringe holder; (2) a needle and syringe; or (3) a needle only.

TECHNIQUES

EQUIPMENT

- Alcohol pads to cleanse the skin and gauze pads to apply pressure after completion of the procedure
- Local anesthetic is optional.
- Beveled hypodermic needles
    - A 23-gauge needle is preferred and typically the one to start with. If inadequate material is obtained, a 22-gauge needle can be used especially for lesions with minimal stroma (i.e., lymphoma, melanoma) or a 25-gauge needle for rubbery or fibrous masses (i.e., fibroadenoma).
    - The length of the needle is typically 5/8 in to 1½ in, which is just long enough to reach the target. Shorter needles are easier to manipulate because they will not bend.
- A slip-tip syringe is best as it is easy to handle and provides a good seal. A Luer lock syringe may also be used, but it can be difficult to remove the needle. A 10-mL syringe is preferred as it allows the hand to be closer to the target and only 2 to 4 mL of suction is needed for aspiration. For larger cystic lesions, a 20-mL syringe may be advantageous.
- A syringe holder allows for one-handed grip and application of suction leaving the other hand free to stabilize the target.
- Glass slides and cover slips
- Slide holder for air-dried slides

- Ninety-five percent ethanol (EtOH) in a jar for fixation of slides or spray fixative. If the jar is not slotted for separating slides, using paper clips on alternating slides can achieve the same goal.
- There are different rapid stains that can be used for adequacy checks including toluidine blue, rapid hematoxylin and eosin, rapid Papanicolaou for fixed slides, and Giemsa and Diff-Quik for air-dried slides.
- Needle rinses can be performed in RPMI (cell block or flow cytometry for lymphoma), 10% buffered formalin (cell block), or CytoLyt (thin prep).

FINE NEEDLE ASPIRATION USING NEEDLE, SYRINGE, AND SYRINGE HOLDER[1,2]

- Carefully palpate the mass to estimate the size and depth as well as assess the structures nearby to avoid (i.e., major blood vessels, bone, and lung especially with small breasts).
- Fix the mass firmly in place with the fingers.
  - For large lesions, use the thumb and opposing finger (**FIG 1**).
  - For smaller lesions, place the forefinger and middle finger on top of the mass and then spread them apart, stretching the skin (**FIG 2**).
- Plan the angle of the needle at the entrance point of the skin and determine the depth of penetration.
  - If the needle enters at 90 degrees to the mass, the needle should penetrate the skin on top of the mass (**FIG 3A,B**).
  - If the needle enters at a 30- to 45-degree angle, which is oftentimes more comfortable and practical, compensate for the acute angle by penetrating the skin adjacent to the mass and not on top of the mass (**FIG 4A,B**).
  - When entering at 90 degrees, penetrating too deep with the needle can potentially result in a pneumothorax. If this is a concern (e.g., mass near the chest wall), a 30- to 45-degree angle is preferred.
  - To stabilize the instrument, rest the barrel of the syringe on the forefinger of the palpating hand or use the thumb to stabilize the syringe as you enter the mass. Once the needle is in the mass, the thumb can be removed (**FIG 4A**).
- Extracting material
  - For cystic lesions, applying suction without back and forth movement is sufficient.
  - For solid masses, 15 to 20 excursions are made before suction is released and the needle is removed from the mass. If blood is seen at the hub, the number

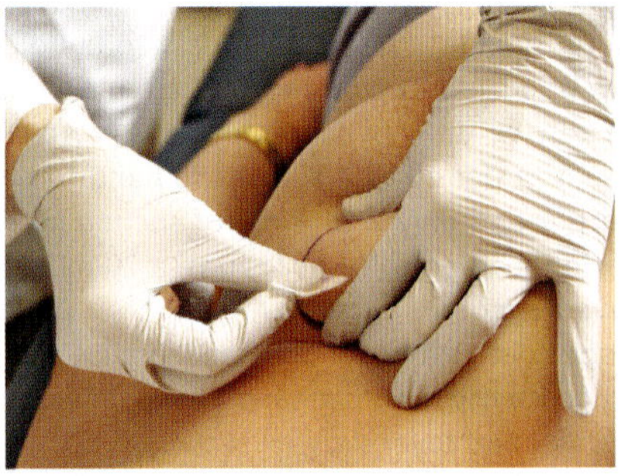

FIG 1 ● Fixation of a large mass using the thumb and opposing finger.

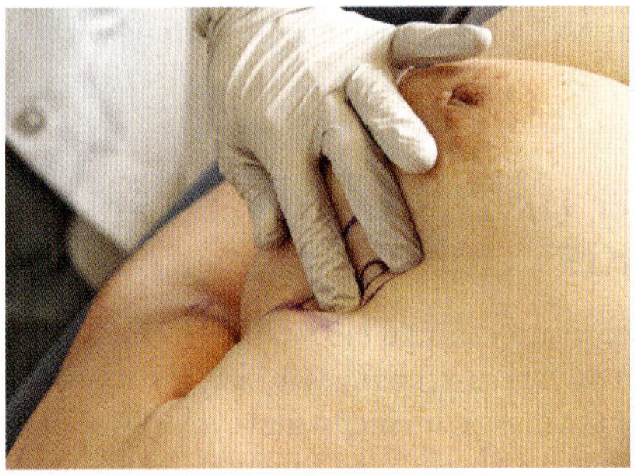

FIG 2 ● Fixation of smaller mass using forefinger and middle finger.

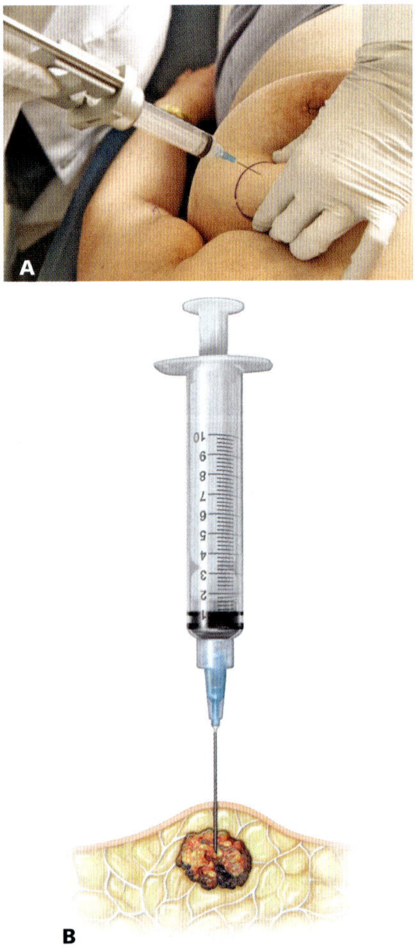

B

FIG 3 ● **A,B.** Needle entering 90 degrees to the mass should penetrate the skin on top of the mass.

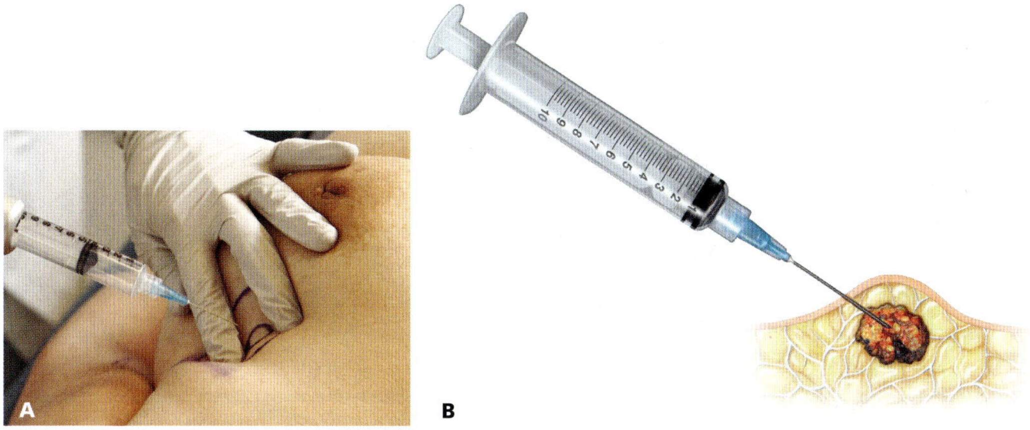

FIG 4 • **A,B.** Needle entering 30 to 45 degrees to the mass should penetrate the skin adjacent to the mass and not on top of the mass.

of excursions should be limited and suction released before reaching 15 to 20. Always release the suction before pulling the needle out of the patient; otherwise, all the material will flow into the barrel of the syringe, which will be very difficult to extract (**FIG 5**).

- Adequate sampling
    - To sample different areas of a well-defined large lesion, it is preferable to make separate passes to sample different areas. This is also preferable in well-defined lesions. In ill-defined targets, especially fibrocystic changes of the breast, it is best to redirect while sampling in a fanlike fashion. To avoid tearing the tissue and causing bleeding, the needle should be retracted to the surface of the target (but still in the patient) before redirecting (**FIG 6**).
    - Typically, two to three passes are adequate. Additional passes are performed if the target is large or the sample is inadequate. However, typically more than three passes is not recommended as often times the yield of diagnostic material decreases with each subsequent pass due to blood. The first pass is traditionally the best.
- Zajdela's technique, which uses only the needle without a syringe or syringe holder (**FIG 7A**). This technique is ideal for small targets as it increases sensitivity to the difference in consistencies between normal breast tissue and the lesion that cannot be appreciated as well with a syringe and syringe holder. In addition, it is less bloody. However, this technique often yields less material than when suction is used, and there is a risk of overflow of material if the lesion is cystic. A syringe (without the plunger) can be used if needed (**FIG 7B**).

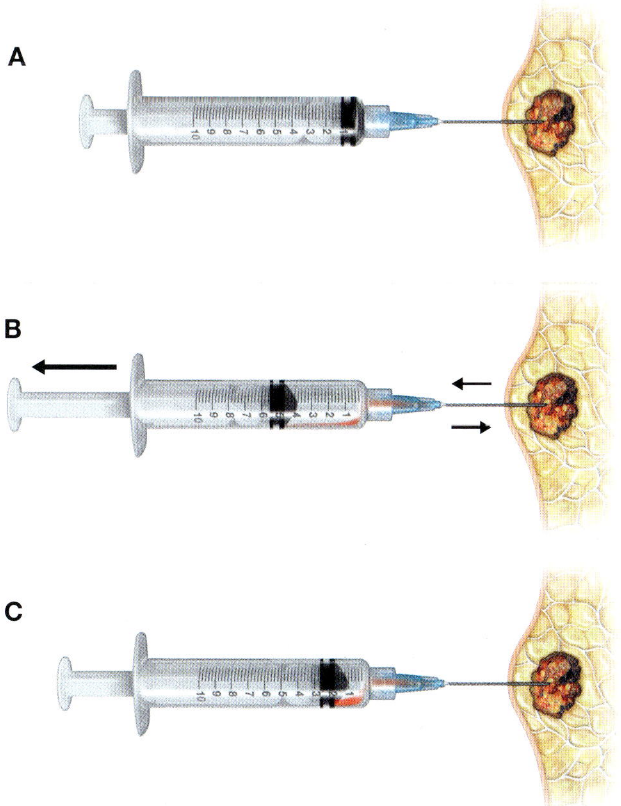

FIG 5 • **A.** Needle placed in mass. **B.** Withdraw plunger creating 2 to 4 mL of vacuum/suction and perform 15 to 20 excursions. **C.** Release the plunger/suction before pulling needle out of the patient.

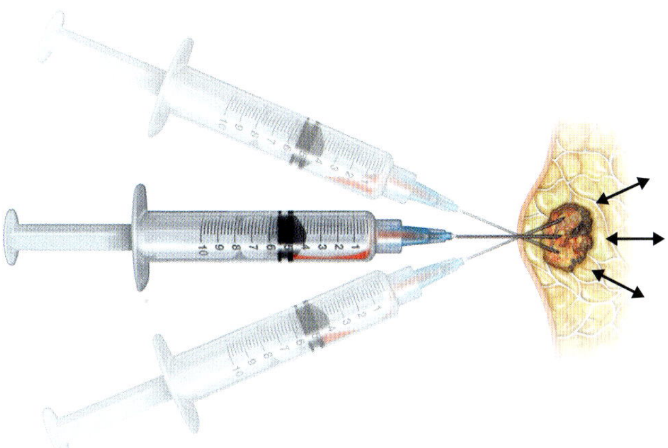

FIG 6 • To sample different areas, redirect the needle in a fanlike fashion.

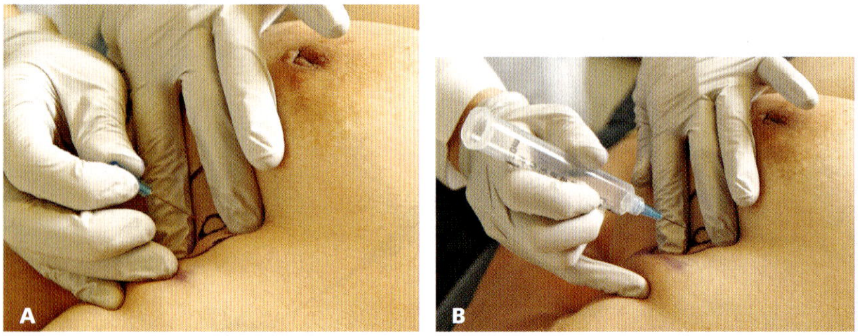

FIG 7 • Zajdela's technique using only a needle **(A)** or a needle and a syringe without the plunger **(B)**.

PREPARING SLIDES[1,2]

- Expulsion of material
  - The needle is first disconnected from the syringe (**FIG 8**). The plunger is then pulled back all the way before reattaching the needle (**FIG 9A,B**). If using the Zajdela technique with the needle and syringe, disconnect the needle from the syringe before putting the plunger back into the syringe.
  - With the tip of the needle on the slide (bevel down), the plunger is forcefully pushed so that all the material is on one slide (**FIG 10A,B**). If there is abundant material, the plunger can be pushed slowly so that only a small amount of material is placed on each slide. The slides should be labeled with patient identifiers (i.e., name and birth date) with a pencil.
  - If there is remaining material in the hub, it can be rinsed for cytocentrifugation (in CytoLyt) or cell block (10% buffered formalin or RPMI) (**FIG 11**). If additional smears are desired, the flip technique can be used where the needle is secured in the rubber top of a Vacutainer tube. The hub is then flicked repeatedly onto a slide. Droplets of the material on the slides can then be smeared. (**FIG 12**).
- Smearing techniques
  - Rest the edge of a second slide on top of the slide that contains the aspirate material (**FIG 13**).

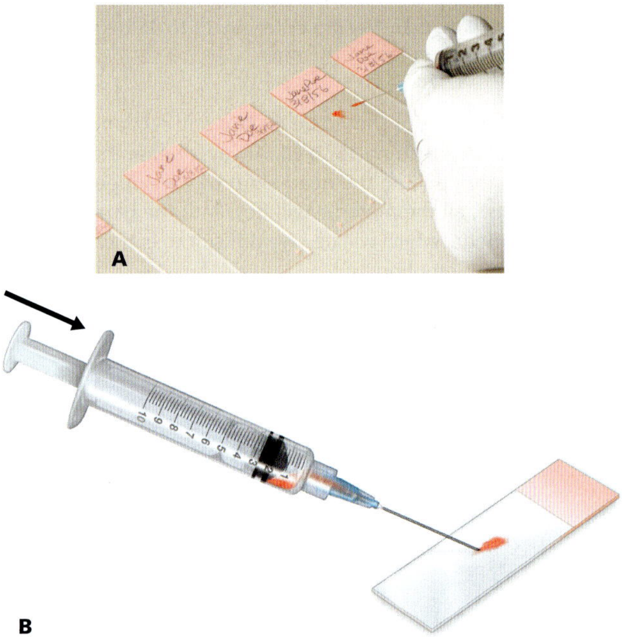

FIG 10 • **A,B.** With the tip of the needle on the slide (bevel down), the plunger is forcefully pushed so that all the material is on one slide. If there is abundant material, the plunger can be pushed slowly so that only a small amount of material is placed on each slide.

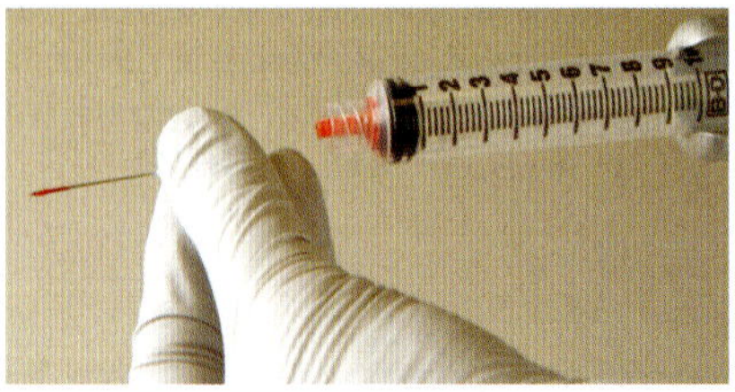

FIG 8 • Disconnect needle from syringe.

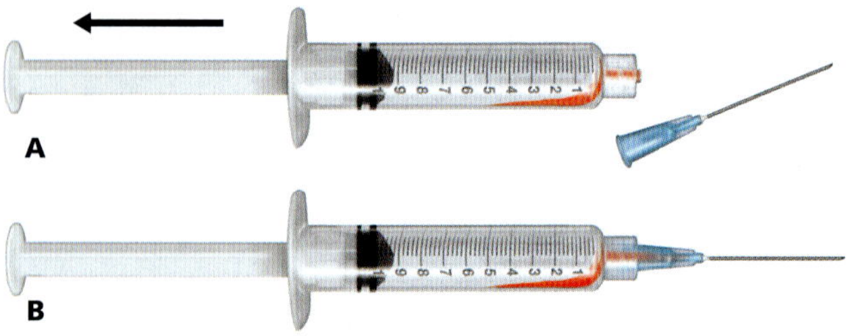

FIG 9 • **A,B.** The plunger is pulled back all the way **(A)** before reattaching the needle **(B)**.

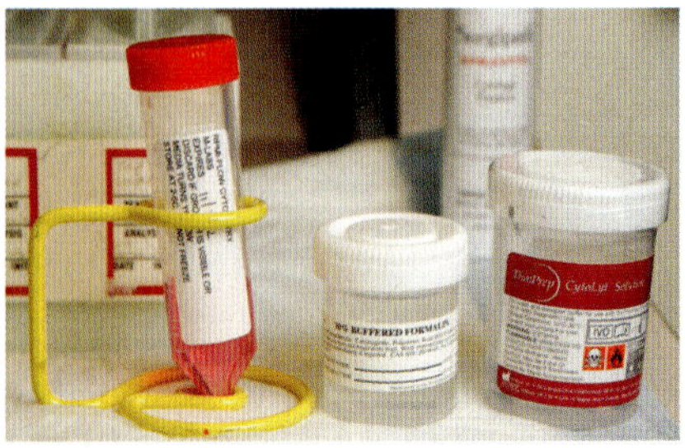

FIG 11 • The needle can be rinsed in RPMI, 10% buffered formalin, or CytoLyt.

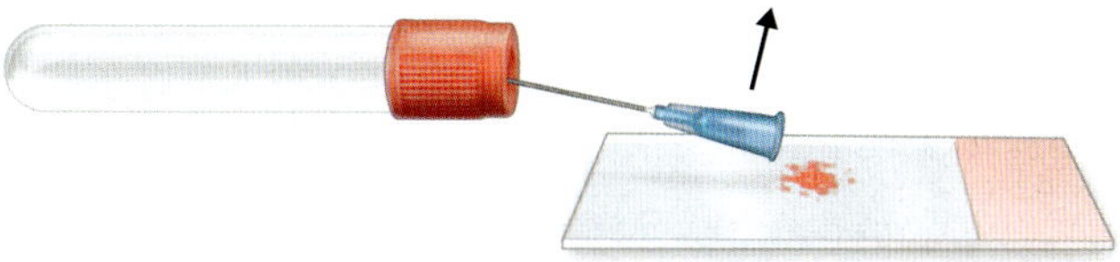

FIG 12 ● Secure the needle in the rubber top of a Vacutainer tube. Flick the hub repeatedly onto a slide.

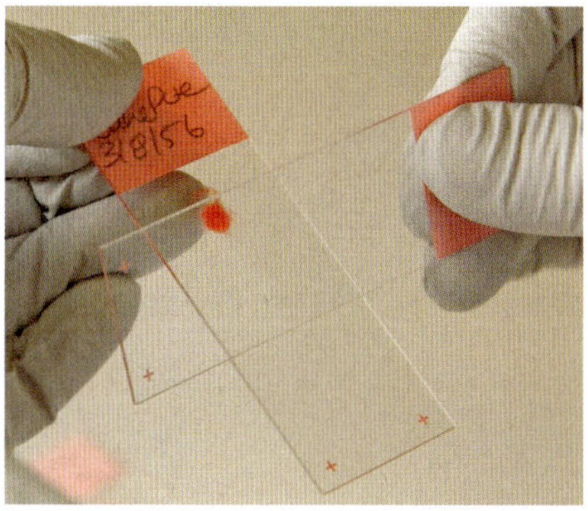

FIG 13 ● Rest a slide on top of the slide that contains the aspirate material.

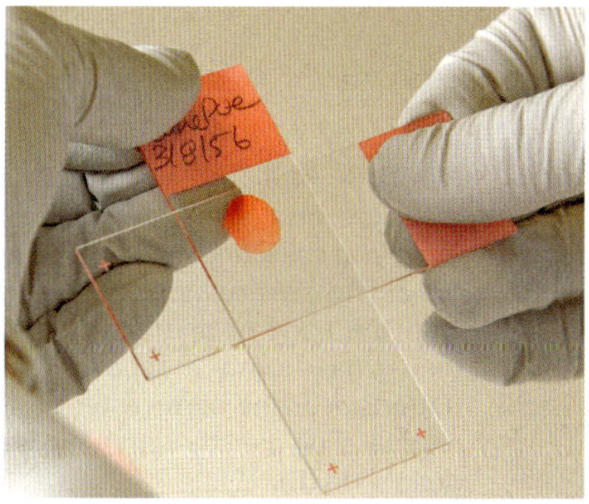

FIG 14 ● Rotate the top slide so that it is parallel to the bottom slide.

  - Rotate the top slide so that it is level with the bottom slide (**FIG 14**).
  - Keeping both slides level, apply light pressure and slide the top slide over the bottom slide (**FIG 15**).
  - The end product should be a slide with material in an oval configuration of even thickness (**FIG 16**). Virtually, all the material should be on the bottom slides. Microscopically, the cells should be well preserved with intact cytoplasm. If too much pressure is applied, there will be crushed nuclei and few cells with preserved cytoplasm. If the slides are not maintained level to each other, the material will be scraped and lost and distortion will be present.

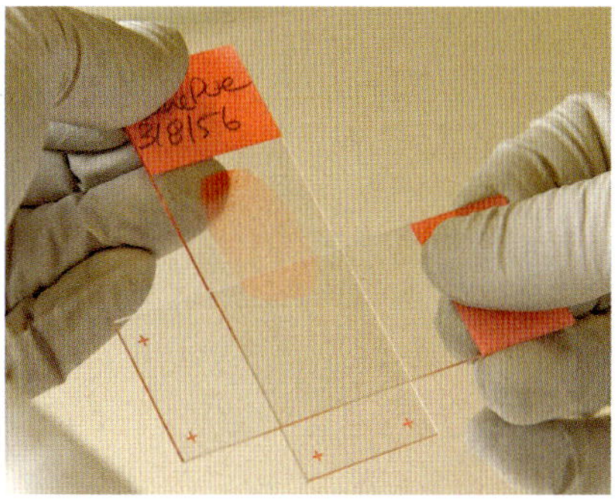

FIG 15 ● Apply light pressure and slide the top slide over the bottom slide.

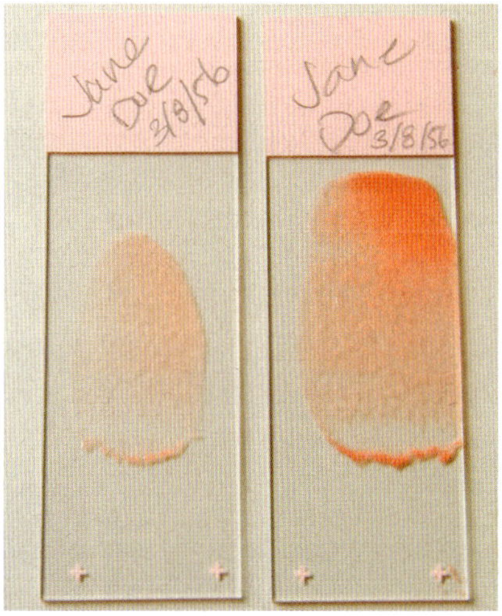

FIG 16 ● End product with material in an oval configuration.

- Other techniques
  - Place a clean slide exactly parallel to the bottom slide containing the aspirate material and slide apart. The material will be present on both slides (also produces good smears) (**FIG 17A,B**).
  - For bloody aspirates, tilt the slide and allow the blood to drain into collecting media (**FIG 18A,B**). The particulates remaining on the slide is then scraped with the edge of another slide and then smeared onto a separate slide (**FIG 18C,D**). Alternatively, the particulates on the original slide can be smeared directly with a separate clean slide (**FIG 18E**).

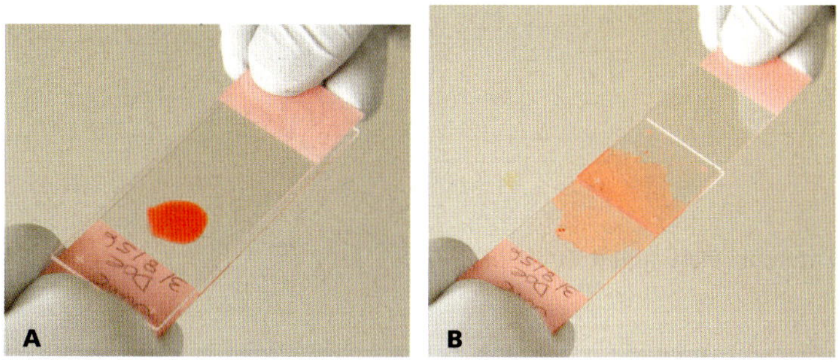

FIG 17 ● **A,B.** Place a clean slide exactly parallel to the bottom slide containing the aspirate material and slide apart.

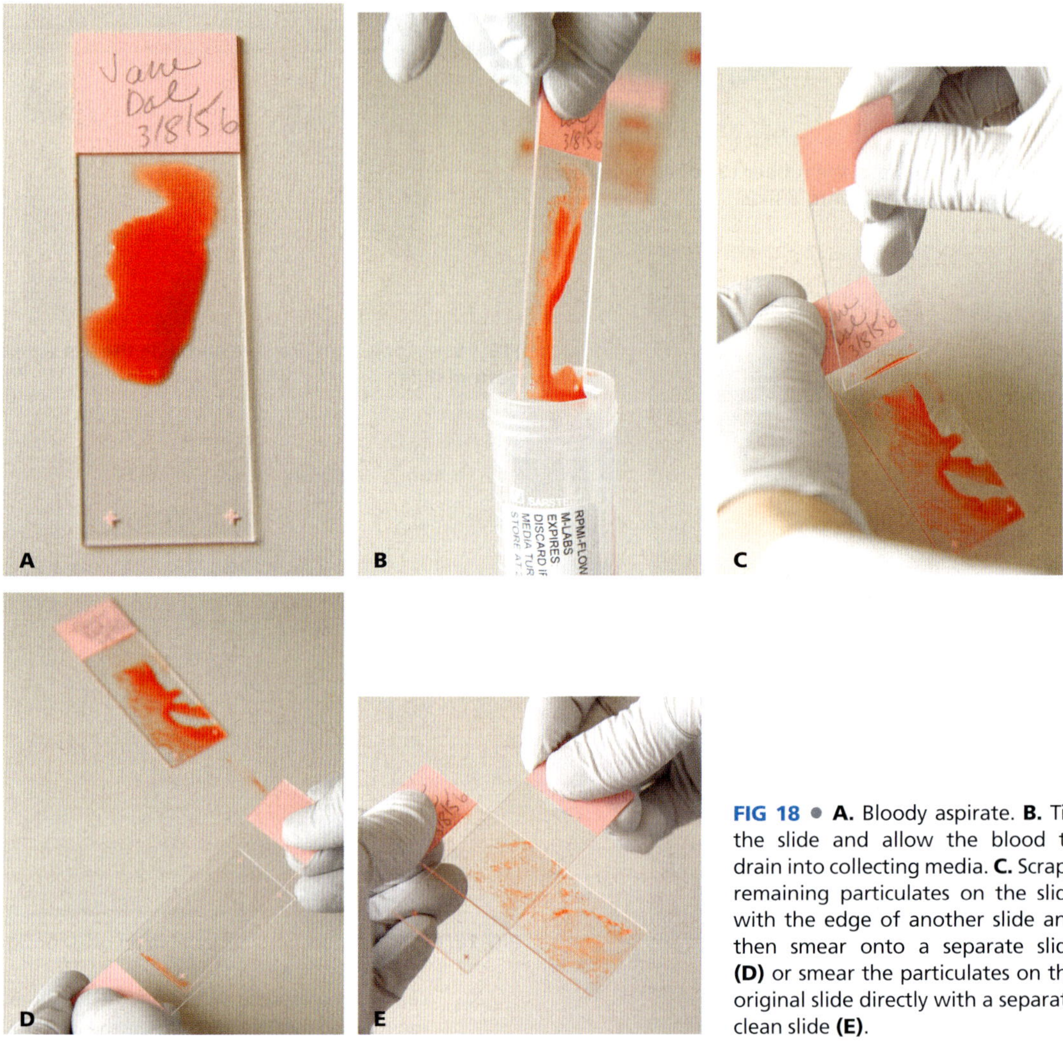

FIG 18 • **A.** Bloody aspirate. **B.** Tilt the slide and allow the blood to drain into collecting media. **C.** Scrape remaining particulates on the slide with the edge of another slide and then smear onto a separate slide **(D)** or smear the particulates on the original slide directly with a separate clean slide **(E)**.

FIX SLIDES

- The slides should be immersed in 95% EtOH or fixed by spray fixation (**FIG 19**). This should be done as quickly as possible after smearing the slides to prevent air-dry artifact. Alternatively, slides may be left to air dry without fixation. Ideally, both air dried and fixed slides should be made for cytologic evaluation.

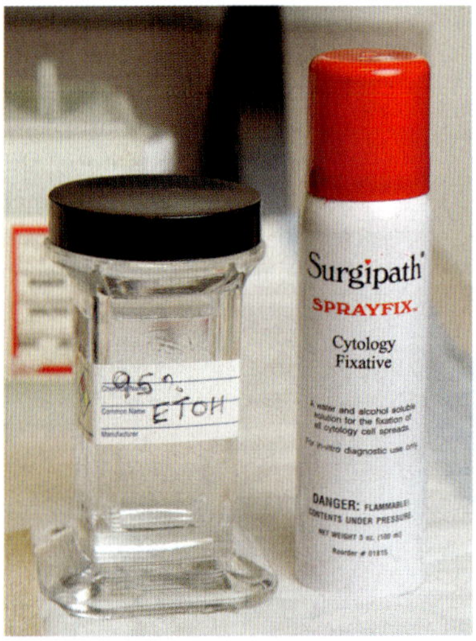

FIG 19 • Fix slides immediately in 95% liquid EtOH or spray fix.

PEARLS AND PITFALLS[3]

Indications	▪ Palpable masses: A brief history and focused physical examination should be performed. ▪ Diagnostic: primary neoplasms (benign vs. malignant), tumor recurrence, secondary or metastatic tumors, inflammatory diseases (uncommon), atypical epithelial lesions (require additional studies) ▪ Therapeutic: evacuation of simple cysts
Major diagnostic pitfalls	▪ False negative: small focus of carcinoma arising in a background of a predominantly benign lesion (i.e., fibrocystic change), carcinoma arising in a complex proliferative lesion (i.e., papilloma), well-differentiated carcinomas, rare tumor types, extensively necrotic or cystic carcinomas, sampling error, inadequate smears ▪ False positive: fibroadenoma, papilloma/papillary lesions, atypical ductal hyperplasia, pregnancy-associated/lactational changes, fat necrosis, collagenous spherulosis, skin adnexal tumors
Major limitations	▪ Inability to distinguish between invasive and in situ carcinoma ▪ Accuracy is often dependent on the size of the lesion (less sensitive if <0.5 cm). ▪ Low accuracy in tumors with a predominant necrotic/cystic component ▪ Lack of specific diagnosis for majority of benign lesions ▪ Need for biopsy (core or excisional) of all lesions with an "atypical" diagnosis ▪ Ability to perform hormone receptor and *HER-2/neu* analysis can only be done with accuracy if an adequate sample is obtained.

POSTOPERATIVE CARE

- Pressure should be applied to the site for a few minutes to assure hemostasis, and then a sterile dressing is applied.

OUTCOMES

- 80% to 100% sensitivity, with a specificity of over 99%
- 3% to 5% false-negative and 0.5% to 2% false-positive rate
- Implementing the "triple test" is essential (correlation of clinical, radiologic, and cytologic findings)

COMPLICATIONS

- Low complication rate and most complications are minor
- Pain
- Bleeding/hematoma
- Infection
- Vasovagal reaction
- Pneumothorax
- Epithelial displacement/tumor seeding
- Artifacts occurring after aspiration may interfere with radiographic interpretation and histologic evaluation of surgical resection (epithelial displacement can mimic invasive carcinoma).

REFERENCES

1. Dusenbery D. The technique of fine needle aspiration of palpable mass lesions of the head and neck. *Otolaryngol Head Neck Surg.* 1997;8(2):61–67.
2. Ljung BM. Pathology FNA technique video. PathLab.org Web site. http://www.pathlab.org/FNA_Cytology_Technique_Pathlab.org_Pathology_UK_Video_Cytology_Books_Media_News.html. Accessed February, 2008.
3. Ali SZ, Parwani AV. *Breast Cytopathology.* New York, NY: Springer; 2007.

Chapter **2**

Wire Localized Breast Biopsy

Michael S. Sabel

DEFINITION

- The wire-localized excisional biopsy (or needle-localized biopsy) is used to obtain tissue for the diagnosis of a nonpalpable, image-detected abnormality. There are various methods for localizing breast lesions for excision, including wire localization, cutaneous markers, and radiocolloid occult lesion localization (ROLL). Wire localization is the most frequently used method and is described in this chapter.
- It is preferable to use image-guided biopsy as a first step (stereotactic biopsy or ultrasound or magnetic resonance imaging [MRI]-guided biopsy), as this avoids surgery in patients with benign disease and allows for a definitive oncologic operation in patients with malignant disease. Thus, the wire-localized excisional biopsy should be limited to patients who failed image-guided biopsy or are not suitable candidates. Wire-localized lumpectomy is a similar procedure for patients who have already been diagnosed with breast cancer, where the goal is a complete excision of the cancer with an adequate margin of surrounding normal tissue. For wire-localized lumpectomy, often, two wires are needed to "bracket" the cancer in order to assure complete removal.

PATIENT HISTORY AND PHYSICAL FINDINGS

- A bilateral breast exam should be performed in all patients for whom wire-localized breast biopsy is being contemplated for two reasons. First, to assess whether or not the lesion is truly nonpalpable. If the abnormality is palpable, then wire localization will not be necessary. If an abnormality is palpated, it is critical to review with the radiologist to be sure that the palpable abnormality corresponds to the imaging abnormality being recommended for biopsy. The second reason for bilateral breast examination is to make sure there are no other palpable occult abnormalities that may also require biopsy.
- For patients with biopsy-proven cancer who are to undergo wire-localized lumpectomy, a thorough history and physical examination is necessary to make sure they are suitable candidates for breast conservation therapy (BCT). Contraindications to BCT include prior radiation, collagen vascular disease, first or second trimester of pregnancy, multicentric cancer, or widespread calcifications (see Chapter 5, Lumpectomy).

IMAGING AND OTHER DIAGNOSTIC STUDIES

- The preoperative imaging is essential to the procedure. Prior to the decision to perform a wire-localized breast biopsy, the breast imaging should be reviewed to determine whether the patient is a suitable candidate for an image-guided biopsy, as this is the preferable first step. The patient's allergies, medications (specifically aspirin or anticoagulants), or the presence of a bleeding diathesis should be reviewed. Contraindications to stereotactic core needle biopsy include an inability to adequately visualize the target lesion or an inability of the patient to remain in the position required for the procedure. Some patients may exceed the weight limit for the stereotactic table. Other factors that may preclude stereotactic core needle biopsy include higher breast density; lesions close to the skin, chest wall, or axilla; or the presence of breast implants.
- Prior to coming to the operating room (OR), the patient undergoes needle localization under image guidance. After local anesthesia, a rigid introducer needle with a hooked wire within it is directed toward the site of the abnormality using biplanar mammography (**FIG 1A**) or ultrasound (**FIG 1B**). The rigid needle is then removed, leaving the wire secured by the hook so it is not easily withdrawn or redirected (**FIG 2A,B**).
- In many cases, a wire-localized excision is recommended after an image-guided core needle biopsy–demonstrated atypia (lobular carcinoma in situ [LCIS], atypical ductal hyperplasia [ADH], atypical lobular hyperplasia [ALH], or flat epithelial atypia [FEA]). It is also often recommended after a needle biopsy of papilloma or radial scar. In these cases, a fraction may upstage to in situ or invasive cancer.[1–6] It is good to review the pathology and indications for the biopsy prior to the procedure.

SURGICAL MANAGEMENT

Preoperative Planning

- Performing a breast exam after the localization will be difficult, as the wire will be secured by a variety of methods that will preclude physical exam. These should not be removed until the patient is positioned in the OR to minimize the chance of dislodging the wire during transport.
- Prior to taking the patient back to the OR, the localization films should be reviewed. Specifically, the surgeon should note the proximity of the abnormality to the wire, the direction of the wire from the point of skin entry, and how far the lesion is from the skin, as this may impact the degree of sedation (if any).
- Although the risk of infection after breast surgery is low, it tends to be higher than average for a clean surgical procedure, and several studies have shown that antibiotic prophylaxis significantly reduces the risk of postoperative infection.[7]

Positioning

- The patient should be positioned supine. Often, the localization wire is placed laterally, so the ipsilateral arm may need to be at 90 degrees.
- Once the patient is on the OR table and positioned, the tape and dressings securing the wire should be removed carefully as not to dislodge the wire. A gentle breast exam can be performed at this point to see if the lesion is palpable. In addition, light palpation while watching the external portion of the wire can give the surgeon an idea of what direction the wire is heading.

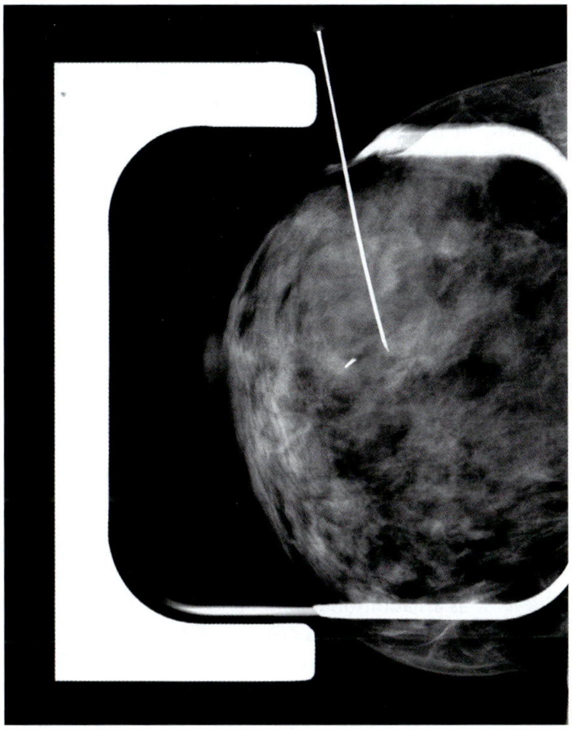

A

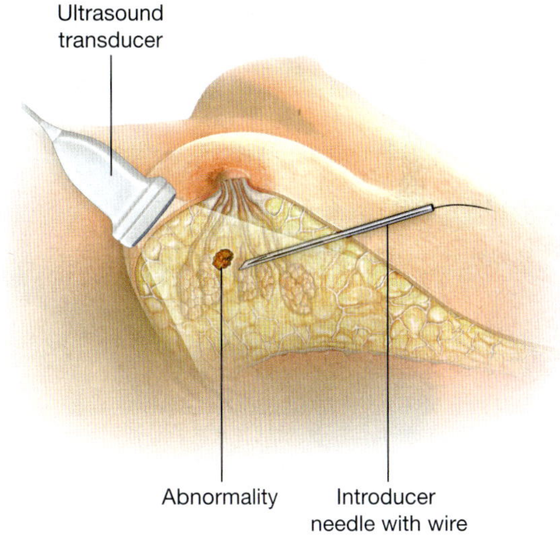

B

FIG 1 • Placement of the rigid needle using biplanar mammography **(A)** or ultrasound **(B)**.

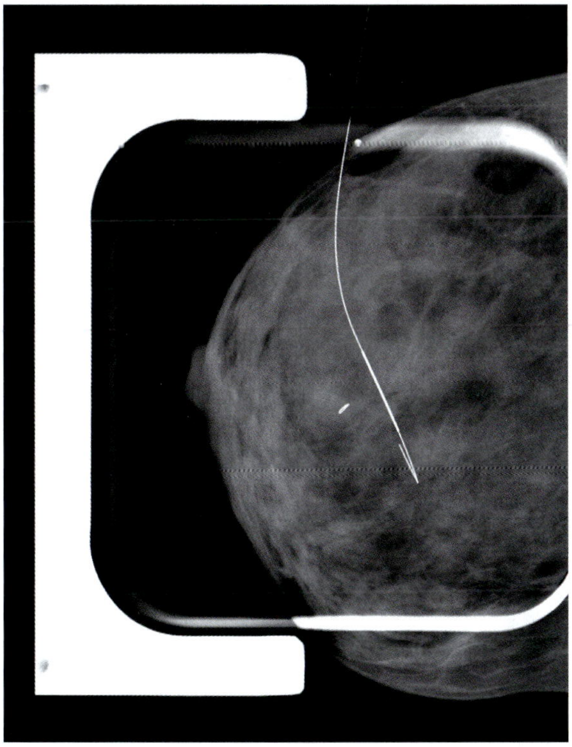

A

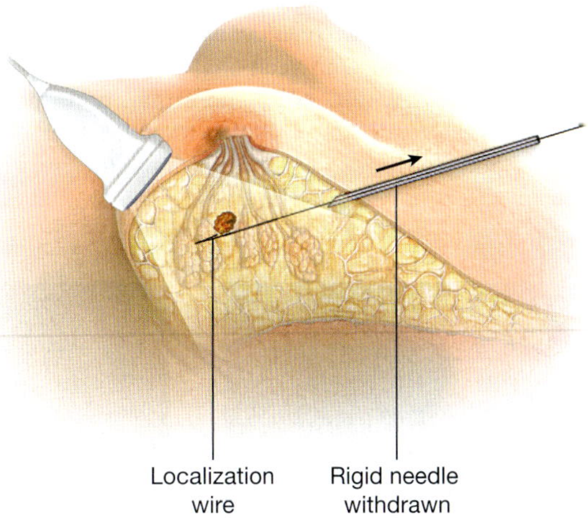

B

FIG 2 • **A,B.** The rigid needle is withdrawn, leaving the wire in the location of the abnormality.

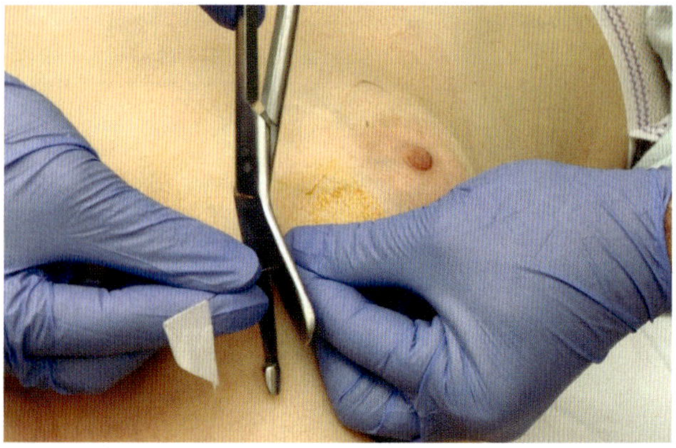

- The localization wire is often quite long and with a significant portion outside of the skin. The case will be facilitated by cutting the wire to a more workable length. Care must be taken not to advance the wire or pull the wire back (or out). It is also important not to cut the wire so close to the skin that it disappears. Secure the wire at the level of the skin prior to cutting with a wire cutter (**FIG 3**).

FIG 3 • The wire is secured at the level of the skin while excess wire is cut. It is important not to dislodge the wire as well as to leave an adequate amount.

ANTICIPATING THE LOCATION OF THE ABNORMALITY

- After the dressings have been removed, the surgeon uses the site and direction of the wire along with the craniocaudal (CC) and lateral–medial (LM) views to determine the location of the abnormality in the breast. A small BB is usually placed at the site where the wire enters the skin, so it is possible to estimate how far through the breast tissue the wire extends. Remember, the breast is compressed during the mammography but not on the OR table, so the measurement on the film may not be exact. It is often helpful to identify the nipple on the mammogram as an additional landmark.
- The CC view (**FIG 4A**) demonstrates both the anterior–posterior and the lateral–medial location of the abnormality but gives no information regarding the superior–inferior location. With a laterally placed wire, the CC view can be used to estimate how deep the lesion is and how medial (especially when also using the nipple as an additional landmark).
- The LM view (**FIG 4B**) demonstrates the anterior–posterior orientation as well as the superior–inferior but gives no information regarding the lateral–medial location. Again, with a laterally placed wire, the deviation from the skin BB to the hook of the wire can be used to assess whether the wire is heading superiorly or inferiorly.
- Using both views, the surgeon should also note where the abnormality is in relation to the wire. Typically, the radiologist attempts to place the reinforced portion of the wire in close proximity to the lesion. It is crucial to know the relative proximity of the wire to the lesion and in what direction the wire sits relative to the lesion.

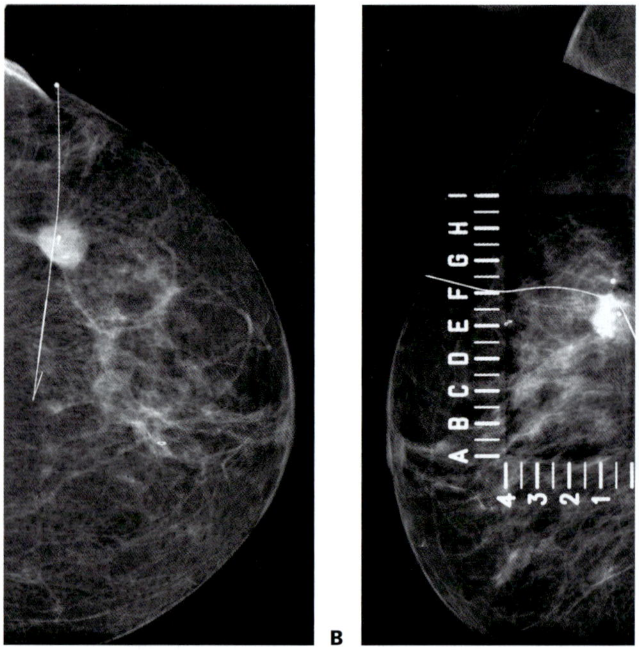

FIG 4 • The localization films show the relationship between the skin, the wire, and the abnormality. In the CC view **(A)**, the *dot* shows the entry point in the skin. The film shows the lesion to be posterior and lateral, but this film does not reveal the anterior–posterior position. The hook and reinforced portion of the wire are distal (medial) to the lesion. In the LM view **(B)**, you can again see the lesion is posterior, but now you can see that it sits superiorly. It may seem like the wire travels through the breast for some distance but most of that is external. The *white dot* shows where it enters the skin.

SKIN INCISION AND IDENTIFICATION OF THE WIRE

- Using both the preoperative imaging and examination of the breast, the surgeon can estimate the direction of the wire and the distance to the reinforced portion of the wire. Using a water-soluble marker, an incision should be marked out (**FIG 5**). For lesions close to where the wire enters the skin, the incision can be planned at the entry site. Otherwise, the incision should be placed directly over the predicted site of the mammographic abnormality.
- When marking the incision, it should be kept in mind that if this lesion is malignant, you may be returning for a reexcision lumpectomy or a mastectomy. Therefore, the incision should be placed in a way that does not compromise that. For lesions near the nipple–areolar complex, a circumareolar incision is cosmetically appealing, but excessive tunneling is discouraged as this will also complicate a reexcision lumpectomy if cancer is present.
- The incision should be kept small at first, as it can be lengthened later if need be (**FIG 6**). As these are typically performed with just local anesthesia or light sedation, the skin is anesthetized prior to any incision.

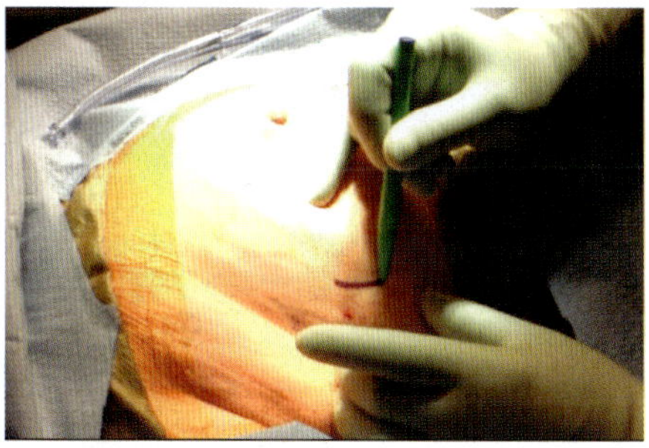

FIG 5 ● An incision is marked out over the anticipated site of the abnormality, keeping in mind a reexcision lumpectomy or mastectomy should the pathology return as malignant.

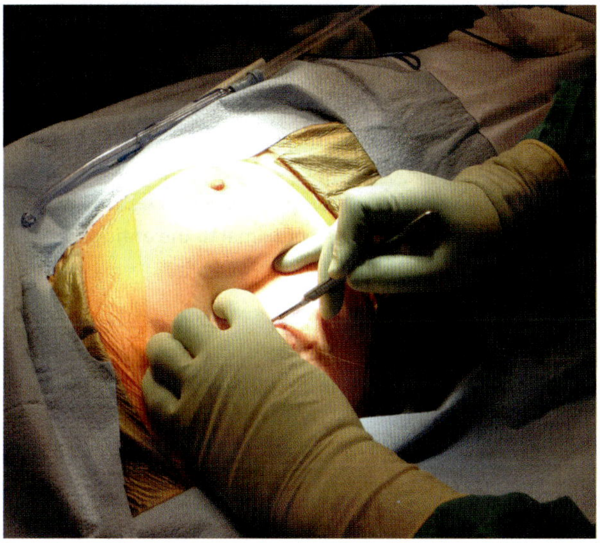

FIG 6 ● A small incision is made in the skin after infiltration of local anesthesia.

EXCISION

- The goal of the wire-localized excisional biopsy is to make the diagnosis while removing as little breast tissue as possible. If the CC and LM views suggest that the lesion is deep to the incision, the dissection is continued posteriorly so as to avoid removing excessive tissue anterior to the lesion and wire (**FIG 7A**). For more superficial lesions, flaps should be elevated shortly after incision but kept thick enough to avoid concavity at the site (**FIG 7B**).

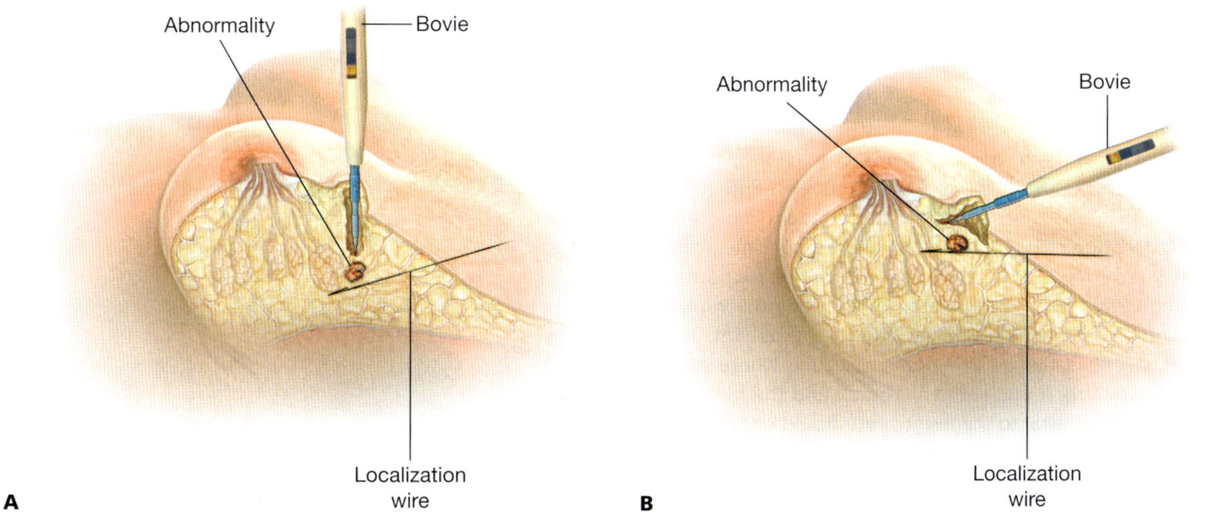

FIG 7 ● The subcutaneous fat and breast parenchyma are divided with cautery. For deep lesions **(A)**, dissect a fair distance to avoid taking excessive tissue anterior to the lesion (causing concavity). For superficial lesions **(B)**, thick flaps should be elevated shortly after incision.

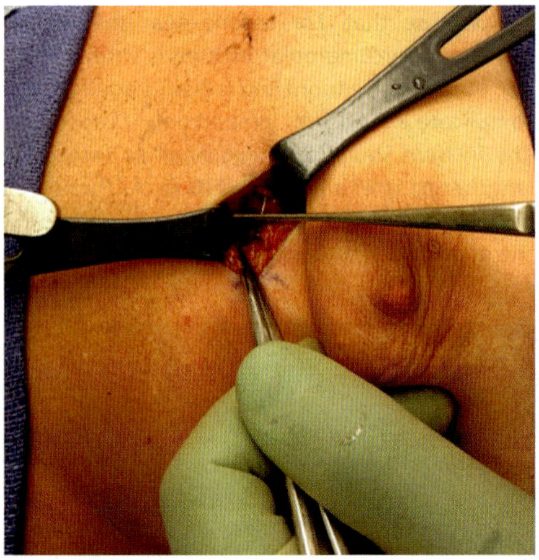

FIG 8 ● The wire is identified proximal to the anticipated site of the abnormality.

- If the incision does not pass through the entry site of the wire, the next step is to identify the shaft of the wire proximal to the lesion. Dissection is carried down to the wire, taking care not to land on top of the abnormality but rather on the wire proximal to the abnormality (FIG 8).
- Once the wire is identified, it is grasped with a hemostat on the specimen side, and the shaft of the wire is retracted into the wound. Take care to secure the wire adequately so it is not dislodged (FIG 9A,B).
- At the point where the wire enters the breast, grasp the tissue with an Allis clamp. Be careful to grasp above or below the wire and not the wire directly, as retraction on the clamp may dislodge the wire (FIG 10).
- Dissection then continues parallel to the wire, maintaining a circumference of approximately 1 cm of breast tissue around the wire. This is modified based on the size of the abnormality and the relationship between the wire and the lesion. For example, for a lesion sitting approximately 1 cm anterior to the wire, a larger margin is taken anteriorly, whereas a smaller margin can be taken deep to the wire.
- For mammographic masses, palpation along the wire will often allow the surgeon to identify the abnormality and proceed with excision, simplifying the procedure.
- Dissection continues until you are confident you are past the location of the abnormality and the specimen can be transected (FIG 11). Often, the wire will be encountered during this step, so take care not to divide the wire, potentially leaving the hooked end in the patient. If the wire is identified at this point, visualize where on the wire you are. If you are at the hook and the films show the hook is distal to the lesion, you should be fine. If you encountered the reinforced portion of the wire, grasp the remaining tissue in the direction of the wire and continue the dissection until you are past the hook.

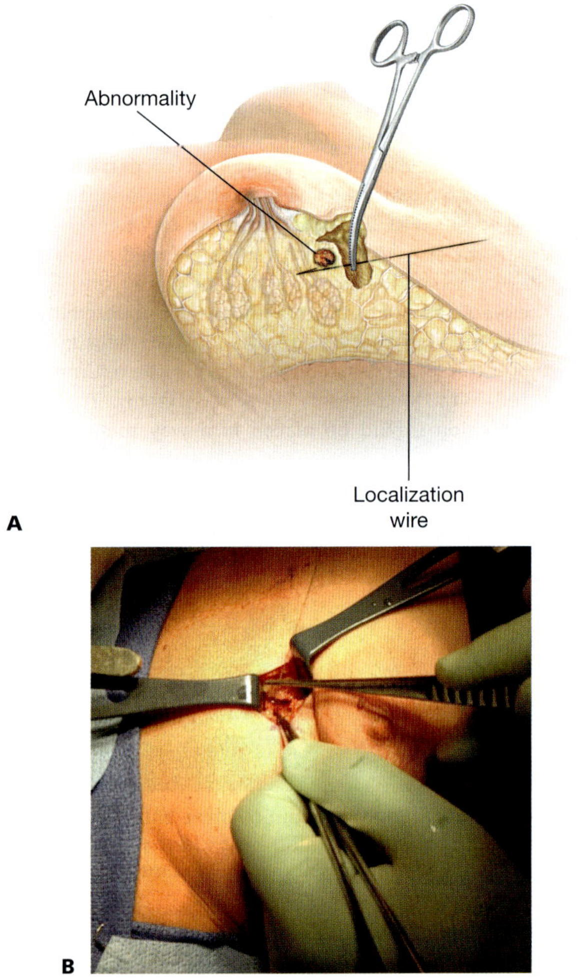

FIG 9 ● **A.** The wire is secured at the breast with a hemostat. **B.** Forceps are then used to pull the external portion of the wire through the skin and out of the wound.

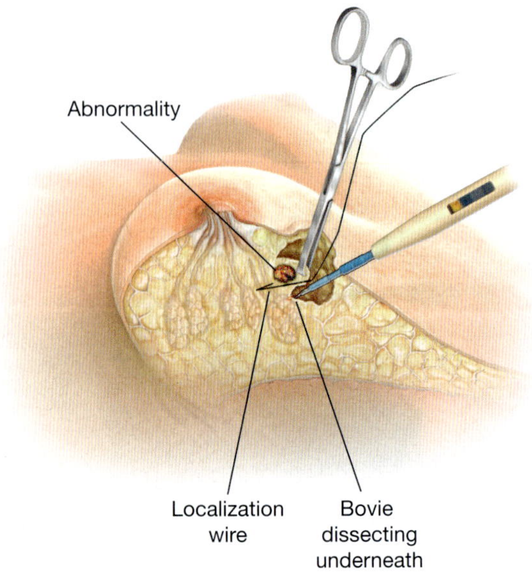

FIG 10 ● An Allis clamp is used to grasp the breast tissue (do not grab the wire) and dissection continues parallel to the wire in all directions.

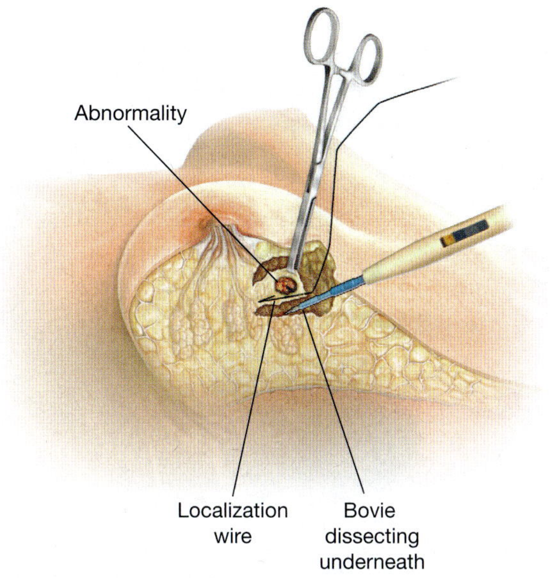

FIG 11 ● Once the circumferential dissection is past where you estimate the lesion to be, the specimen is transected, taking care not to divide the wire (and leave the hook).

ORIENTATION

- Immediately upon removing the lesion, maintain the orientation and place 2-0 silk sutures for the pathologist. If this returns as cancer, this allows for simple reexcision of any involved margin as opposed to a reexcision of the entire cavity. It is often preferable to place one or two orienting sutures before complete removal of the specimen.

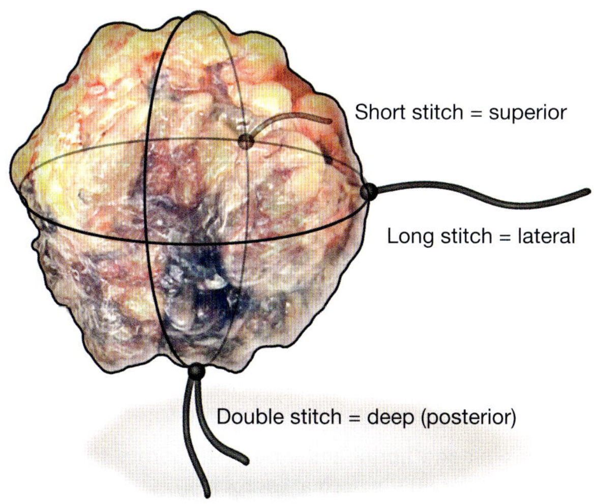

- Three sutures are recommended to orient the mass correctly for the pathologist and avoid errors.[8] We recommend placing a short suture superiorly, a long suture laterally, and a double suture deep posteriorly (**FIG 12**).
- It is also often beneficial to place radiopaque clips on the specimen to allow for orientation of the lesion on the specimen mammograms. For example, if the wire enters laterally, placing a single clip superiorly and a double clip posteriorly allows you to orient the specimen on the films (**FIG 13A,B**). In the case of a wire-localized lumpectomy for cancer, this allows for reexcision of a potentially close margin. For a biopsy, if the abnormality is not within the specimen, this may help the surgeon identify in what direction additional tissue should be sampled.

FIG 12 ● The lesion is oriented with three marking sutures prior to sending to radiology for specimen mammography.

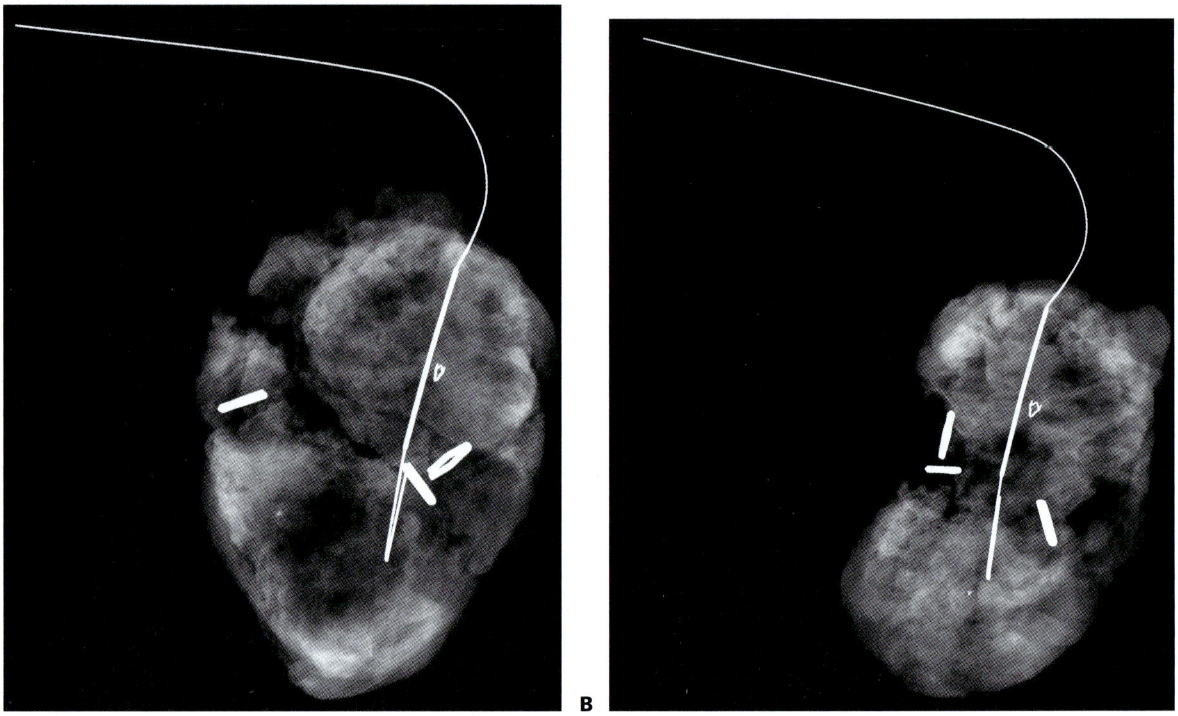

FIG 13 ● **A,B.** Specimen mammography shows the clip and wire to be completely removed.

SPECIMEN RADIOGRAPHY AND ADDITIONAL TISSUE

- Specimen radiography is performed to confirm that the area of concern has been removed (**FIG 13A,B**). The specimen mammogram should demonstrate the presence of the microcalcifications of concern or the presence of a clip placed within the specimen. It should also show that the entire wire has been removed. If the wire becomes separated from the specimen, send both to radiology to document its removal.
- If the lesion is identified on specimen radiography, the wound can be closed. If the lesion is not present, then additional tissue should be excised and sent to radiology. It may be clinically evident what area needs further excision based on exposure of the wire during the dissection. The use of radiopaque clips on the specimen, as well as other landmarks on the original mammograms, may also help identify where to excise additional tissue.
- If a second specimen fails to identify the lesion, it becomes a judgment call whether to continue or abandon the procedure. For ultrasound-visible lesions, intraoperative ultrasound may be able to identify the abnormality. In the case of a clip that should have been in the specimen, sometimes these can get dislodged and suctioned out. Filtering and x-raying the fluid in the suction canister can sometimes reveal a dislodged clip. Otherwise, it may be prudent not to continue and plan on reimaging and, if necessary, returning to the OR rather than taking an excessive amount of breast tissue.

CLOSURE

- Once the biopsy is complete, hemostasis is assured and the wound is irrigated with saline.
- For an excisional biopsy, the surgeon should *not* try to reapproximate the breast tissue. The cavity will fill with seroma and fibrin, and ultimately, fibrous tissue, which will maintain the normal contour.
- The incision is closed with absorbable deep dermal sutures, followed by either a subcuticular stitch or tissue adhesive. Drains should not be used.

PEARLS AND PITFALLS

Indications	■ Image-guided biopsy is the preferred approach to the nonpalpable abnormality. Review the case with the radiologist to confirm whether this is an option.
Placement of incision	■ Keep in mind that if malignant, the patient may need a reexcision lumpectomy or mastectomy. Orient your incision with this in mind.
Identifying the wire	■ Take care not to move or dislodge the wire during the positioning, prepping, and draping of the patient. ■ Identify the wire early and secure it while bringing it into the wound so that it does not become dislodged during the procedure.
Excision	■ Grasp the tissue, not the wire, while excising the lesion so as not to accidently pull the wire out. ■ During dissection, palpate the area to identify the mass or if you are too close to the wire.
Specimen mammography	■ Three orientation sutures are necessary to avoid error. ■ Clips can help orient the specimen on the mammography so as to guide a reexcision.
Closure	■ Do not try to reapproximate the breast tissue or place a drain.

POSTOPERATIVE CARE

- After a breast biopsy, the patient should be placed in a breast binder or supportive brassiere. This helps sustain hemostasis and relieves tension on the skin closure imposed by the weight of the breasts. The patient should be encouraged to wear the support bra day and night for 1 week after surgery.

OUTCOMES

- In experienced hands, the failure rate of wire-localized biopsy is low, although published reports suggest the wire localization failure rate can range from 0% to 20%. Factors associated with failure include lesion type and size, distance from the wire, breast shape and size, and volume of excised tissue.[9–11]

COMPLICATIONS

- Seroma
- Hematoma
- Infection (cellulitis or abscess)
- Pneumothoraces (rare)
- Retained wire fragments
- Failure to identify abnormality

REFERENCES

1. Lewis JA, Lee DY, Tartter PI. The significance of lobular carcinoma in situ and atypical lobular hyperplasia of the breast. *Ann Surg Oncol.* 2012:19(13):4124–4128.
2. Nguyen CV, Albarracin CT, Whitman GJ, et al. Atypical ductal hyperplasia in directional vacuum-assisted biopsy of breast microcalcifications: considerations for surgical excision. *Ann Surg Oncol.* 2011;18:752–761.
3. Peres A, Barranger E, Becette V, et al. Rates of upgrade to malignancy for 271 cases of flat epithelial atypia (FEA) diagnosed by breast core biopsy. *Breast Cancer Res Treat.* 2012;133(2):659–666.
4. Douglas-Jones AG, Denson JL, Cox AC, et al. Radial scar lesions of the breast diagnosed by needle core biopsy: analysis of cases containing occult malignancy. *J Clin Pathol.* 2007;60:295–298.
5. Jaffer S, Nagi C, Bleiweiss IJ. Excision is indicated for intraductal papilloma of the breast diagnosed on core needle biopsy. *Cancer.* 2009;115:2837–2843.
6. Cheng TY, Chen CM, Lee MY, et al. Risk factors associated with conversion from nonmalignant to malignant diagnosis after surgical excision of breast papillary lesions. *Ann Surg Oncol.* 2009;16:3375–3379.
7. Bunn F, Jones DJ, Bell-Syer S. Prophylactic antibiotics to prevent surgical site infections after breast cancer surgery. *Cochrane Database Syst Rev.* 2012;(1):CD005360. doi:10.1002/14651858.CD005360.pub3.
8. Molina MA, Snell S, Franceschi D, et al. Breast specimen orientation. *Ann Surg Oncol.* 2009;16:285–288.
9. Jackman RJ, Marzoni FA Jr. Needle-localized breast biopsy: why do we fail? *Radiology.* 1997;204(3):677–684.
10. Abrahamson PE, Dunlap LA, Amamoo MA, et al. Factors predicting successful needle-localized breast biopsy. *Acad Radiol.* 2003;10(6):601–606.
11. Kouskos E, Gui GP, Mantas D, et al. Wire localization biopsy of nonpalpable breast lesions: reasons for unsuccessful excision. *Eur J Gynaecol Oncol.* 2006;27(3):262–366.

Chapter 3 Subareolar Duct Excision

Amy C. Degnim

DEFINITION

- Subareolar duct excision is defined as the surgical removal of lactiferous ducts in the immediate subareolar space. The terms "major duct excision" or "central duct excision" refer to excision of the entire bundle of ducts contained within the central nipple stalk; microdochectomy refers to selective excision of a single abnormal duct.

ANATOMY

- The lactiferous ducts drain converging ducts from lobes of the breast gland and serve as a conduit for milk egress via the nipple during lactation (**FIG 1**). Most women have approximately 7 to 20 ducts that are distinct and functional sources of milk during lactation. At the base of the nipple, the lactiferous ducts widen centrally in a spindle shape over a short distance. This region is called the lactiferous sinus and can expand in lactation to 8 mm as a reservoir for milk. Surrounding the lactiferous ducts is a system of smooth muscle fibers that contract in response to nipple stimulation and oxytocin release, facilitating milk flow through the nipple.[1]

PATIENT HISTORY AND PHYSICAL FINDINGS

- Subareolar duct excision is undertaken in cases of abnormal nipple discharge for two purposes:
  - To obtain diagnostic biopsy tissue and rule out malignancy
  - To provide resolution of the bothersome discharge
- Abnormal, or "pathologic," nipple discharge is characterized by the following features:
  - Discharge from a single duct
  - Spontaneous discharge
  - Clear or bloody discharge
- The history should be focused on questions to determine the laterality and quality of the discharge as well as whether it is spontaneous or only occurs with manual expression.
- Physical exam should include a thorough examination of both breasts and axillae.
- In addition, a detailed examination is necessary for both nipple–areolar complexes and the subareolar tissues.
- Inspect the nipples for crusting, bloodstained ducts, or any visible protuberances or nodules.
- The deep tissue of the areolae should be palpated carefully for any small nodules and to determine if subareolar pressure results in nipple discharge.
- The nipple itself should be palpated by rolling the nipple between the thumb and forefinger in order to best detect any small nodules located centrally within the nipple stalk. This should be performed first for the breast without discharge to set a normal comparison to the breast that is symptomatic.
- If no discharge has been identified up to this step of the examination, then attempt should be made to elicit discharge from both nipples, by applying pressure to the areola at the base of the nipple, then grasping the base of the nipple between the thumb and forefinger and drawing upward with gentle pressure.
- Throughout the examination, for any nipple discharge observed, its location (o'clock position) and quality of the fluid should be noted.

IMAGING AND OTHER DIAGNOSTIC STUDIES

- All women with abnormal nipple discharge should undergo diagnostic mammogram and ultrasound. Prior to the imaging studies, the imaging team should be informed about the symptom of nipple discharge and which breast is affected.
- Because nipple discharge can be associated with underlying malignancy, the primary purpose of diagnostic imaging is to look for possible signs of malignancy. Another goal of imaging is to evaluate the subareolar tissues for any findings that would explain the presence of nipple discharge.
- Generally, subareolar ducts are not visible with ultrasound unless they are abnormally dilated. A small nodule visualized within a dilated subareolar duct indicates a likely diagnosis of intraductal papilloma (**FIG 2**).

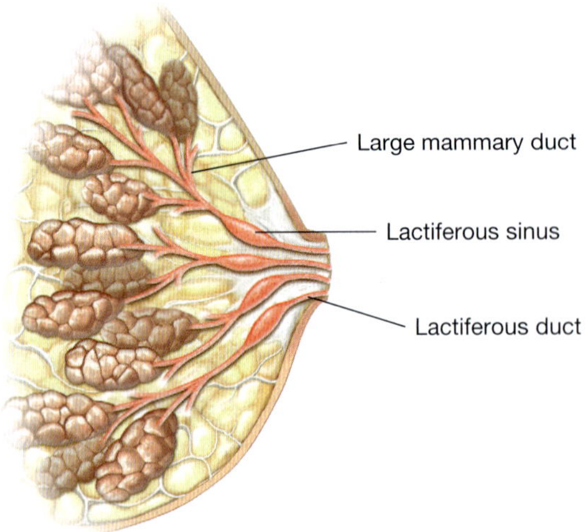

FIG 1 • Normal anatomy of subareolar lactiferous ducts and sinuses.

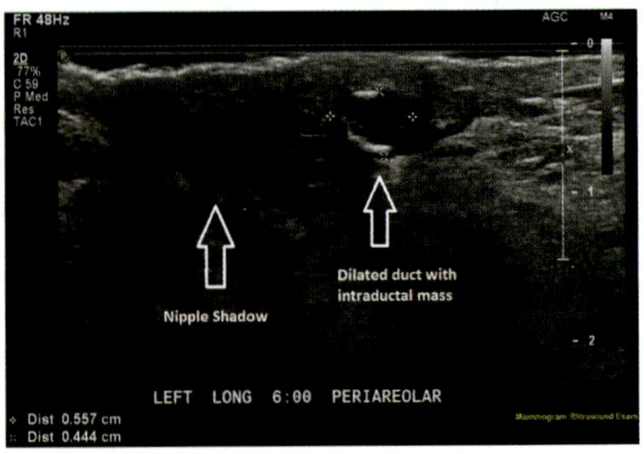

FIG 2 • Ultrasound of a subareolar nodule.

- Evaluation with magnetic resonance imaging (MRI) is controversial. It detects more lesions than standard imaging for women with nipple discharge but is imperfect in ruling out malignancy associated with nipple discharge.[2]
- Ductography can be considered as a diagnostic test. This is a radiographic procedure that entails cannulation of the duct with abnormal discharge, then injection of contrast dye with immediate mammographic imaging. This procedure can identify and map out abnormal ducts and identify some intraductal filling defects, but it does not provide diagnostic tissue. For these reasons, it is not a required component of the evaluation and is intentionally avoided in some practices. Although it may help to localize the etiology of the discharge, it cannot reliably exclude malignancy or eliminate need for duct excision.[3]
- Another approach to diagnostic evaluation is via ductoscopy, a microendoscopic procedure to directly visualize the duct(s) with discharge. This requires special equipment and skill, with a learning curve for technical success. Ductoscopy can help to identify lesions and guide excision but has not been proven in large numbers of women to improve diagnosis to the point that duct excision can be avoided.[4,5]

DIFFERENTIAL DIAGNOSIS

- Intraductal papilloma
- Duct ectasia
- Carcinoma, either invasive or ductal carcinoma in situ
- Paget's disease

NONOPERATIVE MANAGEMENT

- Nonoperative management can be considered for cases of nipple discharge when
  - The discharge occurred on only one occasion and was not reproducible on examination
  - Both mammogram and ultrasound show no abnormalities.[6,7]
  - In this case, 3-month follow-up history and physical examination is recommended.
- Alternately, if imaging identifies a benign-appearing lesion and percutaneous core biopsy confirms a benign intraductal papilloma with complete or near complete removal by imaging, then observation is also appropriate with follow-up imaging in 3 months.

SURGICAL MANAGEMENT

- Subareolar duct excision removes the lactiferous ducts under the nipple, the primary connection between the nipple and the milk-producing lobules of the breast, so patients must be counseled that lactation from the operated breast should not be possible after surgery.
- Selective and focused excision of the single abnormal duct may be performed in an attempt to preserve other ducts for future lactation, but due to the very close proximity of the remaining ducts, scar tissue from the operation may still impair future lactation.
- In women who are past childbearing age, a plan to remove the entire bundle of subareolar ducts is preferred because future lactation is not needed, and this approach reduces the chance of recurrent discharge from another duct and need for repeat operation in a field of scar tissue.
- The patient should be informed of the possibility of a diagnosis of malignancy yet reassured that benign findings are most likely.

Preoperative Planning

- For subareolar mass lesions that are nonpalpable and identified only by imaging, preoperative localization with either a wire or a radioactive seed should be performed to ensure intraoperative guidance to the target.
- Before surgery, patients should be counseled that they may experience continued discharge in the first few weeks postoperatively, as postoperative fluid in the subareolar space may discharge via the nipple duct until healing is complete. This should resolve completely by 4 to 6 weeks.

Positioning

- The patient should be positioned supine.
- The ipsilateral arm is generally positioned at approximately 90 degrees, although the arm could also be tucked based on the patient's body habitus and preferences of the anesthesia team.

Approach

- The general approach is to dissect under the areola toward the nipple, isolate and excise the central duct bundle, and follow any abnormal ducts to complete removal, along with simultaneous excision of any nonpalpable lesions identified on preoperative imaging.

TECHNIQUES

INCISION PLANNING

- In general, incisions are placed at the areolar edge.
- An incision at the inferior areolar edge is preferred if possible for better cosmesis, especially if the involved duct is located centrally on the nipple surface and the imaging does not demonstrate any abnormalities (**FIG 3**).
- Otherwise, incisions can be placed along the areolar border in the o'clock position of the abnormality, for either a peripherally located duct with discharge or if there is an imaging abnormality a few centimeters from the nipple.

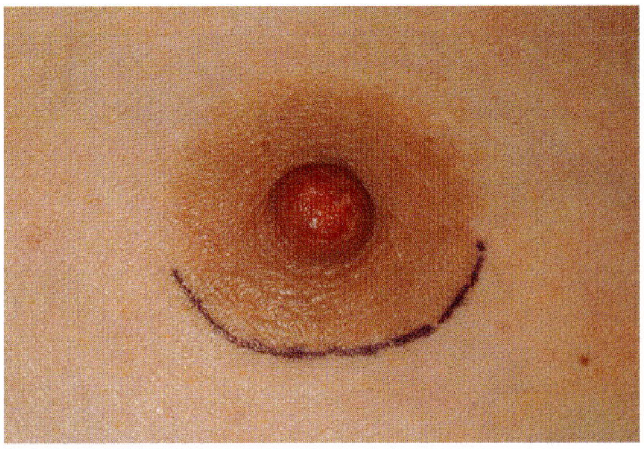

FIG 3 • Incision at inferior areolar border.

- The length of the incision should be large enough that the surgeon has adequate visualization of the subareolar space without requiring excess retraction and ischemia of the areolar edge. Depending on the areolar size, the incision may go up to 50% of the circumference of the areola, but a shorter incision is preferred when possible to help preserve blood supply to the nipple and areolar dermis.
- Prior to incision, correct surgical site and plan should be confirmed with the operative team.

DUCT CANNULATION

- Once the field is prepped and draped, attempt should be made to cannulate the involved duct.
- A fine lacrimal duct probe (4-0) should be held ready in the dominant hand for cannulation prior to expressing the nipple discharge.
- The nipple should be grasped between the thumb and forefinger of the nondominant hand at the nipple base and drawn upward gradually (**FIG 4**). If no discharge is seen, increasing pressure can be applied to a reasonable degree. The goal is to elicit a single tiny drop of fluid at the skin surface; a smaller drop of fluid will be more helpful in identifying the location of the abnormal duct (**FIG 5**).
- The nipple should be pulled away from the breast gently in order to elongate the subareolar lactiferous sinus and improve the chance of cannulation (**FIG 6**).
- The lacrimal duct probe should be gently probed along the nipple skin surface at the site of the expressed fluid. The goal is to find the opening rather than make a false passage; the probe will slide easily into the duct once it is in the right location (**FIG 7**).

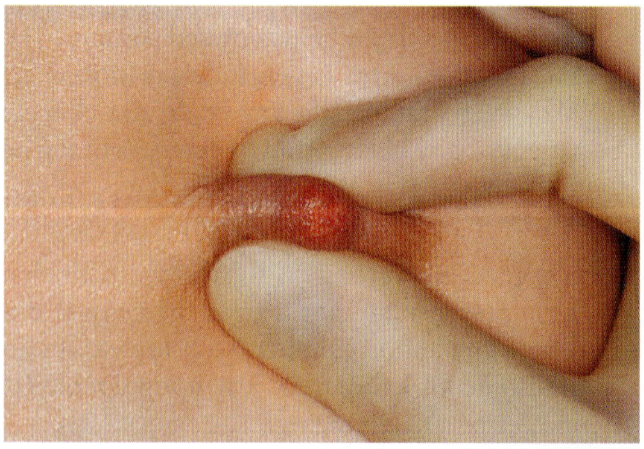

FIG 4 ● Manual expression of nipple discharge.

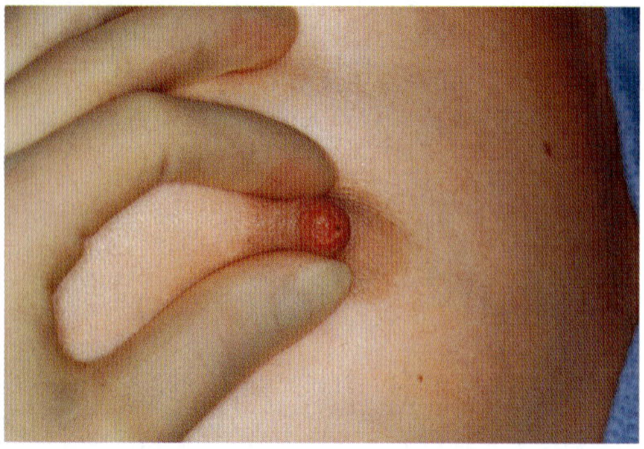

FIG 5 ● Visible tiny drop of fluid at nipple surface.

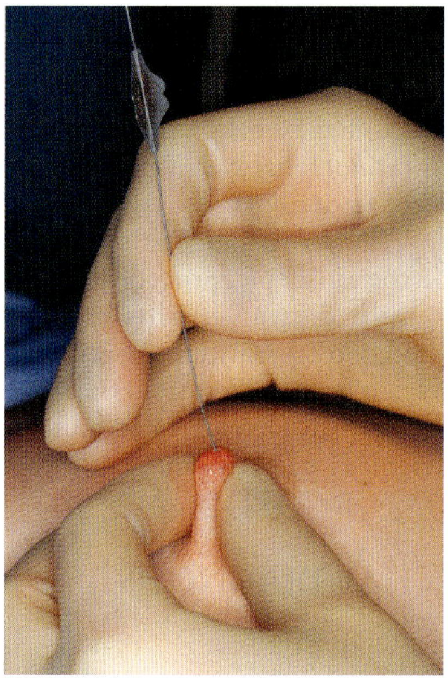

FIG 6 ● Cannulation technique.

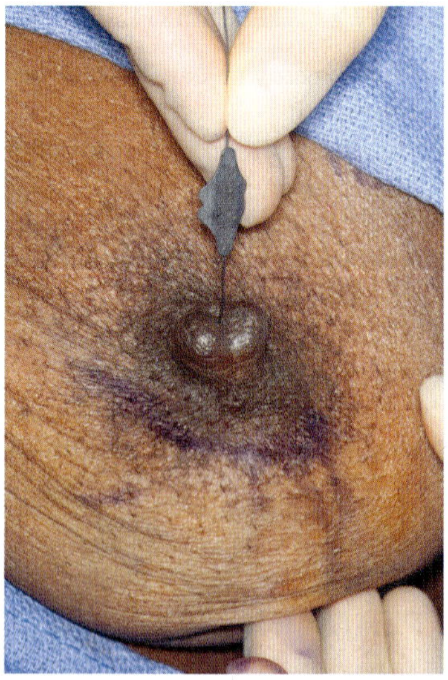

FIG 7 ● Cannulated duct with probe advanced.

- The probe should be gently advanced as far as it will easily go. If it does not pass greater than 1 cm beyond the nipple skin surface, then the depth of the cannulation should be noted as a sign that there may be a very superficial obstructing mass lesion.
- If no discharge is identified or if the duct cannot be cannulated despite several attempts, the procedure should proceed to incision.

INCISION

- Prior to incision, local anesthetic can be used but should not be injected directly into the area of the subareolar ducts. If used, it should be injected intradermally directly at the planned incision site (no more than 1 mL) and additionally in a peripheral fashion into the four quadrants of the breast to create a local field block.
- The skin should be incised sharply with a scalpel, taking care to maintain a blade angle that is perpendicular to the skin.
- The incision should be deepened a few millimeters into the subcutaneous fatty tissue (**FIG 8**).

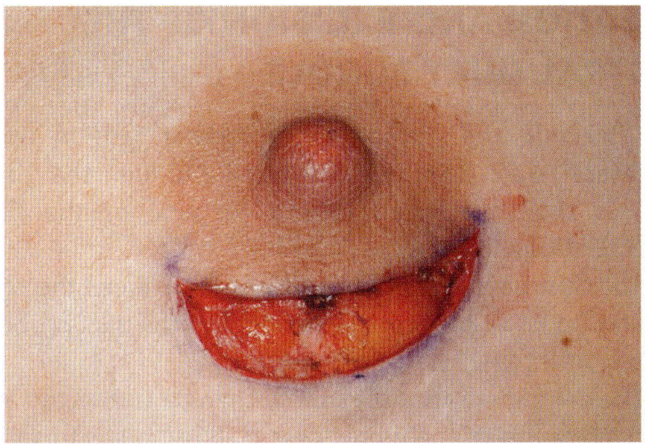

FIG 8 ● Incision into subcutaneous tissue.

ELEVATION OF THE AREOLAR SKIN FLAP

- The areolar skin edge is then retracted superiorly (skin hooks or sutures could be used), and dissection proceeds in the direction of the nipple toward the central duct bundle (**FIG 9**).
- Care should be taken to perform the dissection at a depth to preserve some subcutaneous fatty tissue under the areolar skin, as this will help to protect the viability of the areolar skin and nipple. Similarly, the lateral edges of the dissection field should narrow as the central duct bundle is approached (**FIG 10**).
- Attention should be paid to the location of dissection and its proximity to the nipple, looking closely for the ducts, which appear as narrow vertical tubular or strand-like structures. The ducts may be visibly discolored (**FIG 11**).

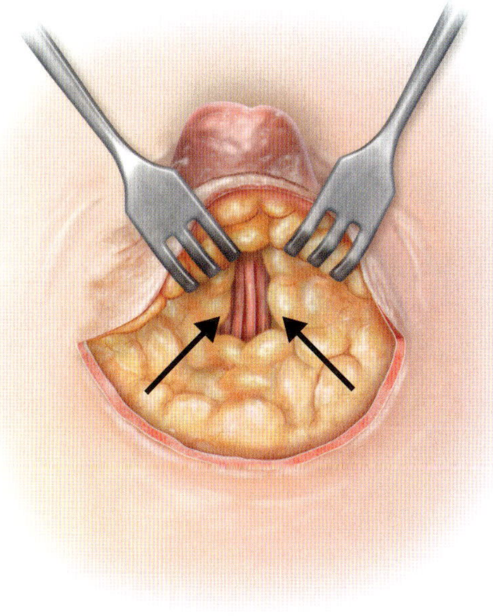

FIG 10 ● Narrowing the dissection field toward the nipple.

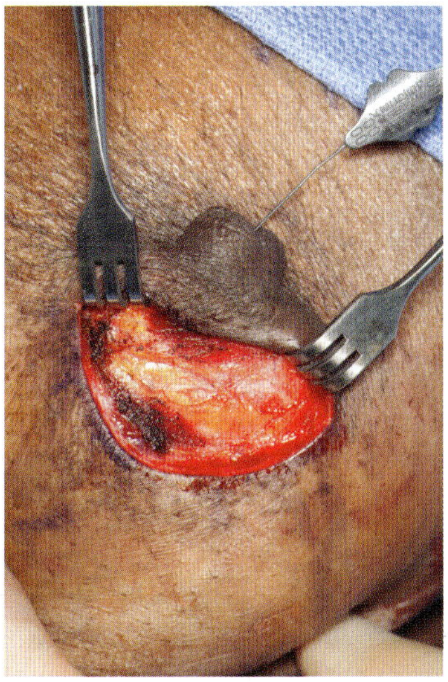

FIG 9 ● Retraction of the skin flap.

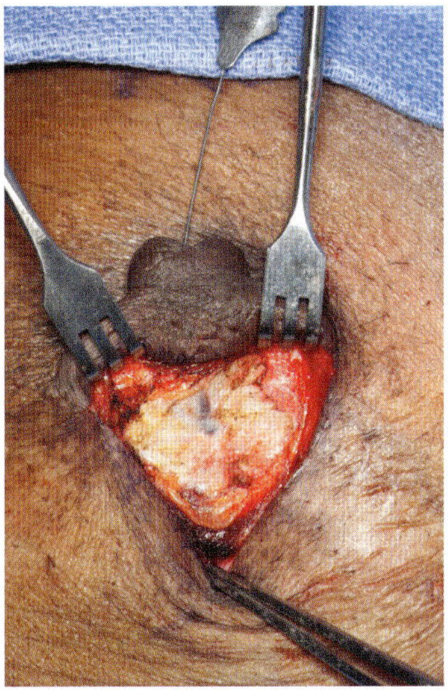

FIG 11 ● A visibly abnormal duct with discolored intraluminal fluid.

ISOLATION AND EXCISION OF THE CENTRAL DUCT BUNDLE

- Dissection then proceeds in vertical fashion on the lateral sides of the duct bundle under the nipple. This should proceed to the far side of the nipple (**FIG 12**).
- The duct bundle should be palpated between the thumb and finger to confirm the presence of the duct probe and any other small palpable nodules.
- The central duct bundle should then be transected at the deep aspect of the nipple dermis. If using electrocautery, the "cutting" mode should be chosen at a low energy setting to minimize thermal damage to the nipple dermis.
- As the duct bundle is transected, the cannulating probe will be identified. It may be withdrawn if it becomes difficult to maintain its position in the duct (**FIG 13**).
- The duct bundle should be retracted away from the breast, dissecting circumferentially around the duct bundle to a depth of approximately 4 to 5 cm or farther along a particular grossly abnormal duct (**FIG 14**).
- The tissue specimen should be transected at its base and oriented for the pathologist (**FIG 15**).
- The open wound should be palpated for any abnormalities, and the nipple dermis should be palpated between the thumb and finger to ensure that there are no any superficial nodules present that were not excised. In the event of a small nodule within the nipple dermis, a tiny skin incision in the nipple can be made to remove the lesion.

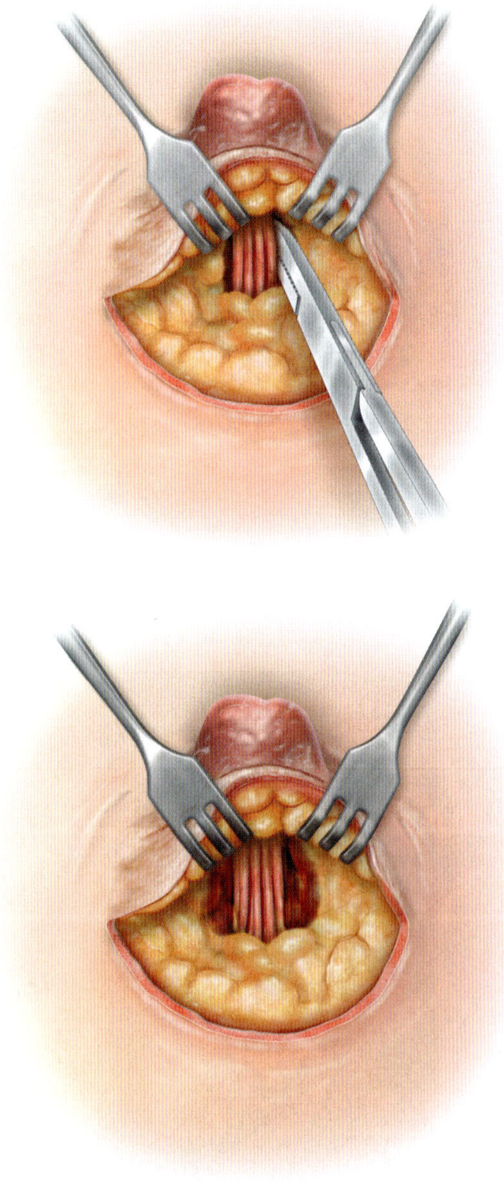

FIG 12 • Vertical dissection along both sides of the duct bundle.

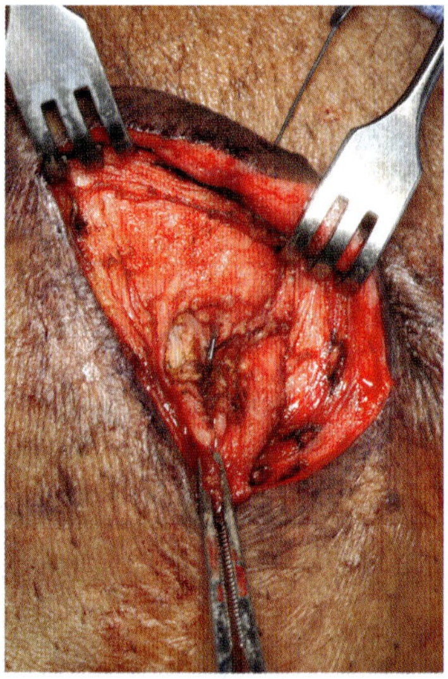

FIG 13 • Transection of the ducts just deep to the nipple dermis.

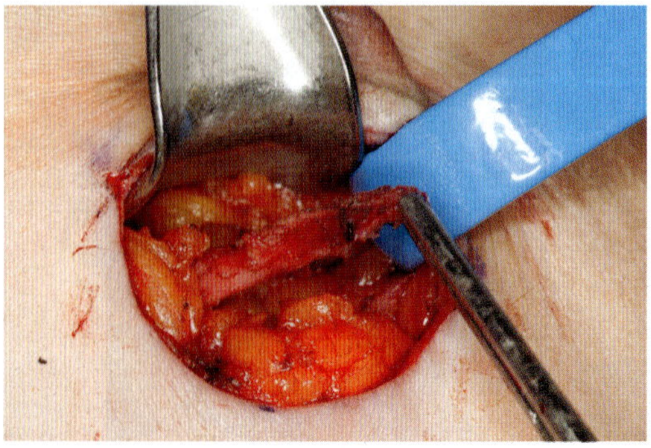

FIG 14 • Dissection of ducts deeper into the breast parenchyma.

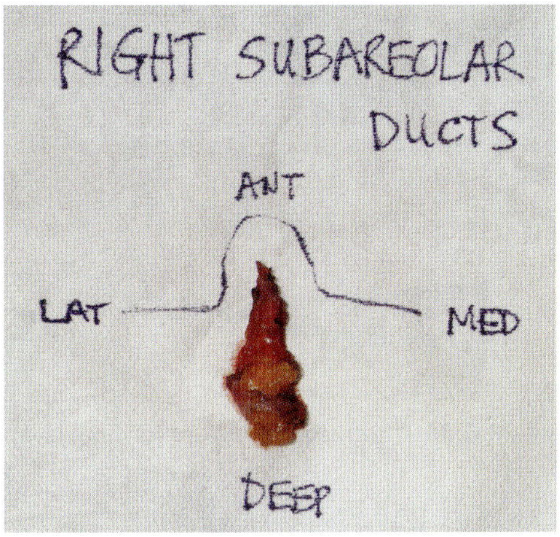

FIG 15 ● Orientation of the specimen.

CLOSURE

- After hemostasis, the parenchymal and subcutaneous tissue defect in the subareolar region must be closed in order to avoid nipple retraction in the healing phase. If there is a solid buttress of tissue underlying the nipple–areolar complex, the nipple will be less likely to retract.
- The parenchymal closure may be performed as a simple direct approximation of tissues, in whatever orientation results in least tension and absence of skin dimpling (**FIG 16**). If the defect is larger, it may require a small local tissue advancement flap or undermining of the breast gland from the skin. In that case, it is preferable to avoid further dissection under the areolar skin and obtain donor tissue from the other side of the cavity.
- If the nipple is effaced, it may be helpful to place a purse-string stitch in the deep dermis around the nipple base to recreate the normal nipple shape and prevent nipple retraction in the healing phase (**FIG 17**).
- The skin should be closed in two layers, with buried interrupted sutures in the deep dermis and subcutaneous tissue, followed by a running intradermal stitch in the skin edge. Care should be taken to place the deep dermal sutures so that the areolar skin edge is at or slightly above the breast skin edge (but not lower) (**FIG 18**), or the nipple–areolar complex will have a sunken-in appearance. If the areola is small, resulting in an incision with greater curvature, the final layer of skin closure should use multiple shorter bites (**FIG 19**).

A

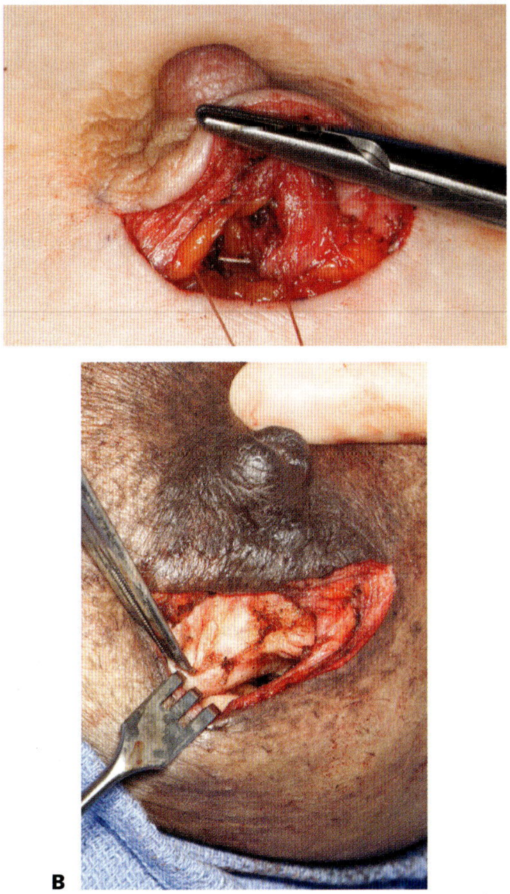

B

FIG 16 ● Closure of the deep tissue. **A.** Medial-to-lateral closure, **(B)** superior-to-inferior closure.

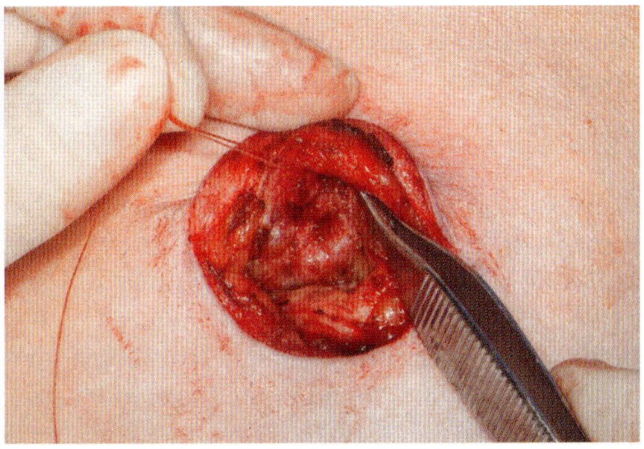

FIG 17 ● Purse-string suture in the deep dermis of the nipple.

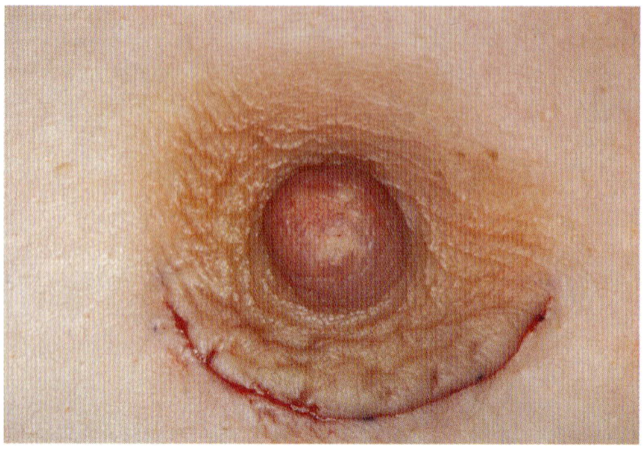

FIG 18 ● Appearance after closure of the deep dermal layer of incision, with the areolar edge at or above the breast skin.

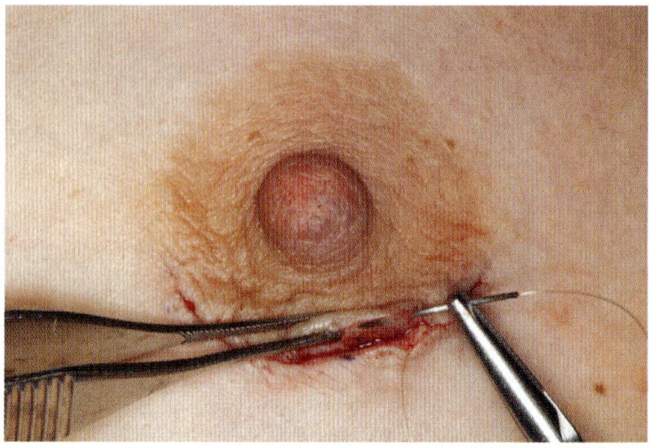

FIG 19 ● Intradermal suture for final layer of closure.

- Adhesive dressings on the dermis of the nipple itself should be avoided. If an incision was required in the nipple dermis for an intradermal nodule, the nipple incision should be closed with fine interrupted nonabsorbable sutures.
- Dressings that create excess pressure on the nipple should also be avoided. If a pressure dressing is desired, it should have a "donut" opening for the nipple.

PEARLS AND PITFALLS

Preoperative counseling	■ Preoperative counseling should address ■ Focused duct excision versus excision of the entire duct bundle ■ Inability to lactate after surgery from the operated breast ■ Likely pathologic findings ■ Possible nipple discharge in the postoperative healing period
Incision planning	■ Inferior areolar edge is preferred.
Subareolar dissection	■ Be careful to preserve subcutaneous fat under the areolar skin and to limit dissection to as narrow a field as possible to reduce risk of skin necrosis.
Closure	■ Proper closure of the deep and superficial tissues under the nipple–areolar complex is critical to avoid nipple retraction with healing, and consider a purse-string stitch to reestablish normal nipple projection.

POSTOPERATIVE CARE

- The incision should be kept clean and dry.
- Clothing that creates excess pressure on the nipple should be avoided, and patients may choose to use a donut-type foam dressing to relieve any pressure on the nipple.
- Showering is permitted.
- If any nonabsorbable sutures were placed in the nipple skin, they are removed at 1 week.

OUTCOMES

- Subareolar duct excision for abnormal nipple discharge is highly successful, with resolution of discharge in the vast majority. Recurrent discharge is reported in the range of less than 5%.[8]
- Pathology findings are most often benign (papilloma or duct ectasia), but malignancy is found in the range of 0% to 20%.[8,9]
- The likelihood of successful lactation after duct excision is not well characterized.

COMPLICATIONS

- Bleeding and infection are possible complications after every surgical procedure but are rare with this procedure. Avoidance of antiplatelet therapies and anticoagulants per surgical routine will help to minimize risk of bleeding, and a single preoperative dose of intravenous antibiotics is recommended prophylactically.
- Skin necrosis is also rare but devastating if it occurs; for this reason, careful attention should be paid to preserving blood supply to the areolar tissue and limiting the extent of dissection under the areolar skin, with focused excision of the central ductal tissue.

ACKNOWLEDGMENTS

Sincere thanks to Marilyn Churchward for assistance with manuscript preparation.

REFERENCES

1. Fritsch H, Kühnel W. *Color Atlas of Human Anatomy: Internal Organs*. Vol 2. 5th ed. New York, NY: Thieme; 2008:418.
2. Morrogh M, Morris EA, Liberman L, et al. The predictive value of ductography and magnetic resonance imaging in the management of nipple discharge. *Ann Surg Oncol*. 2007;14(12):3369–3377.
3. Dawes LG, Bowen C, Venta LA, et al. Ductography for nipple discharge: no replacement for ductal excision. *Surgery*. 1998;124: 685–691.
4. Fisher CS, Margenthaler JA. A look into the ductoscope: its role in pathologic nipple discharge. *Ann Surg Oncol*. 2011;18:3187–3191.
5. Khan SA, Mangat A, Rivers A, et al. Office ductoscopy for surgical selection in women with pathologic nipple discharge. *Ann Surg Oncol*. 2011;18:3785–3790.
6. Gray RJ, Pockaj BA, Karstaedt PJ. Navigating murky waters: a modern treatment algorithm for nipple discharge. *Am J Surg*. 2007;194:850–855.
7. Sabel MS, Helvie MA, Breslin T, et al. Is duct excision still necessary for all cases of suspicious nipple discharge? *Breast J*. 2012;18(2):157–162.
8. Morrogh M, Park A, Elkin EB, et al. Lessons learned from 416 cases of nipple discharge of the breast. *Am J Surg*. 2010;200:73–80.
9. Kooistra BW, Wauters C, van de Ven S, et al. The diagnostic value of nipple discharge cytology in 618 consecutive patients. *Eur J Surg Oncol*. 2009;35:573–577.

Chapter 4

Cryoablation of Breast Fibroadenomas

Cary S. Kaufman

CRYOABLATION TREATMENT FOR BREAST FIBROADENOMAS—OVERVIEW

- Cryoablation is a minimally invasive, innovative treatment for breast fibroadenomas. The treatment is performed in an office setting rather than an operating room, resulting in a cost-effective and patient-friendly procedure with little to no scarring. Published reports demonstrate that cryoablation as primary treatment for breast fibroadenomas is safe and effective and at long-term follow-up, demonstrates progressive resolution of the treated area, with excellent patient and physician satisfaction (Table 1).
- About 80% of the approximately 1.3 million biopsies performed annually in the United States reveal benign conditions, primarily benign tumors or fibrocystic change. The most common benign breast tumor is a fibroadenoma.[1–3]
- Although not life threatening, benign breast tumors can cause fear, anxiety, and discomfort in the patient, and definitive treatment is often desired.[3–5]
- Fibroadenomas consist of a proliferation of epithelial and connective tissue elements within the lobular region of the breast. They are usually sharply demarcated from the adjacent breast tissue and give the clinical and imaged appearance of being encapsulated.[5]
- They often grow to a size of 2 to 3 cm and are multiple in 20% of women.[4,6–9]
- Approximately 10% of women will experience a fibroadenoma in their lifetime. Although most common in young women, fibroadenoma occurs in every age-group from adolescents to octogenarians.[1,2,7,10,11]

DIFFERENTIAL DIAGNOSIS

- These benign breast tumors have a classic physical examination: rubbery texture, smooth and well defined, circular to oval, and freely moveable within the breast.
- Other breast lesions that may have similar clinical presentations include phyllodes tumors, juvenile fibroadenomas, breast cancer (particularly medullary carcinomas), or breast cysts. Diagnosis is resolved by imaging and core needle biopsy.
- Cryoablation has only been proven effective for biopsy-proven fibroadenomas (Table 2).[12–16]

Table 1: Potential Advantages for Cryoablation in the Treatment of Fibroadenoma

Reasons to consider ablation techniques:
Small puncture incision
A procedure not surgery
Less scarring
Minimal discomfort
Less invasive
Less expensive

PATIENT HISTORY AND PHYSICAL FINDINGS

- Patients with small- to medium-sized single tumors that are not too close to the skin or nipple are appropriate candidates for cryoablation. Indications and contraindications are listed in Table 3.
- The target lesion must be clearly visible with ultrasound and not be within 1 cm of the skin or immediately deep to the nipple.
- A histologic diagnosis using a core biopsy should demonstrate a classic fibroadenoma without atypia. Other histologic lesions are not appropriate for cryoablation.
- Tumors should be measured in three dimensions and the longest dimension used to calculate freezing time (**FIG 1**).
- It is important to discuss with the patient the process of cryoablation and the progressive resorption of the residual necrotic debris over time (**FIG 2**).
- The candidate should not currently have breast cancer in the ipsilateral breast and be otherwise healthy. She should not be pregnant, breastfeeding, or have breast implants.

IMAGING AND OTHER DIAGNOSTIC STUDIES

- If the patient is in the mammography screening age-group, a pretreatment screening mammogram should be obtained and be normal except for the fibroadenoma (**FIG 3**).
- There are classic imaging findings of fibroadenoma on both ultrasound and mammography, but histology is needed for an accurate diagnosis[1,3,9,17] (**FIGS 3** and **4A,B**, ultrasound and mammogram of a fibroadenoma).
- The differential diagnosis includes the larger and faster growing juvenile fibroadenomas and phyllodes tumors.[1,7,9]
- Large-core needle biopsy is the diagnostic method of choice because of the need to differentiate between benign and malignant tumors in general and fibroadenoma from phyllodes tumor in particular.[1,9]

MANAGEMENT OPTIONS

- There are three treatment options for a confirmed fibroadenoma: (1) serial observation ("watchful waiting"), (2) surgical removal, and (3) cryoablation. Surgery for fibroadenoma provides definitive treatment while confirming the diagnosis and eliminating patient anxiety and future monitoring. Drawbacks to surgical excision include patient discomfort, anesthetic and surgical recovery, skin incision and potential scarring as well as operating room costs.[18]
- On the other hand, many women choose serial observation with the advantages of no surgical pain, avoidance of the operating room and anesthesia, less cost, and only a minimal scar from the large-core needle biopsy. Drawbacks to conservative management include ongoing patient anxiety regarding the presence and potential growth of a lump, the inconvenience of serial office visits, and the confusion of physical examination and mammography evaluations caused by the mass effect.[7,19]

Table 2: Published Reports of Cryoablation for Fibroadenomas

Author	Fibroadenomas (n)	Mean Size (cm)	Freeze Time (min)	Skin Injury	Any Growth @ 1 y	Still Palpable @ 1 y	Volume Decr (%) @ 1 y	Cosmesis by Patient @ 1 y	Satisfied Patient @ 1 y
Edwards[a]	310	1.8	N/A	0%	None	33%	97%	92%	100%
Nurko[b]	444	1.8	22	0%	None	35%	71%	82%	88%
Hahn[c]	23	<3.0	10	4%	None	22%	76%	96%	96%
Kaufman[d]	70	2.1	15	6%	None	25%	89%	100%	97%
Total/average	847	1.9	16	3%	None	29%	83%	93%	95%

[a]*From Edwards MJ, Broadwater R, Tafra L, et al. Progressive adoption of cryoablative therapy for breast fibroadenoma in community practice.* Am J Surg. *2004;188:221–224.*
[b]*From Nurko J, Mabry CD, Whitworth P, et al. Interim results from the FibroAdenoma Cryoablation Treatment Registry.* Am J Surg. *2005;190(4):647–651.*
[c]*From Hahn M, Pavlista D, Danes J, et al. Ultrasound guided cryoablation of fibroadenomas.* Ultraschall Med. *2013;34(1):64–68.*
[d]*From Kaufman CS, Littrup PJ, Freman-Gibb LA, et al. Office-based cryoablation of breast fibroadenomas: 12-month followup.* J Am Coll Surg. *2004;198:914–923.*

Table 3: Indications and Contraindications for Cryoablation for Fibroadenomas

Inclusion criteria for fibroadenoma cryoablation:
1. Lesion must be sonographically visible.
2. Diagnosis of fibroadenoma must have histologic confirmation.
3. Lesion size must be <3 cm in largest diameter.

Contraindications for cryoablation:
1. Pathology suggestive of phyllodes tumor or malignancy
2. Poor ultrasound visualization
3. Pathologic diagnosis of fibroadenoma nonconcordant with imaging or physical examination

Note: After cryoablation, patients should be followed with ultrasound assessment and physical examination at 6, 12, 18, and 24 months postprocedure.

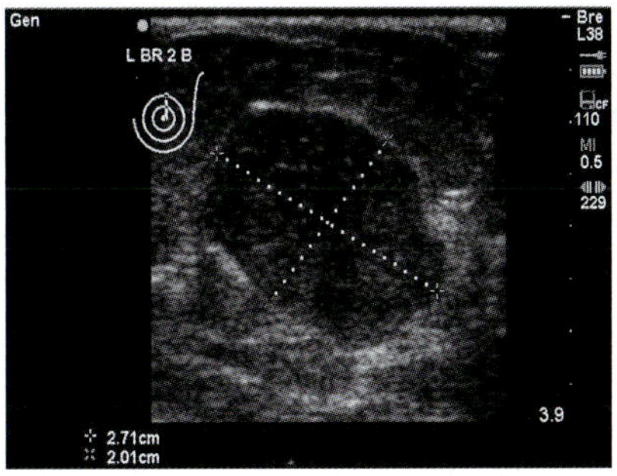

FIG 1 • Ultrasound of fibroadenoma prior to treatment. Size, position, and two orthogonal views are taken.

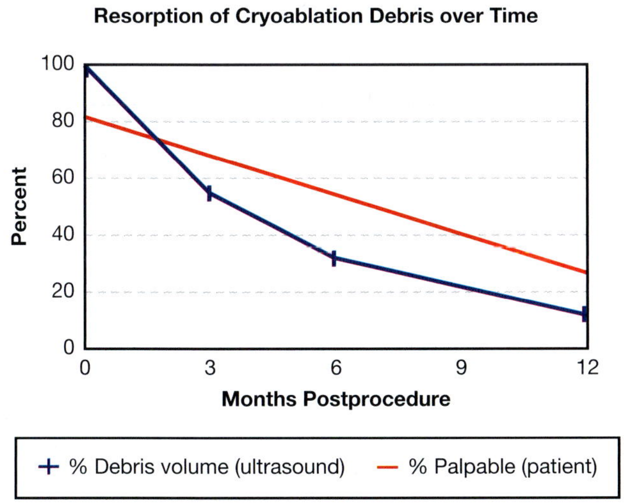

FIG 2 • Postcryoablation resolution of palpable and ultrasound-visible cryolesion over the first year. Most cryolesions fully dissolve over the year, but tumors larger than 2 cm will take longer to resorb.

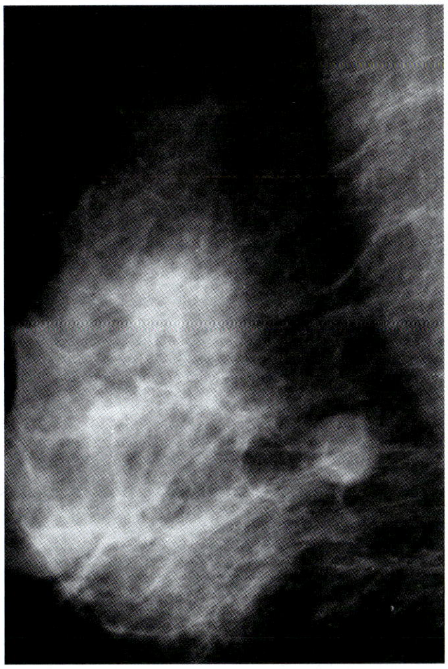

FIG 3 • Mammogram demonstrating oval fibroadenoma.

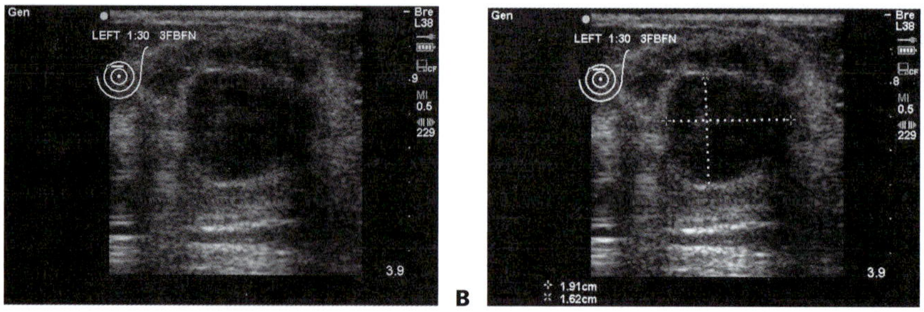

FIG 4 • **A,B.** Classic ultrasound image of fibroadenoma demonstrating well-defined borders and homogeneous solid mass with edge shadowing.

- Cryoablation for fibroadenoma has the advantage of being an office-based procedure with no need for systemic anesthesia, minimal discomfort, skin incision similar to the core biopsy site, and the expectation of lower overall costs of treatment compared with surgical excision. Drawbacks include slow progressive resorption of residual palpable debris.
- Multiple reports in the United States and Europe of favorable outcomes make cryoablation for fibroadenoma an attractive alternative for patients.[12–16,20] As a result of these reports, the American Society of Breast Surgeons has produced a statement in support of cryoablation as an acceptable alternative method of treatment of fibroadenoma.[21]

POSITIONING AND PROCEDURE DESCRIPTION

- Prior to the procedure, the cryoablation machine should be prepared, which typically includes filling the Dewars with liquid nitrogen.
- Cryoablation is an office-based sterile procedure with preparation similar to that of an ultrasound-guided core needle biopsy. Have a sterile cryoprobe available and a sterile field setup with equipment similar to that needed for core needle biopsy. In addition to the sterile instruments, multiple syringes of sterile saline should be available for injections to distance the skin away from the cryoprobe during the procedure.
- The cryoprobe should be tested just prior to use. A backup probe should be available in case the probe tests defective. During the test, no air bubbles should be discharged from the tip of the probe.
- Most cryoablation devices have an automated treatment program that is based on the longest tumor dimension to calculate treatment times. To initiate the automated treatment protocol on the cryoablation device, enter the fibroadenoma size measurement into the cryomachine.
- Note the distance beyond the fibroadenoma that the probe must extend for the symmetric distribution of the freezing.
- Identify the ideal skin entry site to create a cryoprobe pathway along the long axis of the fibroadenoma with adequate circumferential distance for the cryoprobe iceball to be entirely within the breast and away from the skin.
- Inject local anesthetic in the skin and along the path toward the fibroadenoma. Infiltrate some local anesthetic deep to and around the periphery of the target lesion. Some local is valuable beyond the target for the "past-pointing" of the cryoprobe beyond the tumor.
- Use a no. 11 scalpel blade to make a 3-mm entry site for the cryoprobe.
- Carefully place the tested cryoprobe along the desired track into and through the fibroadenoma (**FIG 5A**). This may take some time to be sure the cryoprobe lies within the center of the fibroadenoma. Before a final pathway is chosen, be sure that the cryoprobe lies in the mid-center

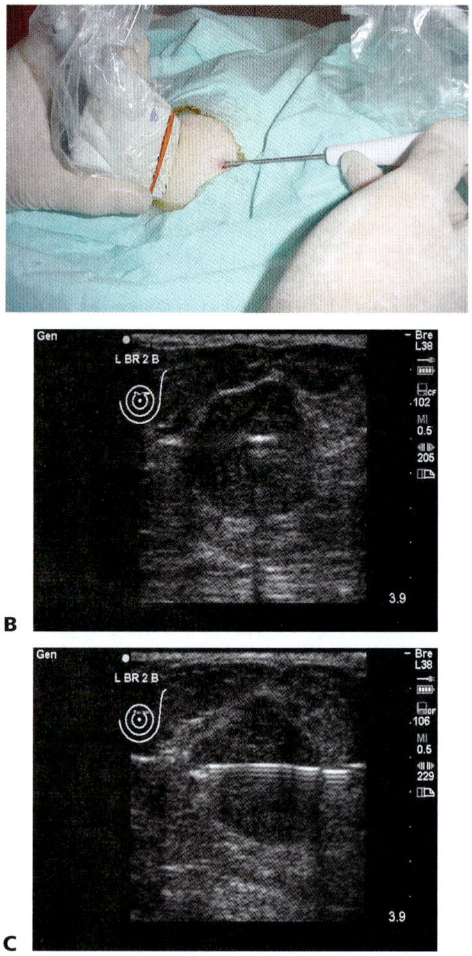

FIG 5 • **A.** Ultrasound examination of probe placement to confirm central location within fibroadenoma. **B.** Ultrasound view of probe in tumor via transverse image. **C.** Ultrasound view of probe in tumor via longitudinal image.

of the target lesion. Move your targeting ultrasound in all directions to confirm cryoprobe central placement both longitudinally and transversely (**FIG 5B,C**, two orthogonal ultrasound views of position of cryoprobe within fibroadenoma).

- Some fibroadenomas are very dense, causing the cryoprobe to deviate off the desired central pathway. It may take repeated efforts to place the probe in the center of a very rubbery tumor.
- One method to facilitate central probe position is to obtain a core needle biopsy just prior to placing the probe. If the core needle biopsy is obtained from the desired central pathway, it will be easier to place the treatment cryoprobe in the same path.
- Once the cryoprobe has adequately been placed and the distal "past-pointing" has been measured, you are ready to initiate the cryoablation sequence.
- Press the start button and use the ultrasound unit to document the development of the iceball. Obtain multiple measurements, especially iceball size, at the end of each of the three phases of treatment: first freeze, thaw, and second freeze (**FIG 6A,B**).

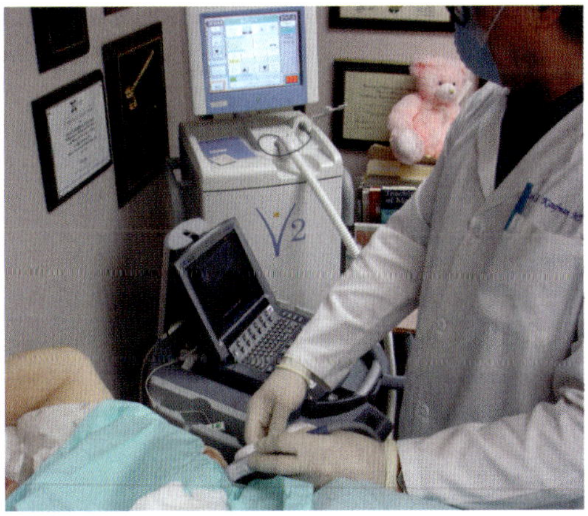

A

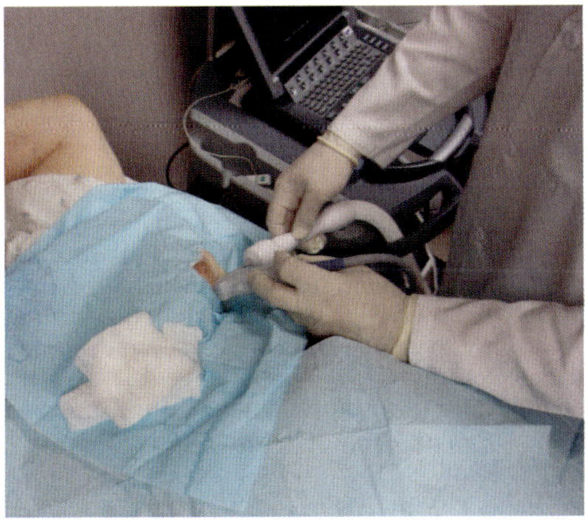

B

FIG 6 • **A.** During procedure, surgeon holds both cryoprobe and ultrasound transducer. Continuous visualization of both cryoablation machine and ultrasound image is required. **B.** Ongoing ultrasound monitoring of skin bridge is necessary. Avoid pressing skin too close to iceball formation with ultrasound transducer.

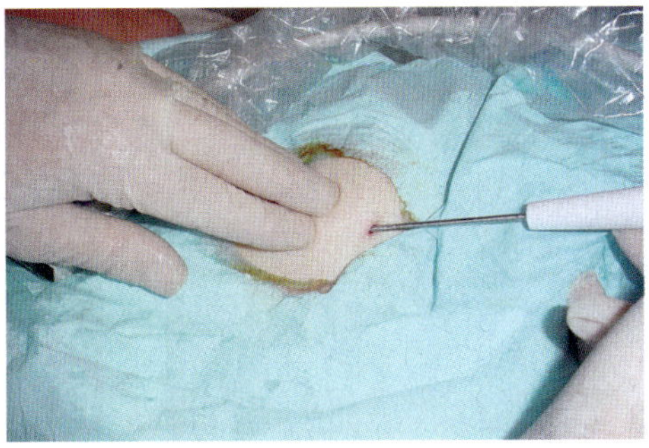

A

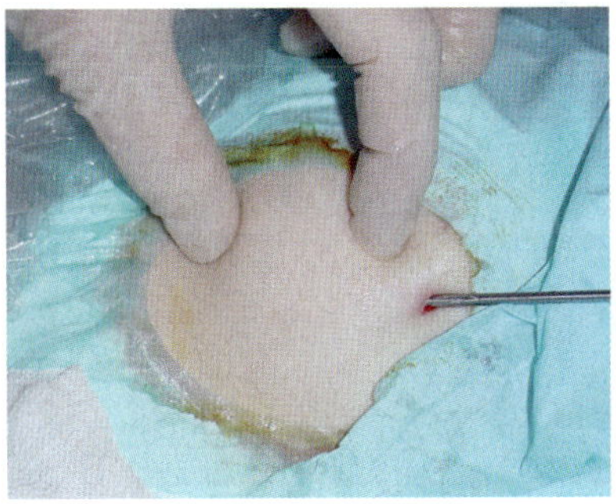

B

FIG 7 • **A.** Use of palpation over iceball to confirm skin is moveable and not frozen to iceball, which can cause skin damage. **B.** Palpation of iceball during cryoablation confirming skin not attached to iceball.

- During the procedure, continuously monitor the skin bridge to be sure skin does not get frozen and attached to the iceball. Freely inject saline between the iceball and the skin to "lift" the skin away from the developing iceball. Skin that becomes attached to the iceball may be injured and result in scar.
- Tips to avoid skin injury during cryoablation include the following: (1) Touch and move the skin horizontally overlying the iceball formation to confirm there is a large subcutaneous portion of mobile fat separating the iceball from the skin. Repeated movement of the skin overlying the iceball confirms it is not becoming attached (**FIG 7A,B**). (2) Avoid continuous pressure of the monitoring ultrasound transducer pushing the skin down onto the developing iceball narrowing the distance between the iceball and the skin; (3) move the distal end of the cryoprobe toward the posterior (chest wall) direction so that the distance from the developing iceball to the skin is maximized. (4) If you wish more distance from the iceball to the skin, inject saline between the skin and iceball to lift the skin away from the iceball development. This can be done repeatedly as needed. Avoid adherence of the skin to the iceball at all times.
- The treatment consists of two high freeze cycles separated by a thaw cycle. Each cycle is usually the same length of time, for example or e.g., 8 minutes each for a total treatment time of 24 minutes.
- The cryoablation device will freeze high for the first and second freeze cycles. During the freezing, continuous ultrasound monitoring will visualize an iceball growing as it envelopes the target lesion. At the end of the first freeze, the iceball will be much larger than the targeted tumor (**FIG 8A–D**).

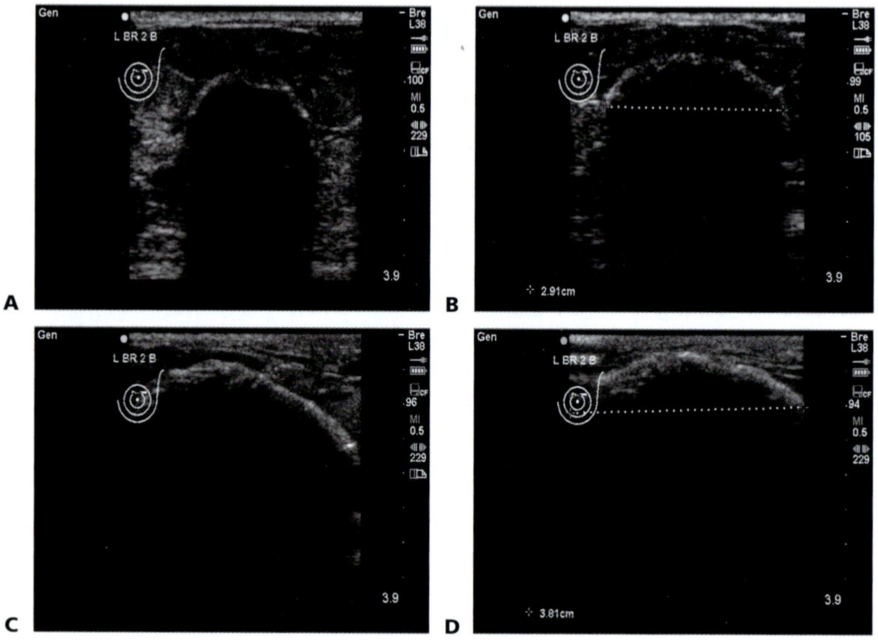

FIG 8 ● Serial Ultrasound Images of Cryoablation. **A.** During initial iceball development. **B.** Transverse view of iceball at the end of first freeze cycle. **C.** Longitudinal view of iceball at end of second freeze cycle. **D.** Transverse view of iceball after cryoprobe removal.

- When the automated cryoablation machine reaches the end of the second freeze, it will automatically go into a warming mode. The cryoprobe cannot be removed while it is frozen. The tip of the probe will warm after about 30 seconds of warming so that the cryoprobe may be gently removed.
- At the end of the procedure, the patient will still be able to feel a firm frozen area, which is the iceball (**FIG 9**) that will thaw within an hour, but there will still remain a palpable mass, which is the residual necrotic debris. It will take several months for the debris to be resorbed.
- A Steri-Strip is placed on the entry wound similar to a core needle biopsy dressing. Careful not to place a tight adhesive bandage on the area because it will swell significantly over the next 2 days and blisters can develop. (see "Postoperative Care").

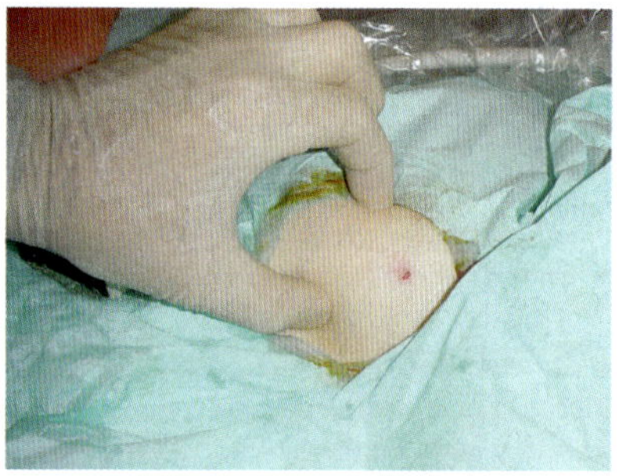

FIG 9 ● Immediate posttreatment palpation of iceball.

PEARLS AND PITFALLS

Lesion location	■ If the target lesion is close to the chest wall, then after placement of the probe during the initial icing phase, lift directly up off the chest wall with the probe in the tumor. This will allow the iceball to form without attachment to the pectoralis major. After the iceball is adequately formed, about 2 minutes into the freezing, you can release the traction away from the chest wall. ■ If the lesion is located close to the skin but away from the nipple, then after placing the probe into the tumor and confirming satisfactory position, inject lidocaine in the space between the skin and the tumor. Try to spread your fluid within the remaining space between the skin and the tumor. After you have over 1 cm of fluid in the ultrasound "window," proceed with freezing. Be ready to inject further saline/lidocaine during the freezing period for the first 4 minutes. Thereafter, the iceball will be unlikely to get too much bigger until the second freeze. ■ On concern during treatment is that there is a progressive iceball enlargement, and frequent skin reassessment must be made to avoid freeze injury. An easy way to tell if the iceball is getting too close to the skin is to examine the mobility of the skin over the iceball. If the skin has much movement, (similar to the skin of your hand over your knuckles) then the iceball is not too close. If there is limited horizontal movement of the skin, inject more fluid. If there is no skin movement, stop the procedure until you can inject more fluid and create a better bridge.

Patient selection	■ Avoid freezing lesions immediately deep to areola and close to the true nipple, especially if the patient is a young woman who wishes to breastfeed in the future. During the cryoablation, the immediate surrounding tissues may be injured or destroyed. This usually is not a problem within the body of the breast, because a small surrounding margin of normal breast tissue is often removed with fibroadenoma excision. But when the immediate surrounding tissue includes major milk ducts, one must be cautious in treating that patient. There is little experience of treating these patients and later determining the ability of these women to breastfeed. ■ There is anecdotal data on cryoablation of nonfibroadenomas. Although early in our experience, other lesions were treated with success, the current acceptable indications for cryoablation are for treatment of fibroadenomas. In the small series of nonfibroadenoma patients, they responded similar to the fibroadenoma cryoablated patients. However, a clinician would have little clinical support if there were complications on a nonfibroadenoma patient. We would refrain from treating those patients. ■ **Treating fibroadenomas during pregnancy.** There is little data on cryoablation during pregnancy. Rapidly growing or painful lesions should consider surgery during pregnancy, whereas others may wait.
Multiple tumors	■ For two tumors close together in the same quadrant, both less than 2 cm, it is possible to place the probe through both lesions at one time and treat both simultaneously. If they cannot be treated simultaneously, then using the same probe in the same quadrant would be reasonable if the entry site were unchanged. If there are two separate punctures to be made or if the lesions are in different quadrants of the same breast, then two separate probes would be optimal. When treating fibroadenomas of both breasts, two separate probes should be used.
Unable to place probe without undue force	■ Some fibroadenomas are very dense and seem to forbid entry of the cryoprobe. The best approach is to reevaluate your entry site and your options to "hold" the tumor in place while you advance the probe into it. One must be cautious to avoid past-pointing and pushing through the tumor once the probe enters it fully. One technique is to start the probe into the lesion, and then use your opposite hand to manually brace the tumor while you advance the probe slowly with your dominant hand. A slow twisting of the probe may allow the cryoprobe to enter the lesion. Use plenty of lidocaine. If it seems impossible to enter the lesion, consider temporarily removing the cryoprobe and using a spring-loaded core needle to take a few "bites" of the tumor at the planned site of cryoprobe entry. By creating a small-bore hole with the needle biopsy device, the cryoprobe may be able to enter the tumor more easily. Care to keep the cryoprobe sterile while you use the core biopsy tool.

POSTOPERATIVE CARE

- Bandage dressing over the entry site is very important to absorb some fluid that may drain out of the entry site. The treatment is essentially a burn of the interior of the breast. As with other burns, the area will swell over the next 2 to 3 days. A dressing over the area must accommodate the skin stretching and tissue swelling; otherwise, there will be blistering of the skin where tape or other adhesive dressings are placed.
- The entry site is closed with a Steri-Strip. Over the Steri-Strip can be placed a couple 2 × 2 gauze pads and then all covered with a Tegaderm-like adhesive waterproof dressing. Be careful not to stretch the adhesive dressing over the gauze because the tissue will swell. Stretch the skin and lay the unstretched dressing over the gauze so that the swelling of the skin over the next couple days will not create blistering at the corners of the dressing from a sheer effect that occurs with tissue swelling under a tight Tegaderm-like plastic. Do not stretch the Tegaderm-like plastic dressing on the skin but rather stretch the skin as you place the unstretched Tegaderm-like dressing over the gauze.
- Immediately after the procedure, patients have a cold firm spot on their breast, which is numb. They typically are able to drive themselves home after a few minutes of relaxation while getting dressed, since no sedation is necessary.
- Inform the patient that her tissue will swell significantly over the next few days, which may also be tender. Local treatments of ice packs and ibuprofen will aid in decreasing the swelling. Patients who are warned of the swelling and local tenderness will less likely be alarmed when it occurs.
- Sometimes, surrounding tissue is damaged and swells more than expected. If the lesion was on the chest wall, cryoablation of pectoralis muscle will be more painful than breast tissue ablation. Supportive pain medicine will allow this to resolve. In other patients, there is significant swelling in and around the cryoablated tissue. This is more likely with longer ablations or larger areas of normal breast tissue ablated. This occurs with cancer ablations due to longer treatment times. With tissue swelling, one must be cautious of skin taping or Steri-Strips during these first few days. Due to the swelling, there may be a sheering force on the skin by the tape, and skin blisters may occur. This is strictly due to tape applied too tight for the amount of tissue swelling that may occur. Avoid tape close to the cryoablation area. Pain may be due to blisters forming under the tape.
- Due to the complete destruction of all cells within the cryoablation target, all blood cells will lyse and exude their hemoglobin into the tissues. The entire treated area will turn a deep shade of red-purple merging to yellow green over the next week to 10 days. An informed patient will not be alarmed when these color changes occur. By 2 weeks, all the color is gone (**FIG 10A–C**).
- The patient is advised to call the office as needed for the first 5 days to let us know of the changes that have been described.

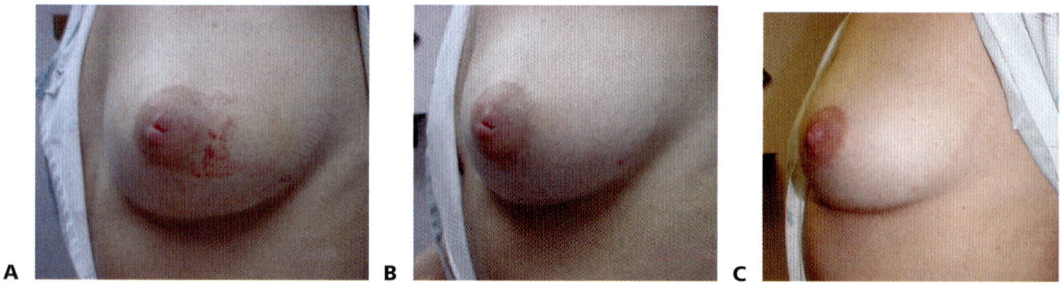

FIG 10 • **A–C.** Clinical images of patient postcryoablation at 1 week, 1 month, and 6 months. Note, the ecchymosis extends in a larger area than the fibroadenoma due to the lysis of blood cells in the area but resolves promptly.

It is not likely at all to have a significant posttreatment hemorrhage or infection. However, patients might think both of these events might be happening due to the typical changes postcryoablation.

- After these initial changes, the patient will be able to feel a firm oval mass at the site of the cryoablation zone. It will not be very tender but will be larger than the patient's original lesion or, if it was nonpalpable prior to cryoablation, it is now palpable to the patient. Knowing this change in physical exam will occur is helpful to prevent the patient's concern when they first palpate the area after the initial swelling is gone.

Long-Term Postprocedure Management

- After the initial healing period, the patient enters a long-term resolution phase. During this time, the patient will have very slow resolution of the residual mass left by the necrotic central cryoablative zone. Typically, there is little pain in the area. Properly informed patients express little concern when feeling the persistent cryonecrotic mass over several months as it resolves (**FIG 2**).
- Follow-up office visits. Some clinicians treat the patients and simply advise the patients of expected local changes in the breast and do not follow their patients in the office. This is not the advised method of follow-up, but some clinicians just wait for patients to call or return as needed. This method creates unnecessary anxiety in the patient and likely decreases patient satisfaction. We recommend regular follow-up exams for 1 year after cryoablation.
- As time goes on, patients are seen less frequently to confirm the residual mass is decreasing as well as to reassure the patient that all is well. The first posttreatment visit is about 2 to 4 weeks after the cryoablation. Next visit is 2 months later. Next visit is 3 to 4 months after that. Thereafter, every 3 to 6 months until the lesion has disappeared.
- With each visit, the area is examined with or without focal ultrasound measurements. With each exam, note the size of the residual cryonecrosis and reassure the patient of slow and progressive absorption.
- Most patients are younger than 40 years and not candidates for routine mammographic screening. If they are older than 40 years, preferably, their most recent mammogram was just prior to their cryoablation. Routine screening may follow. The first mammogram postcryoablation will have imaging changes from the procedure. If the imager is unaware of the treatment, they will note increased density and mass effect with indistinct margins in the area of the previously benign-appearing lesion. The unaware imager may consider the image BIRADS 4 and suggest a biopsy. However, clarifying the treatment events will modify the reading to either BIRADS 3 or 2, suggesting serial follow-up imaging.[22,23]
- The speed of resorption of the residual cryoablation debris relates to the original size of the target lesion. For tumors less than 2 cm, the area normally disappears within 1 year posttreatment. For those larger than 2 cm, it may take longer than a year. Almost all lesions over 2 cm are not palpable by 2 years. Ultrasound visualization of the residual cryoablated tissue remains visible for longer periods but that is similar to surgical scar seen by ultrasound. Ultrasound identification of the treated area is difficult to find by 3 years.
- Long-term (over 3 years) imaging changes vary from no evidence of treatment to residual scar similar to surgical biopsy changes. Mammograms may occasionally show focal calcifications in the area or radiating fibrosis, but the most common mammographic image is fatty replacement of the treatment area.[22] Ultrasound imaging most often demonstrates nonspecific breast tissue with some areas of hypoechoic scar over time. The iceball is usually at least 30% larger than the treated lesion then slowly resorbs. The tissue within the iceball becomes firm and much more noticeable than the prior tumor. Nonpalpable tumors become palpable immediately. Over the first 1 to 2 months, these areas will start to decrease in firmness. It will not be until about 6 months before they dissolve. Continue to reassure the patient that the firmness they feel is normal and expected. Anxiety of finding a new mass when none was present previously can readily undo the benefits of the procedure.
- Some patients may have a persistent firm mass for 6 to 9 months. If the cryoprobe was placed accurately and the treatment given properly, these patients will need to wait for the expected resolution of the palpable mass. For lesions over 2 cm, it will take over 6 months before their lesions start to noticeably decrease in size. Signs of a successful cryoablation include no growth in the palpable mass after the first month, and that after 6 months, there seems to be a slight softening of the mass, although it is difficult to notice. There should be no progressive measurable growth in the "mass." Reassurance is necessary for both the doctor and the patient during this time. By 9 months, it is clear that the cryolesion is getting smaller and the firmness is decreasing. By 12 months, there is noticeable change, even if the

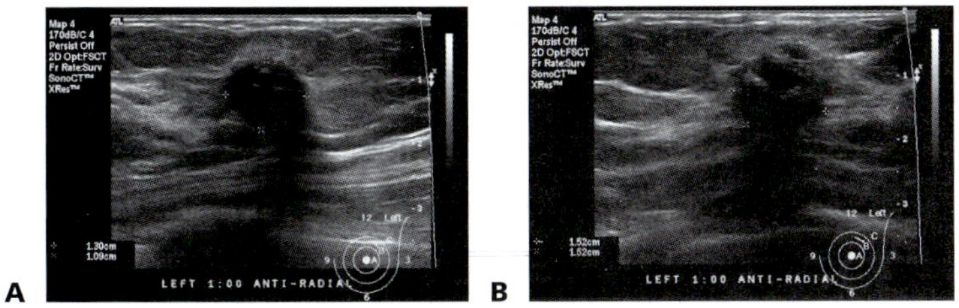

FIG 11 • **A,B.** Ultrasound images of cryoablation site 4 years after treatment. Site is smaller and has residual scar of necrotic debris where lesion had previously been.

lesion is not gone. Progressive decrease in size is noticeable on ultrasound and palpation (**FIG 2**).

- The ultrasound picture of cryoablated tissue is similar to surgical scar. There is typically an irregular hypoechoic shadowing mass, noticeably more suspicious on ultrasound than prior to cryoablation, but smaller than original lesion. The clues of normalcy are that there is no progressive growth but slow and progressive decrease in overall size. These lesions are followed but not biopsied unless there is growth (**FIG 11A,B**).

OUTCOMES

- Many reports have demonstrated the effectiveness of cryoablation of fibroadenomas. These reports are consistent in their results in properly chosen patients. After treatment, clinical and imaging evidence of the lesion slowly resorbs until the area disappears. Imaging evidence of the targets also disappears (Table 2).
- After initial positive reports of this technique, a Current Procedural Terminology (CPT) code was assigned to this process. Many payers reimbursed for this procedure. However, due to limited use of this method of treatment, many payers reversed their acceptance of payment and reclassified this procedure as investigational. Yet, the data supporting this method of treatment as acceptable has been repeated in the peer-reviewed literature in many sites. The few negative comments are mostly reports of slow resorption of the treated lesion.

COMPLICATIONS

- Most complications can be prevented, or said another way, most complications are iatrogenic. These include choosing a patient who has too narrow a window between the skin and the lesion, making skin injury more likely.
- Other complications include blistering on the skin due to swelling of the skin under adhesive from Steri-Strips or the Tegaderm-like dressing.
- Although ecchymosis and swelling is expected, significant hemorrhage and infection is quite rare.

REFERENCES

1. Smith BL. Fibroadenomas. In: Harris JR, Hellman S, Henderson IC, et al, eds. *Breast Diseases*. Philadelphia, PA: JB Lippincott; 1991:34–37.
2. Haagensen CD. *Diseases of the Breast*. 3rd ed. Philadelphia, PA: WB Saunders; 1986.
3. Greenberg R, Skornick Y, Kaplan O. Management of breast fibroadenomas. *J Gen Intern Med*. 1998;13(9):640–645.
4. Dixon JM, Dobie V, Lamb J, et al. Assessment of the acceptability of conservative management of fibroadenoma of the breast. *Br J Surg*. 1996;83(2):264–265.
5. Houssami N, Cheung MN, Dixon JM. Fibroadenoma of the breast. *Med J Aust*. 2001;174(4):185–188.
6. Yilmaz E, Sal S, Lebe B. Differentiation of phyllodes tumors versus fibroadenomas. *Acta Radiol*. 2002;43(1):34–39.
7. Isaacs JH. Benign neoplasms. In: Marchant DJ, ed. *Breast Disease*. Philadelphia, PA: WB Saunders; 1997:66–67.
8. Rosen PP. Fibroepithelial neoplasms. In: Rosen PP, ed. *Rosen's Breast Pathology*. New York, NY: Lippincott-Raven Press; 1996:143–155.
9. Hughes LE, Mansel RE, Webster DJT. Fibroadenoma and related tumours. In: *Benign Disorders and Diseases of the Breast: Concepts and Clinical Management*. Philadelphia, PA: WB Saunders; 2000:73–94.
10. Kaufman CS, Bachman B, Littrup PJ, et al. Office-based ultrasound-guided cryoablation of breast fibroadenomas. *Am J Surg*. 2002;184(5):394–400.
11. Hindle WH. Fibroadenoma. In: Hindle WH, ed. *Breast Care: A Clinical Guidebook for Women's Primary Health Care Provider*. New York, NY: Springer-Verlag; 1999:191–193.
12. Kaufman CS, Littrup PJ, Freman-Gibb LA, et al. Office-based cryoablation of breast fibroadenomas: 12-month followup. *J Am Coll Surg*. 2004;198:914–923.
13. Kaufman CS, Littrup PJ, Freeman-Gibb LA, et al. Office-based cryoablation of breast fibroadenomas with long-term follow-up. *Breast J*. 2005;11(5):344–350.
14. Kaufman CS, Bachman B, Littrup PJ, et al. Cryoablation treatment of benign breast lesions with 12 month follow-up. *Am J Surg*. 2004;188:340–348.
15. Edwards MJ, Broadwater R, Tafra L, et al. Progressive adoption of cryoablative therapy for breast fibroadenoma in community practice. *Am J Surg*. 2004;188:221–224.
16. Nurko J, Mabry CD, Whitworth P, et al. Interim results from the FibroAdenoma Cryoablation Treatment Registry. *Am J Surg*. 2005;190(4):647–651.
17. Stavros AT, Rapp CL, Parker SH. *Breast Ultrasound*. Hagerstown, MD: Lippincott Williams & Wilkins; 2003.
18. Sperber F, Blank A, Metser U, et al. Diagnosis and treatment of breast fibroadenomas by ultrasound-guided vacuum-assisted biopsy. *Arch Surg*. 2003;138(7):796–800.
19. Foxcroft L, Evans E, Hirst C. Newly arising fibroadenomas in women aged 35 and over. *Aust N Z J Surg*. 1998;68(6):419–422.
20. Hahn M, Pavlista D, Danes J, et al. Ultrasound guided cryoablation of fibroadenomas. *Ultraschall Med*. 2013;34(1):64–68.
21. American Society of Breast Surgeons. Statement on use of ablative techniques for benign tumors. ASBS Web site. https://www.breastsurgeons.org/new_layout/about/statements/PDF_Statements/Fibroadenoma.pdf. Accessed June 2, 2014.
22. Kaufman CS. Mammographic appearance of fibroadenoma disappears after cryoablation. Scientific paper presented at: RSNA Annual Meeting; December 4, 2002; Chicago, IL.
23. Brenner RJ, Pfaff JM. Mammographic changes after excisional breast biopsy for benign disease. *AJR Am J Roentgenol*. 1996;167(4):1047–1052.

Chapter 5 Lumpectomy for Breast Cancer

Michael S. Sabel

DEFINITION

- Lumpectomy is defined as the complete excision of a breast tumor with an adequate margin of surrounding normal tissue. Lumpectomy plus breast irradiation are the essential components of successful breast conservation therapy (BCT). Lumpectomies for nonpalpable cancers require wire localization. Other terms for lumpectomy include partial mastectomy, tumorectomy, or tylectomy.

PATIENT HISTORY AND PHYSICAL FINDINGS

- For BCT to be successful, it must be possible to (1) obtain negative surgical margins around the tumor while still maintaining a cosmetically acceptable result and (2) safely deliver radiation therapy. A thorough history and physical examination is necessary to carefully select patients for BCT. Absolute contraindications to BCT are listed in Table 1.
- A thorough history should be performed prior to treatment, including a detailed past medical history, present medications and allergies, and a personal and family history of cancer.
- Prior radiation to the breast is a contraindication to BCT. For patients who may have had chest wall radiation for indications other than a prior breast cancer (such as mantle radiation for Hodgkin disease), it may be helpful to obtain the prior records and review the fields treated. These patients may be eligible for a partial breast irradiation technique (Chapter 7).
- Patients with a history of autoimmune or collagen-vascular diseases, such as scleroderma, lupus, or dermatomyositis, may have abnormal reaction to radiation therapy, which significantly compromises the cosmetic outcome. For some types of collagen-vascular disease, such as Raynaud phenomenon, rheumatoid arthritis, or Sjögren's syndrome, the response to radiation is not as severe and these patients may be considered for BCT.
- A detailed family history is critical to assess the risk of a future breast cancer, and consider genetic counseling and testing. High-risk patients may want to consider bilateral mastectomy as they are at considerable risk of a second primary cancer. The data is mixed regarding the local recurrence rate among patients with a known or suspected BRCA 1 or 2 mutations who opt for BCT. Some, but not all, studies suggest an increased risk.[1,2] The decision to pursue BCT in known BRCA1/2 carriers should be made following extensive discussion with a genetic counselor.
- Patient age, nodal status, histologic tumor type, tumor grade, and extensive intraductal component (EIC) are not contraindications to BCT as long as negative margins can be obtained.
- If an adequate lumpectomy can be performed, prior breast augmentation with breast implants are not an absolute contraindication, and radiation can be delivered to the augmented breast using standard techniques and doses. However, capsular contraction is a risk. If the tumor is close to the implant, preventing negative margins (cancers sometimes invade the fibrous capsule around the implant), the implant may need to be removed.
- A complete, bilateral breast examination should focus on both assessing the cosmetic implications of lumpectomy and identifying additional areas of concern to rule out multicentric disease. Any additional suspicious masses should be biopsied, and cancer ruled out, prior to proceeding with BCT.
- The size of the mass relative to the size of the breast, location of the mass, proximity to the skin and amount of skin needed to be resected, and symmetry of the breasts should be noted. For some patients with a large tumor relative to the size of the breast, neoadjuvant chemotherapy may be considered to downstage the primary tumor. For other patients in whom a poor cosmetic outcome with standard lumpectomy is predicted, an oncoplastic approach should be considered (Chapter 6).
- A detailed examination of the bilateral axillary, supraclavicular, and cervical lymph nodes should be undertaken, and any suspicious lymphadenopathy worked up prior to surgery.

Table 1: Absolute Contraindications to Breast Conserving Surgery

Unable to receive radiation therapy
Previous chest wall irradiation
Need to deliver radiation during pregnancy
Scleroderma or active systemic lupus erythematosus
Multicentric disease
Diffuse suspicious calcifications on mammography
Inability to achieve adequately negative margins

IMAGING AND OTHER DIAGNOSTIC STUDIES

- All patients require bilateral mammographic evaluation, with appropriate magnification views, within 3 months of surgery (**FIG 1**). The tumor size, the presence of microcalcifications, and the extent of calcifications outside of the mass should be noted. Some patients with palpable cancers may still require wire localization of the calcifications to assure complete removal at the time of lumpectomy.
- Any additional areas of abnormality should be worked up and biopsied to rule out multicentric cancer. Multicentric disease is typically a contraindication to BCT; however, patients with two tumors close enough that they can be removed in one specimen with an acceptable cosmetic outcome can still be considered candidates for BCT.
- The use of magnetic resonance imaging (MRI) to determine eligibility for BCT has been increasing. Although MRI may more accurately determine the extent of the tumor or identify multicentricity, particularly in women with dense breast tissue (for whom mammography is less sensitive), its use is

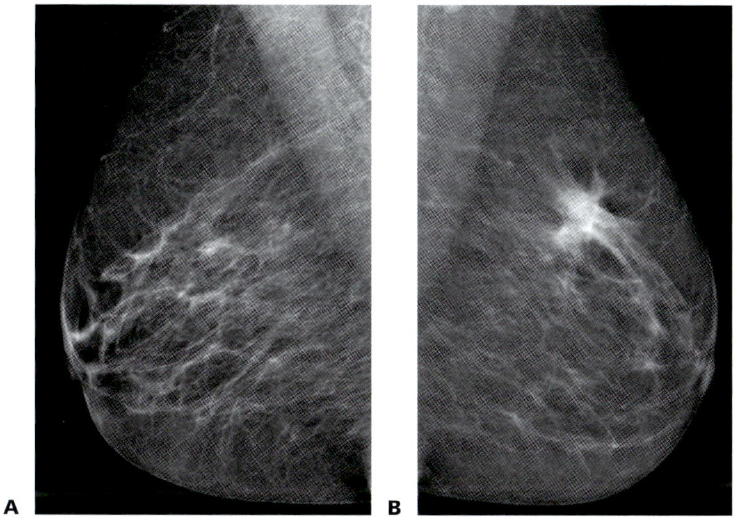

FIG 1 • Bilateral mammogram demonstrating a left breast cancer. **A.** Right breast. **B.** Left breast.

controversial. MRI is highly sensitive but has limited specificity and is limited in its ability to visualize ductal carcinoma in situ (DCIS). Studies have shown that the use of MRI appears to increase the mastectomy rate without decreasing re-excision or local recurrence rates.[3] The need for MRI should be evaluated on a case-by-case basis.

- Accurate histologic assessment of the primary tumor, including histologic subtype and hormone receptor status, is necessary in evaluating the breast cancer patient for suitability for BCT. This is best accomplished through a core needle biopsy rather than fine needle aspiration biopsy or excisional biopsy.

SURGICAL MANAGEMENT

Preoperative Planning

- Prior to taking the patient back to the operating room, the presence of the palpable cancer should be confirmed with the patient. In the preoperative area, the mass should be examined in both the upright and supine positions.
- With the patient in the supine position, the mass should be carefully marked.
- Although the risk of infection after breast cancer surgery is low, it tends to be higher than average for a clean surgical procedure, and several studies have shown that antibiotic prophylaxis significantly reduces the risk of postoperative infection.[4]

Positioning

- Lumpectomy is often performed in conjunction with a sentinel lymph node biopsy. Therefore, the patient should be positioned supine with the ipsilateral arm at 90 degrees.
- If intraoperative analysis of the sentinel lymph node and possible axillary lymph node dissection is planned, the ipsilateral arm should be prepped into the sterile field. Otherwise, the ipsilateral arm can be secured.
- If sentinel lymph node biopsy is to be performed in conjunction with lumpectomy, then the blue dye should be injected at this point. The skin is prepped with alcohol and either isosulfan or methylene blue dye is injected peritumoral (see Chapter 8, Sentinel Lymph Node Biopsy for Breast Cancer) (**FIG 2**).

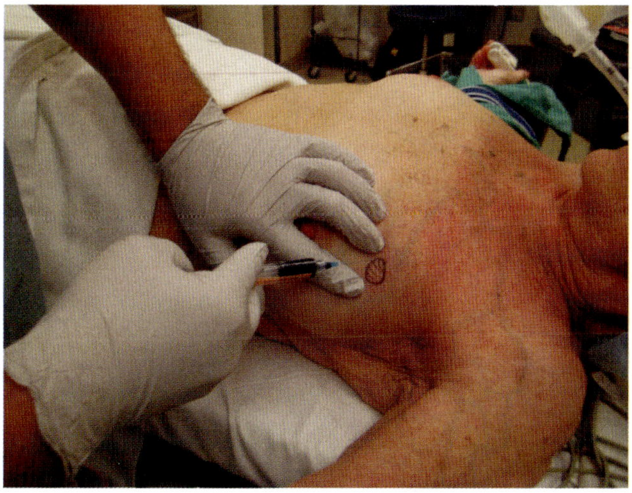

FIG 2 • Peritumoral injection of blue dye prior to lumpectomy for performance of sentinel lymph node (SLN) biopsy.

PLACEMENT OF INCISION

- The skin incision should be placed directly over the palpable mass (**FIG 3**). One should avoid excessive tunneling. This may compromise the margins and make a reexcision for close or positive margins unnecessarily difficult.
- When there is adequate distance between the skin and the tumor, skin does not need to be removed. However, when the tumor is close to the skin, an ellipse of skin over the tumor should be removed with the lumpectomy specimen.
- In the upper hemisphere of the breast, curvilinear incisions following the Langer lines (the normal lines of tension in the skin) are ideal. In the lower hemisphere, the incisions can either be circumareolar or radial (**FIG 4**). For smaller tumors in relatively larger breasts, where there is adequate breast parenchyma, curvilinear incisions are acceptable. However, when skin or a fair amount of tissue is to be removed, curvilinear incisions will collapse the breast inferiorly so that the nipple points downward. In this situation, radial incisions will result in less distortion of the nipple–areolar complex.
- All incisions must be planned with an eventual mastectomy in mind should attempts at breast conservation fail (**FIG 5**). The incision size needs to be adequate to remove the mass and surrounding margin. Using a small incision for cosmetic benefit results in excessive manipulation of the tumor and involved margins that require reexcision.

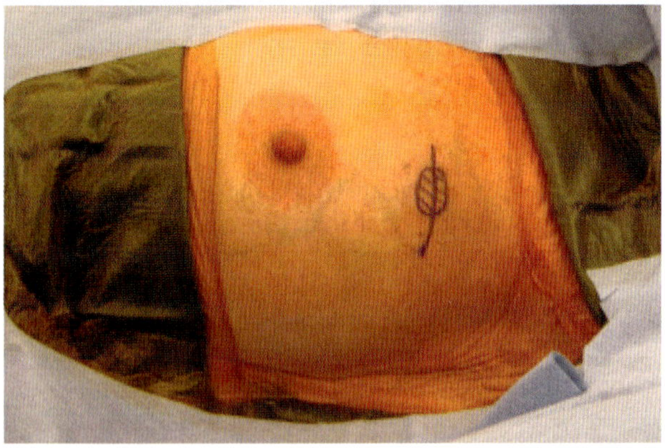

FIG 3 • Placement of incision within the Langer lines of the breast directly over the palpable cancer. The incision is planned large enough to remove the cancer without excess manipulation.

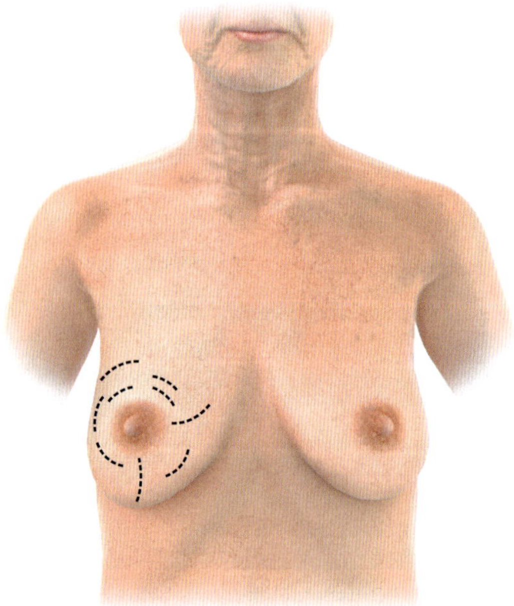

FIG 4 • Potential lines of excision for breast lumpectomy. In the upper hemisphere of the breast, curvilinear incisions are best, keeping within the Langer lines of the skin. In the lower hemisphere, either curvilinear or radial incisions are acceptable.

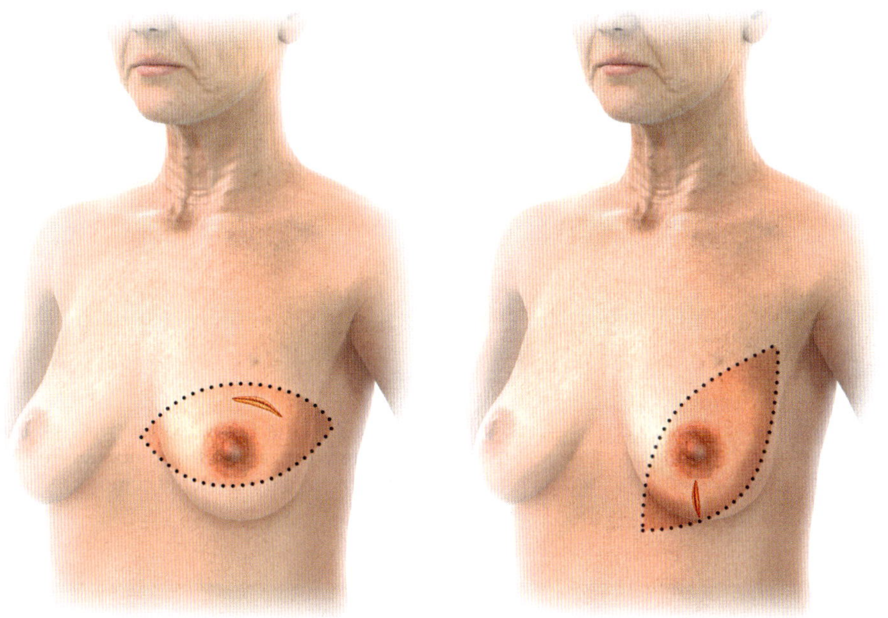

FIG 5 ● Potential mastectomy incisions if breast conservation fails. Lumpectomy incisions should be planned with a possible mastectomy in mind should negative margins not be attainable.

SKIN INCISION AND RAISING OF FLAPS

- An incision is made in the skin going just deep to the dermis. For lesions closer to the skin, skin flaps should be immediately elevated in all directions over the mass (**FIG 6**). Adequate subcutaneous fat should be left on the flaps, which should get progressively thicker as the flaps are elevated (approximately 45 degrees). Excessively thin flaps lead to excessive retraction and concavity with radiation and should be avoided by excising the skin over the mass.
- For deep-seated tumors, after dividing the skin, the breast tissue may be divided straight down to approximately 1 cm over the mass before beginning the dissection around the tumor (**FIG 7**).

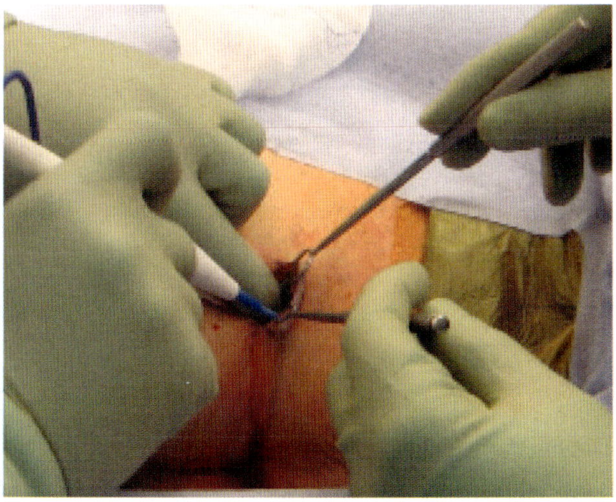

A

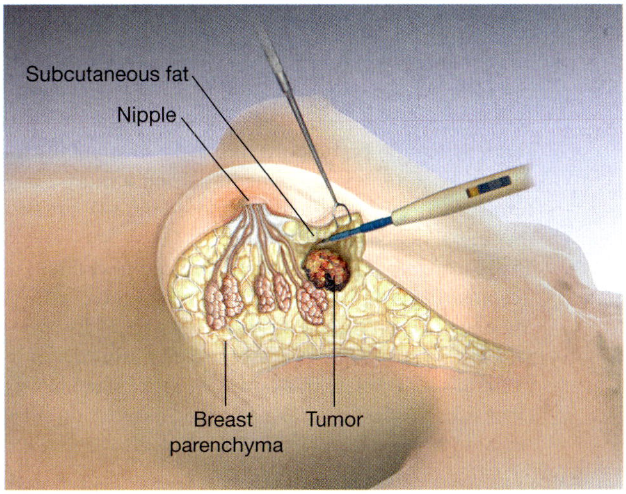

B

FIG 6 ● Raising of flaps over the tumor. Excessively thin flaps should be avoided. The flaps should get thicker as they are elevated.

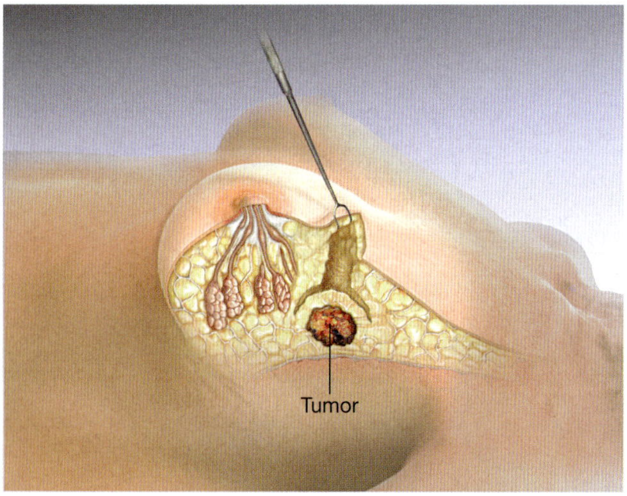

FIG 7 • The breast parenchyma is divided until approximately 1 cm above the tumor before dissecting around the tumor for a deep-seated tumor.

EXCISION

- The excision is then carried out with the goal of maintaining 1-cm grossly free margins around the mass. This is best accomplished by retracting the mass with the index finger of the nonoperative hand so you are constantly aware of the margin and maintaining a 1-cm rim of normal breast tissue or fat as dissection continues toward the chest wall (**FIG 8A,B**).
- The tissue is divided circumferentially around the mass. Once it is free, it can usually be elevated out of the wound (**FIG 9**). The skin incision must be large enough so that the resected portion can be easily brought out; struggling to deliver a mass through a small incision leads to excessive manipulation and positive margins on final pathology.
- Before the lesion is completely removed from the body, the specimen should be oriented with 2-0 silk sutures. Orientation is critical so that if reexcision for close or positive margins are needed, this can be limited to just the involved margin (as opposed to reexcising the entire cavity). Three sutures are necessary to orient the mass correctly for the pathologist and avoid errors (**FIG 10**).[5] At this juncture, we recommend placing a short 2-0 silk suture at the superior margin and a long silk suture at the lateral margin (**FIG 11**).
- The specimen is now completely removed by dividing the deep margin (**FIG 12**). For lesions close to the chest wall, the deep margin should include the fascia of the pectoralis major muscle. In rare cases, excision of some of the pectoralis is necessary to assure a negative deep margin. Once excised, a third double-stranded orientation suture is placed at the deep margin (**FIG 13**).

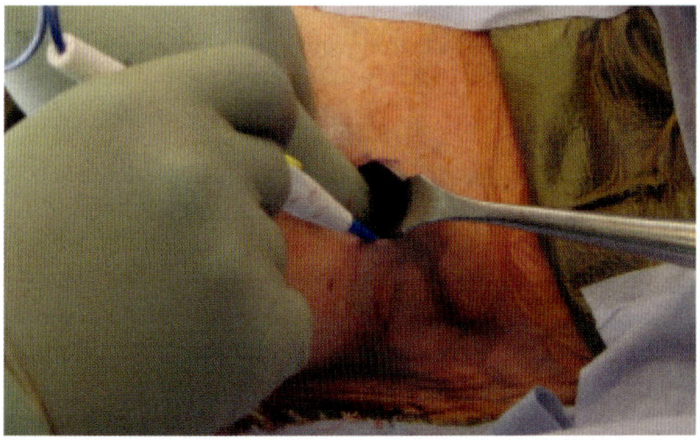

A

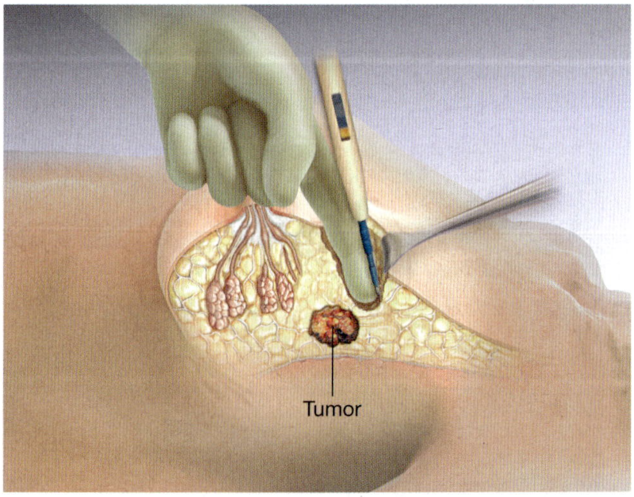

B

FIG 8 • With the tumor retracted with the index finger, the surgeon dissects around it, maintaining 1 cm of normal breast tissue around the tumor.

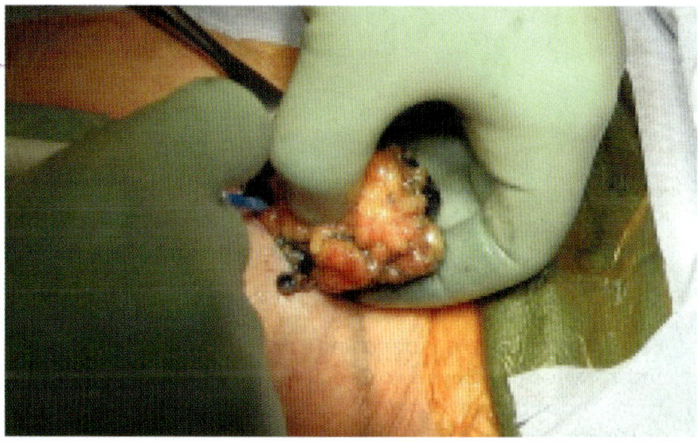

FIG 9 ● The entire tumor is excised circumferentially and delivered from the wound.

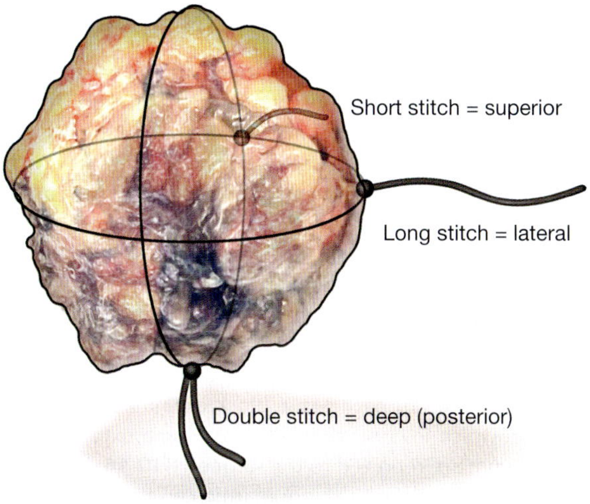

FIG 10 ● Three suture marking system for lumpectomy specimens. A 3-0 silk short stitch is placed superiorly, a long stitch is placed laterally, and a double stitch is placed deep (posteriorly).

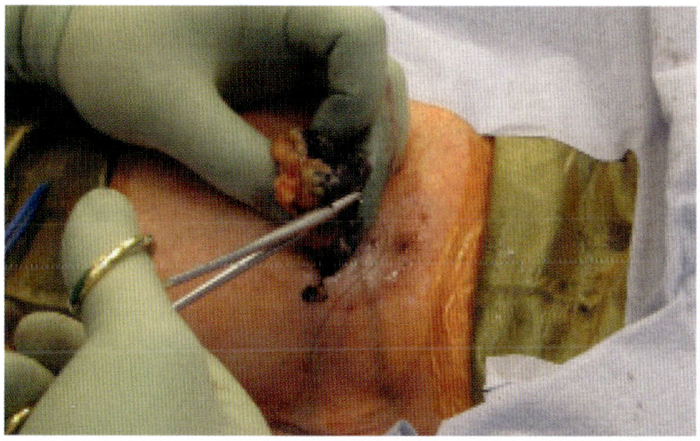

FIG 11 ● Marking sutures are placed prior to complete excision of the specimen so as not to lose the orientation.

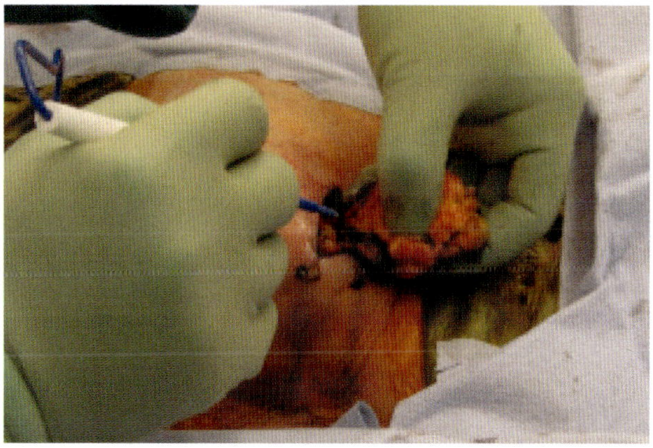

FIG 12 ● The posterior tissue is divided last, completing the lumpectomy.

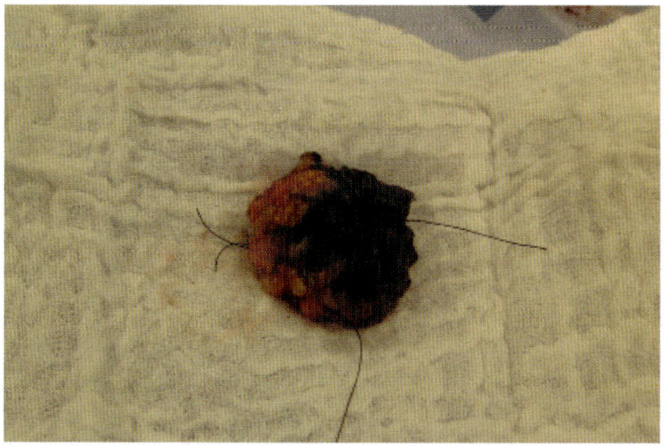

FIG 13 ● Lumpectomy specimen with marking sutures.

INTRAOPERATIVE MARGIN ANALYSIS

- Without intraoperative margin analysis, reexcision rates to obtain negative margins can be as high as 30% to 50%. Intraoperative margin analysis is highly recommended to minimize reexcision rates to as low as 10%.[6] After orientation, the margins of the specimen are inked using six colors and then sectioned at 2- to 3-mm intervals (**FIG 14**).
- After gross examination of the margin status, sections are taken for each suspicious margin (**FIG 15**). Sections 6- to 7-μm thick are cut on a −20°C cryostat and stained with a rapid hematoxylin and eosin technique (with two levels of each tissue block examined). Any margins in which invasive or in situ carcinoma extend to within 2-mm are reported to the surgeon (**FIG 16**).
- A reexcision of the close margin can then be performed by grasping the top of the margin with an Allis clamp and excising back another 0.5 to 1 cm around the hemisphere in need of reexcision (**FIG 17A,B**). The new margin should be appropriately marked for the pathologist (**FIG 18**).

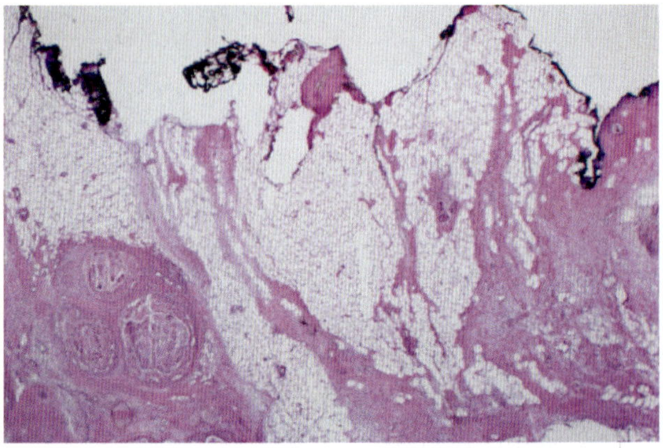

FIG 16 • DCIS is identified close to the margin. This information is relayed to the surgeon so a reexcision of that margin can be performed.

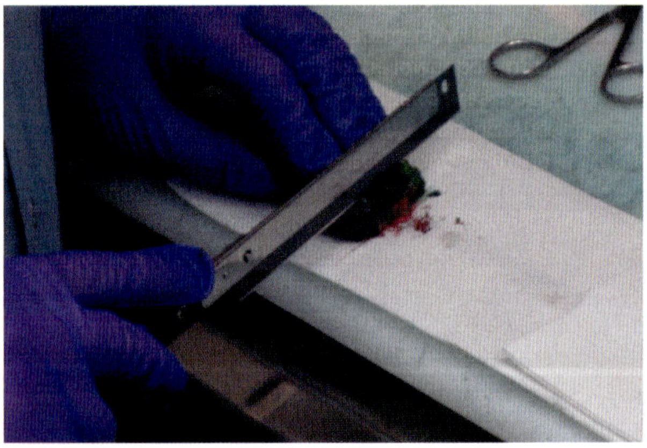

FIG 14 • The specimen is inked with six colors and sectioned for intraoperative margin analysis.

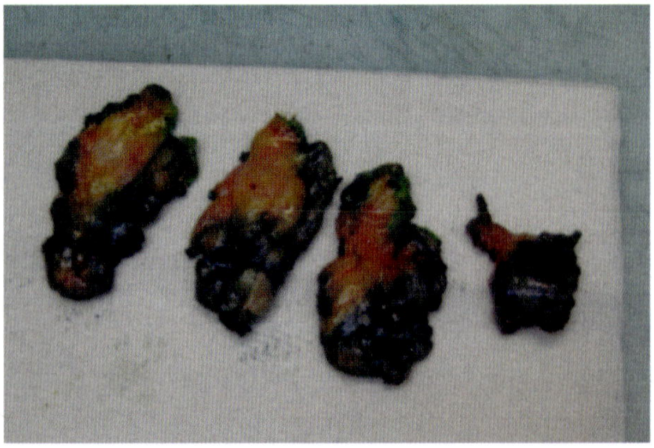

FIG 15 • The sections are grossly examined for involved margins.

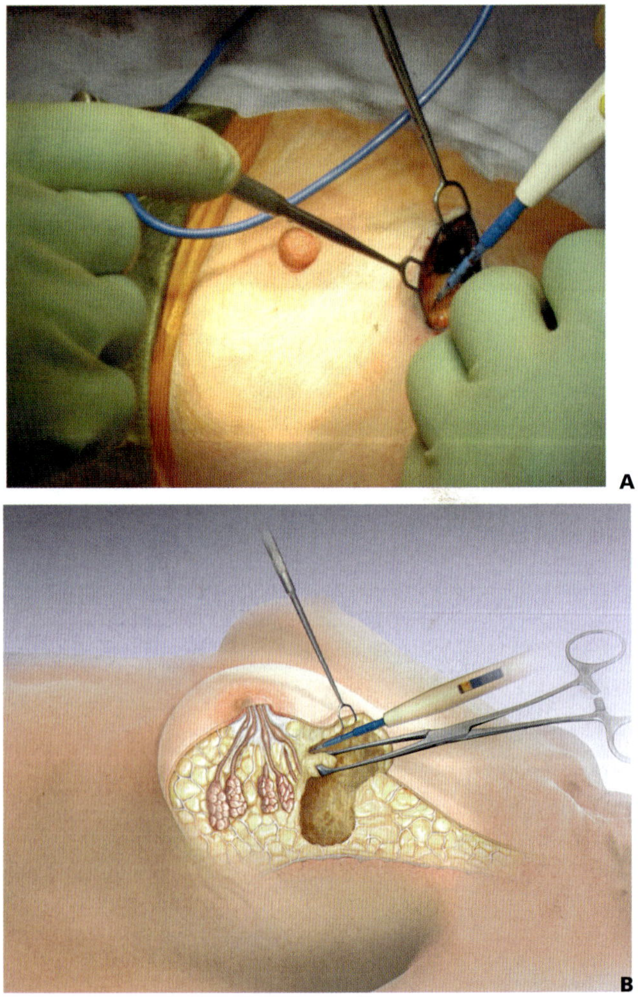

FIG 17 • **A.** An additional inferior margin is obtained based on the intraoperative margin analysis. **B.** The top of the cavity is grasped with an Allis and the entire hemisphere is excised approximately 1 cm back from the cavity.

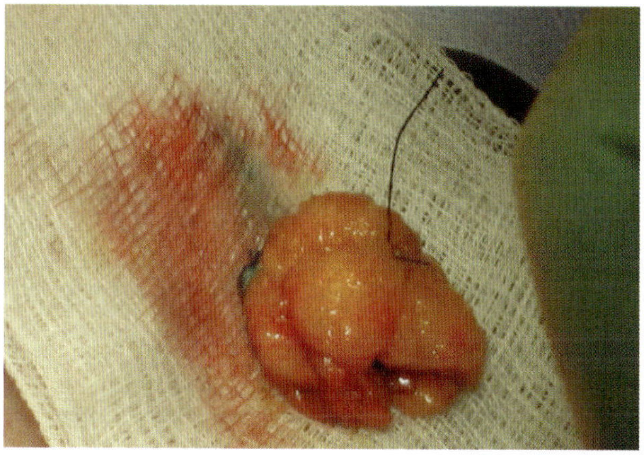

FIG 18 • A marking stitch designating the new, true margin after reexcision.

CLOSURE

- Once the lumpectomy is complete, hemostasis is assured and then surgical clips are placed within the cavity at the six anatomic locations (anterior, posterior, medial, lateral, superior, and inferior) (**FIG 19**). This helps in the planning of radiation therapy, particularly for a boost or for partial breast irradiation.
- For the standard lumpectomy, the surgeon should *not* try to reapproximate the breast tissue. The cavity will fill with seroma and fibrin, and ultimately fibrous tissue, which will maintain the normal contour. For large defects, oncoplastic techniques can be considered, which are discussed in Chapter 6.
- The incision is closed with absorbable deep dermal sutures, followed by either a subcuticular stitch or tissue adhesive (**FIG 20**). Drains should not be used.

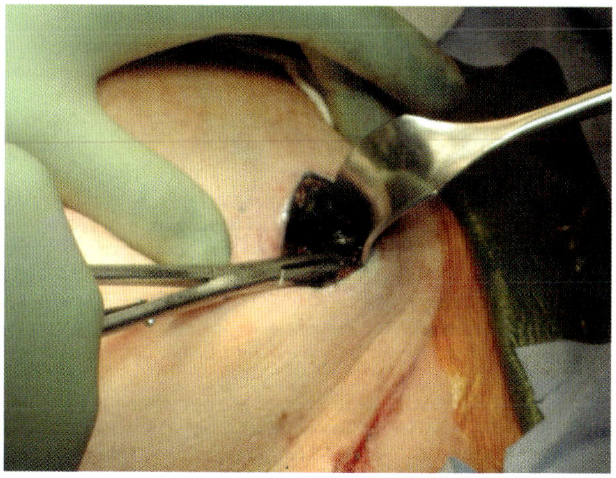

FIG 19 • Clips are placed around the lumpectomy cavity to aid in the delivery of radiation.

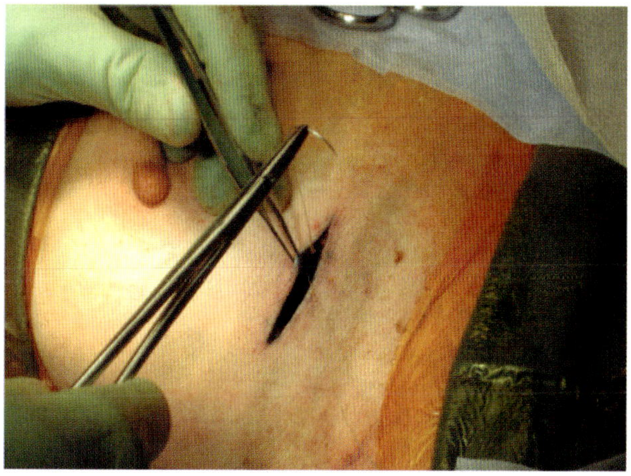

FIG 20 • The skin is reapproximated with absorbable deep dermal sutures.

PEARLS AND PITFALLS

Indications	■ A complete history and physical and review of the breast imaging should take place to assure the patient is a suitable candidate for BCT. ■ Suspicious lesions on exam or imaging should be biopsied prior to proceeding with BCT.
Placement of incision	■ Incisions should be created, keeping in mind a possible mastectomy should BCT fail. ■ In the inferior portion of the breast, radial incisions can give superior cosmetic outcomes compared to curvilinear incisions. ■ Make the incision large enough to remove the tumor without excessive manipulation. This decreases the close/positive margin rate and the need for reexcision.
Raising of flaps	■ Thin flaps will lead to excessive retraction and concavity after radiation. Avoid them by excising the skin over the tumor with the lumpectomy. ■ Flaps should get progressively thicker as they are raised.
Excision	■ Maintain at least 1 cm of grossly normal margins around the mass throughout the excision. ■ Intraoperative margin analysis can greatly reduce reexcision rates, leading to lower mastectomy rates and improved cosmetic outcome.
Orientation	■ Three orientation sutures are necessary to avoid error. ■ Place two sutures before complete excision of the tumor to avoid losing the orientation.
Closure	■ Do not try to reapproximate the breast tissue or place a drain.

POSTOPERATIVE CARE

- After a lumpectomy, the patient should be placed in a breast binder or supportive brassiere. This helps sustain hemostasis and relieves tension on the skin closure imposed by the weight of the breasts. The patient should be encouraged to wear the support bra day and night for 1 week after surgery.

OUTCOMES

- Long-term recurrence rates after lumpectomy and radiation therapy range from 5% to 22%, compared with 4% to 14% for mastectomy. Survival rates are equivalent.[7]
- Among women undergoing lumpectomy and radiation, excellent or excellent/good cosmetic results were noted at 3 years in 73% and 96%, respectively.[8] This is primarily driven by the volume of breast tissue resected, with scores higher among women with less than 35 cm^3 resected compared to women with greater than 85 cm^3.[9,10]

COMPLICATIONS

- Seroma
- Hematoma
- Infection (cellulitis or abscess)
- Altered sensation to the nipple
- Close or positive margins
- Poor cosmetic outcome

REFERENCES

1. Haffty BG, Harrold E, Khan AJ, et al. Outcome of conservatively managed early-onset breast cancer by BRCA1/2 status. *Lancet*. 2002;359:1471–1477.
2. Pierce LJ, Phillips KA, Griffith KA, et al. Local therapy in BRCA1 and BRCA2 mutation carriers with operable breast cancer: comparison of breast conservation and mastectomy. *Breast Cancer Res Treat*. 2010;121(2):389.
3. Houssami N, Hayes DF. Review of preoperative magnetic resonance imaging (MRI) in breast cancer: should MRI be performed on all women with newly diagnosed early stage breast cancer? *CA Cancer J Clin*. 2009;59(5):290–302.
4. Bunn F, Jones DJ, Bell-Syer S. Prophylactic antibiotics to prevent surgical site infection after breast cancer surgery. *Cochrane Database Syst Rev*. 2012;(1):CD005360. doi: 10.1002/1465858.CD005360.pub3.
5. Molina MA, Snell S, Franceschi D, et al. Breast specimen orientation. *Ann Surg Oncol*. 2009;16:285–288.
6. Sabel MS, Jorns JM, Wu A, et al. Development of an intraoperative pathology consultation service at a free-standing ambulatory surgical center: clinical and economic impact for patients undergoing breast cancer surgery. *Am J Surg*. 2012;204(1):66–77. doi:10.1016/j.amjsurg.2011.07.016.
7. Clarke M, Collins R, Darby S; Early Breast Cancer Trialists' Collaborative Group (EBCTCG). Effects of radiotherapy and of differences in the extent of surgery for early breast cancer on local recurrence and 15 year survival: an overview of the randomized trials. *Lancet*. 2005;366(9503):2087–2106.
8. de la Rochefordière A, Abner AL, Silver B, et al. Are cosmetic results following conservative surgery and radiation therapy for early breast cancer dependent on technique? *Int J Radiat Oncol Biol Phys*. 1992;23(5):925–931.
9. Harris JR, Levene MB, Svensson G, et al. Analysis of cosmetic results following primary radiation therapy for stages I and II carcinoma of the breast. *Int J Radiat Oncol Biol Phys*. 1979;5(2):257–261.
10. Beadle GF, Silver B, Botnick L, et al. Cosmetic results following primary radiation therapy for early breast cancer. *Cancer*. 1984;54(12):2911–2918.

Chapter 6 Oncoplastic Breast Surgery

Kristine E. Calhoun Benjamin O. Anderson

DEFINITION

- Breast-conserving therapy was first introduced as a treatment option for women with breast cancer beginning in the 1970s, with multiple clinical trials having since demonstrated equivalency in terms of overall survival between lumpectomy with radiation and mastectomy.[1,2]
- For breast conservation to be effective, the cancer must be resected with adequate surgical margins while simultaneously maintaining the breast's shape and appearance. Unfortunately, satisfying these dual goals may prove to be challenging.[3]
- In a traditional lumpectomy, the skin is opened, the tumor removed, and the wound closed without any specific effort being made to obliterate the internal cavity. Closing the remaining fibroglandular tissue may result in cosmetic defects if alignment of the breast tissue is suboptimal. Although such an approach may work well for smaller tumors, declivity of the skin and/or displacement of the nipple–areolar complex (NAC) may be the end result if the lesion removed from the breast is sizable.
- In 1994, Werner P. Audretsch was one of the first to advocate the use of "oncoplastic surgery" for repair of partial mastectomy defects by combining the techniques of volume reduction with immediate flap reconstruction.[4] Although initially used to describe partial mastectomy combined with large myocutaneous flap reconstruction using the latissimus dorsi or the rectus abdominis muscles, oncoplastic surgery currently refers to a series of surgical approaches that use partial mastectomy and breast flap advancement to address tissue defects following wide resection.
- The most widely used techniques, which will be described in this chapter, include the parallelogram mastopexy lumpectomy, batwing mastopexy lumpectomy, lateral segmentectomy lumpectomy, donut mastopexy lumpectomy, reduction mastopexy lumpectomy, and the central lumpectomy.[3,5]

ANATOMY

- One of the fundamental challenges for the oncoplastic breast surgeon is to determine how the individual cancer is distributed within the breast and to assess whether the lesion can be resected as a single en bloc fibroglandular resection.
- The modern anatomic analysis of ductal anatomy suggests that the number of major ductal systems is probably fewer than 10. The size of ductal segments can be incredibly variable, with some presenting as a narrow "pie slice" of tissue; in other cases, a single ductal segment can occupy up to 25% of the total breast volume.[6]
- Not all ducts pass radially from the nipple to the periphery of the breast, as some travel directly back from the nipple toward the chest wall. Single ductal segments may radiate to the sternal (medial) and clavicular (superior) aspects of the breast, with two or three ductal branches layered on each other, creating a fuller pad of fibroglandular tissue in the axillary (lateral) and abdominal (inferior) aspects of the breast.[7] Although the ductal branches appear to interdigitate with each other within the breast parenchyma, the segments do not communicate with each other via ductal anastomoses.
- In contrast to breast ductal anatomy, the fibroglandular tissue of the breast has a rich anastomotic circulatory bed, which allows oncoplastic resection and mastopexy fibroglandular advancement to be safely performed with minimal threat to tissue viability. This well-collateralized breast vasculature allows the surgeon to remodel large amounts of fibroglandular tissue within the skin envelope without major risk of breast devascularization and subsequent necrosis.
- The axillary and internal mammary arteries are the most common origins of the arterial blood supply of the breast. By maintaining communication with one of these two arterial connections, adequate blood supply to the breast parenchyma is maintained during tissue advancement and mastopexy closure.

PATIENT HISTORY AND PHYSICAL FINDINGS

- Patients should undergo standard preoperative history and physical, with special attention given to any prior breast surgical history, including the placement and location of breast implants.
- Tissue biopsy, preferably using core needle sampling, should be performed and conclusive proof of malignancy documented, with mandatory internal review of all external pathology slides required at our institution.
- Every effort should be made to make the tissue diagnosis by needle sampling, as an excisional biopsy scar may complicate the placement of the subsequent lumpectomy incision.

IMAGING AND OTHER DIAGNOSTIC STUDIES

- Patients considered for oncoplastic lumpectomy should undergo a standard preoperative breast imaging workup, which typically includes a combination of mammography and ultrasound, with or without breast magnetic resonance imaging (MRI). Although mammography may underestimate the extent of disease, especially if ductal carcinoma in situ (DCIS) is present, it is still warranted and is often the initial diagnostic study.[8]
- Although still controversial, the use of MRI may contribute greatly to the surgeon's ability to preoperatively determine the extent of disease present, especially for more mammographically subtle or occult cancers. Compared with mammographic and ultrasound images, the extent of disease seen on MRI may correlate best with the extent of tumor found at pathologic evaluation.
- Although sensitivity is high, MRI has a low specificity of 67.7% in the diagnosis of breast cancer before biopsy.[9] Up to one-third of MRI studies will show some area of enhancement

that needs further assessment but ultimately prove to be histologically benign breast tissue.[3]

- For cancers containing both invasive and noninvasive components, a combination of imaging methods (mammography with magnification views, ultrasonography, and/or MRI) may yield the best estimate of overall tumor size.[10]

SURGICAL MANAGEMENT

- The indications, as well as the contraindications, for oncoplastic surgery are the same as those of traditional breast-conserving surgery. In general, such techniques are only offered to those otherwise believed to be breast preservation candidates, including patients with single quadrant disease and individuals who can tolerate and have access to postsurgical radiation therapy.
- The techniques described in this chapter are easily learned and implemented by breast surgeons, even those lacking formal plastic surgery training.

Preoperative Planning

- While planning oncoplastic resections, as with traditional lumpectomy, the surgeon needs to accurately identify the area requiring removal, which is often aided by the use of preoperatively or perioperatively placed localization wires.
- Single wire localization for larger breast lesions may be more likely to result in positive margins, because the surgeon lacks landmarks to determine where the true boundaries of nonpalpable disease are located. For such scenarios, multiple bracketing wires may assist the surgeon in achieving complete excision at the initial intervention (**FIG 1**).

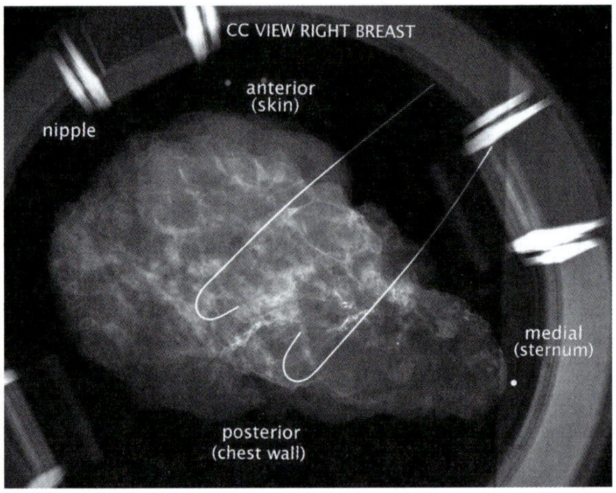

FIG 1 • Multiple bracketing wires used to perform a wire localized excision of a larger lesion.

Positioning

- Before the procedure, consideration should be given to marking skin landmarks with the patient in the upright sitting position.
- Relevant landmarks to be identified include the inframammary crease, the anterior axillary fold at the pectoralis major muscle, the posterior axillary fold of the latissimus dorsi muscle, the sternal border of the breast, and the periareolar circle. Identifying these structures with the patient in the sitting position is very important to the final cosmetic outcome, because these sites may be challenging to accurately locate once the patient is anesthetized and lying supine on the operating room (OR) table.

Approach

- The patient should be supine on the OR table with the arms abducted.
- It is preferable to have both breasts prepped and draped into the field so that visual comparison with the patient in a beach chair position is possible as the wound is closed. Such an approach allows the surgeon to identify areas of unsightly tugging or dimpling inadvertently created during closure so that they can be addressed at that time.
- Multicolored inking can help orient the specimen and is best performed by the operating surgeon (**FIG 2**).

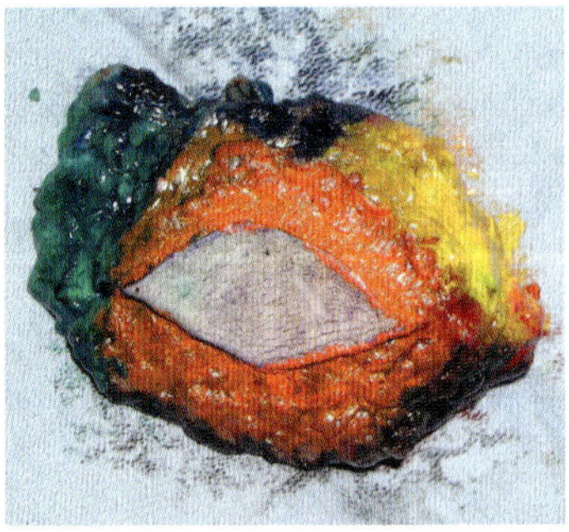

FIG 2 • Multiple ink colors are used to orient the lumpectomy specimen.

PARALLELOGRAM MASTOPEXY LUMPECTOMY

- The most basic of the oncoplastic techniques, this involves removal of the skin island located directly superficial to the known disease and is most commonly used for superior pole or lateral cancers.[11]
- For upper inner quadrant lesions, the skin island excisions should be small or performed using a simple reapproximation of breast tissue and skin without removal of any skin island.[12]
- Removal of the overlying parallelogram of skin avoids excessive, redundant skin from being left behind after excision and helps prevent declivity.
- Be cautious when designing the skin ellipse, because removal of too broad of an island can cause substantial shifting of the NAC.
- A rounded parallelogram with two equal length lines is drawn, thus marking the skin island to be excised in conjunction with the underlying target lesion and surrounding tissues (**FIG 3**). For lesions in the upper breast, incisions should be curvilinear, whereas lesions

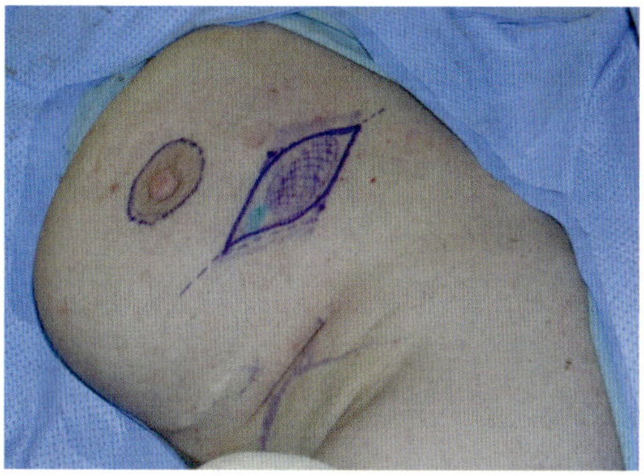

FIG 3 • The rounded parallelogram, with two equal line lengths, to excise a skin island en bloc with the tumor.

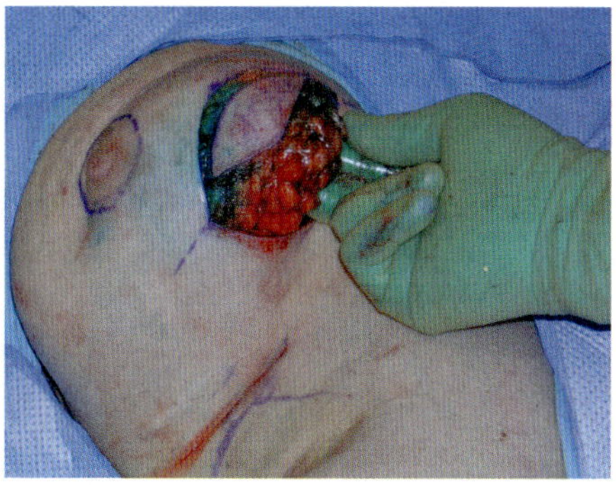

FIG 5 • The lumpectomy specimen is lifted off the pectoralis muscle.

located within the lower breast, including the 3 o'clock and 9 o'clock positions, should have a radially placed parallelogram.

- The proposed skin incision is made to breast parenchyma (**FIG 4**).
- After excision of the skin island, short-distance mastectomy-type skin flaps are raised along both sides of the wound.
- Dissection is carried down to the chest wall, the breast gland is lifted off the pectoralis muscle (**FIG 5**), and a standard tumor resection is performed.
- Four to six marking clips are typically placed at the base of the defect within the surrounding fibroglandular tissue.
- Once resection is complete and hemostasis obtained, the fibroglandular tissue at the level of the pectoralis fascia is undermined so that breast tissue advancement can be performed over the muscle (**FIG 6**).
- The margins of the residual cavity are then shifted together by the advancement of breast tissue over muscle and the defect is sutured at the deepest edges using 3-0 absorbable suture. The direction of tissue advancement can be adjusted depending on the location of the fibroglandular defect and the excess tissue that can be shifted to close it. The goal of the mastopexy is to perform as complete of a closure over the pectoralis muscle as possible to discourage communication between the anterior skin and the deeper tissues (**FIG 7**).
- The superficial tissue layer is closed with interrupted subdermal absorbable sutures (we use 3-0 sutures), whereas the skin is closed by absorbable subcuticular sutures (we use 4-0 sutures) in routine fashion (**FIG 8**).

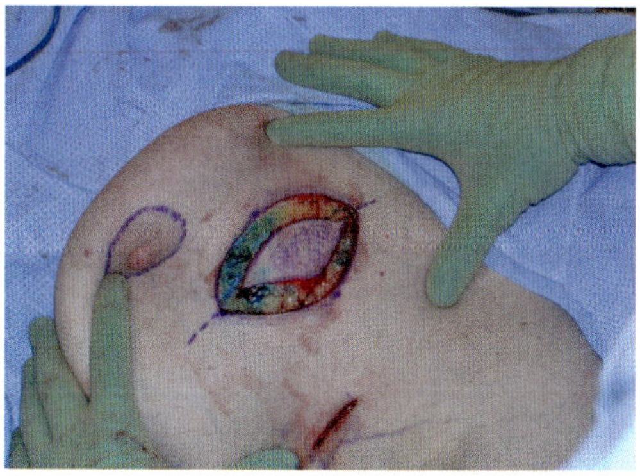

FIG 4 • The skin of the rounded parallelogram is divided with a scalpel down to the breast parenchyma.

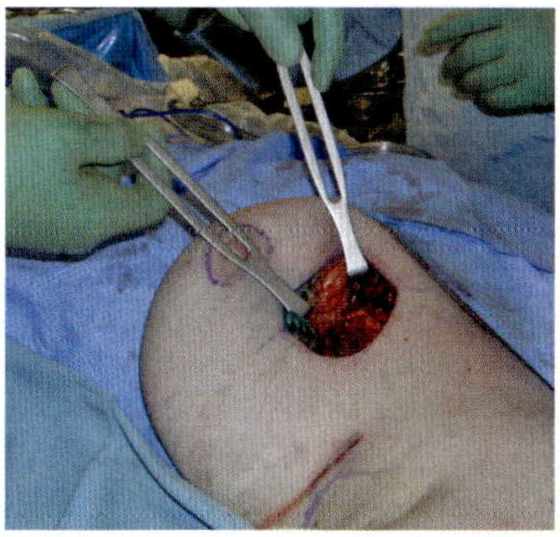

FIG 6 • The fibroglandular tissue is elevated off the pectoralis fascia in order to advance it over the muscle.

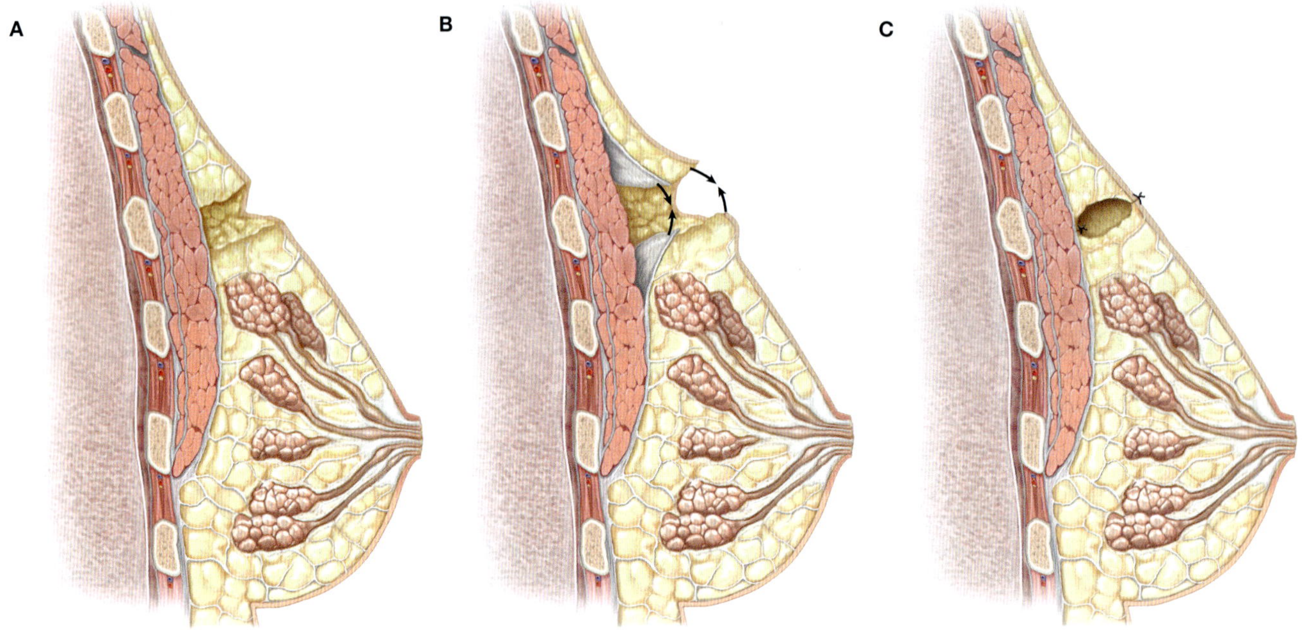

FIG 7 • **A–C.** The fibroglandular tissue is advanced over the pectoralis muscle to separate the deeper tissues from the overlying skin.

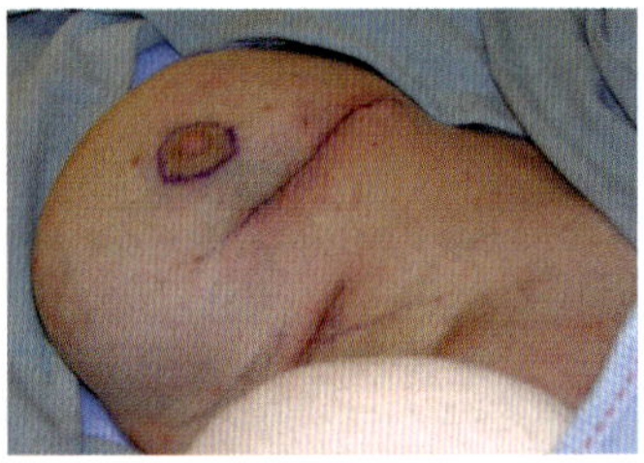

FIG 8 • Closure of the rounded parallelogram.

BATWING MASTOPEXY LUMPECTOMY

- For cancers adjacent to or deep to the NAC, but without direct involvement of the nipple, lumpectomy can be performed without sacrifice of the nipple itself.
- The batwing approach simultaneously preserves NAC viability as well as the breast mound by using mastopexy closure to close the resulting fibroglandular defect of the full-thickness resection.
- Two similar semicircle incisions are made with angled "wings" on each side of the areola (**FIG 9**). The two half circles are positioned to allow them to be reapproximated to each other at wound closure.
- Removal of these skin wings allows the semicircles to be shifted together without creating redundant skin folds at closure (**FIG 10**).
- Fibroglandular tissue dissection is carried down deep to the known cancer. In most situations, this dissection is carried down to the chest wall, with the breast gland lifted off the pectoralis muscle in a fashion similar to that for the parallelogram lumpectomy (**FIG 11**).
- Following full-thickness resection of the targeted lesion, some mobilization of the fibroglandular tissue for

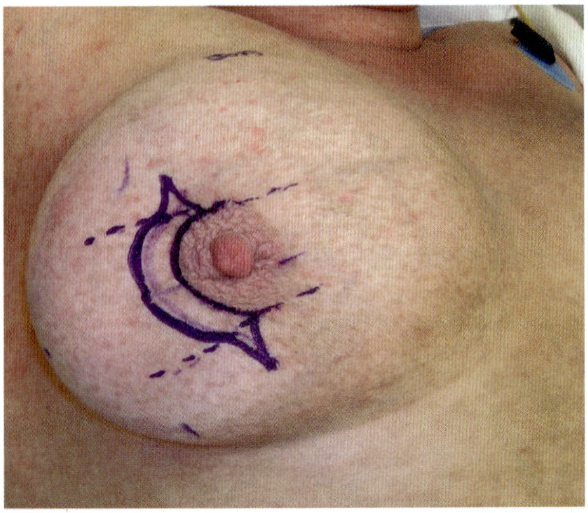

FIG 9 • Planned incision for a batwing mastopexy. Two semicircular incisions with angled wings on each side of the areola.

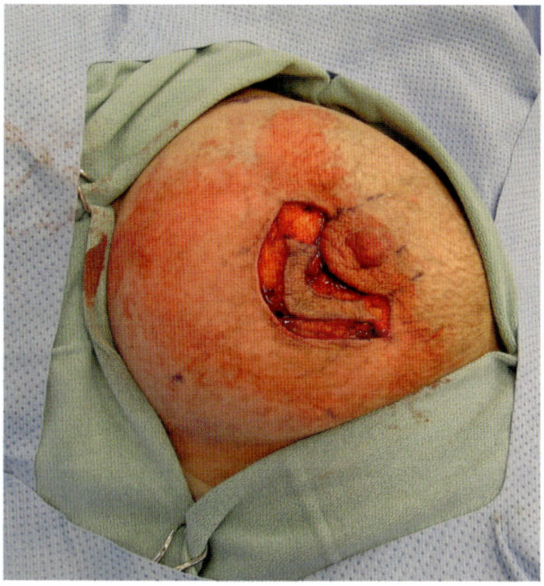

FIG 10 ● The skin is incised for a batwing mastopexy.

mastopexy closure may be required. The breast tissue is elevated off of the chest wall at the plane between the pectoralis muscle and breast gland and the remaining fibroglandular tissue is then advanced to close the resulting defect.

- We typically secure the fibroglandular tissue to itself but do not place anchoring stitches into the chest wall, thereby allowing the reapproximated breast tissues to move on the chest wall and adjust to find its most natural way to settle in for final healing. It is important to remember that what looks perfect on the chest wall when the patient is supine on the OR table may not sit as well when she sits upright and the breast becomes pendulous.
- The superficial layer is closed in the same fashion as the parallelogram mastopexy lumpectomy (**FIG 12**).
- As this procedure can cause some lifting of the nipple, it may create asymmetry when compared to the contralateral breast. If desired, a contralateral lift can be performed. Although this can be performed concurrently at the time of lumpectomy, it may be preferable after adjuvant radiation has finished and the treated breast has "declared" its new size and shape.

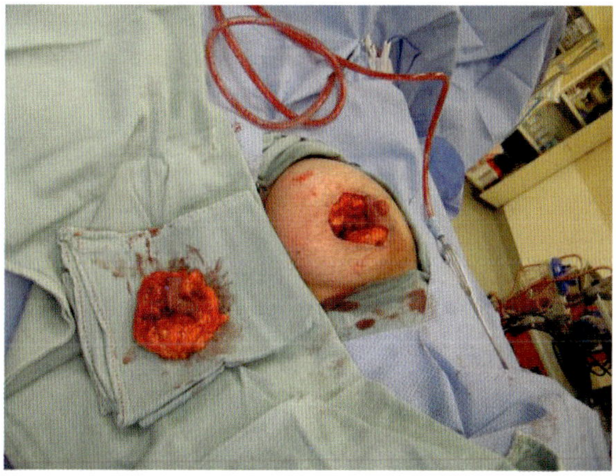

FIG 11 ● The excision is carried down to the chest wall and excised off of the underlying pectoralis muscle.

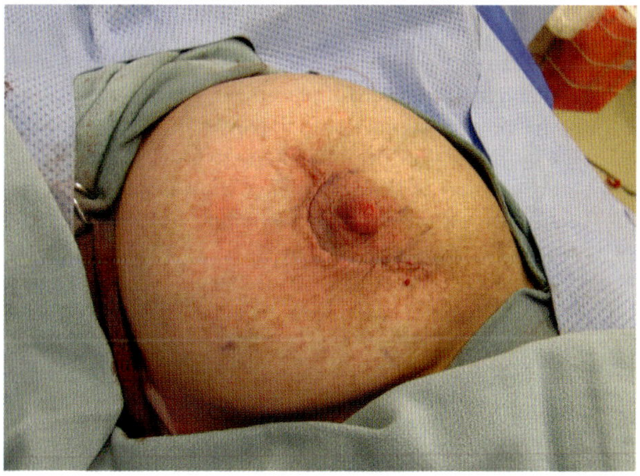

FIG 12 ● The semicircles are shifted together without creating redundant skin folds at closure.

LATERAL SEGMENTECTOMY

- A variation of the parallelogram lumpectomy, the lateral segmentectomy is especially useful for lesions located within the lower breast, including the 3 o'clock and 9 o'clock positions.
- The skin parallelogram is placed radially and, at the corner of the parallelogram which comes closest to the nipple, the design should be positioned such that the closed incision after resection will approach the NAC tangential to the periareolar line (**FIG 13**). This reduces deviation

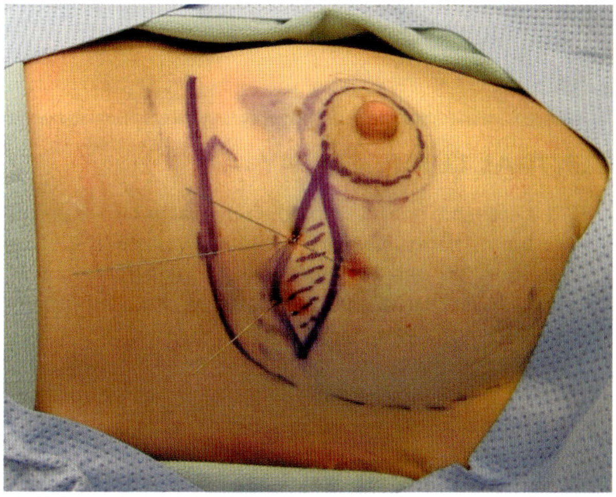

FIG 13 ● A parallelogram for a lateral segmentectomy, placed radially so that when closed, the incision will approach the NAC tangential to the periareolar line.

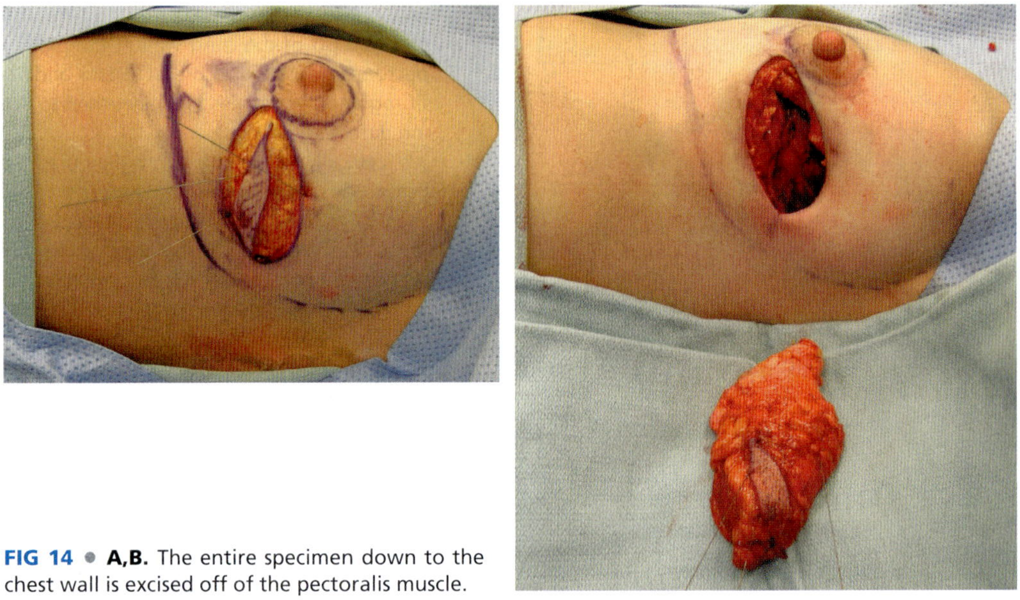

FIG 14 • **A,B.** The entire specimen down to the chest wall is excised off of the pectoralis muscle.

of the NAC toward the lesion, a condition that can result from scar contraction.

- This radial approach gives more projection to the nipple, avoiding the downward displacement, which can be caused by a purely horizontal scar in the lower pole of the breast.
- The proposed skin incision is made to breast parenchyma.
- After excision of the skin island, short-distance mastectomy-type skin flaps are raised along both sides of the wound.
- Dissection is carried down to the chest wall, the breast gland is lifted off the pectoralis muscle, and a standard tumor resection is performed (**FIG 14**).
- Four to six marking clips are typically placed at the base of the defect within the surrounding fibroglandular tissue.
- Once resection is complete and hemostasis obtained, the fibroglandular tissue at the level of the pectoralis fascia is undermined so that breast tissue advancement can be performed over the muscle.
- The margins of the residual cavity are then shifted together by the advancement of breast tissue over muscle and the defect is sutured at the deepest edges using 3-0 absorbable suture.
- The superficial tissue layer is closed with interrupted subdermal absorbable sutures (we use 3-0 sutures), whereas the skin is closed by absorbable subcuticular sutures (we use 4-0 sutures) in routine fashion (**FIG 15**).

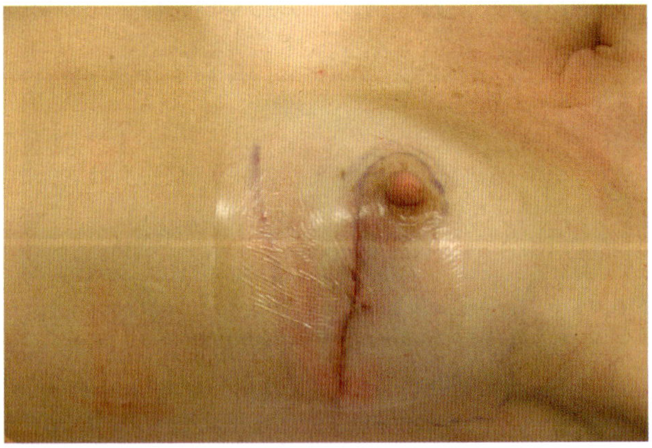

FIG 15 • The lateral segmentectomy incision after closure.

CENTRAL LUMPECTOMY

- The cosmetic impact of nipple removal, which is an unfortunate necessity when cancer involves the NAC, likely accounts for the common use of mastectomy among these individuals despite the existence of the alternative option of central lumpectomy.
- Although central lumpectomy removes the NAC and underlying central tissues, it typically leaves behind a significant breast mound.
- The cosmetic outcome with central lumpectomy can range from good to outstanding, depending on the woman's body habitus, and may be better tolerated than mastectomy and subsequent reconstruction, particularly in women with large breasts where total mastectomy may create prominent asymmetry.
- In central lumpectomy, the incision can be made in the pattern of a large parallelogram, which encompasses the entire NAC. Angling the incision along the lay of the breast when the patient is upright may lead to a more natural position of the scar.
- After excision of the skin island, short-distance mastectomy-type skin flaps are raised along both sides of the wound.

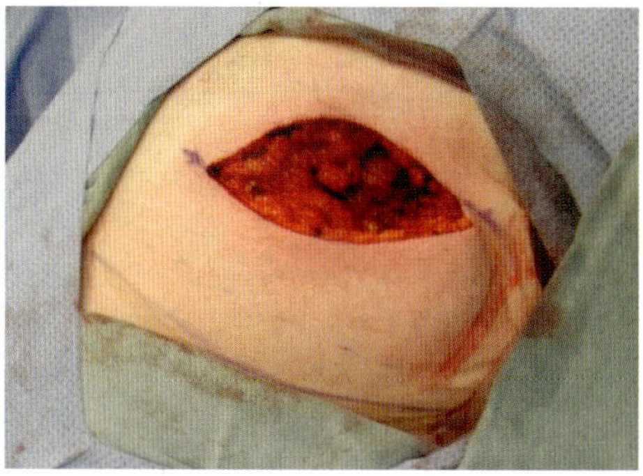

FIG 16 ● The central segmentectomy cavity after excision of the tumor down to the underying pectoralis muscle.

- Dissection is carried down to the chest wall, the breast gland is lifted off the pectoralis muscle, and a standard tumor resection is performed (**FIG 16**).
- Four to six marking clips are typically placed at the base of the defect within the surrounding fibroglandular tissue.
- Once resection is complete and hemostasis obtained, the fibroglandular tissue at the level of the pectoralis fascia is undermined so that breast tissue advancement can be performed over the muscle.
- The margins of the residual cavity are then shifted together by the advancement of breast tissue over muscle and the defect is sutured at the deepest edges using 3-0 absorbable suture. The superficial tissue layer is closed with interrupted subdermal absorbable sutures (we use 3-0 sutures), whereas the skin is closed by absorbable subcuticular sutures (we use 4-0 sutures) in routine fashion (**FIG 17**).

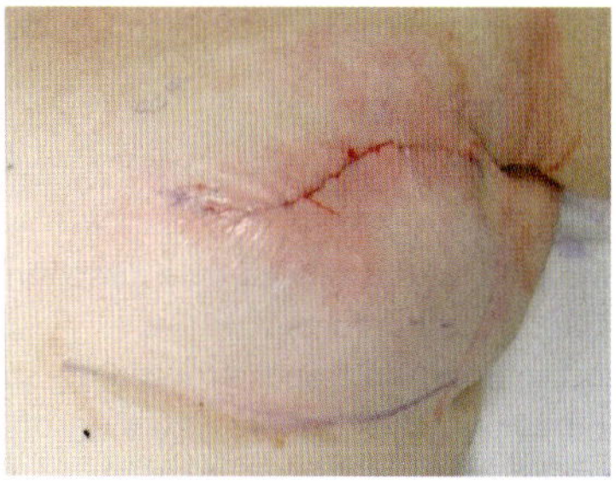

FIG 17 ● The breast tissue is advanced over the muscle and the skin closed in routine fashion.

REDUCTION MASTOPEXY LUMPECTOMY

- For cancers in the lower pole of the breast, traditional lumpectomy using circumareolar incision may result in unacceptable downturning of the nipple due to scar contracture after radiotherapy.
- This unpleasant cosmetic outcome can be prevented by using the technique of reduction mastopexy lumpectomy, especially for resection of lesions in the lower hemisphere of the breast between the 4 o'clock and 8 o'clock positions.
- A reduction mammoplasty keyhole pattern incision is made (**FIG 18A,B**) and the skin above the areola is de-epithelialized in preparation for skin closure.
- A superior pedicle flap is created by inframammary incision and undermining of the breast tissue off the pectoral fascia to mobilize the NAC and underlying tissues (**FIG 19**).
- For cancers located in the inferolateral or inferomedial quadrants, the keyhole pattern can be rotated slightly to allow for a more lateral or medial excision while at the

A

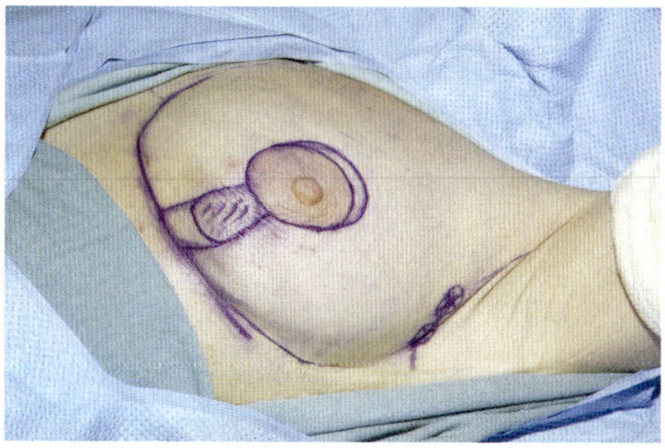

B

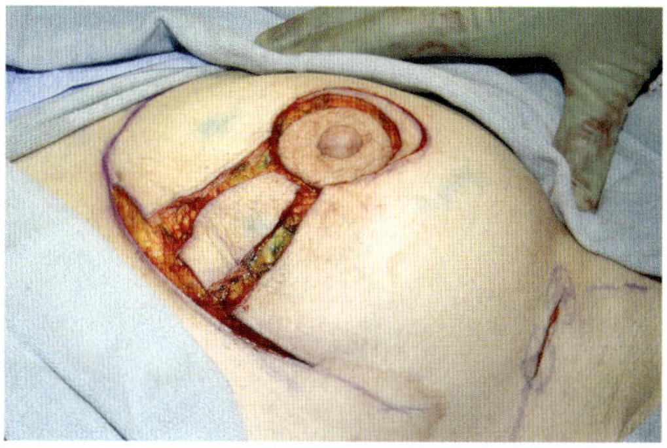

FIG 18 ● **A,B.** Planned incision for a reduction mastopexy, including a keyhole pattern inferiorly and de-epithelialization above the areola.

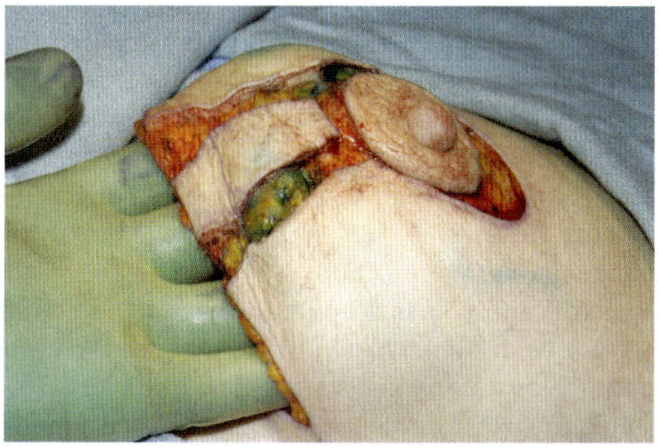

FIG 19 ● Through the inframammary incision the breast tissue is elevated off the pectoralis fascia to mobilize the NAC and underlying tissues.

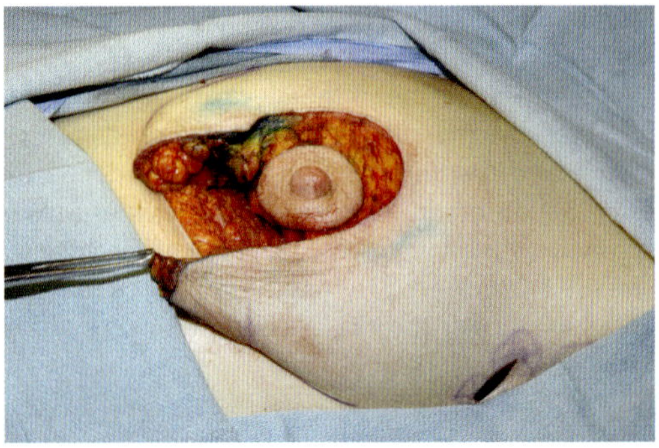

FIG 20 ● The resultant cavity after a full-thickness excision of the tumor.

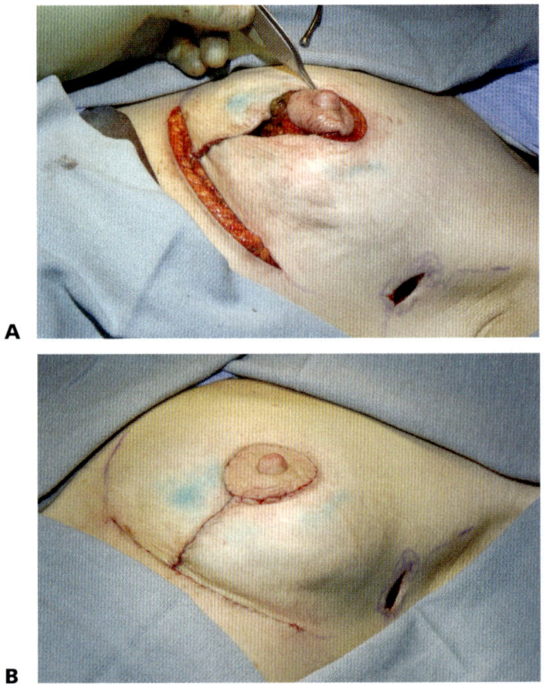

FIG 21 ● **A,B.** The NAC is recentralized and the medial and lateral flaps are undermined and re-approximated, resulting in the classic inverted T scar.

same time, the NAC is moved in a direction opposite to that of the surgical defect.[12]

- Commencing inferiorly and proceeding superiorly beneath the tumor, full-thickness excision of the lesion is accomplished, with at least a 1-cm macroscopic margin of normal tissue, and the skin overlying the lesion is removed (**FIG 20**).
- Recentralization of the NAC is performed to recreate a harmonious breast size and shape. The medial and lateral breast flaps are undermined and sutured together to fill the excision defect, leaving a typical inverted T scar (**FIG 21A,B**).
- Uplifting of the NAC by virtue of removal of the superior skin island helps restore a youthful appearance to the breast but can create mild asymmetry in comparison to the contralateral breast (**FIG 22**).
- For patients with macromastia, consistent positioning of the breast for radiotherapy may be difficult, resulting in dosing inhomogeneity and suboptimal treatment.[13] These patients can benefit from reduction mastopexy lumpectomy using a unilateral or bilateral approach.

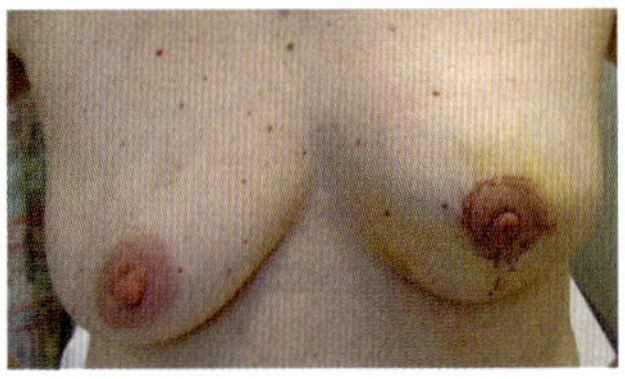

FIG 22 ● The reduction mastopexy can result in asymmetry compared to the contralateral breast that may require a contralateral reduction in the future.

DONUT MASTOPEXY LUMPECTOMY

- The donut mastopexy lumpectomy is best used for segmentally distributed cancers located in the upper or lateral breast to achieve resection of long, narrow segments of breast tissue.
- This technique avoids a visible long radial scar placed against Kraissl's or Langer's lines while allowing for adequate margin resection.
- Two concentric lines are placed around the areola and a periareolar "donut" skin island is excised, with only a periareolar scar visible after this operation (**FIG 23**).
- De-epithelialization by separating this skin island from the underlying tissues is performed, taking care to avoid full devascularization of the areolar skin.

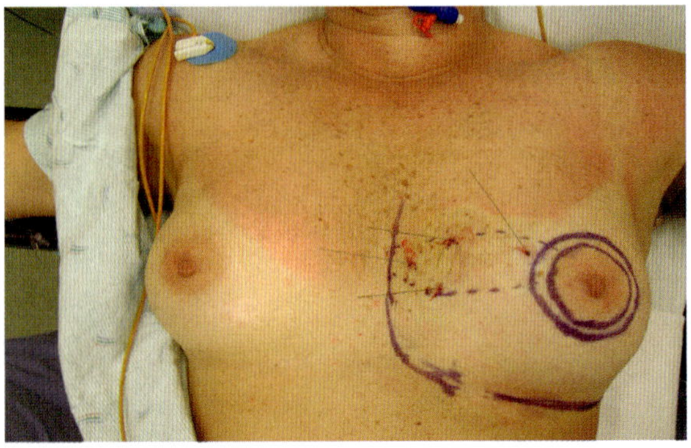

FIG 23 ● Two concentric circles are drawn around the areola, with approximately 1 cm between them.

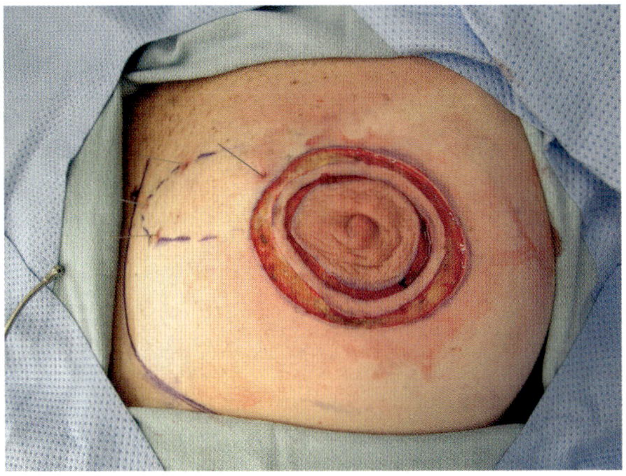

FIG 24 • The donut mastopexy incision.

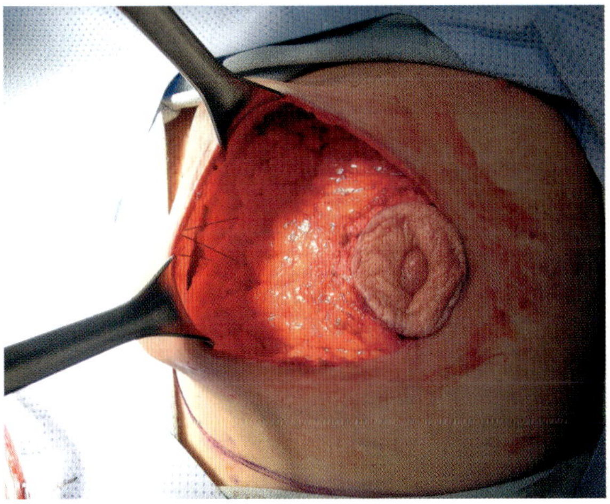

FIG 25 • A skin flap is developed off of the tumor-bearing quadrant.

- The width of the donut skin island should be approximately 1 cm but is somewhat dependent on the size of areola and expected extent of excision (**FIG 24**).
- Removal of this tissue ring is required to allow for both adequate access and exposure to the breast tissue and closure of the skin envelope around the remaining fibroglandular tissue that will reduce tissue volume overall.
- A skin envelope is created in all directions around the NAC.
- The quadrant of breast tissue containing the target lesion is fully exposed using the same dissection used for a skin-sparing mastectomy (**FIG 25**).
- The full-thickness breast gland is then separated from the underlying pectoralis muscle and delivered through the circumareolar incision.
- The tumor-bearing segment of breast tissue is resected in a wedge-shaped fashion (**FIG 26**), with the width of tissue excision balanced against the difficulty that will be created by virtue of an oversized segmental defect.
- The remaining fibroglandular tissue is returned to the skin envelope; the peripheral apical corners of the fibroglandular tissue are secured to each other and then anchored to chest wall (**FIG 27**). This anchoring maintains proper orientation of the mobilized fibroglandular tissue within the skin envelope during the initial phases of healing.
- A purse string using absorbable 3-0 suture is placed around the areola opening at a size that reapproximates the original NAC.
- Interrupted inverted 3-0 absorbable sutures are placed subdermally around the NAC, at which time the purse-string suture is tied and then 4-0 subcuticular sutures are used to close the wound (**FIG 28**).
- Uplifting of the NAC may create mild asymmetry in comparison to the untreated breast, so if desired, a contralateral lift can be performed to achieve symmetry (**FIG 29**).

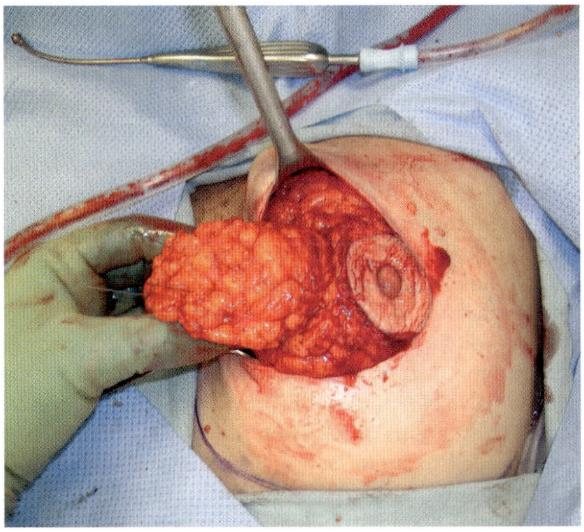

FIG 26 • A wedge-shaped excision of the tumor-bearing tissue is performed down to the underlying pectoralis muscle.

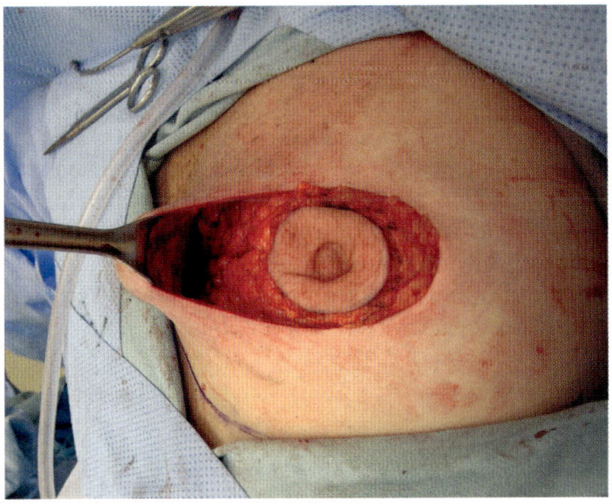

FIG 27 • The fibroglandular tissue is reapproximated to fill the defect and anchored to the chest wall.

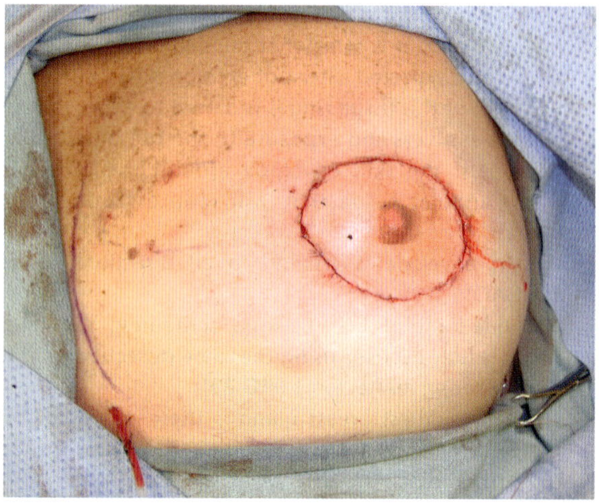

FIG 28 • The circimareolar incision is closed in standard fashion.

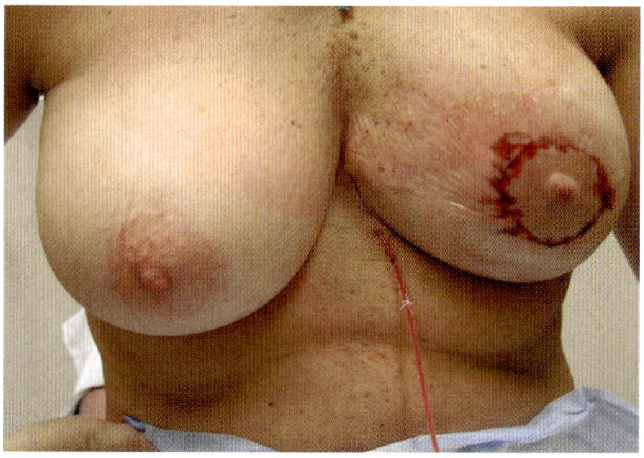

FIG 29 • As with the reduction mastopexy, the donut mastopexy will result in asymmetry that may require a contralateral lift and/or reduction.

PEARLS AND PITFALLS

Indications	▪ The same contraindications exist as with traditional lumpectomy: ▪ Multicentric disease ▪ Radiation contraindication ▪ Inability to obtain negative surgical margins
Nipple areolar uplifting and asymmetry	▪ May occur with some techniques, namely the batwing, reduction, and donut mastopexy lumpectomies ▪ Contralateral reduction and/or lift may be necessary.
Seroma formation	▪ More common with larger volume resections ▪ Consider small drain placement for a short time period.
Inadequate margins	▪ Will need to be addressed again surgically ▪ With limited involvement, reexcision likely is feasible. ▪ Multiple involved margins may require mastectomy to clear.
Long-term outcomes	▪ Appear to have superior cosmetic results with similar local recurrence rates

POSTOPERATIVE CARE

- Drains are rarely required in standard partial mastectomy cases, as any seroma will generally be reabsorbed.
- With more extensive dissections, such as the donut mastopexy lumpectomy, fluid accumulation can become more pronounced and may require postoperative aspiration on occasion. A 15-Fr round Blake drain left overnight will help avoid excessive fluid accumulation in the dissected breast that might distort the oncoplastic closure.
- Drains are typically removed either prior to discharge if kept overnight or on postoperative day 1 in the clinic.

OUTCOMES

- As with traditional lumpectomy, the main goal of all the oncoplastic approaches remains negative surgical margin resection.
- Excision of calcified lesions, masses, and the intended targeted lesion should be confirmed with specimen radiography during surgery.
- Additional oriented margins can be resected prior to mastopexy closure when the radiograph suggests inadequate resection may have occurred, hopefully eliminating the need for a delayed reexcision.
- Some centers use intraoperative analysis with frozen section or cytology to aid in decisions regarding the resection of additional segments of tissue.
- If subsequent reexcision is needed for inadequate surgical margins following the initial resection, use of the same incision is preferred.
- When the positive margin involves a minority of the specimen, the entire biopsy cavity does not need to be reexcised with only the involved margins of the previous biopsy cavity taken.
- When all the margins of resection are involved, mastectomy may be needed to attain satisfactory surgical clearance. In this instance, it may be technically challenging to include both the initial oncoplastic incision and the NAC in a subsequent total mastectomy and consultation with the plastic surgeon in the event that immediate postmastectomy reconstruction is mandatory.

- Although there are few large volume studies of long-term outcomes specifically addressing oncoplastic approaches in breast conservation, the results that are available are promising. One investigation from Europe followed 148 women for a median of 74 months (range 10 to 108 months) and only 2 were lost to follow-up. Among the remaining 146 individuals, there were only 5 (3%) women who suffered an ipsilateral in-breast cancer recurrence after 5 years and all had either T2 or T3 tumors at presentation.[14]
- Although additional studies are needed, it seems reasonable to presume that oncoplastic approaches, which often results in wider margins of resection than the traditional segmental mastectomy, will continue to be a sound option for breast conservation therapy.

COMPLICATIONS

- When using oncoplastic approaches, surgeons without formal training must determine which procedures they are comfortable performing without plastic surgery consultation or intraoperative collaboration.[3]
- In addition to standard potential postsurgical complications, wound infection, fat necrosis, and delayed healing in the more advanced reduction mastopexy lumpectomy have all been reported with oncoplastic resections.[15]
- The blood supply of the external nipple arises from underlying fibroglandular tissue using major lactiferous sinuses rather than the collateral circulation from surrounding areolar skin, so nipple necrosis may occur if dissection extends high up behind the nipple.[3]

REFERENCES

1. Veronesi U, Cascinelli N, Mariani L, et al. Twenty-year follow-up of a randomized study comparing breast-conserving surgery with radical mastectomy for early breast cancer. *N Engl J Med*. 2002;347:1227–1232.
2. Fisher B, Anderson S, Bryant J, et al. Twenty-year follow-up of a randomized trial comparing total mastectomy, lumpectomy, and lumpectomy plus irradiation for the treatment of invasive breast cancer. *N Engl J Med*. 2002;347:1233–1241.
3. Anderson BO, Masetti R, Silverstein MJ. Oncoplastic approaches to partial mastectomy: an overview of volume-displacement techniques. *Lancet Oncol*. 2005;6:145–157.
4. Audretsch WP. Reconstruction of the partial mastectomy defect: classification and method. In: Spear SL, ed. *Surgery of the Breast: Principle and Art*. 2nd ed. Philadelphia, PA: Lippincott Williams & Wilkins; 2006:179–216.
5. Chen CY, Calhoun KE, Masetti R, et al. Oncoplastic breast conserving surgery: a renaissance of anatomically-based surgical technique. *Minerva Chir*. 2006;61:421–434.
6. Love SM, Barsky SH. Anatomy of the nipple and breast ducts revisited. *Cancer*. 2004;101:1947–1957.
7. Cooper AP. *On the Anatomy of the Breast* (Special Collections, Scott Memorial Library, Thomas Jefferson University). London, United Kingdom: Longman, Orme, Green, Brown, and Longmans; 1840. http://jdc.jefferson.edu/cooper/. Accessed April 12, 2012.
8. Holland R, Faverly DRG. The local distribution of ductal carcinoma in situ of the breast: whole-organ studies. In: Silverstein MJ, ed. *Ductal Carcinoma in Situ of the Breast*. 2nd ed. Philadelphia, PA: Lippincott Williams & Wilkins; 2002:240.
9. Bluemke DA, Gatsonis CA, Chen MH, et al. Magnetic resonance imaging of the breast prior to biopsy. *JAMA*. 2004;292:2735–2742.
10. Silverstein MJ, Lagios MD, Recht A, et al. Image-detected breast cancer: state of the art diagnosis and treatment. *J Am Coll Surg*. 2005;201:586–597.
11. Kraissl CJ. The selection of appropriate lines for elective surgical incisions. *Plast Reconstr Surg*. 1951;8:1–28.
12. Grisotti A. Conservation treatment of breast cancer: reconstructive problems. In: Spear SL, ed. *Surgery of the Breast: Principles and Art*. Philadelphia, PA: Lippincott-Raven Publishers; 1998:137–153.
13. Masetti R, Di Leone A, Franceschini G, et al. Oncoplastic techniques in the conservative surgical treatment of breast cancer: an overview. *Breast J*. 2006;12:S174–S180.
14. Rietjens M, Urban CA, Rey PC, et al. Long-term oncological results if breast conservation treatment with oncoplastic surgery. *Breast*. 2007;16:387–395.
15. Iwuagwu OC. Additional considerations in the application of oncoplastic approaches. *Lancet Oncol*. 2005;6:356.

Chapter 7

Brachytherapy Catheter Insertion for Breast Cancer

Peter D. Beitsch

DEFINITION

- Breast conservation therapy (BCT) requires postlumpectomy radiation.
- Radiation can be given to the entire breast as whole breast irradiation (WBI) or to the area at the highest risk of recurrence—the breast tissue surrounding the lumpectomy cavity—by accelerated partial breast irradiation (APBI).
- APBI can be delivered from an external source (3-D conformal) or an internal source (brachytherapy).

DIFFERENTIAL DIAGNOSIS

- Brachytherapy can be delivered via multiple inserted catheters (interstitial multicatheter; **FIG 1**) or via a single insertion/multiple catheter device (**FIGS 2–4**) (see videos 1 and 2 in the accompanying eBook).

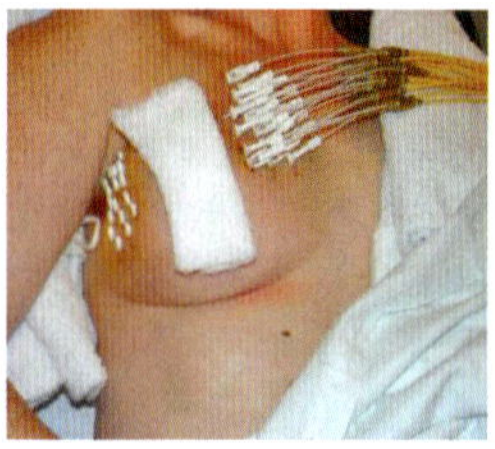

FIG 1 • Multiple catheter interstitial brachytherapy.

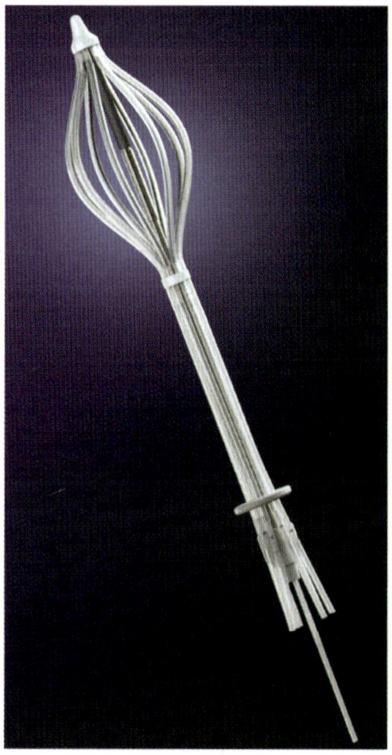

FIG 2 • Strut-adjusted volume implant (SAVI)—single insertion multicatheter strut-based device. ©Cianna Medical, Inc.

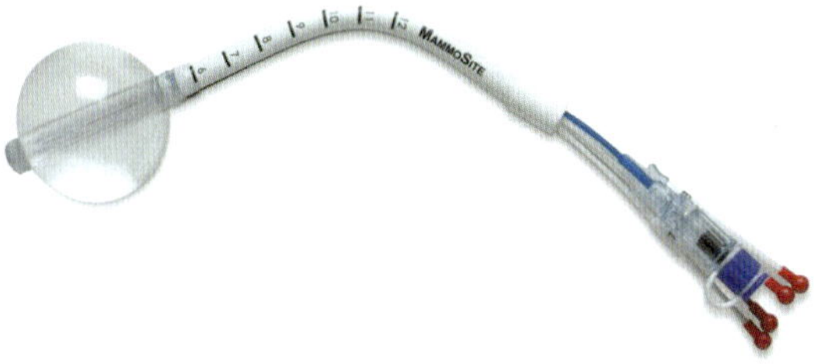

FIG 3 • MammoSite ML—single insertion multicatheter balloon device.

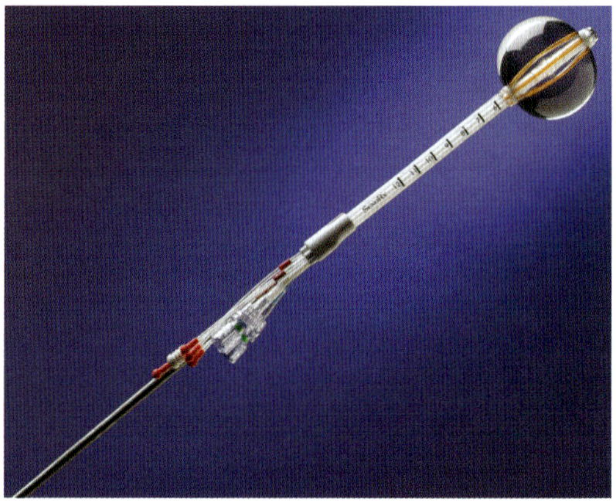

FIG 4 • Contura—single insertion multicatheter balloon device.

- Radiation oncologists usually perform the multiple catheter insertions and surgeons insert the single insertion/multiple catheter devices (which is the focus of this chapter).

PATIENT HISTORY AND PHYSICAL FINDINGS

- Patient selection for APBI is critically important (not everyone is a candidate).
- The American Society of Breast Surgeons[1] and the American Brachytherapy Society[2] have published guidelines for patient selection (Table 1).
- The American Society of Radiation Oncology (ASTRO) has published a consensus statement on patient selection for APBI (Table 2).[3]

IMAGING AND OTHER DIAGNOSTIC STUDIES

- Controversy exists whether all patients undergoing APBI should get preoperative advanced breast imaging (magnetic resonance imaging [MRI] or positron emission mammography); however, most surgeons only do so selectively.
- Ultrasound skills by the surgeon are helpful for insertion but are not mandatory.

Table 1: Patient Selection Guidelines for Accelerated Partial Breast Irradiation

Criteria	American Brachytherapy Society	American Society of Breast Surgeons
Age	≥50	≥45
Histology	IDC	IDC, DCIS
Tumor size	≤3 cm	≤3 cm
Node status	N0	N0
Margins	Negative	Negative

IDC, invasive ductal carcinoma; DCIS, ductal carcinoma in situ.

Table 2: American Society of Radiation Oncology Consensus Statement on Patient Selection for Accelerated Partial Breast Irradiation

	"Suitable"	"Cautionary"	"Unsuitable"
Definition	*Off clinical trial*	*Limited clinical data*	*Only on trial*
Age	≥60 y	50–59 y	<50 y
T size	≤2 cm	2–3 cm	>3 cm
Nodes	Neg	—	Pos
Histology	IDC	ILC or DCIS	—
Margins	Neg (>2 mm)	Close (<2 mm)	Pos
Path features	No EIC or LVI	EIC or focal LVI	>3 cm EIC/DCIS
Grade	Any	—	—
Multicentricity	Unifocal	—	—
ER status	Pos	Neg	—

IDC, invasive ductal carcinoma; ILC, invasive lobular carcinoma; DCIS, ductal carcinoma in situ; EIC, extensive intraductal component; LVI, lymphovascular invasion; ER, estrogen receptor.

SURGICAL MANAGEMENT

- Brachytherapy devices are routinely placed in the surgeon's office.
- Cavity evaluation devices (CEDs) (**FIG 5**) can be inserted at the time of the lumpectomy as a "space holder" until exchanged in the office for the brachytherapy device.

Preoperative Planning

- Preoperative consultation with the radiation oncologist will be helpful in facilitating postoperative treatment scheduling.
- Postlumpectomy placement in the office begins with the preoperative plan for the lumpectomy including
  - Location of incisions (do not perform sentinel lymph node biopsy through the lumpectomy incision)
  - Use of oncoplastic techniques (minimal flap rearrangement is okay but major flap movement with obliteration of the lumpectomy cavity negates the use of APBI)
  - Thicker wound closure if possible (more tissue between skin and cavity may require skin resection and multilayer closure)

Positioning

- Operative: No changes needed for CED placement.
- Office: Generally, brachytherapy devices are placed from lateral to medial to minimize the nontherapeutic radiation that other parts of the body receive as the brachytherapy seed travels into and out of each of the catheters.

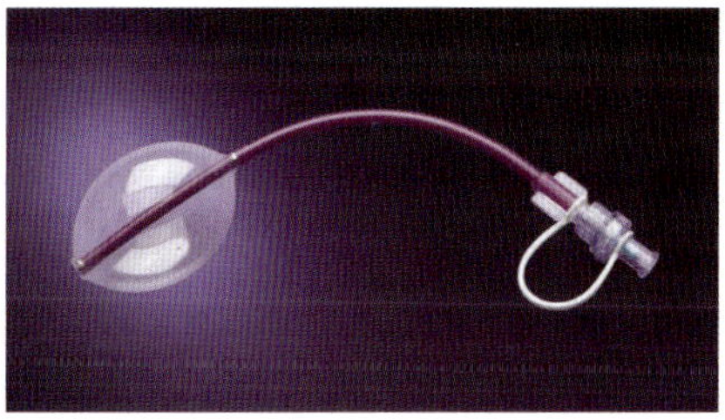

FIG 5 • Cavity evaluation device.

OPERATIVE PLACEMENT OF A CAVITY EVALUATION DEVICE

First Step

- After lumpectomy but before closure, a small skin nick is made laterally or inferiorly and the CED is tunneled from the skin nick into the lumpectomy cavity (**FIG 6**).

Second Step

- Inflate the balloon with enough saline to fill the cavity (**FIG 7**).

Third Step

- Deflate the balloon and close the lumpectomy wound.

Fourth Step

- Reinflate the balloon and note the volume used. This will assist in choosing the correct size of brachytherapy device to be placed in the office.
  - There is no need to suture the CED to the skin as the inflated balloon will hold it in place.

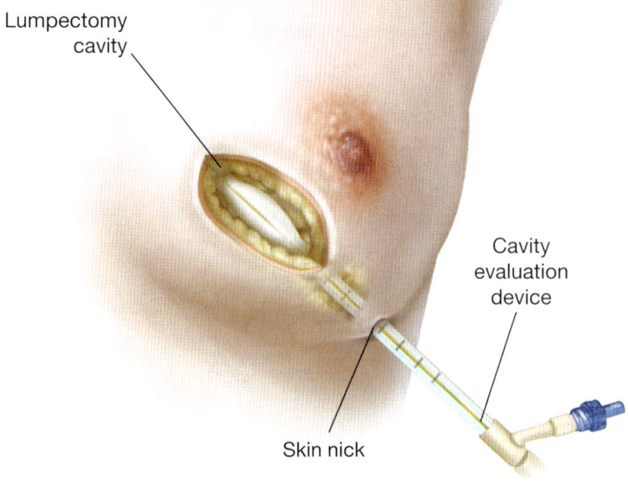

FIG 6 • Operative placement of CED.

TECHNIQUES

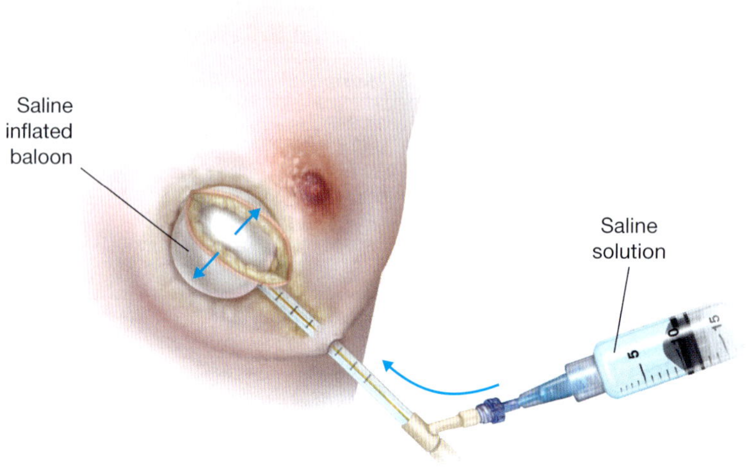

FIG 7 • Inflating the CED.

OFFICE EXCHANGE OF CAVITY EVALUATION DEVICE FOR BRACHYTHERAPY DEVICE

First Step

- Review the pathology to ensure negative margins and negative sentinel node(s) and confirm with the radiation oncologist that the patient is a candidate for APBI.

Second Step

- Prep and drape the CED and the surrounding breast tissue with Betadine or chlorhexidine and sterile drape or towels (**FIG 8**).
  - Inject local anesthetic around the skin nick.

Third Step

- Deflate the CED (noting the volume used) and remove it, immediately placing the brachytherapy device through the same track into the lumpectomy cavity (**FIG 9**).

Fourth Step

- Inflate the balloon with the same amount of saline or expand the struts until they engage the cavity walls.

Fifth Step

- Sterilely dress the entrance site of the device.

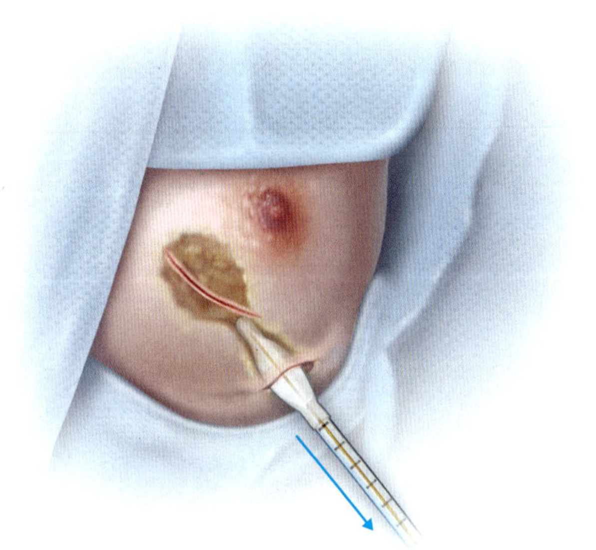

FIG 8 • Prep and drape the CED and surrounding breast.

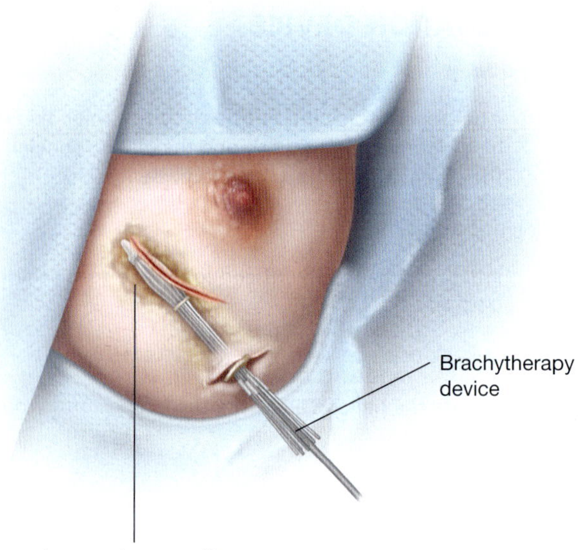

FIG 9 • Exchange of brachytherapy device for CED through same track without need for ultrasound.

OFFICE PLACEMENT OF BRACHYTHERAPY DEVICE WITH ULTRASOUND GUIDANCE

First Step

- Review the pathology to ensure negative margins and negative sentinel node(s) and confirm with the radiation oncologist that the patient is candidate for APBI.

Second Step

- Examine the lumpectomy cavity with ultrasound to determine the best size of brachytherapy device and the best approach to place the device (**FIG 10**).
  - The approach is particularly important for the strut-based device because it is elliptical and should be placed along the long axis of the lumpectomy cavity (balloon devices will expand and make the lumpectomy cavity conform to the balloon).
  - Plan incision ~2 cm from the edge of the cavity.

Third Step

- Inject local anesthetic into the skin nick site and the track that leads to the lumpectomy cavity (**FIG 11**).

Fourth Step

- Sterilely prep and drape the site and place the ultrasound transducer into a sterile drape onto the field.
  - If a sterile transducer cover is not available, you can clean the transducer with alcohol swab and use sterile gel, but the hand using the ultrasound will no longer be sterile and therefore that hand cannot touch any of the instruments or brachytherapy device.

Fifth Step

- Use a no. 11 blade and make an approximately 12-mm incision (**FIG 12**).

Sixth Step

- The trocar is inserted into the cavity under ultrasound guidance (the lumpectomy seroma may partially evacuate at this time) (**FIG 13A,B**).

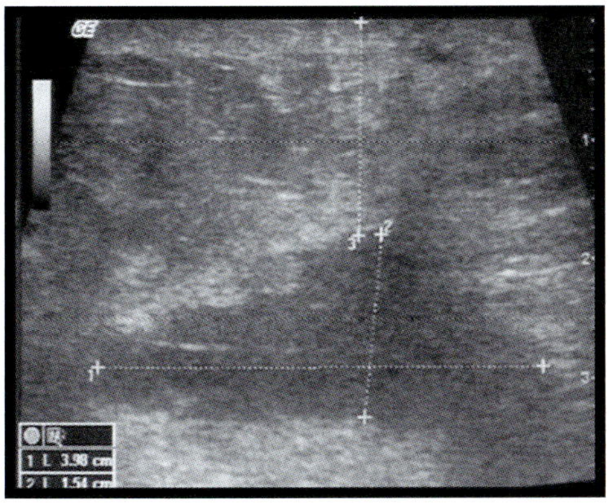

FIG 10 ● Ultrasound examination of the lumpectomy cavity.

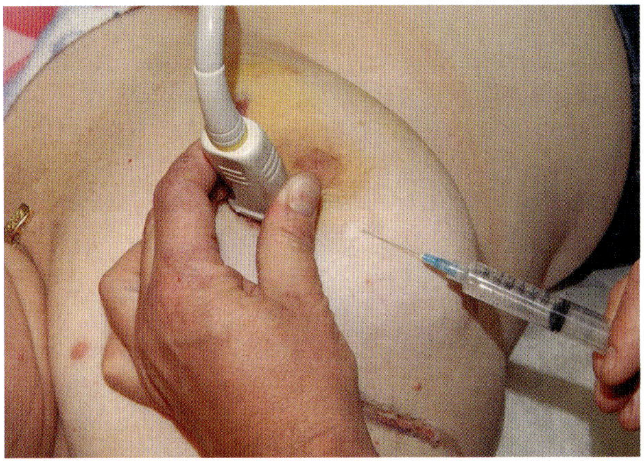

FIG 11 ● Local anesthetic at the insertion site.

Seventh Step

- Insert the brachytherapy device through the trocar track into the lumpectomy cavity (**FIG 14**).

Eighth Step

- Inflate the balloon until you meet resistance or deploy the struts until they engage the cavity walls (**FIG 15**).

Ninth Step

- Examine the device placement with ultrasound (**FIG 16**).

Tenth Step

- Remove the center stiffener rod and replace with a catheter cap to keep fluid out of the catheter (**FIG 17**).

Eleventh Step

- Sterilely dress the device entrance site (**FIG 18**).

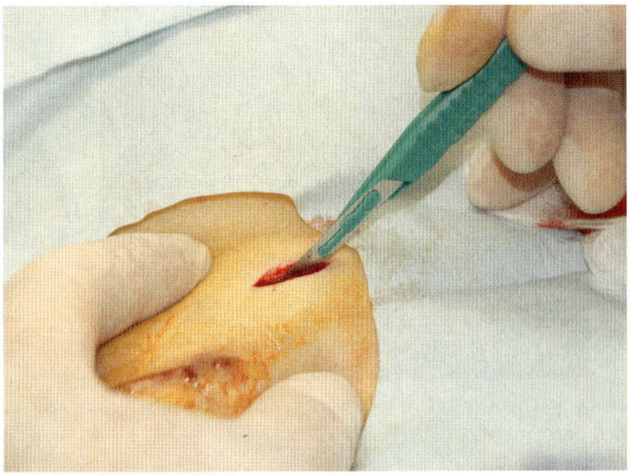

FIG 12 ● Skin incision at insertion site.

A

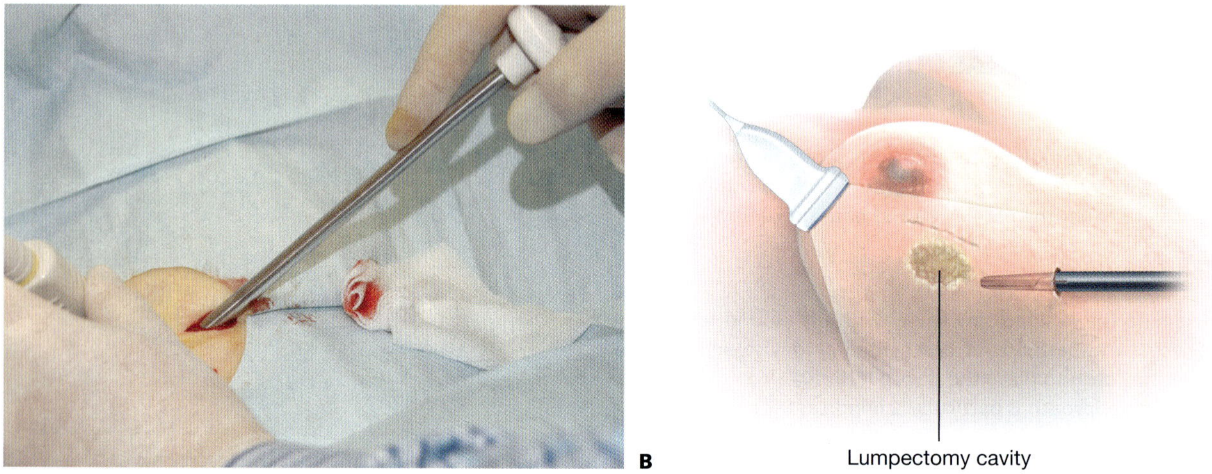

B

FIG 13 ● **A,B.** Trocar insertion into lumpectomy cavity under ultrasound guidance.

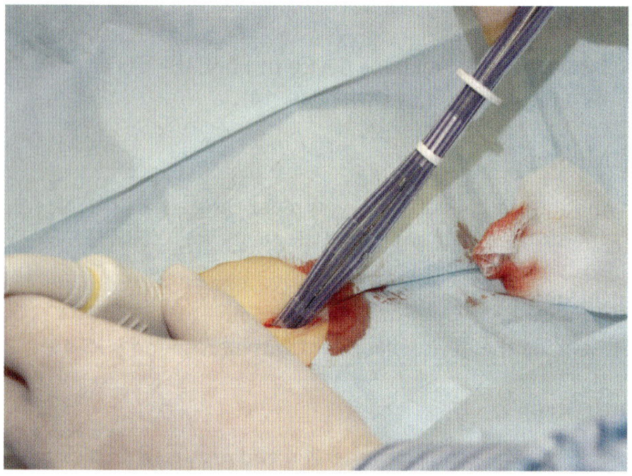

FIG 14 ● Brachytherapy device placement into cavity under ultrasound guidance.

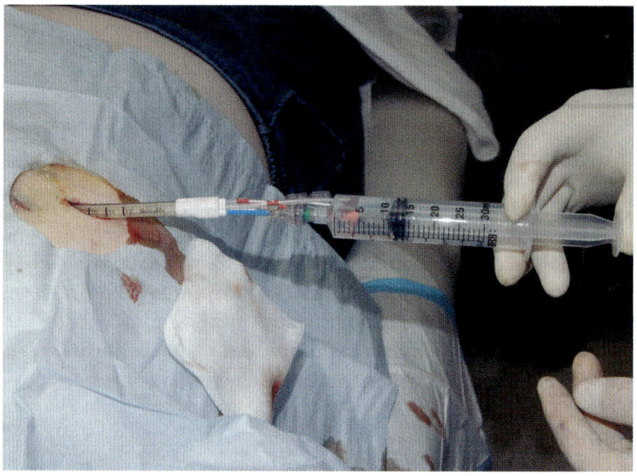

FIG 15 ● Inflating the brachytherapy device balloon.

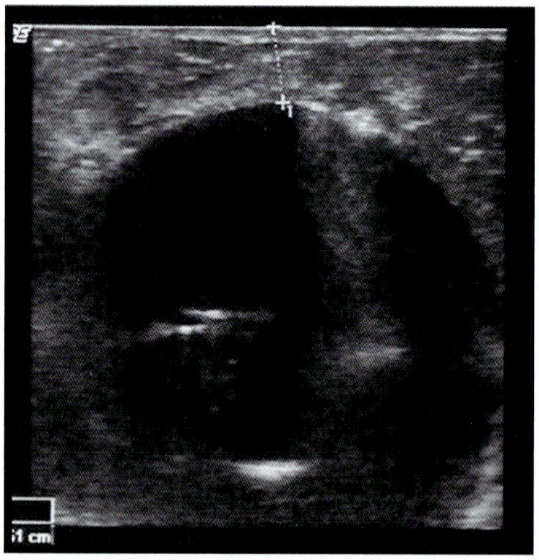

FIG 16 ● Ultrasound examination of the brachytherapy device placement.

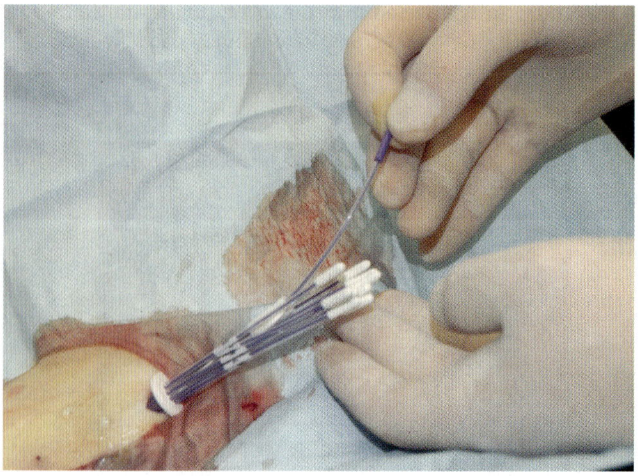

FIG 17 ● Replacing the center catheter cap.

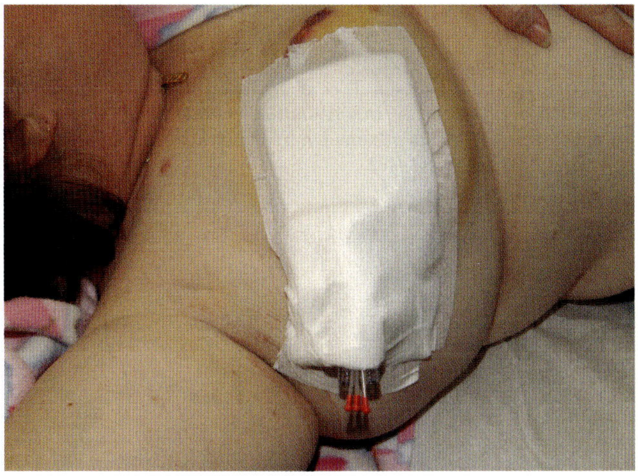

FIG 18 ● Sterile dressing around the brachytherapy device.

PEARLS AND PITFALLS

Poor conformance of balloon device to cavity wall	▪ If there is a pocket of fluid or air between the balloon and lumpectomy cavity wall (as seen by ultrasound), gently massage the breast to evacuate the fluid/air.
Drainage through track	▪ There is often fluid that will drain out through the track of the CED or device. Warning your patient about this will often save a phone call at bedtime (usually occurs when patient lays down for bed).
Delay in device placement after lumpectomy	▪ As the lumpectomy wound heals, the cavity will become fibrotic and eventually obliterates. This can vary between patients, but it is generally best to place the device within 4 weeks of the lumpectomy.
Avoiding radiation recall	▪ If the patient is going to be receiving chemotherapy, it is best to wait a minimum of 3 weeks after the last APBI treatment to prevent radiation recall (poorly understood phenomena of noninfectious erythema overlying the lumpectomy cavity).
Minimizing skin radiation	▪ Although the newer devices have multiple catheters that allow much better tailoring of the radiation to minimize radiation to normal structures (skin, lungs, ribs, heart, pectoral muscle), it is still best to create as much distance between the skin and the brachytherapy device as possible, so you may need to excise skin overlying the breast cancer and close the cavity in multiple layers.

POSTOPERATIVE CARE

- Postinsertion care includes daily dressing changes, no showering (sponge baths only until device removed).
- Most surgeons place the patient on antibiotics while the device is in.
  - Cephalexin, Bactrim DS, and ciprofloxacin are commonly used.
- Typically, the radiation oncologist will remove the device after the last treatment and Steri-Strip the opening.

OUTCOMES

- APBI has local recurrence rates of 2% to 5% at 5 years—similar to WBI.[4–7]
- Overall survival and breast cancer–specific survival are also equivalent to similarly staged patients who receive WBI.
- True recurrences (tumor bed) are usually treated with mastectomy, but elsewhere, recurrences (presumably new primaries) may be treated with lumpectomy and APBI.

COMPLICATIONS

- Early complications[4]
  - Infections—~9% (no catheter explant due to infection)
  - Seromas—~30%
    - Painful seromas—~13%
- Late complications
  - Cosmesis—excellent/good, 90%; and fair/poor, 10%
  - Fat necrosis—~2%

REFERENCES

1. American Society of Breast Surgeons. Consensus statement for accelerated partial breast irradiation. https://www.breastsurgeons.org/statements/PDF_Statements/APBI.pdf. Accessed July 28, 2013.
2. Keisch M, Arthur D, Patel R, et al. American Brachytherapy Society Breast Brachytherapy Task Group. American Brachytherapy Society Web site. http://www.americanbrachytherapy.org/guidelines/abs_breast_brachytherapy_taskgroup.pdf. Accessed July 28, 2013.
3. Smith BD, Arthur DW, Buchholz TA, et al. Accelerated partial breast irradiation consensus statement from the American Society

for Radiation Oncology (ASTRO). *Int J Radiat Oncol Biol Phys.* 2009;74(4):987–1001.

4. Vicini FA, Beitsch P, Quiet C, et al. Five-year analysis of treatment efficacy and cosmesis by the American Society of Breast Surgeons MammoSite Breast Brachytherapy Registry Trial in patients treated with accelerated partial breast irradiation. *Int J Radiat Oncol Biol Phys.* 2011;79(3):808–817.
5. Shah C, Antonucci JV, Wilkinson JB, et al. Twelve-year outcomes and patterns of failure with accelerated partial breast irradiation versus whole-breast irradiation: results of a matched-pair analysis. *Radiother Oncol.* 2011;100:210–214.
6. Swanson TA, Vicini FA. Overview of accelerated partial breast irradiation. *Curr Oncol Rep.* 2008;10:54–60.
7. Polgár C, Fodor J, Major T, et al. Breast-conserving treatment with partial or whole breast irradiation for low-risk invasive breast carcinoma-5-year results of a randomized trial. *Int J Radiat Oncol Biol Phys.* 2007;69(3):694–702.

Chapter 8 Sentinel Lymph Node Biopsy for Breast Cancer

Anees B. Chagpar

DEFINITION

- Sentinel node biopsy is a minimally invasive means to accurately stage the axilla in breast cancer patients.

PATIENT HISTORY AND PHYSICAL FINDINGS

- As always, a complete history and physical exam is warranted. If the patient has obvious clinically enlarged axillary lymph nodes on physical exam, ultrasound, and/or fine needle aspiration (FNA) or core needle biopsy may provide diagnostic information. If the biopsied node is positive, one could proceed to neoadjuvant chemotherapy and/or axillary dissection if primary surgery is planned. Alternatively, if the biopsied node is negative, sentinel node biopsy is still indicated for definitive evaluation.

IMAGING AND OTHER DIAGNOSTIC STUDIES

- Lymphoscintigraphy is commonly performed in conjunction with sentinel lymph node (SLN) biopsy for breast cancer, although it is not absolutely necessary.[1] Depending on how the radionucleotide tracer is injected, lymphoscintigraphy may show drainage to the internal mammary nodes (see Chapter 9). If patients have had previous sentinel node biopsy and/or axillary node dissection, repeat sentinel node biopsy may be considered for staging ipsilateral recurrent or new primary disease. In this circumstance, alternative drainage patterns are possible, and therefore, preoperative lymphoscintigraphy may be useful.[2]

SURGICAL MANAGEMENT

- Sentinel node biopsy is indicated for staging of patients with invasive breast cancer or those with ductal carcinoma in situ undergoing mastectomy.

Preoperative Planning

- Timing of sentinel node biopsy vis-à-vis neoadjuvant chemotherapy is controversial; some opt to perform this procedure prior to initiation of neoadjuvant chemotherapy so as to most accurately stage the axilla, whereas others will do a sentinel node biopsy after completion of neoadjuvant chemotherapy so as to potentially spare patients who have had a pathologic complete response to the morbidity of a complete axillary dissection.

Positioning

- Patients are positioned supine. A roll may be placed under the ipsilateral shoulder so as to elevate the latissimus dorsi muscle. Care should be exercised to ensure that the arm is supported on folded sheets so as to avoid a brachial plexus stretch injury (**FIG 1**).
- Intravenous lines, pulse oximeter devices, and blood pressure cuffs should be placed on other extremities if possible.

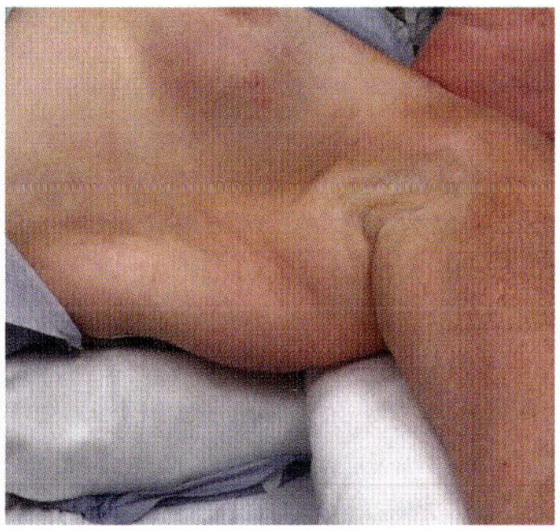

FIG 1 • Patient positioned with roll under ipsilateral latissimus and folded sheets to support arm.

TECHNIQUES

INJECTION OF RADIOACTIVE TRACER AND/OR BLUE DYE

- Use of dual tracer has been shown to be associated with higher identification and lower false-negative rates[3]; however, particularly in patients undergoing skin-sparing mastectomy, surgeons may wish to forego blue dye, as the dye may discolor the skin and make it more difficult to evaluate for skin ischemia or necrosis.
  - In general, the radioactive tracer used is technetium Tc 99m sulfur colloid. For patients not undergoing lymphoscintigraphy, the tracer can be injected in the preoperative holding area. However, injection of this material is painful, and adequate counts can often be obtained with intradermal injection after induction of anesthesia. The radiotracer can be injected peritumoral, intradermal (in the skin over the location of the cancer), or periareolar (four intradermal injections around the areola). If injection is done on the same day as the operative procedure, a dose of 0.5 mCi is adequate. If injection is done the day prior to surgery, 2.5 mCi should be used.
- Both isosulfan and methylene blue dye have been used for SLN biopsy; they vary in their color, complication profile, and cost. Isosulfan blue is a more azure blue (which is easier to distinguish from venous structures) but is associated with less than 1% risk of anaphylaxis[4] and is significantly more costly than methylene blue. Methylene blue is darker, associated with a higher rate of skin necrosis, but is far cheaper.[5]

In general, 5 mL of these tracers are used; if methylene blue is chosen, it should be diluted 1:2 with saline.

- Blue dye may be injected peritumoral or using a subareolar approach. The latter allows for lymphatic mapping of multiple tumors and those which are not easily identifiable[6] (**FIG 2**). For patients undergoing breast conservation, the subareolar approach may leave the patient with a "blue breast" for some time.

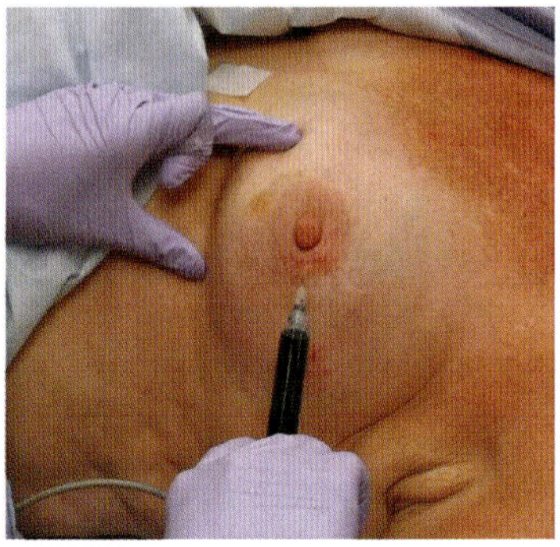

FIG 2 ● Subareolar injection of blue dye.

PREPPING AND DRAPING

- The arm is prepped circumferentially along with the breast. The arm is draped into the field and kept free such that the surgeon may move the arm in a sterile fashion during the case (**FIG 3**).

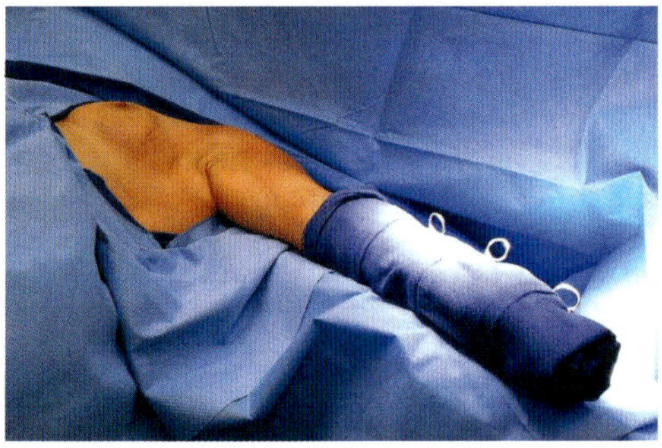

FIG 3 ● Patient draped with breast and axilla in the field; the ipsilateral arm is draped in the sterile field.

INCISION

- Identification of the area of maximal radioactivity in the axilla using a handheld gamma probe allows one to position the incision over the sentinel node.
- Landmarks of the pectoralis and latissimus dorsi muscle are used to fashion an incision for an axillary dissection of which the sentinel node incision would be a segment (**FIG 4**). A lazy S incision will allow for optimal cosmesis and will allow for extension superiorly and inferiorly if needed for maximal visualization. Alternatively, if a conventional mastectomy is planned, the sentinel node biopsy can often be performed through the lateral aspect of the same incision.
- Local anaesthetic may be used for preemptive analgesia. The incision is taken down through skin, subcutaneous tissue, and clavipectoral fascia.

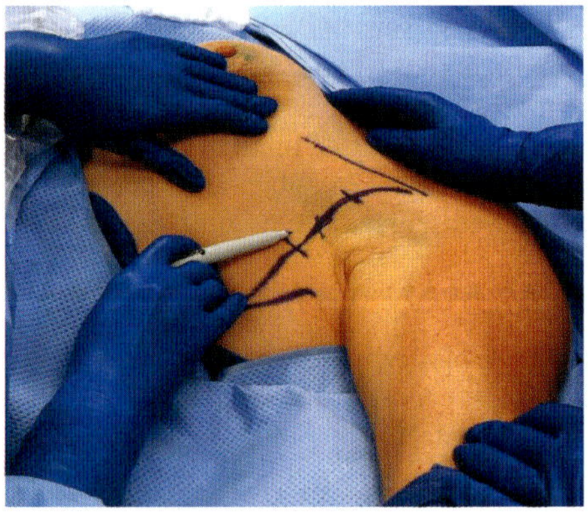

FIG 4 ● Incision planning. The pectoralis and latissimus dorsi muscle borders are identified. An "X" marks the area of maximal radioactivity. A lazy S incision is fashioned for a potential axillary dissection going through the X. A smaller segment (marked by the crosshatch lines) delineates the incision for the sentinel node biopsy.

IDENTIFICATION OF SENTINEL NODES

- Care is taken to remove the hottest node, and any node with radioactive counts greater than 10% of the ex vivo counts of the hottest node. In addition, all blue nodes and those at the end of a blue lymphatic channel are also removed (**FIG 5**).
- Palpation is critical to identify any clinically suspicious lymph nodes; these should also be removed regardless of whether they are blue or hot, as tracers may not have travelled to positive lymph nodes if lymphatics are obstructed with tumor.
- Although some have argued that the procedure can be terminated after three SLNs have been removed,[7] others have argued that all nodes that fit the earlier mentioned criteria be removed.[8] On average, however, two sentinel nodes are identified.

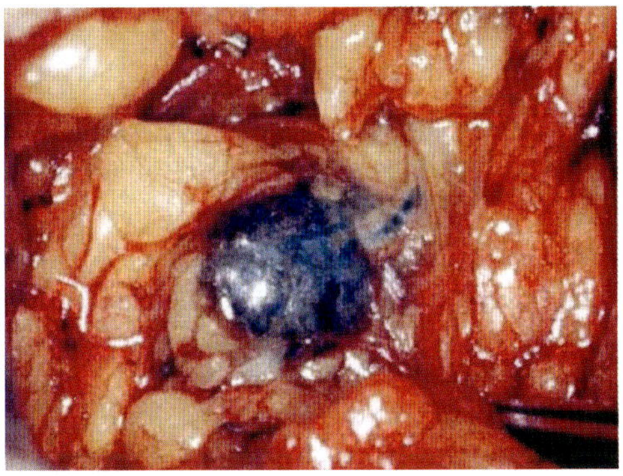

FIG 5 ● Blue SLN at the end of a blue lymphatic channel.

INTRAOPERATIVE EVALUATION

- Intraoperative evaluation with either touch preparation cytology or frozen section has been found to have a high specificity and fairly high sensitivity (FIG 6).
- Some surgeons may opt to forego intraoperative evaluation if they do not intend to complete the axillary node dissection at the same operative setting given the findings of the sentinel node biopsy. For patients who fit the American College of Surgeons Oncology Group Z0011 criteria, completion axillary node dissection may be avoided if only one to two sentinel nodes are positive and whole breast irradiation after partial mastectomy is planned.[9]

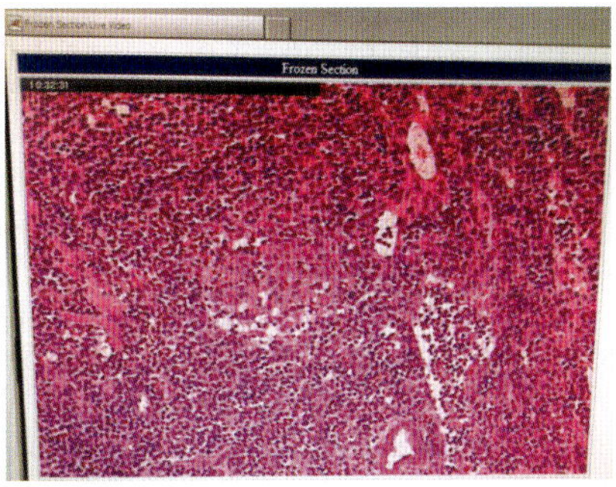

FIG 6 ● Intraoperative frozen section results.

CLOSURE

- In general, if axillary node dissection is not performed, no drains are required. The incision is closed in standard fashion with subdermal and subcuticular sutures followed by Steri-Strips. If, however, an axillary dissection is indicated, the incision can be extended (as planned in the earlier discussion).

POSTOPERATIVE CARE

- After sentinel node biopsy alone (i.e., without axillary dissection), patients can go back to usual activities. No special exercises are required nor is there any need for lymphedema compression garments.

OUTCOMES

- Outcomes after sentinel node biopsy alone are outstanding, with no detriment in survival or local recurrence. Morbidity is low, especially compared to axillary dissection.

COMPLICATIONS

- Bleeding/hematoma
- Infection
- Seroma
- Numbness/paresthesia
- Lymphedema
- Allergic reaction to isosulfan blue dye
- "Blue breast" from blue dye injection
- Skin or fat necrosis from methylene blue dye

REFERENCES

1. McMasters KM, Wong SL, Tuttle TM, et al. Preoperative lymphoscintigraphy for breast cancer does not improve the ability to identify axillary sentinel lymph nodes. *Ann Surg*. 2000;231:724–731.
2. Port ER, Fey J, Gemignani ML, et al. Reoperative sentinel lymph node biopsy: a new option for patients with primary or locally recurrent breast carcinoma. *J Am Coll Surg*. 2002;195:167 172.
3. Chagpar AB, Martin RC, Scoggins CR, et al. Factors predicting failure to identify a sentinel lymph node in breast cancer. *Surgery*. 2005;138:56–63.
4. Albo D, Wayne JD, Hunt KK, et al. Anaphylactic reactions to isosulfan blue dye during sentinel lymph node biopsy for breast cancer. *Am J Surg*. 2001;182:393–398.
5. Simmons RM, Smith SM, Osborne MP. Methylene blue dye as an alternative to isosulfan blue dye for sentinel lymph node localization. *Breast J*. 2001;7:181–183.
6. Chagpar A, Martin RC III, Chao C, et al. Validation of subareolar and periareolar injection techniques for breast sentinel lymph node biopsy. *Arch Surg*. 2004;139:614–618.
7. Zakaria S, Degnim AC, Kleer CG, et al. Sentinel lymph node biopsy for breast cancer: how many nodes are enough? *J Surg Onc*. 2007;96:554–559.
8. Chagpar AB, Scoggins CR, Martin RC, et al. Are 3 sentinel nodes sufficient? *Arch Surg*. 2007;142:456–459.
9. Giuliano AE, McCall L, Beitsch P, et al. Locoregional recurrence after sentinel lymph node dissection with or without axillary dissection in patients with sentinel lymph node metastases: the American College of Surgeons Oncology Group Z0011 randomized trial. *Ann Surg*. 2010;252:426–432.

Chapter 9

Internal Mammary Sentinel Node Biopsy

A. Marilyn Leitch

DEFINITION

- Internal mammary node dissection is performed for both diagnostic and therapeutic purposes. This surgery is generally performed in conjunction with breast cancer surgery as part of nodal staging. In modern times, this usually involves removal of lymph nodes from one or two parasternal interspaces as part of a sentinel node staging procedure. In the first descriptions of internal mammary node dissection, the entire internal mammary nodal chain was resected including the adjacent ribs.[1] With the advent of sentinel lymph node mapping, it is possible to perform a more minimally invasive procedure to resect in a directed fashion internal mammary nodes that are demonstrated to have lymphatic drainage from the breast. Internal mammary sentinel node drainage is identified on lymphoscintigraphy in 10% to 22% of mapping studies. Internal mammary drainage is more likely to be identified if the radionucleotide is injected in the peritumoral region rather than subareolar. The technique described here to retrieve sentinel nodes can also be used to surgically biopsy small suspicious internal mammary nodes identified on preoperative imaging with computed tomography (CT) scan or breast magnetic resonance imaging (MRI).

PATIENT HISTORY AND PHYSICAL FINDINGS

- The breast cancer patient should have a careful evaluation with a complete history and physical examination as well as appropriate imaging studies. The patient's history should focus on specific breast complaints including how long the patient has been aware of the cancer in her breast, associated symptoms and signs, and focal chest wall pain. It is important to ascertain the patient's medical history to assess the patient's risk for surgery related to intercurrent medical conditions. Prior surgery such as sternotomy, coronary artery bypass graft, thoracotomy, and breast augmentation should be noted, as these may complicate the performance of internal mammary node dissection. Past history should include annotations about prior radiation to the chest wall such as mantle radiation for Hodgkin's disease. The patient should be queried about prior trauma to the anterior chest wall.
- Physical examination includes the full examination of the breast to document any palpable mass lesion, including the size and location with respect to the quadrant of the breast and its distance from the nipple. The nodal basin should be carefully examined including the cervical, supraclavicular, axillary basins, as well as the palpation of the parasternal region. If there are any evident abnormal nodes, these should be further evaluated with imaging including mammography and ultrasound. Needle biopsy of suspicious nodes can be undertaken preoperatively in order to plan the therapeutic intervention.

IMAGING AND OTHER DIAGNOSTIC STUDIES

- The standard imaging workup for a newly diagnosed breast cancer patient would include mammography and ultrasound of the breasts. Many patients will have an MRI performed as well. This study permits visualization of the internal mammary nodal chain. If an abnormal lymph node is identified, it can be biopsied with a needle or targeted for excision at the time of surgery (**FIG 1A,B**).
- CT scanning of the chest is not routine for the workup of that early-stage breast cancer. However, if a CT scan of the chest or positron emission tomography (PET)-CT is performed for other indications, internal mammary node enlargement may be identified (**FIG 2A,B**). If the patient has palpable fullness in the parasternal region, a CT scan should be ordered to evaluate for internal mammary nodal metastases.
- In order to identify the internal mammary nodal drainage in the sentinel node procedure, it is critical to inject a radiolabeled tracer for mapping of the pathways to the internal mammary nodes. To maximize the chance of identifying internal mammary lymphatic drainage, it is important to perform the injections of technetium sulfur colloid in the peritumoral region rather than performing a subareolar injection only. Lymphoscintigraphy can be performed to have a visual representation of the location of the internal mammary drainage (**FIG 3A–D**). The area of radioactivity in the parasternal region can be marked on the skin by the nuclear medicine technician at the time of scanning (**FIG 4A,B**). This increases the efficiency of identifying the appropriate interspace for exploration for the sentinel node. Most commonly, there will be one interspace that demonstrates a hot spot. However, more than one interspace may demonstrate a radioactive focus. The most common areas of drainage are the 2nd and 3rd interspaces.

SURGICAL MANAGEMENT

Preoperative Planning

- The lymphoscintigraphy should be reviewed prior to going into the operating room. It is important to consent the patient specifically for the internal mammary exploration. Knowing from the lymphoscintigraphy that there is internal mammary lymphatic drainage, the surgeon can convey to the patient that this pathway can be pursued if the patient is agreeable. If it is the practice of the surgeon not to perform lymphoscintigraphy prior to surgery, then the interspaces can be examined intraoperatively with the gamma probe to identify foci of increased radioactivity in the parasternal interspaces. It remains important to consent the patient for the possibility of an internal mammary exploration with its potential complications.

Positioning

- The patient is positioned supine with the arms abducted to 90 degrees on padded arm boards. The skin prep of the chest wall should cross to the contralateral breast so that the sternum and parasternal regions are draped into the field of operation.

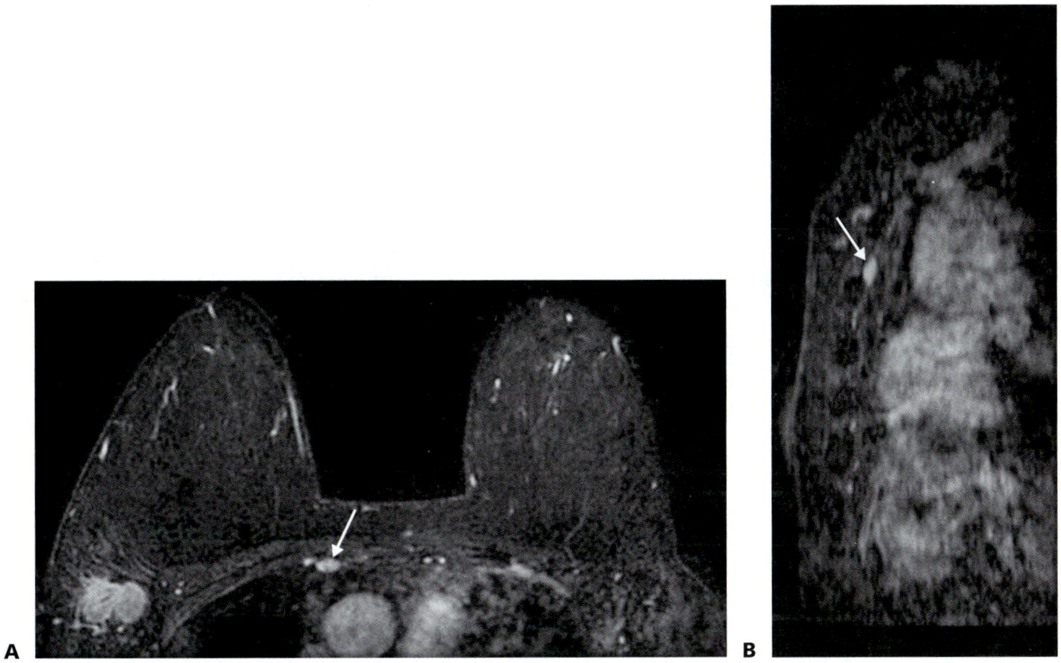

FIG 1 • **A.** Abnormal right internal mammary lymph node and right axillary lymphadenopathy seen on breast MRI axial T1 postcontrast subtraction series. **B.** Breast MRI. Sagittal T1 reconstruction demonstrating the abnormal internal mammary node. (Courtesy of Stephen Seiler, MD, University of Texas Southwestern Medical Center.)

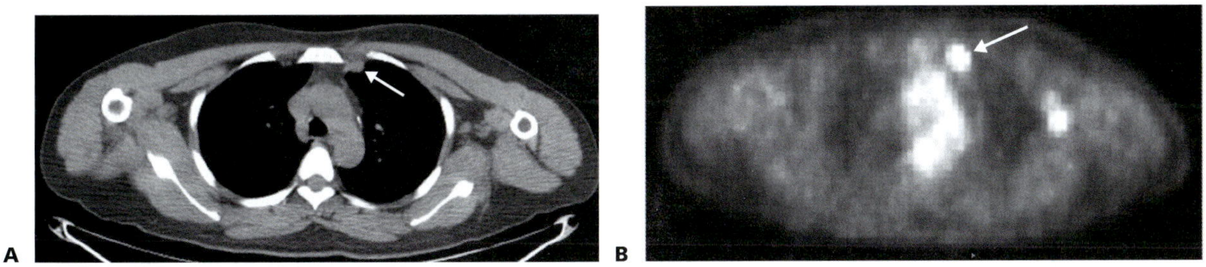

FIG 2 • **A.** Chest CT scan demonstrating enlarged left internal mammary node. **B.** PET scan image shows fluorodeoxyglucose (FDG) uptake in the left internal mammary node. (Courtesy of Stephen Seiler, MD, University of Texas Southwestern Medical Center.)

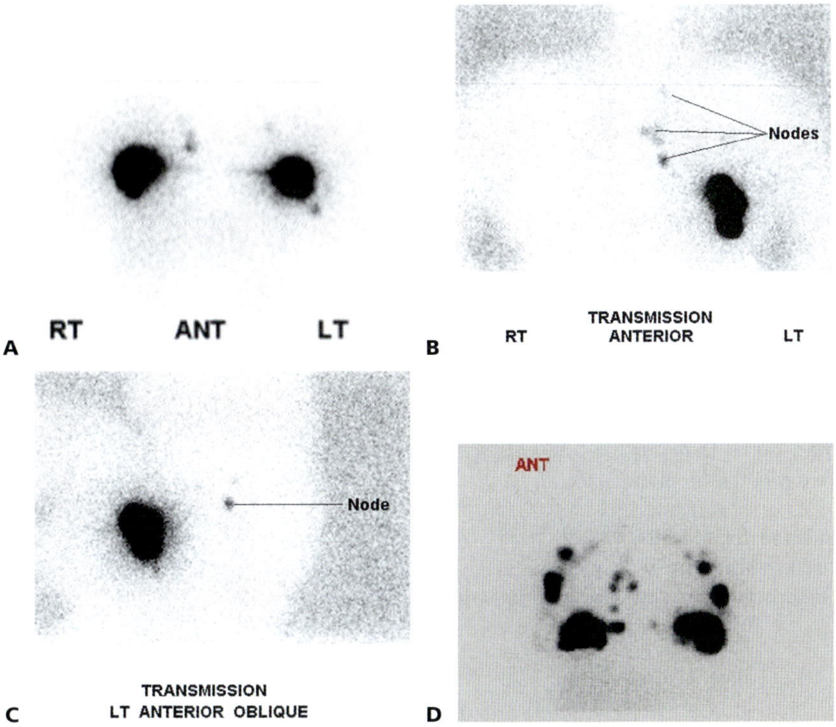

FIG 3 • **A.** Lymphoscintigraphy of bilateral breasts demonstrating internal mammary nodal drainage on the right in the anterior projection. **B.** Anterior projection of lymphoscintigraphy showing radioactive uptake in two interspaces with faint uptake base of neck. In this view, the axillary node is faint. **C.** Left anterior oblique projection shows the axillary uptake more intensely. **D.** Lymphoscintigraphy (anterior projections) with lymphatic drainage to multiple internal mammary nodes.

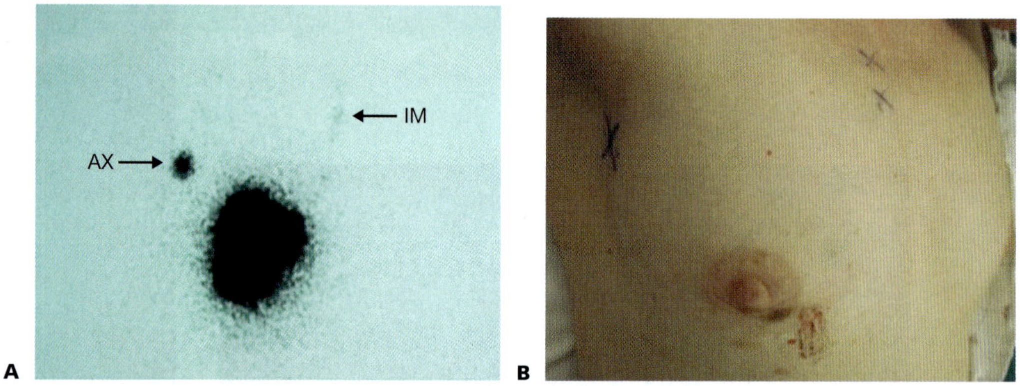

FIG 4 ● **A.** Lymphoscintigraphy demonstrating intense radioactivity in the right axillary node basin and very faint radioactivity in the internal mammary basin. **B.** Note "X" marks placed by the nuclear medicine technician to guide gamma probe examination.

INCISION AND INITIAL IDENTIFICATION OF AREA OF INTERNAL MAMMARY SENTINEL NODE

- Placement of the incision is governed by the procedure planned for resection of the breast tumor. For patients having breast-conserving surgery, the incision for the primary tumor is placed overlying the primary lesion. If the primary lesion is near to the area of internal mammary drainage, then it may be feasible to explore the interspaces via the partial mastectomy incision. However, if the primary lesion is distant from the parasternal region, then the incision for exploration of the interspace is placed overlying the area of focal radioactivity.
- If the patient is undergoing a mastectomy, the standard mastectomy incision is used for accessing the parasternal interspaces (**FIG 5**). When reconstruction is planned, the mastectomy incision is generally more limited with the skin-sparing technique. However, the parasternal region can be generally accessed via these incisions with retraction of skin flaps, unless there is nipple preservation with the incision placed in the inframammary line. In this circumstance, the incision location would be determined in a similar fashion as patients having breast-conserving surgery.
- It is much easier to identify the area of focal radioactivity in the interspaces after the breast is removed or after the partial mastectomy is completed. This reduces the amount of background radioactivity, which increases the ease of identifying radioactivity in an internal mammary node. In order to find an internal mammary sentinel node, it is imperative to have a strong signal that can be picked up by the gamma probe to direct the incision placement.
- Lymphazurin blue, which is often injected for identification of the sentinel nodes in the axilla, should be injected prior to beginning any resective procedure in the operating room. Lymphazurin blue alone will not be successful in identifying the internal mammary sentinel nodes. However, once the area of radioactivity is identified and exploration is begun, blue lymphatics or staining of the sentinel nodes may be identified but not with the frequency that it is seen in the axillary nodes. As with the radioactive tracer, the blue dye is more likely to be identified in the internal mammary nodes if the injection is peritumoral.
- After the blue dye is injected, the axillary sentinel node exploration is then begun. (Refer to Chapter 8 for more information on sentinel node dissection.) In most cases, there will be an axillary sentinel node identified in those patients who also have internal mammary drainage.
- The mastectomy or partial mastectomy is then performed.

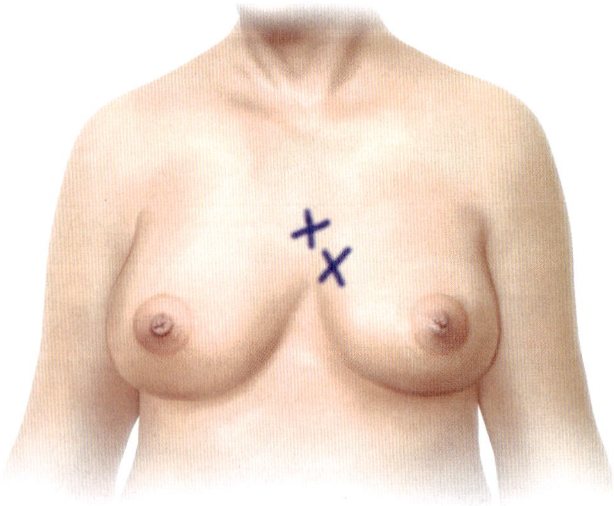

FIG 5 ● Skin sparing mastectomy incision with edge retracted to expose parasternal interspace.

EXPLORATION OF THE PARASTERNAL INTERSPACES

- Using the gamma probe, the **parasternal interspaces** are examined in sequence from superior to inferior. In patients having a standard or skin-sparing mastectomy incision, the skin edges can be retracted with a Richardson retractor or with Lone Star hooks, which can obviate the need for an assistant to retract. With the pectoralis muscle exposed, the gamma probe is then placed directly on the muscle after palpating the interspace. When an area of focal radioactivity is identified, counts are taken for 10 seconds, two or three times with a background taken a centimeter away to confirm that it is a focal hot spot. Counts are taken at each interspace.
- For the partial mastectomy patients, the initial examination with a gamma probe may have to be done through the skin overlying the interspaces if the partial mastectomy incision is away from this area. Because the skin surface is farther from the node, it can be more technically difficult to identify the hot spot. Each interspace is examined and counts taken as described for the mastectomy. When the focal hot spot is identified, the incision is made overlying the interspace along the axis of the ribs (**FIG 6**). The incision is carried through the skin, the subcutaneous tissue, and any underlying breast tissue down to the pectoralis muscle. A self-retaining retractor is placed to expose the pectoralis muscle widely. Lone Star hook retractors may be used if the thickness of the tissue in this portion of the breast is thin.

A 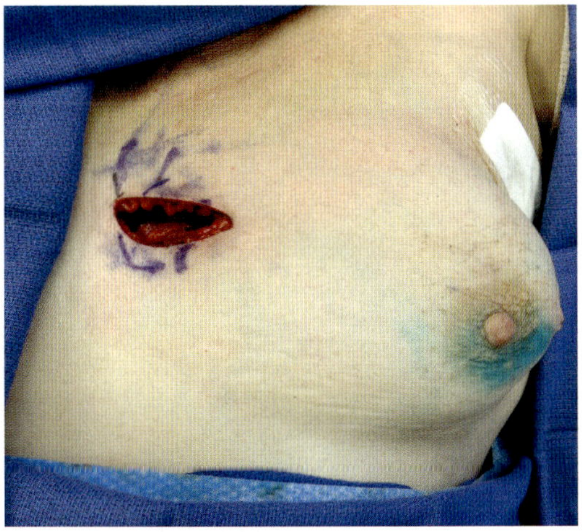

B 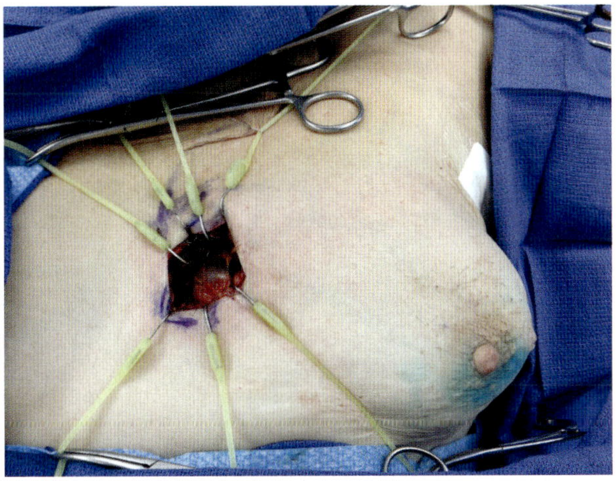

FIG 6 ● **A.** Parasternal incision in conserved breast with exposure of pectoralis muscle. **B.** Lone Star hook retractors placed to retract skin to expose muscle.

DISSECTION THROUGH THE CHEST WALL

- Once the pectoralis major muscle is exposed overlying the radioactive interspace, the fibers of the pectoralis muscle are split along their axis. A small self-retaining retractor or Lone Star hooks are placed to hold the fibers apart (**FIG 7**). Examination is performed again with the gamma probe to confirm that the radioactivity is persistent deep to the pectoralis muscle (**FIG 8**). If there is persistent radioactivity, then the intercostal muscles are incised with electrocautery over a 3- to 4-cm length extending from the sternal edge laterally (**FIG 9A**).

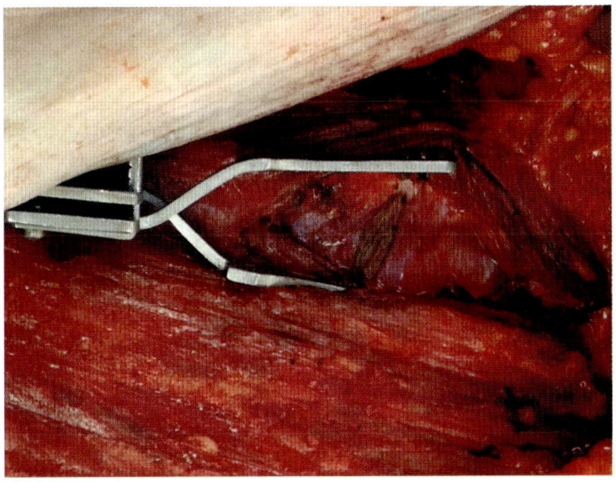

FIG 7 ● Pectoralis muscle fibers split and retracted to expose intercostal muscle.

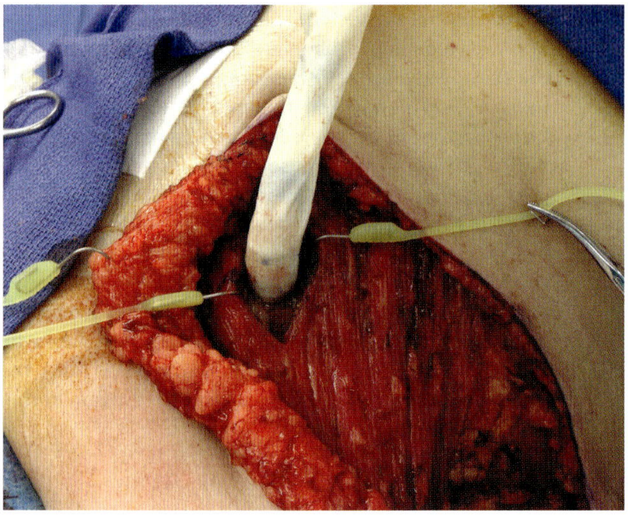

FIG 8 ● Examination is performed again with the gamma probe to confirm that the radioactivity is persistent deep to the pectoralis muscle.

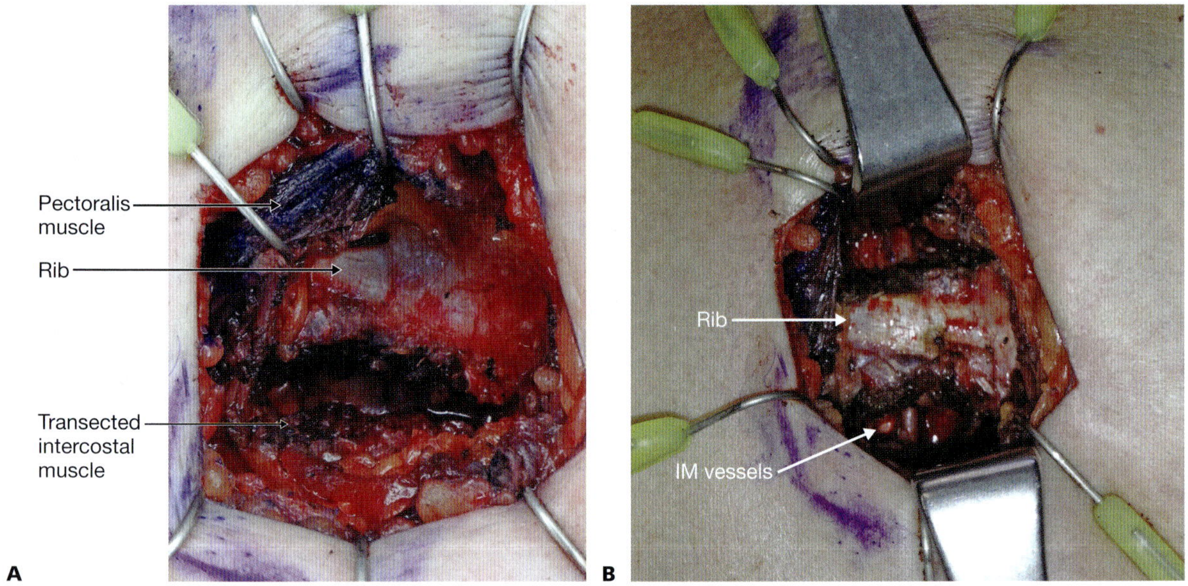

FIG 9 ● Exposure of intercostal space in breast conserving surgery with intercostal muscle divided **(A)**. Two interspaces exposed by dividing intercostal muscle above and below the rib via this limited incision. The internal mammary vessels are medially located in the interspace **(B)**.

DISSECTING IN THE INTERSPACE TO RETRIEVE THE SENTINEL NODE

- A thin, filmy fascia is incised deep to the intercostal muscles to expose a thin plaque of fatty tissue that lies just anterior to the pleura. Again, the gamma probe is used to localize the node that will be in fatty tissue deep to the intercostal muscles. The internal mammary vessels are most medial in the interspace (**FIG 10**)
- The sentinel nodes are often quite small and are yellow to yellow tan in color. Thus, their identification may be somewhat tedious. Frequent use of the gamma probe helps to direct the dissection. Fine instruments are used to tease out the fat around the nodal tissue. A small Kittner may be used to gently tease away the fatty tissue to expose the nodes. Small titanium clips can be used to ligate fine capillaries. It is critical to avoid any bleeding, which can obscure the small operative field. The lymph nodes may be intimately related with the internal mammary vessels, so any branches must be securely ligated in dissecting the node away from these vessels. The pleura will be exposed as the fatty tissue is teased away with the movement of the lung visible through the thin pleura (**FIG 11**).
- When the node is removed, gamma counts are taken of the node to confirm its radioactivity (**FIG 12**). The interspace is again examined with the gamma probe to confirm there is no residual radioactivity. If there is residual activity, further exploration is done to identify any other sentinel nodes in the interspace.

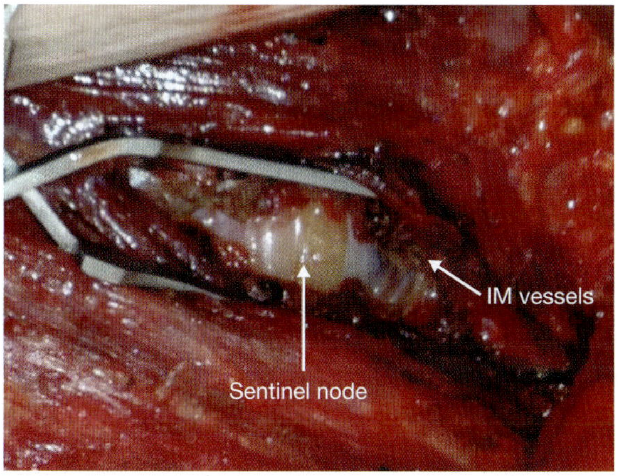

FIG 10 ● Right mastectomy procedure with exposure of interspace showing internal mammary vessels medially and yellow sentinel node lateral to vessels.

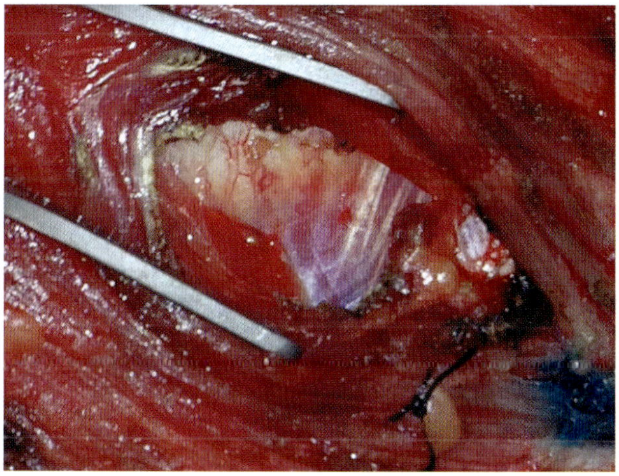

FIG 11 ● Mastectomy site with pectoralis muscle retracted and pleura visible after removal of sentinel node.

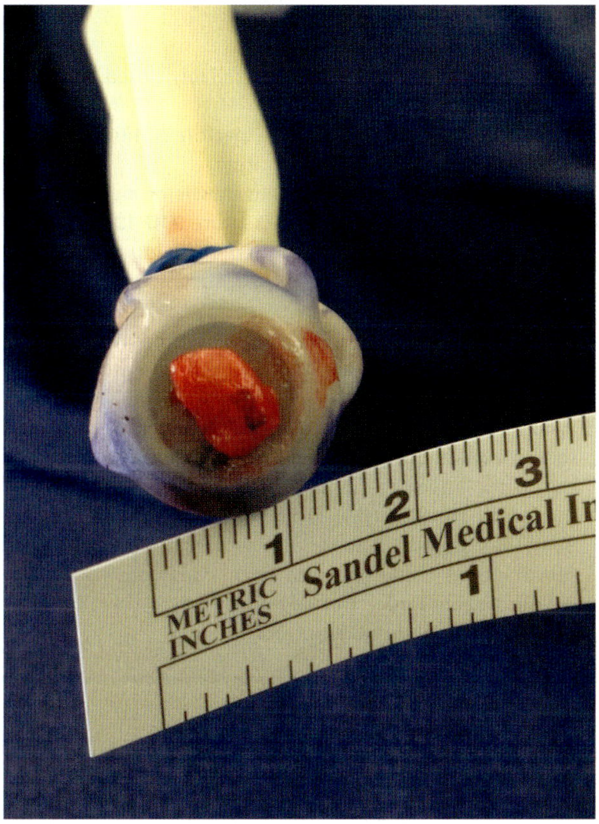

FIG 12 ● Internal mammary node ex vivo on gamma probe to confirm radioactivity in resected specimen.

EXAMINATION OF THE INTERSPACE FOR A PLEURAL TEAR

- The wound is irrigated to clear all blood and loose fat tissue that may obscure the field. Then, irrigation fluid is instilled and left to pool in the interspace. The anesthesiologist can then deliver a sustained breath into the endotracheal tube. The interspace is observed for air bubbles. If air bubbles are seen, a pleural tear can be assumed.
- One can aspirate the fluid and look for the tear. If the tear can be identified, it can be repaired with a 5-0 suture. This is more important if the tear is large. A small red rubber catheter can be put in the opening with repair performed up to it. Prior to tying the suture, the tube can be aspirated with the anesthesiologist giving a sustained breath to the patient to inflate the lung. The tube is removed and the suture tied down.
- If the tear if quite small, attempting repair may enlarge the hole. Fluid can be placed in the interspace and wound closure begun with the anesthesiologist maintaining lung inflation.

WOUND CLOSURE

- The intercostal muscles cannot be reliably closed, as the sutures tear through the muscle.
- Close the posterior fascia of the pectoralis muscle in a running fashion with 3-0 Vicryl suture.
- Then, close the anterior pectoralis muscle or muscle fascia, if present, with a running 3-0 suture (**FIG 13**).
- With mastectomy, a drain is placed overlying the chest wall in the usual fashion. Closed suction bulb is attached. Skin closure is then performed. The dermis is closed with interrupted 3-0 or 4-0 absorbable suture. The skin is closed with a running monofilament absorbable suture.
- Wound closure in the partial mastectomy circumstance should include closure of the divided breast tissue anterior to the interspace to avoid a soft tissue defect over the interspace. This is performed with either a running or an interrupted 3-0 absorbable suture. The dermis and subcutaneous tissue is closed with interrupted 3-0 or 4-0 absorbable suture. The skin is closed with a running monofilament absorbable suture.

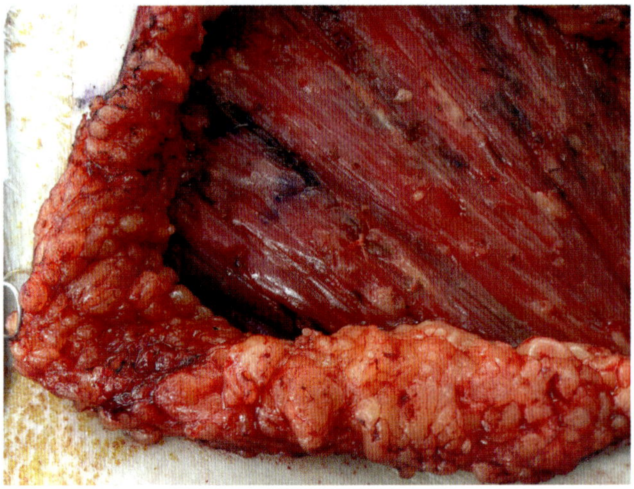

FIG 13 • Closure of the anterior pectoralis muscle or muscle fascia, if present, with a running 3-0 suture.

PEARLS AND PITFALLS

Preoperative planning	■ The injections of the radionuclide for lymphatic mapping should be performed in the peritumoral region rather than subareolar alone in order to identify the lymphatic pathways to the internal mammary nodes.
Placement of incision and exposure	■ Making exposure easier—If free flap breast reconstruction is being done with anastomosis of vessels to the internal mammary vessels, wait to remove the internal mammary sentinel node until the vessel exposure is done with removal of the costochondral cartilage which gives much wider exposure (**FIG 14**). If the patient has breast implants, prepectoral, or subpectoral, be certain that the implant is well retracted from the interspace to permit adequate exposure but also to avoid implant injury. There will be a fibrous capsule to be dissected through to get to the intercostal muscle.

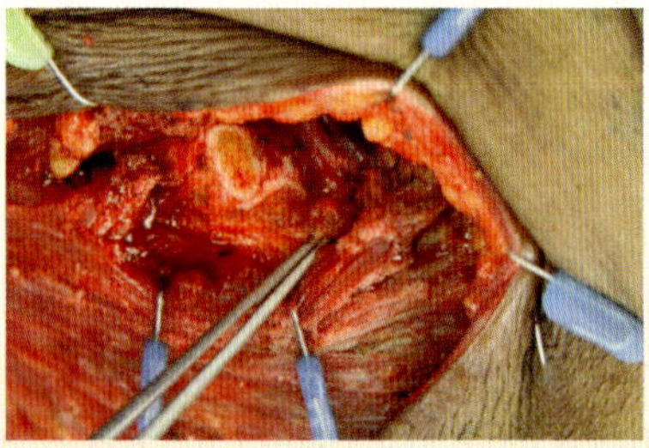

FIG 14 • Removal of the costochondral cartilage.

Exploration of the parasternal interspaces	■ Performing examination with the gamma probe after the breast or breast lesion is removed will make identification of the area of radioactivity in the internal mammary nodal chain easier, because of reduction of background radioactivity.
Dissection through the chest wall	■ Reexamine with the gamma probe at each layer through the chest wall to be certain there is persistent radioactivity in the next layer. There can be an intramammary node medially that picks up radioactivity or background radioactivity may have complicated the exam.
Dissecting in the interspace	■ Avoid excessive bleeding. Dissection must be careful and deliberate with securing of even very small vessels. An obscured field will increase chance of pleural tears or more major vasculature injury. When biopsy is being performed for an abnormal internal mammary node identified on preoperative imaging, it may be necessary to remove the costochondral cartilage to expose and successfully remove the enlarged node.
Closure	■ Know when to stop. When performing the surgery for staging, do not risk major vasculature injury if you are not able to find the node with usual maneuvers. Place a titanium clip to mark the area of increased radioactivity, which can inform radiation planning.

POSTOPERATIVE CARE

- In the recovery room, a chest x-ray should be performed if a pleural tear occurred to be certain there is no significant pneumothorax.
- If the surgeon is early in experience, a chest x-ray may be done as routine postoperatively.
- A small pneumothorax will generally not require therapy, as there is no intrinsic lung injury with ongoing air leak.
- If there is a large pneumothorax causing symptoms, then a chest tube can be placed, which can usually be removed in 1 to 2 days.
- Usual postoperative pain management is acceptable for these patients. They generally do not complain of focal pain in the area of the internal mammary node resection.
- Patients having breast-conserving surgery can be discharged home on the same day if there is no pneumothorax.

OUTCOMES

- Success in identification of the internal mammary sentinel node at surgery varies from 70% to 100%.[2]
- Complications from internal mammary node biopsy are rare, ranging from 0% to 5%. Even when a pleural injury occurs, chest tube drainage is rarely required.
- Recovery from this procedure is similar to that of the mastectomy or breast-conserving surgery performed at the same time.
- Patients who undergo lymphoscintigraphy and biopsy of internal mammary nodes that demonstrate lymphatic drainage have more accurate staging of their breast cancer, which can result in treatment changes. The rate of internal mammary sentinel node positivity ranges from 10% to 24%. Among five series of internal mammary sentinel node biopsy, in approximately 37% of cases, the internal mammary sentinel node was positive when the axillary sentinel node was negative.[3–7]
- The 10-year survival for patients who are internal mammary node positive and axillary node negative is similar to those who are axillary node positive alone as reported by Veronesi and colleagues.[8] In this study, patients with either axillary or internal mammary node metastasis only had a 10-year survival of approximately 54% compared to 30% if both internal mammary and axillary nodes were positive.[8] This indicates the equivalent significance of knowing the internal mammary nodal status as well as the axillary, if there is lymphatic drainage to the internal mammary nodal basin. In a modern series, patients with internal mammary nodal metastases had an overall survival of 97% at 5 years with multimodality therapy.[9]

COMPLICATIONS

- Pleural injury with or without pneumothorax
- Bleeding from injury to internal mammary vessels

REFERENCES

1. Urban JA, Baker HW. Radical mastectomy in continuity with en bloc resection of the internal mammary lymph-node chain; a new procedure for primary operable cancer of the breast. *Cancer*. 1952;5:992–1008.
2. Chen RC, Lin NU, Golshan M, et al. Internal mammary nodes in breast cancer: diagnosis and implications for patient management—a systematic review. *J Clin Oncol*. 2008;26:4981–4989.
3. Caudle AS, Yi M, Hoffman KE, et al. Impact of identification of internal mammary sentinel lymph node metastasis in breast cancer patients. *Ann Surg Oncol*. 2014;21:60–65.
4. Gnerlich JL, Barreto-Andrade JC, Czechura T, et al. Accurate staging with internal mammary chain sentinel node biopsy for breast cancer. *Ann Surg Oncol*. 2014;21:368–374.
5. Estourgie SH, Tanis PJ, Nieweg OE, et al. Should the hunt for internal mammary chain sentinel nodes begin? An evaluation of 150 breast cancer patients. *Ann Surg Oncol*. 2003;10:935–941.
6. Heuts EM, van der Ent FWC, Hulsewé KWE, et al. Results of tailored treatment for breast cancer patients with internal mammary lymph node metastases. *Breast*. 2009;18:254–258.
7. Carcoforo P, Sortini D, Feggi L, et al. Clinical and therapeutic importance of sentinel node biopsy of the internal mammary chain in patients with breast cancer: a single-center study with long-term follow-up. *Ann Surg Oncol*. 2006;13:1338–1343.
8. Veronesi U, Cascinelli N, Greco M, et al. Prognosis of breast cancer patients after mastectomy and dissection of internal mammary nodes. *Ann Surg*. 1985;202:702–707.
9. Dellapasqua S, Bagnardi V, Balduzzi A, et al. Outcomes of patients with breast cancer who present with ipsilateral supraclavicular or internal mammary lymph node metastases. *Clin Breast Cancer*. 2014;14:53–60.

Chapter 10 Simple Mastectomy

Michael S. Sabel Lisa Newman

DEFINITION

- A simple mastectomy, also commonly referred to as a total mastectomy, is the surgical removal of all breast tissue, including the nipple–areolar complex and enough overlying skin to allow closure. A simple mastectomy does not include removal of the axillary contents; when the breast tissue and axillary lymph nodes are removed en bloc, this is referred to as a modified radical mastectomy (MRM) (see Chapter 12). Variations of the simple mastectomy, typically performed in concert with immediate reconstruction include the "skin-sparing mastectomy," where the nipple–areolar complex is removed but the overlying skin is preserved; and the "nipple–areolar sparing mastectomy," where the native skin and nipple–areolar complex are preserved. These are described in Chapter 11.

PATIENT HISTORY AND PHYSICAL FINDINGS

- In clinically early-stage breast cancer, survival is largely driven by risk of distant organ micrometastatic disease and ability to control/eliminate this aspect of the cancer with adjuvant systemic therapy. Locoregional manifestations of disease in the breast and axilla can usually be controlled with surgery and radiation. Multiple prospective, randomized clinical trials have therefore documented survival equivalence between breast-conserving and mastectomy surgery for invasive breast cancer as well as for ductal carcinoma in situ (DCIS). Lumpectomy for a diagnosis of breast cancer is usually followed by breast radiation to sterilize microscopic/occult foci of disease in the remaining breast tissue, thereby reducing the incidence of ipsilateral breast tumor recurrence. Many women will nonetheless undergo total mastectomy as the primary breast surgical option either because of personal preference, medical contraindication to breast radiation, or because of disease features suggesting inability to achieve a margin-negative lumpectomy with a cosmetically acceptable result (e.g., diffuse suspicious-appearing microcalcifications on mammogram, multiple breast tumors not amenable to resection within a single lumpectomy, unfavorable tumor-to-breast size ratio). It is important for the clinician to remember that aesthetic acceptability must be defined by the patient. Total mastectomy is also the conventionally accepted surgical approach for breast cancer prophylaxis in high-risk women such as those with hereditary susceptibility.
- A detailed history and physical examination is imperative on the first consultation with these patients. In addition to the details of their breast cancer diagnosis, the history should cover medical comorbidities, medications, surgeries, allergies, and also any musculoskeletal issues, which could affect operative positioning and/or radiation treatment planning. Prior chest wall irradiation (such as for Hodgkin's lymphoma or as part of breast-conserving treatment for a past ipsilateral breast cancer) is a contraindication to reirradiation and breast conservation for a new or recurrent breast cancer. Connective tissue disorders such as Sjögren's syndrome or scleroderma can result in severe radiation-related toxicity and patients with these medical conditions will typically require mastectomy for management of breast cancer, even if the tumor is detected at a small size that would otherwise have been amenable to breast-conserving surgery. Patients that are unable to raise the arm above shoulder level may have difficulty tolerating the breast radiation tangents.
- All breast cancer patients should have a detailed family cancer history, focusing on both the maternal and paternal sides of the family. Patients with a strong family history, particularly of breast and ovarian cancer, should receive genetic counseling. These patients may want to consider bilateral mastectomies for prevention of second cancers.
- A bilateral breast and lymph node examination, including the axillary, cervical and supraclavicular lymph nodes, is critical. Any patient with clinically evident lymph nodes should undergo further evaluation, including axillary ultrasound and fine needle aspiration (FNA) biopsy.
- Breast examination should focus on the size and location of the tumor, fixation to the underlying musculature or overlying skin, and skin changes, particularly those consistent with inflammatory breast cancer (erythema, swelling, peau d'orange) or locally advanced disease (bulky tumors, tumors with secondary inflammatory changes, or cancers associated with matted nodal disease). These patients may require neoadjuvant chemotherapy in order to downstage the cancer and to improve resectability. A coordinated multidisciplinary approach, including input from medical and radiation oncology specialists promptly following the breast cancer diagnosis, is important for efficient management planning and is vital to the successful treatment of these patients.
- Early-stage breast cancer patients with a clinically negative axillary exam undergoing total mastectomy require axillary staging, which can usually be performed as lymphatic mapping and sentinel lymph node (SLN) biopsy. Mastectomy patients with axillary metastases documented by either needle biopsy or SLN dissection require standard levels 1 and 2 axillary lymph node dissection (ALND) or MRM, and postmastectomy locoregional radiation needs are then determined by the full pathologic extent of disease identified in the breast and axillary contents.
- All patients planning mastectomy should be presented the option of immediate reconstruction and a consultation with a plastic surgeon. Patients who opt for immediate reconstruction may be candidates for a skin-sparing or nipple–areolar sparing mastectomy. If postmastectomy radiation is being considered, this might impact the patient's options and eligibility for immediate reconstruction. Because the axillary nodal status is a strong predictor of postmastectomy radiation benefit, it may therefore be helpful to perform the SLN biopsy prior to the mastectomy surgery in cases where immediate breast reconstruction is planned.

IMAGING AND OTHER DIAGNOSTIC STUDIES

- Breast imaging plays a vital role in the screening and diagnostic workup for breast cancer. Imaging can define the extent of the disease and help assess for any abnormalities in the contralateral breast. Bilateral mammography is essential for any patient with breast cancer. Any suspicious contralateral lesions should be worked up before making the final surgical decision.
- Axillary ultrasound can be performed in many patients with a biopsy-proven invasive cancer to identify suspicious nodes suggestive of regional involvement. Suspicious nodes on axillary ultrasound should undergo an FNA biopsy with ultrasound guidance.
- It should not be assumed that any axillary node that is palpable or suspicious on ultrasound is malignant, as often they may be reactive. They should always be interrogated with FNA biopsy; and if the FNA is negative, then definitive axillary staging should be performed by SLN biopsy. At the time of lymphatic mapping and sentinel node dissection, it is important to excise any palpable/suspicious node, regardless of whether or not the node has any appreciable radiocolloid or blue dye uptake. If local resources permit, intraoperative evaluation of the sentinel node(s) with frozen section analysis can also be useful so that the patient can proceed onto immediate completion of the ALND if metastatic nodal disease in confirmed. When frozen section analyses are available and planned, the patient must be consented preoperatively for possible conversion from total mastectomy to MRM.
- The use of magnetic resonance imaging (MRI) is controversial. For patients undergoing mastectomy, MRI may detect contralateral cancers that were not visualized on mammography. For patients that hope to pursue breast-conserving surgery, a preoperative breast MRI may detect suspicious foci of disease in the breast such that mastectomy may be recommended. MRI usage has therefore been associated with increased rates of bilateral mastectomies. However, MRIs are sensitive but not specific and may lead to false-positive findings that necessitate additional biopsies. Furthermore, the natural history of MRI-detected multifocal/multicentric lesions in the cancerous breast is unclear, as these areas of otherwise occult disease would typically be radiated following lumpectomy for the known cancer. Retrospective and prospective studies of outcome following breast-conserving surgery in patients whose breast-conserving surgery eligibility was planned with versus without breast MRI have failed to demonstrate any significant differences in cancer-related outcomes.[1–3] We do not recommend routine MRI but rather its use should be on a patient by patient basis.
- In the absence of locally advanced disease (skin or muscle involvement, multiple matted nodes), routine staging tests, such as computed tomography (CT) scan of the chest, abdomen and pelvis, or bone scan, are not indicated.

SURGICAL MANAGEMENT

Preoperative Planning

- In the preoperative area, the breast to be removed should be clearly marked and confirmed with the patient.
- Prophylactic antibiotics have been shown to reduce postoperative infections and are indicated.[4] Sequential compression devices should be placed prior to initiation of general anesthesia for venous thromboembolism (VTE) prevention.

Positioning

- The patient should be positioned supine with the arm out laterally, taking care not to abduct the arm greater than 90 degrees as this may cause an injury to the brachial plexus. For a simple mastectomy, it is not necessary to prep and drape the ipsilateral arm into the field. However, if an SLN biopsy with frozen section and possible ALND is planned, it may be reasonable to include the arm using a sterile stockinette and Kerlix wrap. The endotracheal tube should be positioned toward the contralateral side of the mouth from the side of the mastectomy.
- Position the table and lights to allow enough room above the arm for an assistant to stand.
- If an SLN biopsy is to be performed and blue dye is to be injected, this can be done at this time. Either isosulfan blue dye or dilute methylene blue dye can be injected subareolar, periareolar, or peritumoral, according to surgeon preference.
- The chest wall, axilla, and upper arm are prepped into the field. Be sure to prep widely, extending across the midline and onto the abdomen and neck.

CHOICE OF INCISION

- The standard incision for a simple mastectomy is the classic Stewart incision, an ellipse oriented medial to lateral, encompassing the nipple–areolar complex and any prior biopsy scar (**FIG 1**). Alternatively, the modified Stewart incision is angled toward the axilla. It has been suggested that the modified Stewart incision, by excising more of the dermal lymphatics running toward the axilla, may provide better local control.
- In addition to the Stewart and modified Stewart, there are alternate options for a simple mastectomy. The placement and orientation of the incision must be based on the location of the biopsy scar and/or the location of the tumor. For a palpable tumor, particularly one close to the skin, the skin over the tumor should be included in the excised skin. Planning of the skin incision in conjunction with the plastic surgeon can be quite helpful in patients undergoing skin-sparing mastectomy and immediate reconstruction. If the patient has a surgical cancer biopsy incision, this scar should be resected with the underlying mastectomy specimen. Incisions located in proximity to the nipple–areolar complex can be resected within the central skin ellipse that is being sacrificed. Incisions that are located remote from the central nipple–areolar skin can sometimes be resected as a separate ellipse of sacrificed skin, as long as the remaining skin bridge is wide enough to remain viable. The original surgical cancer biopsy scars should not be left intact in the mastectomy skin flaps because of the oncologic concern that this skin

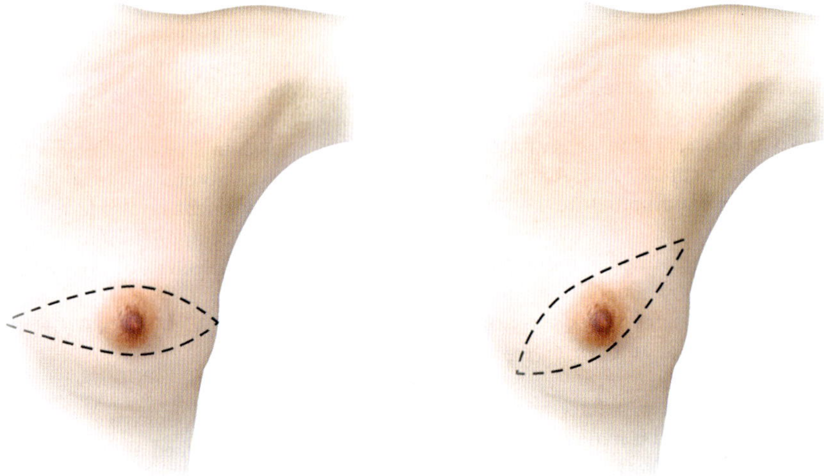

FIG 1 ● Standard incisions for a simple mastectomy. The Stewart incision **(left)** involves a horizontal ellipse that encompasses the nipple–areolar complex and adequate skin to allow a flat closure. The modified Stewart incision is angled toward the ipsilateral axilla.

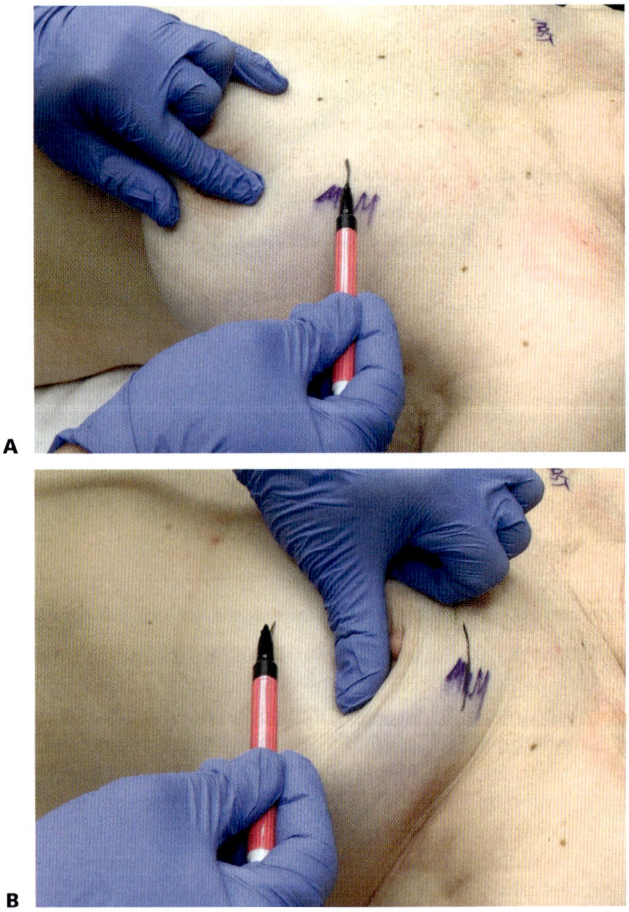

FIG 2 ● With a marking pen held over the nipple, the breast is retracted inferiorly **(A)** and the extent of the superior flap is marked. The breast is then retracted superiorly **(B)** and the inferior extent is marked. This allows the surgeon to estimate how much skin should be excised to eliminate redundancy without undue tension.

may potentially harbor cancer cells (and the mastectomy skin is usually not being radiated, as is the case following lumpectomy); and from a wound healing perspective, the subcutaneous fat deep to the traumatized incisional skin will be less healthy and more likely to necrose. Old surgical biopsy scars that are unrelated to the cancer diagnosis can be left in place. Also, percutaneous needle biopsy scars can be left intact on the skin flaps, as these have not been shown to contribute to risk of local recurrence.

- It is important to remove enough skin so that there is no redundancy but not so much that there is undue tension on the incision. A useful method to determine the placement of the superior and inferior incisions is to hold a marking pen in the air over the nipple and retract the breast inferiorly. Mark this site on the skin and then retract the breast superiorly to mark the inferior extent (**FIG 2A,B**).
- When designing the ellipse, closure will be facilitated by making sure the superior and inferior incisions are of equal length (**FIG 3**). This can easily be assessed using a 3-0 silk suture.

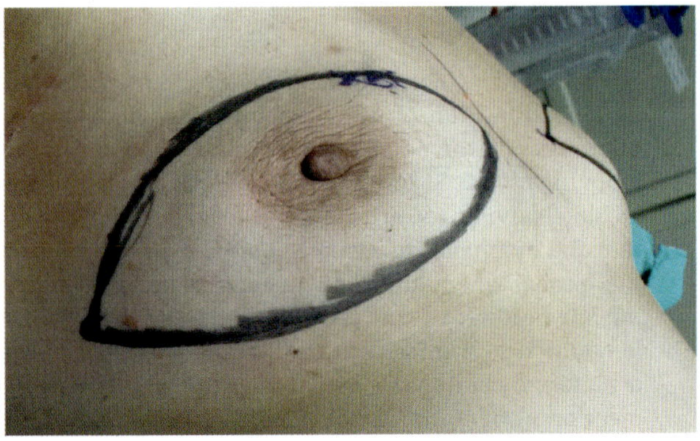

FIG 3 ● Confirming the superior and inferior incisions are of equal length will facilitate closure.

- Before making the incision, mark the boundaries of the breast tissue. Although the breast is an obvious external feature of the human anatomy, its boundaries deep to the skin are less well defined. Lacking any clear-cut capsule to delineate breast tissue from surrounding fat and subcutaneous tissue, the surgeon must identify anatomic landmarks that serve as reasonable and relatively constant structures, beyond which it is unlikely to find significant amounts of breast tissue. These radial boundaries for the skin flaps essentially serve as a picture frame; and once these flaps are completed, the breast is dissected off the pectoralis major muscle en bloc with the pectoralis fascia. The conventionally accepted peripheral mastectomy flap boundaries are as follows: superior margin—clavicle or 2nd rib (identified by palpation); inferior margin—inframammary fold (IMF); medial margin—lateral border of the sternum (identified by palpation); lateral margin—the lateral extent of the breast tissue can be marked externally on the skin surface and the edge of the latissimus dorsi muscle is a useful vertical boundary that can be visually identified from within the mastectomy surgical field (**FIG 4**).

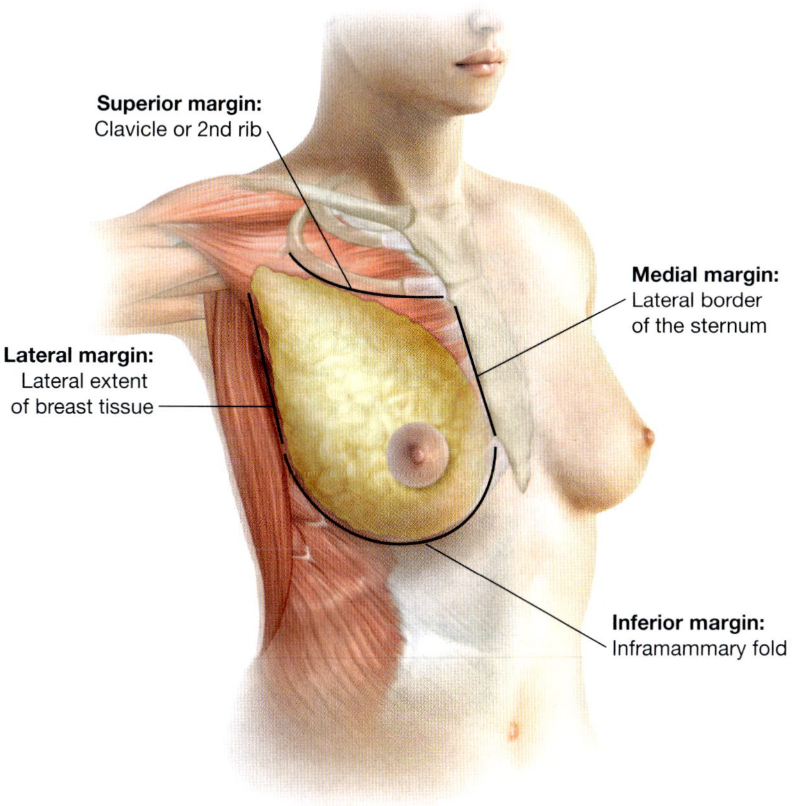

FIG 4 • To assure removal of all breast tissue, the dissection is performed to the clavicle or 2nd rib superiorly, the IMF inferiorly, the lateral border of the sternum medially, and the lateral extent of the breast tissue or edge of the latissimus dorsi muscle laterally.

SKIN INCISION AND CREATION OF FLAPS

- Once the skin incision has been mapped out on the breast, a scalpel is used to cut through the skin and dermis. Cautery is used to then obtain hemostasis. It is important to get into the right plane to raise flaps at the start. The initial incision should extend through full-thickness skin, just barely exposing the subcutaneous fat, and no further. Incising through deeper layers of subcutaneous fat will result in a splaying out of those fatty planes, and these deeper tissues will spuriously appear as anterior margin surfaces when analyzed and inked in the pathology laboratory. The actual anterior margin of the mastectomy specimen (beyond the central ellipse of sacrificed nipple–areolar skin) should be defined by the surgeon via dissection of the appropriate-thickness skin flaps. Failing to leave a small amount of tissue beneath the dermis can lead to ischemia and wound complications, and this can be particularly concerning in cases involving immediate reconstruction. Conversely, an excessively thick skin flap leaves the patient at risk for residual breast tissue on the chest wall, thereby increasing risk of local recurrence.

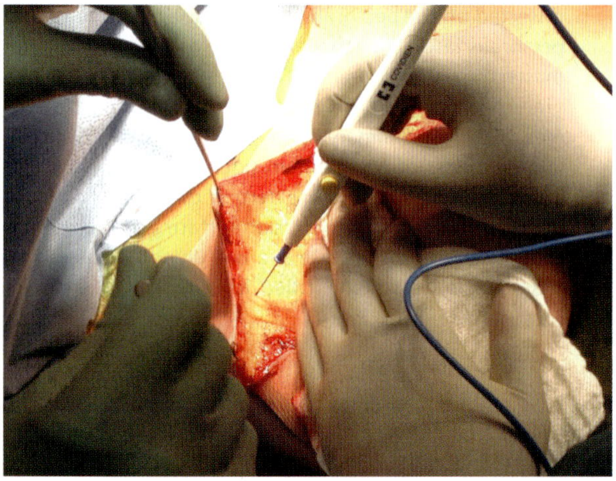

FIG 5 • The surgeon's opposite hand is used to provide adequate tension on the breast tissue to allow elevation of the superior flap in the correct plane.

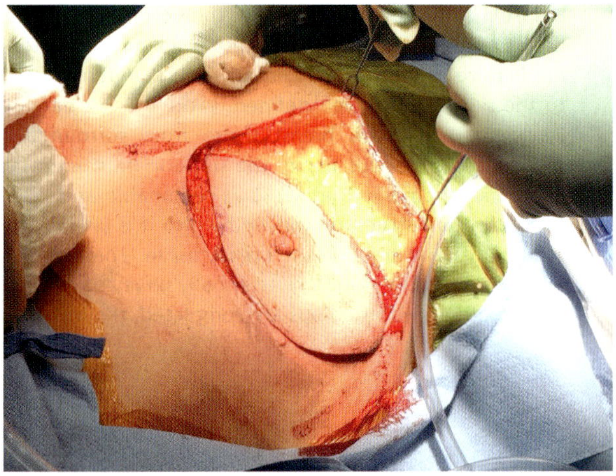

FIG 7 • If done correctly, there will be a small amount of subcutaneous fat beneath the dermis so that the blood supply is preserved.

- Starting with the superior flap, skin hooks are used to elevate the skin and provide appropriate tension for elevation of the flap (**FIG 5**). The key to elevating an appropriate flap is the tension on the breast tissue. Initially, a forceps can be used to get into the right plane; but once that plane is identified, traction with the contralateral hand of the surgeon using a laparotomy pad on the breast tissue will be critical. As the flap elevation proceeds, it is important to reposition the contralateral hand accordingly.
- It is imperative that the assistant holding the skin hooks maintain retraction straight up (**FIG 6**). Often, a resident will retract toward themselves so they have a better view of the dissection. However, this can lead to exposing the dermis and possibly a buttonhole injury to the skin.

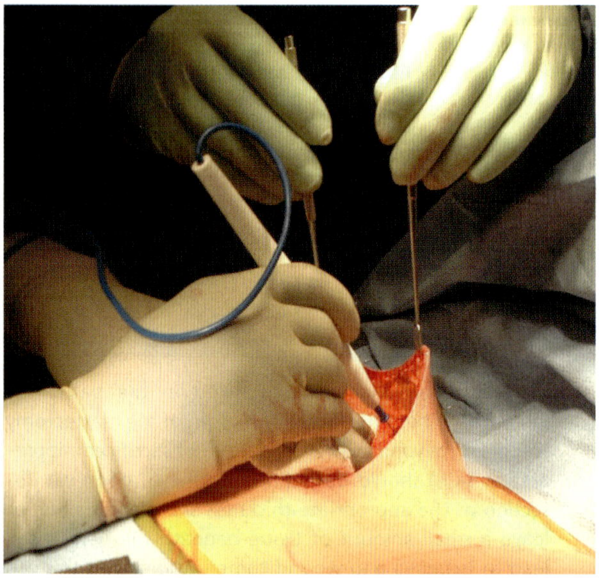

FIG 6 • It is important that the assistant retract straight up while the flap is raised; otherwise, exposure of the dermis or injury of the flap is more likely.

- The correct plane will leave a small amount of subcutaneous fat beneath the dermis so that the blood supply is preserved while not leaving any breast tissue. This plane is often avascular (**FIG 7**). Intermittently inspecting and palpating the flap will assure the correct thickness. Older women (where much of the breast is fatty-replaced) and heavier patients often have a thicker flap of subcutaneous fat separating the skin from the underlying breast parenchyma. In contrast, younger and thin patients may have breast tissue closely abutting the dermis, allowing for a very narrow margin of error while raising the flap.
- Flaps can be elevated using cautery, scissors, or a scalpel. Cautery will help provide hemostasis during the procedure. If sharp dissection is used, pressure on the breast with a laparotomy sponge will help maintain hemostasis.
- The superior flap is complete when you reach the level of the clavicle. At this point, the pectoralis muscle should be identified and the pectoralis fascia divided (scored) along the length of the flap (**FIG 8**).
- At this point, if an SLN biopsy is to be performed, this can usually be performed through this incision. Performing the SLN at this time point allows adequate time for intraoperative analysis if conversion to an MRM is being considered. The lateral edge of the pectoralis muscle is identified and the clavipectoral fascia is identified and divided. This allows access to the fibrofatty tissue of the axilla. The sentinel nodes can now be identified by using the gamma probe or by following any blue-stained lymphatics.
- The medial margin should extend to the lateral edge of the sternum. Going too far medially can lead to excessive dog-earing, which will need excision and thus lengthen the incision. In the case of bilateral mastectomies, going too far medially can accidently connect the two incisions,

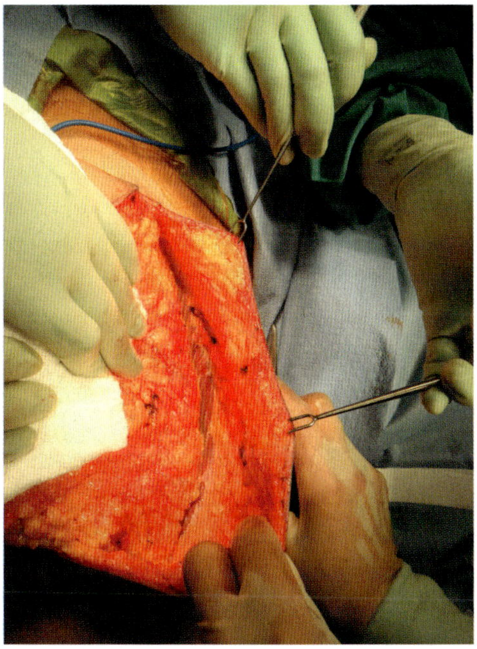

FIG 8 ● At the superior extent (clavicle or 2nd rib), the pectoralis fascia is divided along its length.

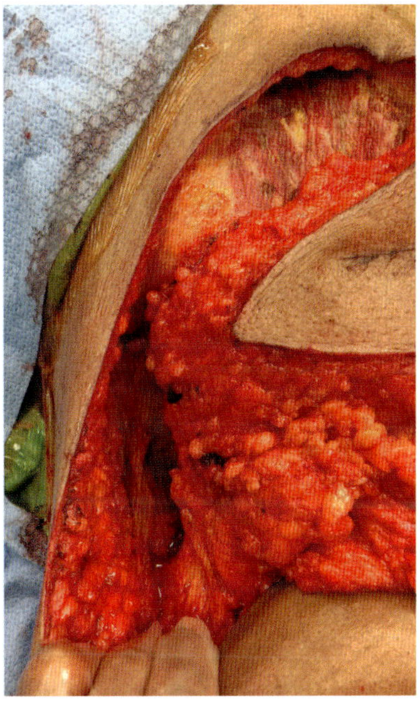

FIG 9 ● Visualization of the edge of the latissimus dorsi muscle assures the completeness of the lateral flap.

potentially contaminating the prophylactic side and complicating reconstruction.

- The inferior flap is then elevated in an identical manner to the level of the IMF. It is important to mark this, as it can easily be lost while elevating the flap. The assistant can provide feedback to the surgeon as the IMF is approached. Elevating past the IMF is not only unnecessary but can also complicate reconstruction, necessitating the plastic surgeon to recreate it to assure symmetry.
- Finally, the lateral margin is developed. As this is not an MRM, it is not necessary to thoroughly mobilize the latissimus dorsi muscle but identifying the edge of these fibers can enhance the completeness of the lateral flap (FIG 9). Avoiding an unnecessary mobilization of the latissimus dorsi muscle in total mastectomy patients undergoing immediate reconstruction is especially important, as creating extra dissection flaps in this lateral tissue can compromise the plastic surgery aesthetics. It is important that the lateral extent of the breast tissue is removed. This includes the axillary tail of Spence, which extends around the superior aspect of the pectoralis muscle to the clavipectoral fascia.

REMOVAL OF THE BREAST TISSUE

- Once the flaps have been completed circumferentially to the appropriate landmarks, it is time to excise the breast tissue and the pectoralis fascia off the pectoralis major muscle. It is important to remove the fascia with the specimen to assure negative margins. Failure to excise the fascia with the specimen may lead to a positive deep margin, increase chest wall recurrence, and prompt the use of postmastectomy radiation.[5] It can be useful to resect a tiny sample of pectoralis muscle fibers (labeled as sample of additional posterior margin) to serve as pathologic documentation that the mastectomy specimen included the pectoralis fascia. Some patients can have diffuse DCIS extending throughout the breast to its posterior surface, but by definition, the noninvasive nature of this disease is such that documenting resection of the pectoralis fascia is consistent with an adequate resection and further local therapy in the form of postmastectomy radiation is unnecessary. Patients with palpable breast tumors abutting the chest wall surface should have a wedge of underlying pectoralis muscle at the site of the tumor resected en bloc with the mastectomy specimen.
- The breast tissue is retracted inferiorly. This is typically done with the contralateral hand but grasping the fascia with a right-angle clamp can facilitate this. The fascia is elevated off the muscle using cautery, moving the cautery back and forth in the direction of the fibers of the muscle (FIG 10). This technique minimizes the damage to the pectoralis muscle.
- Small perforators extending from the pectoralis to the breast should be grasped with a hemostat or forceps and cauterized. There are slightly larger perforators medially. It is best to preserve these if possible. If not, these should be grasped and cauterized or suture

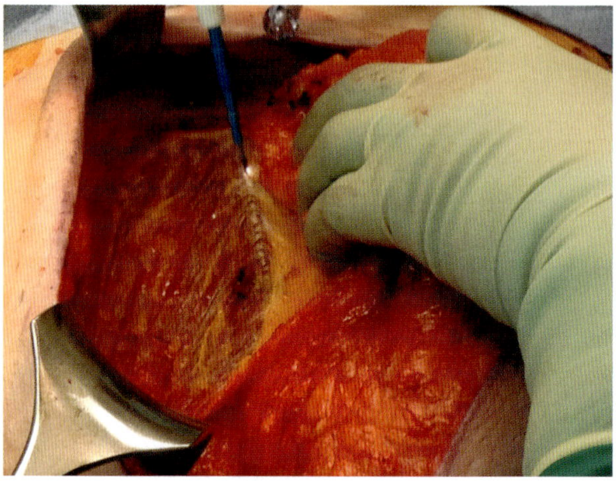

FIG 10 ● Retracting the breast inferiorly, the breast tissue and pectoralis fascia are taken off the pectoralis major. The cautery is moved back and forth in the direction of the fibers of the muscle.

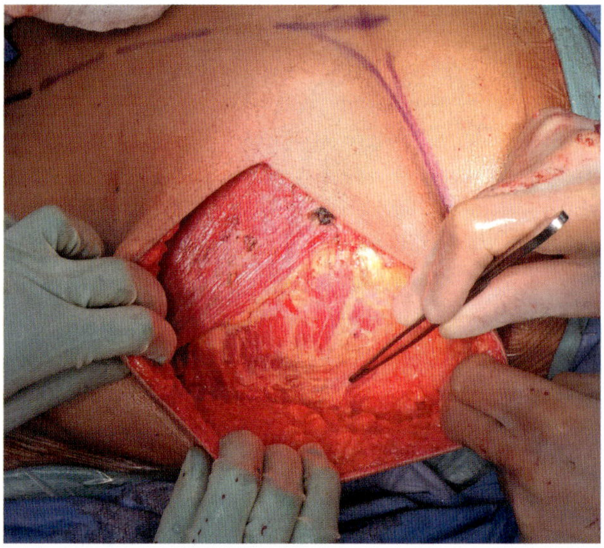

FIG 12 ● As opposed to the pectoralis fascia, which is taken with the breast tissue, the fascia over the serratus anterior is left intact.

ligated (**FIG 11**). If these are accidentally divided, they often retract into the muscle and can be difficult to control. Some patients (especially older and/or less fit patients) will have a weakened, attenuated, and fatty-replaced pectoralis musculature. Caution should be exercised during the lateral retraction of the breast in these cases, as overly aggressive tugging on the breast can result in the muscle being inadvertently avulsed from its costochondral and sternal attachments.

- Dissection of the breast off the pectoralis muscle continues inferiorly toward the IMF and then out laterally. Resecting the pectoralis fascia has oncologic significance; however, fascia overlying the serratus anterior muscle can be left intact (**FIG 12**). Dissecting deep to this fascia and exposing the serratus muscle bed results in unnecessary bleeding and can place the long thoracic nerve at risk for injury, because this important motor nerve is not routinely identified through visual exposure unless the patient is undergoing an ALND.
- Intercostal nerve block: Many mastectomy patients will benefit from intraoperative injection of approximately 5 mL of 0.5% ropivacaine into 2 or 3 intercostal spaces along the surgical field lateral to the pectoralis muscle. The surgeon should notify the anesthesia staff who will then give the patient a few extra deep breaths. At maximal end expiration, the patient is taken off the ventilator while the surgeon injects the long-acting anesthetic just at the inferior edge of the selected rib to block the associated intercostal nerves. Ventilator-assisted respirations then resume. If intercostal nerve blocks as well as incisional long-acting anesthetic injection is planned, then the maximum volume of safe anesthetic delivery (based on body weight of the patient) should be calculated.

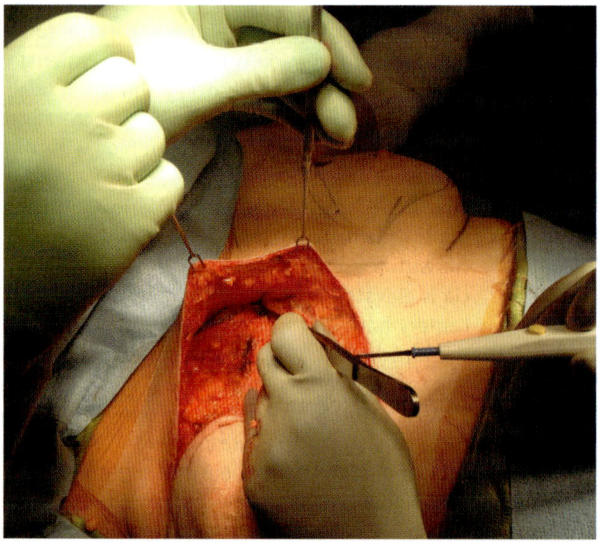

FIG 11 ● Medial perforators are grasped and cauterized.

DRAIN PLACEMENT

- A closed suction drain is placed over the pectoralis major muscle through a separate stab incision and sutured in place with a monofilament suture (**FIG 13**). When inserting the drain through the skin flap, it is useful to be mindful of the location of the latissimus dorsi muscle. Inadvertent insertion of the drain through this muscle can result in excessive bleeding from the tract. In cases where the drain tract does bleed excessively, the best remedy is to simply remove the drain, apply pressure, and replace the drain through a different tract.

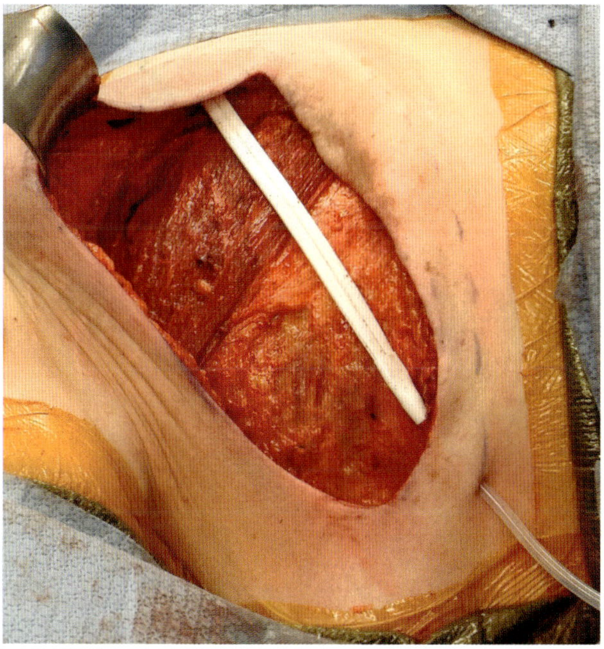

FIG 13 • A flat channel drain is placed over the pectoralis major muscle through a separate stab incision prior to closing.

CLOSURE

- Although excess tension on the incision can lead to wound complications, excess skin will lead to redundant flaps, which can be uncomfortable for the patient; they can be difficult to monitor for recurrence and can interfere with wearing a prosthesis. In cases where postmastectomy radiation and delayed reconstruction is planned, it may be helpful to leave the skin flaps a little looser, but a floppy anterior skin flap will be unsightly and serves as a site for recurrent seroma accumulation. Excess skin can be excised, so that the incision approximates flat on the chest wall. Remember that the patient is lying flat back, but once awake will slouch forward slightly, so a small amount of tension will be released.
- Commonly, the medial and lateral aspects of the incision will "dog ear." Often, these can be easily excised as an ellipse. There are times, particularly in older, heavier women, where excising the lateral dog ear simply moves the dog ear more posteriorly. In these cases, a fish-tail plasty (**FIG 14A–C**) can be useful.[6]
- The dermal layer should be closed with interrupted deep dermal absorbable sutures. Because the Jackson-Pratt (JP) drain will evacuate the postoperative seroma formation, the mastectomy skin flap closure should be subject to minimal tension. A reasonable closure alternative can therefore rely on a few interrupted sutures to line up the appropriate skin closure, followed by a running, continuous absorbable deep dermal suture. The skin can be approximated with an absorbable 4-0 monofilament suture in a running subcuticular closure or a surgical adhesive.

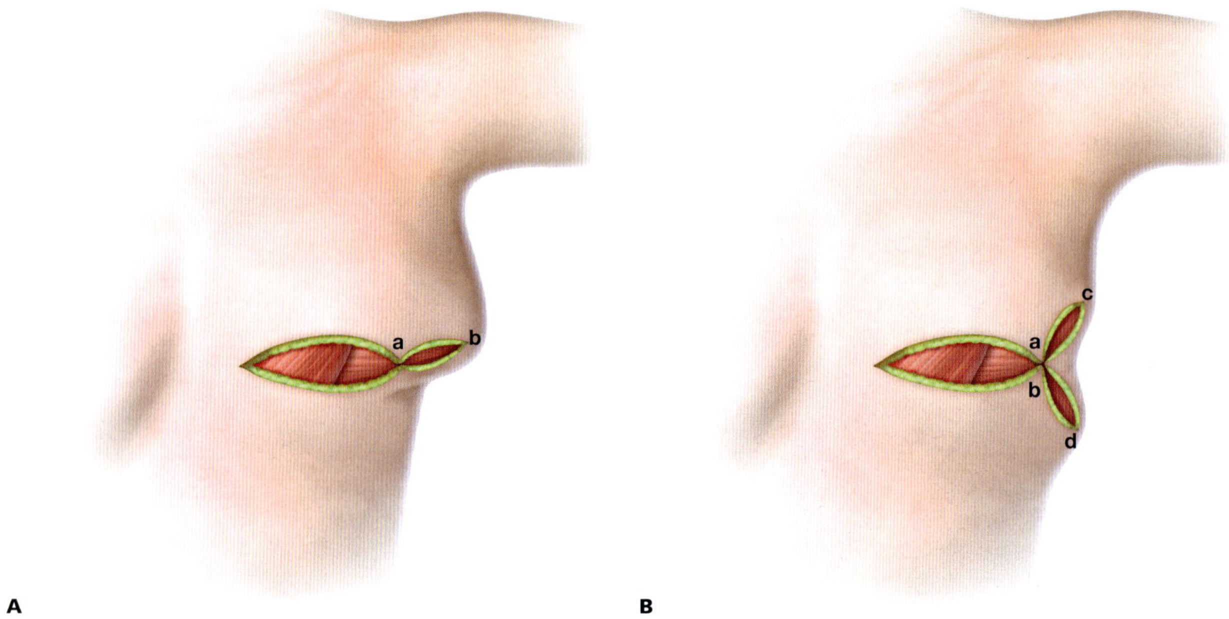

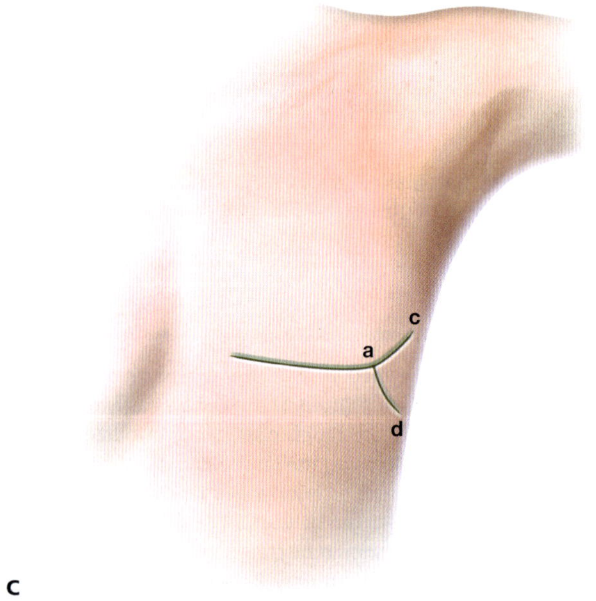

FIG 14 ● For patients with excessive lateral tissue that cannot be excised as a simple ellipse, a fish-tail plasty can be useful. **A.** The skin is reapproximated so the medial aspect closes appropriately. **B.** The lateral corner is brought medially, creating two smaller ellipses superiorly and inferiorly. These two ellipses are then excised separately and the wound is closed **(C)** so that there is a Y extension laterally.

PEARLS AND PITFALLS

Patient expectations	■ Patients who are candidates for breast conservation therapy (BCT) should understand there is no improvement in survival with a mastectomy. ■ All patients undergoing mastectomy should be offered consultation with a plastic surgeon to discuss reconstruction options. ■ Patients may have concerns regarding cosmesis and sexual identity after mastectomy that should be addressed preoperatively. ■ Patients should also understand the potential for redundancy or dog ears after mastectomy and how these can be addressed.

Planning the incision	■ Include the excisional biopsy scar in the ellipse. For palpable tumors, include an adequate amount of skin over the tumor. ■ Plan the ellipse so that it will lie flat, without excess laxity, yet not too tight. ■ Measure the superior and inferior incisions to confirm they are roughly the same length.
Raising the flaps	■ Make sure to start in the right plane with the initial incision and not go too far into the subcutaneous fat. ■ The assistant should hold the skin hooks straight up. Bending the skin backward can inadvertently lead to exposing dermis or "buttonholing." ■ Countertension with the opposite hand is the key to being in the right plane. As you progress, reposition the hand accordingly. ■ Be careful not to pass the IMF while raising the inferior flap.
Removing the breast	■ Retract the breast inferiorly and move the cautery medial to lateral, parallel to the pectoralis major muscle fibers. ■ Remove the fascia of the pectoralis with the specimen. ■ Grasp perforators with a forceps or clamp and coagulate rather than try to directly cauterize. ■ Do not retract the breast laterally with excess force, this will avulse the muscle from the sternum.
Closure	■ Excise excess skin so that the flaps close flat against the chest wall. ■ Medial and lateral dog ears should be excised, but do not keep repositioning a lateral dog ear more posteriorly. A plasty can eradicate a dog ear but can make reconstruction more difficult. A dog ear can always be corrected at a later date under local anesthetic.

POSTOPERATIVE CARE

- A nonadherent dressing can be placed over the incision. Patients can be placed in a breast binder with Kerlix fluffs in order to apply even compression. This will help prevent hematoma but should not be excessively tight.
- Patients do not need to be admitted to the hospital overnight, they may be safely discharged to home. Arranging for a visiting nurse can be helpful for drain management and wound checks.
- The drain can be removed when the output is less than 30 mL/24 hours for 2 days in a row.

OUTCOMES

- Overall, local (chest wall) recurrence after mastectomy is low, ranging from 0.6% to 9.5%, increasing with increasing stage, the presence of nodal metastases, and positive margins after mastectomy. However, local recurrence rates also appear to be decreasing as systemic therapies improve.[7] Local recurrence is also related to the histologic subtype, with luminal subtype tumors (ER/PR positive) less likely to recur than *HER2/neu* overexpressing or triple negative tumors after mastectomy.[8]
- Because local recurrence rates remain higher among patients with node-positive disease or positive margins, postmastectomy radiation therapy (PMRT) should be considered in these situations. PMRT is strongly indicated for patients with positive margins or more than four positive lymph nodes. It should also be considered for patients with one to three positive lymph nodes, particularly, if they have other risk factors for chest wall recurrence.

COMPLICATIONS

- Seroma
- Wound infection
- Hematoma
- Wound dehiscence
- Flap necrosis
- Positive margins

REFERENCES

1. Turnbull L, Brown S, Harvey I, et al. Comparative effectiveness of MRI in breast cancer (COMICE) trial: a randomized controlled trial. *Lancet*. 2010;376(9714):563–571.
2. Peters NH, van Esser S, van den Bosch MA, et al. Preoperative MRI and surgical management in patients with nonpalpable breast cancer: the MONET-randomised controlled trial. *Eur J Cancer*. 2011;47:879–886.
3. Solin LJ, Orel SG, Hwang WT, et al. Relationship of breast magnetic resonance imaging to outcome after breast-conservation treatment with radiation for women with early-stage invasive breast carcinoma or ductal carcinoma in situ. *J Clin Oncol*. 2008;26:386–391.
4. Tejirian T, DiFronzo LA, Haigh PI. Antibiotic prophylaxis for preventing wound infection after breast surgery: a systematic review and metaanalysis. *J Am Coll Surg*. 2006:203(5):729–734.
5. Dalberg K, Krawiec K, Sandelin K. Eleven-year follow-up of a randomized study of pectoral fascia preservation after mastectomy for early breast cancer. *World J Surg*. 2010;34(11):2539–2544.
6. Hussien M, Daltrey IR, Dutta S, et al. Fish-tail plasty: a safe technique to improve cosmesis at the lateral end of mastectomy scars. *Breast*. 2004;13(3):206–209.
7. Yi M, Kronowitz SJ, Meric-Bernstam F, et al. Local, regional, and systemic recurrence rates in patients undergoing skin-sparing mastectomy compared with conventional mastectomy. *Cancer*. 2011;117:916–924.
8. Lowery AJ, Kell MR, Glynn RW, et al. Locoregional recurrence after breast cancer surgery: a systematic review by receptor phenotype. *Breast Cancer Res Treat*. 2012;133:831–841.

Chapter 11 Skin-Sparing and Nipple/Areolar-Sparing Mastectomy

Eleni Tousimis Rache Simmons

DEFINITION

- Skin-sparing mastectomy is defined as removal of the breast tissue while preserving the natural skin envelope for immediate breast reconstruction. This is an effective treatment option for patients with operable breast cancer without skin involvement. By preserving the patient's skin envelope with a smaller incision, it markedly improves the aesthetics of the breast reconstruction. To further enhance cosmesis, the nipple and areola can be preserved at the time of mastectomy in select patients. This is called nipple-sparing mastectomy.

ANATOMY

- As with all types of mastectomy, a thorough understanding of the anatomy of the breast, chest wall, and axilla is necessary. The goal of mastectomy is to remove the breast tissue while maintaining the viability of the skin envelope.
- The breast tissue is encapsulated by the superficial fascia that adheres to the subcutaneous tissue in a lobulated fashion (**FIG 1**). This makes it difficult to remove all of the breast tissue during mastectomy and maintain skin viability.
- The boundaries of the breast (**FIG 2**) are defined by the clavicle superiorly, the sternum medially, the 6th rib inferiorly, and the latissimus dorsi muscle laterally.
- The axillary tail of the breast extends toward the low axilla and is called the axillary tail of Spence. Posteriorly, the breast adheres to the pectoralis major muscle and is separated by the deep fascia of the breast (see **FIG 1**).
- A skin-sparing mastectomy involves preserving the skin envelope while removing the nipple–areolar complex and underlying breast via a small incision (**FIG 3**). Nipple-sparing mastectomy is a total skin-sparing mastectomy with preservation of the nipple–areolar complex.
- When performing a skin-sparing mastectomy, it is important to remove as much breast tissue as possible while maintaining the viability of the skin. This is a balancing act from the oncologic standpoint to remove the majority of the breast tissue but not make the skin flaps so thin, resulting in skin necrosis and flap loss. The anatomic plane that divides the

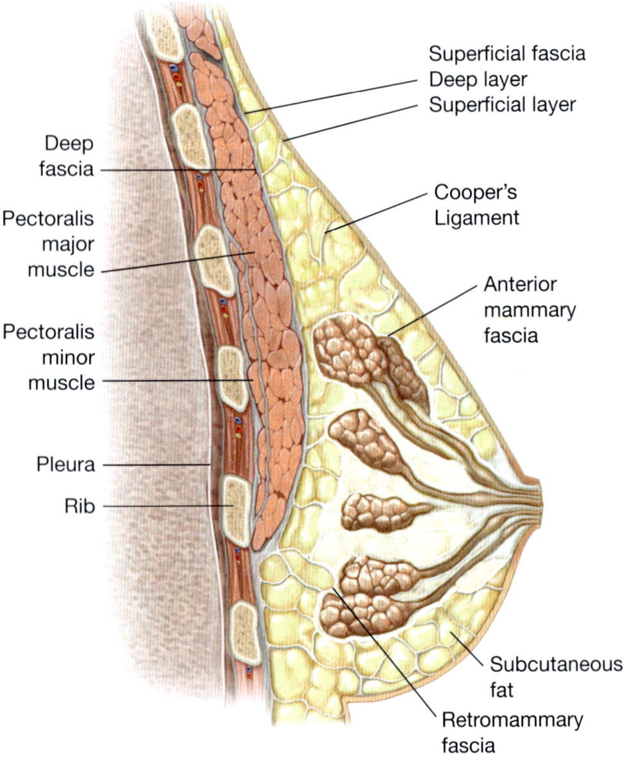

FIG 1 • Cross-section of the breast demonstrating the superficial fascia, including both the superficial and deep layers.

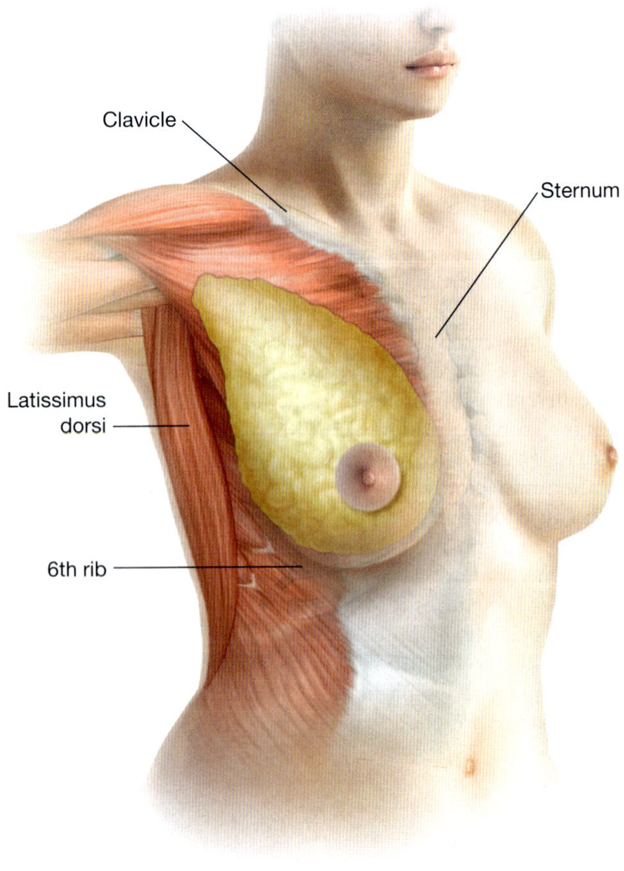

FIG 2 • Anatomic boundaries of the breast.

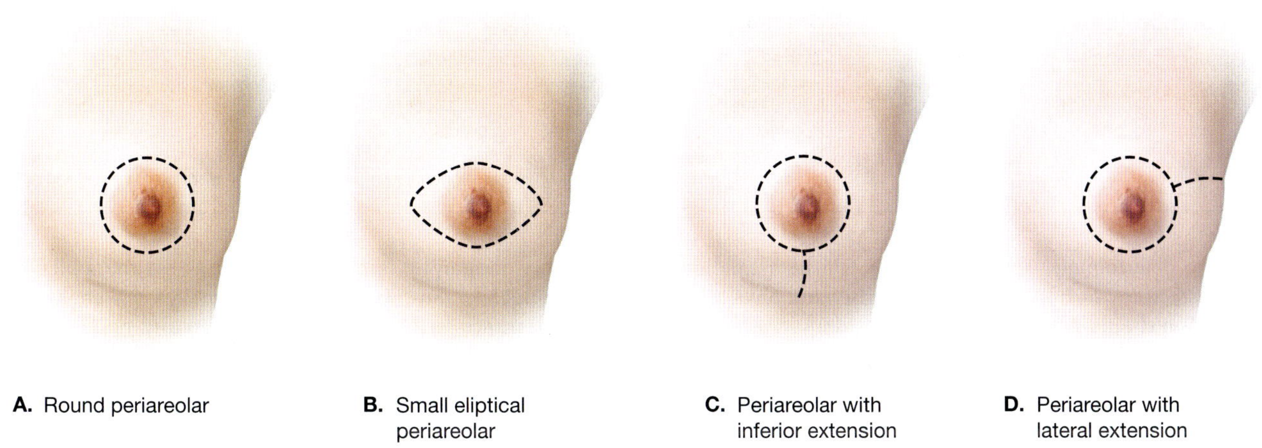

FIG 3 • **A–D.** Surgical incisions used for a skin-sparing mastectomy.

subcutaneous tissue and the underlying breast parenchyma is formed by the superficial fascia of the breast. This is an ill-defined thin layer visualized by a faint white fascial line (see **FIG 1**). The dissection is carefully performed in this plane. The remaining tissue on the skin envelope usually ranges between 2 and 5 mm in thickness depending on the patient's anatomy.

- It is crucial to flap viability to preserve both the subcutaneous venous plexus under the skin as well as the branches of the 2nd intercostal perforator in the upper medial flap as it exits the ribs. This is the largest blood supply to the skin flap (**FIG 4A,B**).
- Once the flaps are created to the clavicle superiorly including the axillary tail of Spence, medially to the sternum, laterally to the latissimus dorsi muscle, and inferiorly to the 6th rib, the breast is then removed posteriorly from the pectoralis major muscle including the underlying deep fascia overlying the muscle. It is important when creating the flap medially not to extend to the contralateral breast.

PATIENT HISTORY AND PHYSICAL FINDINGS

- Patients with operable breast cancer are candidates for either breast conservation therapy (BCT) or skin-sparing mastectomy with or without reconstruction. It is important for patients to understand that the survival between BCT and mastectomy is equal. However, mastectomy does carry a slightly lower locoregional recurrence rate of about 2% versus 5% in 10 years after BCT.[1]
- Another important difference between the two surgical treatment options is that mastectomy usually does not require postoperative radiation therapy. Postmastectomy radiation is recommended for patients with tumors greater than 5 cm in size, patients with positive margins after mastectomy, or select patients with axillary lymph node involvement for locoregional control and to improve survival.[2]

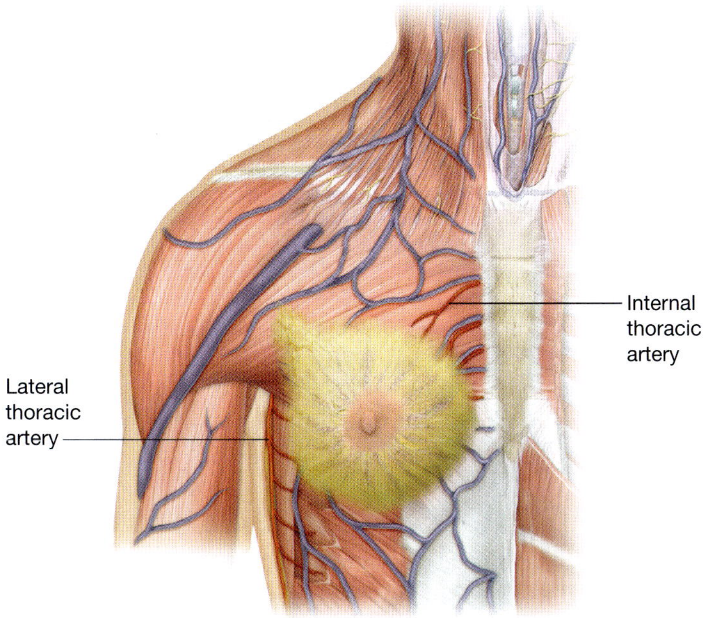

A

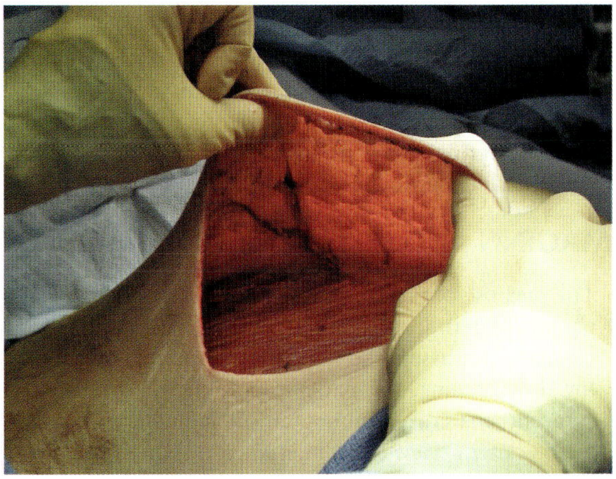

B

FIG 4 • **A.** The blood supply to the breast comes primarily from the lateral (mammary) thoracic artery, the internal (mammary) thoracic artery, and the intercostal arteries. It is crucial to preserve the branches of the 2nd intercostal artery in the upper medial flap to ensure viability. **B.** The subcutaneous venous plexus and branch off the 2nd intercostal artery are seen preserved with the flap.

Table 1: Methods for Examining the Breast and Pathognomonic Signs

Examination	Technique	Grading	Significance
Breast exam	Upright Supine	Symmetry Skin changes Palpable masses Adenopathy Nipple discharge	Cancer causing enlargement Peau d'orange, associated with inflammatory breast cancer, or an underlying tumor pulling on Cooper's ligaments Cancer, benign mass or cyst Lymph node metastasis or reactive lymph nodes Bloody or clear spontaneous unilateral discharge associated with carcinoma risk

- Prior to determining whether a patient will be a candidate for mastectomy or BCT, a thorough history and physical examination should be performed.
- The medical history should focus on the patient's family history of breast cancer in first-degree relatives and ovarian cancer in the family. Patients with a strong family history of breast or ovarian cancer, premenopausal breast cancer, patients with bilateral breast cancer, male family members with breast cancer, or those of Ashkenazi Jewish descent should be recommended for genetic counseling and testing for the BRCA 1 and 2 gene mutations. Also included in the medical history, the surgeon should ask about personal risk factors for developing breast cancer such as early menses, late menopause, a personal history of an atypical breast biopsy, lobular carcinoma in situ (LCIS), a history of previous chest wall radiation for Hodgkin's lymphoma, or use of hormone replacement therapy. Many of these high-risk patients who decide to undergo mastectomy also opt for contralateral mastectomy at the time of mastectomy to decrease their risk of a future breast cancer. Another reason for the recent increased incidence of contralateral prophylactic mastectomy is because of patient's anxiety, fear, and desire to reduce future risk of recurrence and cosmetic symmetry.[3]
- After obtaining a thorough medical history, a detailed physical examination would include examination of the patient in both the upright and supine positions (Table 1). While placing the patient's hands on her hips in the upright position, the patient is visually examined for symmetry, evidence of skin changes, or dimpling. The cervical and axillary areas are palpated for adenopathy and the breasts are examined. The patient is then placed supine with both arms over her head. The breasts are examined again for palpable masses and nipple discharge, and the axillae are palpated again while lowering the arms to the side. The abdomen is then examined for hepatosplenomegaly.

IMAGING AND OTHER DIAGNOSTIC STUDIES

- The purpose of preoperative imaging is to clinically stage the patient, determine operability, assist with surgical decision making, and assess the need for preoperative chemotherapy for downstaging. All patients prior to mastectomy require a recent bilateral mammogram including craniocaudal and medial lateral views. On mammogram, one should look for spiculated masses, tumor size and location, additional tumors, skin involvement, and associated calcifications (**FIG 5**).
- For patients with dense breast tissue or young age, a breast sonogram may be a helpful addition to assess the presence of additional lesions in dense breast tissue and the extent and depth of the tumor.
- Ultrasonography is also helpful to assess the axilla radiographically. Suspicious nodes have a very characteristic appearance with an obliterated hilum and nondistinct borders. An ultrasound-guided fine needle aspiration (FNA) can be performed preoperatively for suspicious nodes (**FIG 6**).

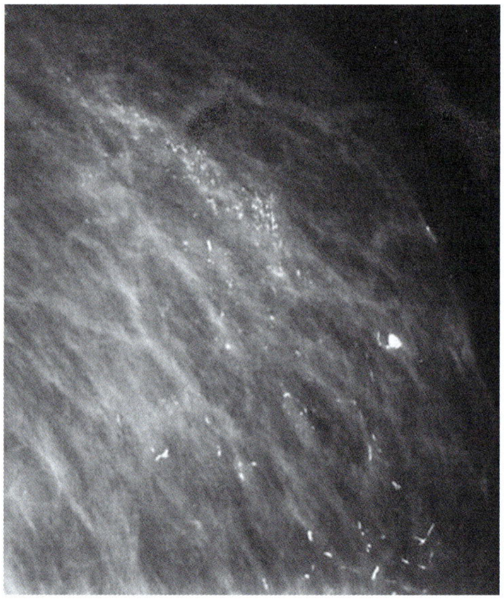

FIG 5 • Magnification mammogram showing pleomorphic calcifications suspicious for carcinoma.

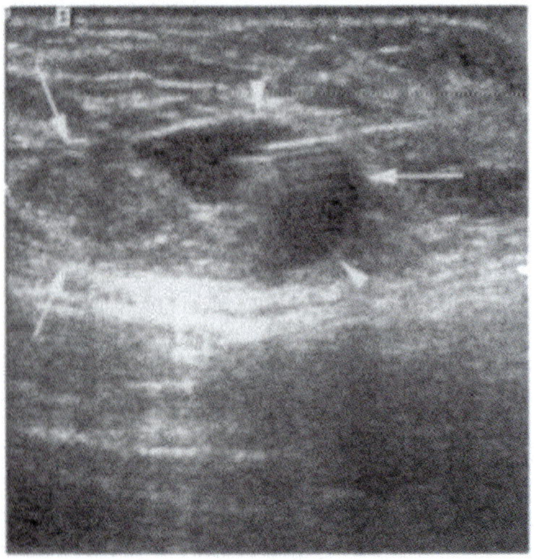

FIG 6 • Ultrasound-guided FNA biopsy of axillary lymph node metastases.

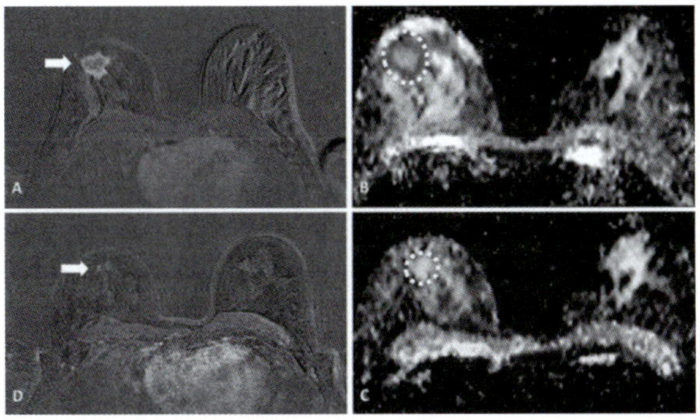

FIG 7 • MRI showing response to chemotherapy before treatment **(A)** and after treatment **(B)**.

- Magnetic resonance imaging (MRI) of the breast is used selectively for patients who are having mastectomy. One indication is for patients with invasive lobular cancer because of a higher incidence of contralateral disease.[4]
- MRI may also be used preoperatively for high-risk patients such as those with the BRCA 1 or 2 mutation, a strong family history, dense breast tissue, difficult breast examinations, large tumors with questionable skin involvement, or those undergoing neoadjuvant chemotherapy. In patients undergoing preoperative chemotherapy, MRI helps to monitor the response to treatment. An MRI is performed before treatment begins and then repeated again after systemic treatment is completed for comparison. The MRI shows a nice relationship of the tumor location to skin distance for treatment planning and choice of surgical incision (**FIG 7**).
- Staging tests to rule out metastatic disease, such as positron emission tomography–computed tomography (PET/CT) or a computed tomography (CT) scan of the chest, abdomen, and pelvis and bone scan should be considered in patients with lymph node involvement and large tumors or those patients with signs or symptoms suggestive of metastases (Table 2).

SURGICAL MANAGEMENT

- Indications for skin-sparing mastectomy include patients who choose mastectomy to reduce their risk of a future local recurrence and patients with the *BRCA* gene mutation, other high-risk patients that have a strong family history of breast cancer, or young age at diagnosis. The patient must have operable breast cancer and not have extensive skin involvement or fungating, ulcerating lesions.
- Indications for nipple-sparing mastectomy include patients who are undergoing prophylactic surgery, *BRCA* gene mutation carriers, and have operable cancers not located close to the nipple. Patients who should not undergo nipple-sparing mastectomy are those patients with very large, ptotic breasts, cancers located directly under the nipple, radiographic evidence of nipple involvement, or those with suspicious nipple discharge or nipple retraction. Patients must be informed that it is not possible to remove all the tissue under the nipple and that there is a reported risk of recurrence in the nipple and nipple necrosis of less than 5%.[5]

Table 2: Indications for Preoperative Positron Emission Tomography–Computed Tomography

Examination	Indications Preoperatively
PET/CT	Tumors >3 cm in size Evidence of lymph node metastasis Symptomatic disease (i.e., bone pain) Locally advanced breast cancer

PET/CT, positron emission tomography–computed tomography.

Preoperative Planning

- All preoperative radiographic studies should be studied prior to surgery to determine tumor location, size, and depth.
- The breast cancer surgeon and patient discuss the optimal type of skin-sparing mastectomy preoperatively and determine whether they are candidates for skin-sparing simple mastectomy or nipple-sparing mastectomy.
- All patients undergoing immediate reconstruction consult with a reconstructive surgeon prior to surgery for preoperative planning. After the reconstructive surgeon examines the patient and determines the optimal reconstruction depending on the patient's body habitus, breast size, and clinical stage, the reconstructive surgeon collaborates with the breast surgeon for the optimal oncologic approach with the best cosmesis.
- Patients with palpable tumors close to skin or those considering nipple-sparing mastectomy with tumors close to the areola may benefit from a preoperative breast MRI to address distance of tumor to the skin or disease below the nipple–areolar complex. This may alter treatment planning such as the use of neoadjuvant chemotherapy to achieve negative margins as well as surgical decision making.

Positioning

- The optimal operative position for all patients undergoing skin-sparing mastectomy is supine with the arms abducted approximately 45 degrees. Care is taken not to hyperextend the arms in anticipation for a long surgery. The arm boards are padded in order to protect the elbows from pressure compression causing a median nerve palsy.
- Compression boots are placed preoperatively and there is no need for additional anticoagulation unless the patient is at high risk for deep vein thrombosis (DVT), including obesity, a personal history of DVT, or cardiac valves requiring prophylaxis.
- Upon induction, if the patient is undergoing immediate breast reconstruction, they should receive a dose of intravenous (IV) antibiotics to cover gram-positive bacteria, usually a first-generation cephalosporin such as cephazolin.
- A Foley catheter is inserted after induction, if a prolonged reconstruction is anticipated.
- Prior to prepping the patient, methylene blue dye is injected subareolar for those surgeons who use both blue dye in addition to radioisotope for identification of the sentinel lymph node (**FIG 8**).
- Once prepped, the patient's arm is wrapped with a free arm dressing in anticipation of an axillary node dissection if axillary metastasis is suspected; otherwise, it is draped outside the field.

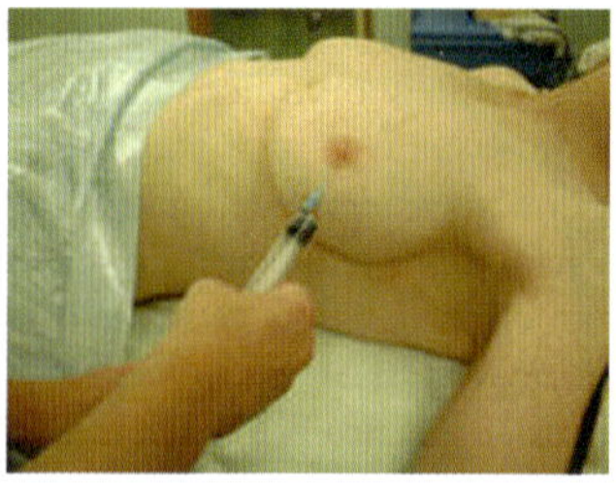

FIG 8 • Patient positioning and preoperative injection of blue dye in a subareolar fashion.

SKIN-SPARING MASTECTOMY

- Prior to surgery, the patient is skin marked by both the reconstructive and breast cancer surgeons. The nipple–areolar complex is removed by a small elliptical skin incision. There are many options of excision depending on breast size and tumor location as well as type of reconstruction (see **FIG 3**).
- The nipple–areolar complex is incised in an elliptical fashion with a no. 15 blade scalpel into the dermis. Skin hooks are placed on the flap and pulled upward by the first assistant. Care is taken to ensure the first assistant pulls directly perpendicular to the chest wall to avoid an inadvertent buttonhole in the flap (**FIG 9**).
- By retracting the breast downward against the upward traction of the skin, the superficial fascial plane is identified. The surgeon uses cautery to create the flaps by dissecting just above the superficial fascia in order to remove as much of the breast tissue as possible. Alternatively, some surgeons may use either the knife or scissors to create the mastectomy flaps. As long as the surgeon is in the correct anatomic plane, it should be relatively avascular.
- As the surgeon progresses further posteriorly, medium-sized Richardson retractors or lighted retractors are used to assist with retraction (see **FIG 15**). Because the skin ellipse opening may be quite small, the flaps are created in a spiral fashion until the pectoralis muscle is identified.
- The surgeon's hand is then used to examine the flaps. If the surgeon is in the proper plane, the flaps will only be a couple of millimeters thick and even throughout. Care is taken to ensure that the axillary tail of the breast has been adequately dissected and removed en bloc with the specimen.
- Next, the breast is removed from the pectoralis muscle. Medium-sized or large Richardson retractors are used to retract the skin superiorly and Kelly clamps may be placed on the superior aspect of the breast to assist with downward traction.
- Electrocautery is then used to separate the breast from the pectoralis muscle by dissecting parallel to the muscle fibers from medial to lateral (**FIG 10**). All perforating vessels are carefully cauterized prior to cutting to prevent retraction into the muscle and subsequent bleeding.
- Once the breast is removed from the chest wall, a silk stitch is used to mark the axillary tail for orientation for the pathologist. The breast is passed off the field for permanent section and attention is paid to the axilla to perform either a sentinel lymph node biopsy or axillary lymph node dissection, depending on the stage of the cancer. This may be performed via the mastectomy incision if there is no tension on the wound. If the axilla is too far away, a separate axillary incision is made.

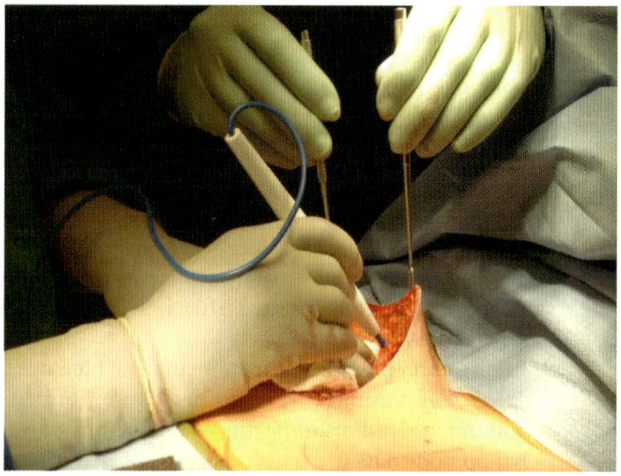

FIG 9 • Skin hooks are placed on the flap and pulled upward by the first assistant. Care is taken to ensure the first assistant pulls directly perpendicular to the chest wall to avoid an inadvertent button hole in the flap.

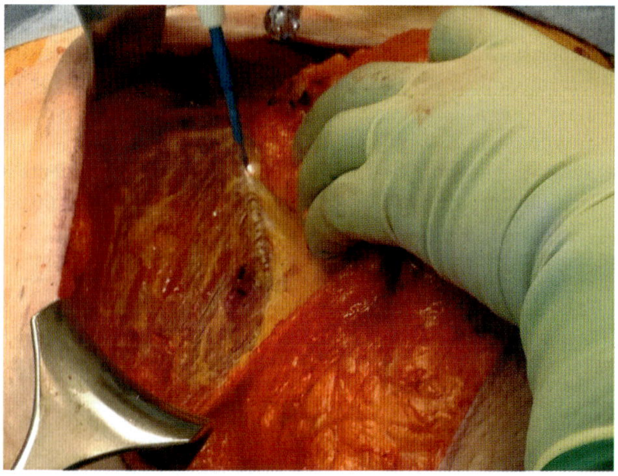

FIG 10 • Electrocautery is used to dissect the breast and pectoralis fascia off the underlying muscle. Cautery is moved parallel to the muscle fibers from medial to lateral.

NIPPLE-SPARING MASTECTOMY

- Nipple-sparing mastectomy is performed similar to skin-sparing mastectomy (**FIG 11**); however, the nipple–areolar complex is spared.This can be done through various approaches (**FIG 12**).
- The most cosmetic approach is via an inframammary fold skin incision (**FIG 13A,B**). The entire flap is created from the inframammary fold inferiorly to the clavicle superiorly. This is a long flap and is therefore best used on women with small to medium-sized breasts. The inframammary fold incision is usually approximately 9 cm in length. It extends from just below the medial aspect of the areola in the inframammary fold to 9 cm laterally. The most challenging technical aspect of this approach is getting sufficient upward traction of the skin in order to create the flap in the appropriate plane.
- Skin hooks are used for upward traction, as in the traditional skin-sparing mastectomy. However, when approaching the nipple–areolar complex, it is best to have the first assistant gently pinch and retract the nipple upward or alternatively place a 2-0 silk stitch through the nipple in order to give upward traction and use a lighted retractor lateral to the nipple–areolar complex in order to visualize the area adequately (**FIGS 14** and **15**).
- The ductal tissue posterior to the nipple is usually more dense and lighter in color (**FIG 16**). Once through this area, the silk stitch can be removed and the lighted retractors are advanced in order to complete the superior aspect of the flaps to the clavicle. The first assistant can apply gentle traction of the skin flap by placing the palm of his or her hand on the superior aspect of the flap and pushing away from the surgeon.
- To create even flaps, it is important that both the first assistant and surgeon apply steady, even traction and avoid readjusting multiple times.
- After the breast is removed from the chest wall, attention is paid to the nipple to take an additional nipple margin.
- The surgeon's finger is placed on the outside of the nipple and the nipple is everted. An Allis clamp is then placed on the tissue inside the nipple and a no. 15 blade scalpel is used to perform a shave biopsy of any residual ductal tissue within the nipple. The tissue is then sent to pathology for frozen or permanent section.
- All patients undergoing nipple-sparing mastectomy are consented preoperatively that if the nipple margin is positive for cancer, then the nipple–areolar complex will be removed. If this is recognized intraoperatively on frozen section, the nipple–areolar complex can be removed at this time. If this is deferred to permanent section, it will be removed postoperatively by the reconstructive surgeon.
- If the skin flaps and nipple–areolar complex appear well vascularized and the nipple margin is negative on

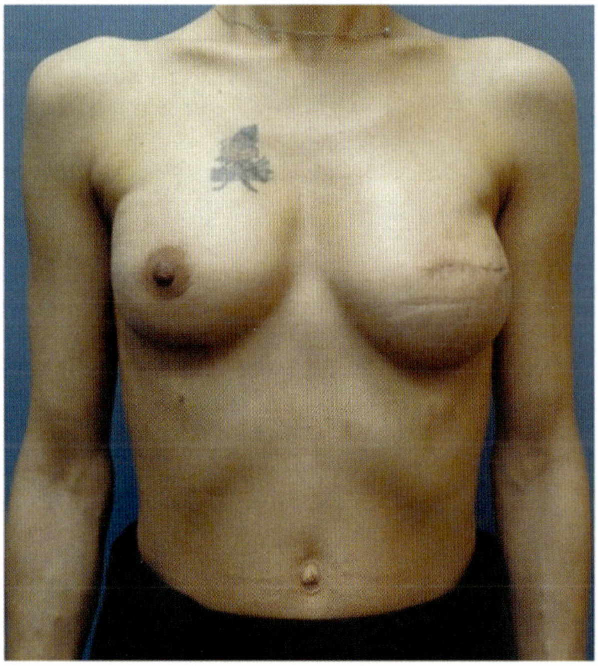

FIG 11 ● Nipple-sparing mastectomy via inframammary skin incision versus skin sparing mastectomy on patient with left centrally located tumor. (Photo courtesy of Sherman J, MD.)

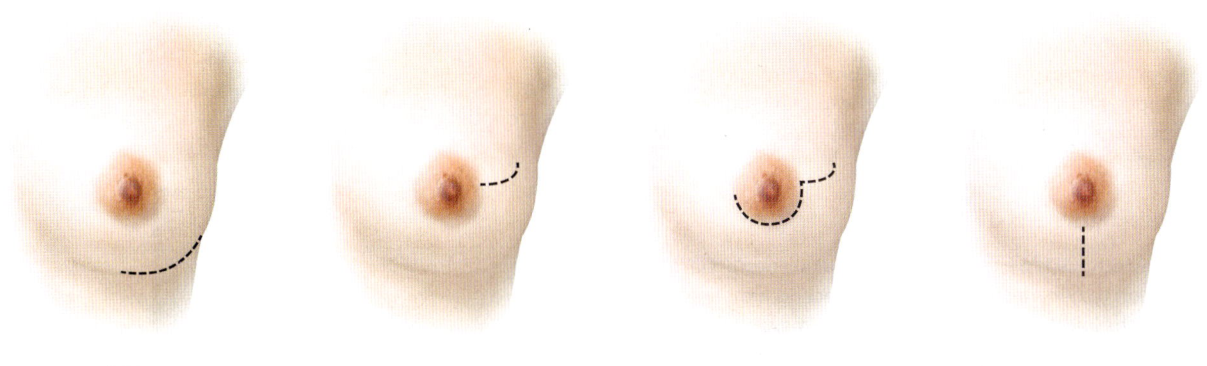

FIG 12 ● Skin incision options for nipple-sparing mastectomy.

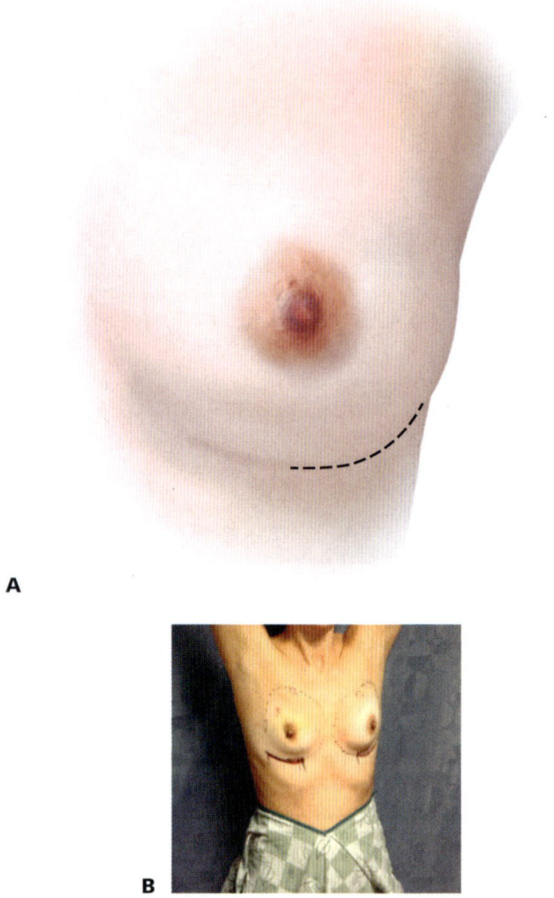

FIG 13 ● **A.** Nipple-sparing mastectomy via inframammary fold skin incision. **B.** Preoperative skin marking for inframammary skin incision. Below medial areola to 9 cm laterally in the inframammary fold.

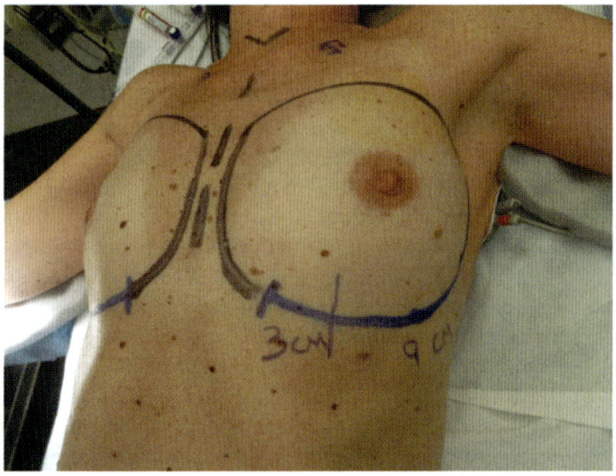

FIG 14 ● Extended incision for more exposure if necessary.

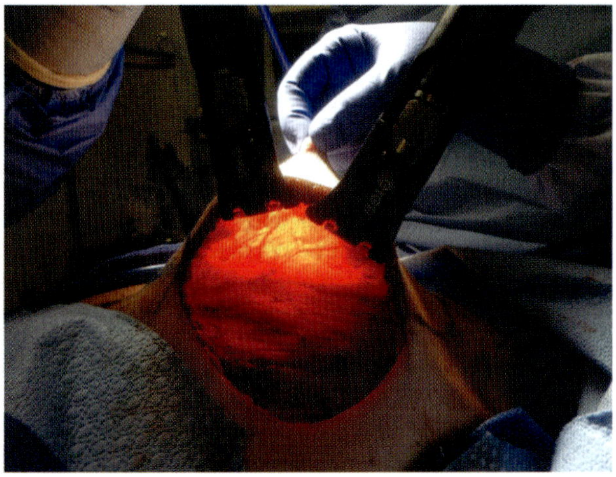

FIG 15 ● Gentle upward traction of the nipple by the first assistant to create plane behind the nipple.

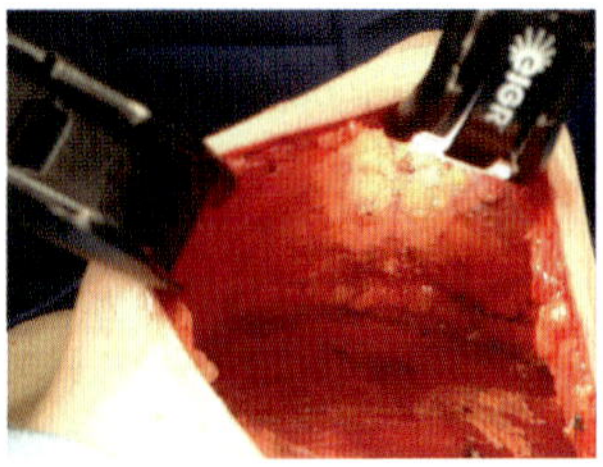

FIG 16 ● Inside of nipple area appears lighter compared to the surrounding tissue.

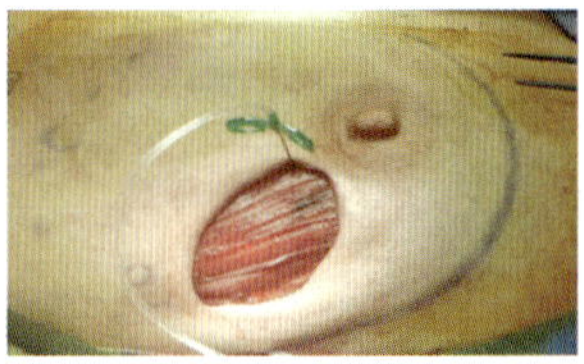

FIG 17 ● Expansion of the tissue expander after a nipple-sparing mastectomy with immediate reconstruction.

frozen section (if obtained), the reconstructive surgeon can proceed (**FIG 17**).

- For patients with ptotic breasts who are not ideal candidates for nipple-sparing mastectomy, we recommend performing a superior circumareolar mastopexy incision with a lateral extension to remove excess skin and achieve a slight lift. Another option for macromastia or significant ptosis is a two-stage procedure suggested by Spear and colleagues[6] where the patient undergoes a primary mammoplasty followed by nipple-sparing mastectomy 3 weeks later (**FIG 18**).

Analgesia after Mastectomy

- Mastectomy is performed under general anesthesia. In addition to general anesthesia, a long acting local anesthetic may be injected into the borders of the mastectomy wound just below the cut edge of the fascia. Postoperatively, patients are given both an oral narcotic as well as vallium to relax the muscle and prevent muscle spasm and tightness.

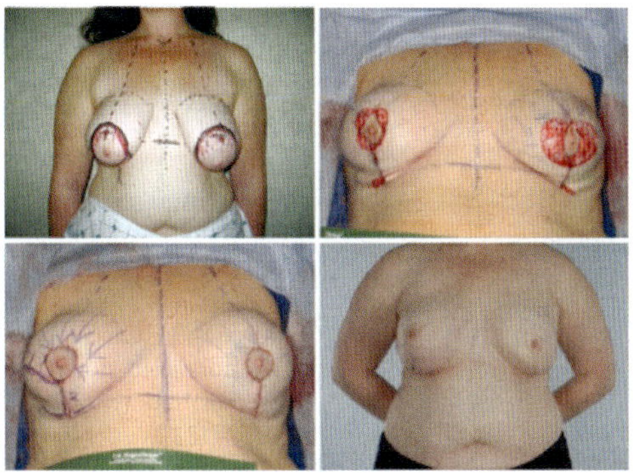

FIG 18 ● Staged nipple-sparing mastectomy following reduction for macromastia or ptotic breasts. (Photo courtesy of Spear S, Rottman S, Seiboth L, et al. Breast reconstruction using a staged nipple-sparing mastectomy following mastopexy or reduction. *Plast Reconstr Surg*. 2012;129:572–581.)

PEARLS AND PITFALLS

Possible Pitfalls of Skin-Sparing Mastectomy	Pearls
Flap necrosis	▪ Identify fascial plan below subcutaneous tissue; stay just above this line to create flap. ▪ Maintain even traction/countertraction in order to create even flaps. ▪ Preserve the subcutaneous venous plexus and the 2nd intercostal perforator to prevent flap necrosis. ▪ Avoid denuding the skin.
Nipple necrosis	▪ Do not denude the nipple. ▪ Avoid too much traction on the nipple for prolonged periods of time. ▪ Avoid cautery under the nipple.
Infection	▪ Treat reconstructive patients with preoperative IV antibiotics and postoperative oral antibiotics until the drains are removed. ▪ Irrigate thoroughly with normal saline after the mastectomy is performed. ▪ Obtain careful hemostasis.

POSTOPERATIVE CARE

- Patients who undergo implant reconstruction are admitted as an inpatient overnight.
- Patients who undergo flap reconstruction are admitted longer depending on the type of flap reconstruction.
- They are maintained on oral first-generation cephalosporin until the Jackson-Pratt (JP) drains are removed.
- The patients are discharged with a surgical bra and the JP drains attached to the bra.
- They may resume showering after 48 hours and are taught how to empty and record the drain output.
- The patient returns in 1 week to have the drains removed if she is draining less than 30 cc per day from each drain and to discuss the pathology report.
- Patients are then referred to medical oncology for adjuvant treatment and a radiation oncologist if indicated.
- When the breast is removed, the sensory innervations to the skin are also removed, resulting in loss of sensation. This resulting band of numbness gets narrower over time but never completely resolves.
- Following mastectomy, patients are seen in follow-up by the breast surgeon every 6 months for 5 years to examine the skin for recurrent disease, then yearly thereafter.
- An instruction book of postmastectomy stretching exercises is given to the patient after the drains are removed to increase mobility and prevent frozen shoulder. For patients who develop decreased mobility after surgery, they are referred to a specially trained physical therapist.

OUTCOMES

- Include functional and prosthetic survivorship data, as applicable.

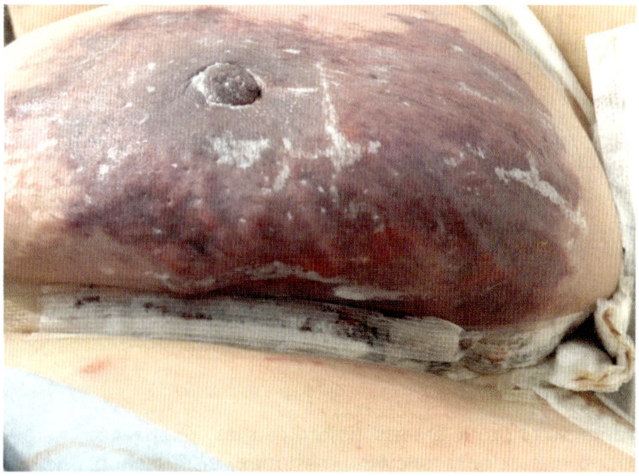

FIG 19 • Nipple and flap necrosis after nipple-sparing mastectomy via inframammary skin incision.

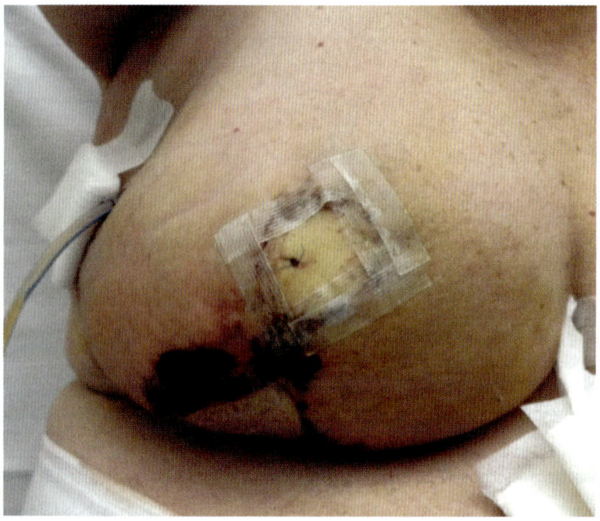

FIG 20 • Inferior flap necrosis after skin-sparing mastectomy with deep inferior epigastric perforator (DIEP) flap reconstruction.

COMPLICATIONS

- Skin flap necrosis (**FIGS 19** and **20**)
- Nipple necrosis
- Infection
- Seroma
- Hematoma

REFERENCES

1. Veronesi U, Cascinelli N, Mariani L, et al. Twenty-year follow-up of a randomized study comparing breast-conserving surgery with radical mastectomy for early breast cancer. *N Engl J Med.* 2002;347(16):1227–1232.
2. Vilarino-Varela M, Chin YS, Makris A. Current indications for post-mastectomy radiation. *Int Semin Surg Oncol.* 2009;6:5.
3. Howard-McNatt M, Schroll RW, Hurt GJ, et al. Contralateral prophylactic mastectomy in breast cancer patients who test negative for BRCA mutations. *Am J Surg.* 2011;202:298–302.
4. Heil J, Buehler A, Golatta M, et al. Do patients with invasive lobular breast cancer benefit in terms of adequate change in surgical therapy from a supplementary preoperative breast MRI? *Ann Oncol.* 2012;23:98–104.
5. Petit JY, Veronesi U, Orecchia R, et al. Risk factors associated with recurrence after nipple-sparing mastectomy for invasive and intraepithelial neoplasia. *Ann Oncol.* 2012;23;2053–2058.
6. Spear S, Rottman S, Seiboth L, et al. Breast reconstruction using a staged nipple-sparing mastectomy following mastopexy or reduction. *Plast Reconstr Surg.* 2012;129:572–581.

Chapter 12 Modified Radical Mastectomy

Tiffany A. Torstenson Judy C. Boughey

DEFINITION

- Modified radical mastectomy (MRM) is a surgical procedure that removes all breast tissue and lymphatic-bearing tissue in the axilla. This operation removes the nipple–areolar complex, skin envelope, and level I and II axillary nodes but spares the pectoralis major muscle. It can also be termed as a total mastectomy with an axillary lymph node dissection.

PATIENT HISTORY AND PHYSICAL FINDINGS

- There has been a huge evolution in types of the mastectomy over the years. We have moved away from the radical mastectomy to more cosmetic pleasing procedures such as simple mastectomy, skin-sparing mastectomy, and nipple-sparing mastectomy. In mastectomy patients with node-positive disease, axillary lymph node dissection is often recommended.
- Patients undergoing an MRM usually have documented lymph node metastases diagnosed preoperatively or surgically and either elect to have a mastectomy or require a mastectomy (i.e., are not candidates for breast-conserving therapy). Patients diagnosed with inflammatory breast cancer should also undergo an MRM after induction chemotherapy according to National Comprehensive Cancer Network (NCCN) guidelines.[1]
- It is crucial to decide from the beginning if these patients are operable candidates and whether neoadjuvant therapy should be considered. A multidisciplinary approach is vital in the treatment success of these patients. Involvement of a medical oncologist and radiation oncologist early in the management of these patients helps treatment planning and to streamline patient care.
- A comprehensive history and physical examination is imperative on the first consultation with these patients. The history should be very detailed and include questions pertaining to medical conditions, medications, surgeries, allergies, and also about any musculoskeletal issues, which could affect operative positioning. It is important to evaluate for any family history of breast or ovarian cancer.
- If there is a strong family history of breast or ovarian cancer, it is essential to offer genetic counseling and possibility of genetic testing.
- Physical examination starts with an inspection of bilateral breasts both with arms at the patient's side and with the arms elevated, noting any asymmetry, nipple retraction, prior scars, or skin changes.
- Palpation of the breasts should always be done both in a sitting and supine position in a circular or vertical pattern. Palpable masses should have bidimensional measurements and should be assessed for chest wall adherence and skin proximity. Any palpable masses that do not correspond to radiologic findings require further testing and tissue biopsy.
- A thorough examination of the lymph node basins should be performed, including the axillary, cervical, supraclavicular, and infraclavicular nodes. If there is adenopathy on palpation, patients should undergo an in-office or radiologic ultrasound. Any suspicious nodes on imaging should undergo a fine needle aspiration or core needle biopsy.
- Imaging and pathologic diagnoses should be shared and explained to the patient. It is helpful to map out the incisions for the patients to see preoperatively. Explain to patients the need for either neoadjuvant or adjuvant chemotherapy as well as likely need for postmastectomy radiation in patients with node-positive disease.
- Neoadjuvant chemotherapy has been shown to be equivalent to adjuvant chemotherapy in terms of survival and can increase rates of breast-conserving therapy.
- Postmastectomy radiation in node-positive disease decreases rates of locoregional recurrence and increases disease-free and breast cancer–specific survival.
- Inquire if patients are seeking immediate reconstruction or desire to go flat chested. If postmastectomy radiation is recommended, patients may not be candidates for immediate reconstruction.
- Allocate enough time to spend with these patients in order to answer all their questions, and be empathetic to their needs during this emotional time. Keep interruptions with pagers and cell phones to a minimum.

IMAGING AND OTHER DIAGNOSTIC STUDIES

- Breast imaging plays a vital role in the screening and diagnostic workup for breast cancer. Imaging can define the extent of the disease and help assess for any abnormalities in the contralateral breast. It is also used as a monitor for local recurrence in patients postoperatively.
- Mammography is the initial imaging test in the breast cancer workup. Mammograms are very sensitive in detecting abnormalities and have been shown to decrease breast cancer mortality approximately by 30%. Screening mammograms should begin yearly in women who are 40 years of age and asymptomatic.[2]
- Diagnostic mammograms should be obtained in any patient being considered for an MRM (**FIG 1**). Spot and magnification views can help aid to focus and distinguish abnormalities. Implant displacement views (Eklund views) should be obtained in women with implants.[2,3] Request films if they were done at an outside institution. An ultrasound should also be performed to further assess the size of the tumor and the proximity of it to the skin and chest wall. Lesions that are suspicious on ultrasound or mammogram should undergo a percutaneous biopsy.
- Axillary ultrasound should be performed in patients with a biopsy-proven invasive cancer. Lymph nodes should be evaluated for their size, shape, and morphology. Suspicious nodes

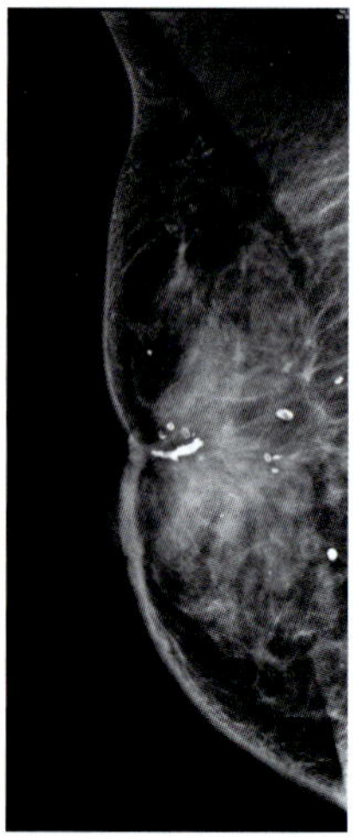

FIG 1 • Mammogram showing a right invasive ductal carcinoma invading the skin and causing skin retraction.

on imaging or clinically palpable nodes should undergo a fine needle aspiration or core needle biopsy with ultrasound guidance (**FIG 2**). Approximately 31% of axillary metastases are diagnosed with ultrasound-guided biopsy.

- Magnetic resonance imaging (MRI) usage is still controversial but can be used as an additional imaging tool for screening, staging of known breast cancers, and evaluating the contralateral breast. MRIs are highly sensitive tests but lack specificity leading to an increased false-positive rate. Studies have also demonstrated an increased rate of mastectomies in patients undergoing MRIs. The decision to order an MRI should be based on the recommended indications and individualized.
- According to NCCN guidelines, positron emission tomography (PET) scans can be used to evaluate for distant metastasis in patients with stage IIIA breast cancer, but this is a category 2B recommendation. Systemic staging is not recommended for patients with early stage breast cancer in the absence of symptoms.[1]
- When a suspicious lesion is identified on imaging, a tissue biopsy is needed to decipher between a benign and malignant process. Percutaneous biopsy is preferred over an excisional biopsy, which can lead to unnecessary surgeries for benign entities. Core needle biopsy is preferred to evaluate histology and differentiate in situ from invasive disease. Most lesions in the breast will need to undergo a core needle biopsy using ultrasound or stereotactic guidance. MRI-guided core needle biopsy can also be performed when lesions are not detected on ultrasound or mammography but these are more technically challenging. If cancer is identified, there should be a detailed pathologic assessment, including subtype and hormone receptor status. In cases with morphologically abnormal lymph nodes on ultrasound, fine needle aspiration biopsy or core biopsy of lymph nodes should be used.
- After any percutaneous biopsy, a marking clip should always be placed. This is extremely important in patients receiving neoadjuvant chemotherapy.

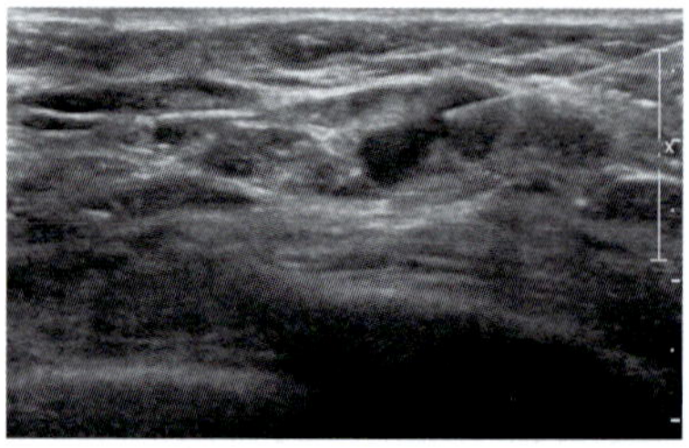

FIG 2 • Ultrasound-guided fine needle aspiration of an axillary lymph node that revealed metastatic carcinoma in a male breast cancer patient who underwent an MRM.

SURGICAL MANAGEMENT

Preoperative Planning

- Preoperatively, patients can be considered for regional anesthesia at the surgeon's and anesthesiologist's discretion. Paravertebral blocks (PVBs) are increasing in popularity for breast surgery and are more commonly favored over epidural blocks. They can be performed as single- or multiple-level injections or as a continuous catheter infusion. PVBs have been shown to shorten recovery times and length of hospital stays, decrease opiate usage, and decrease the incidence of vomiting. It is also hypothesized this type of regional anesthesia may protect the immune system and decrease metastasis.[4]
- PVBs are preferred over epidural blocks because they induce less hypotension, less urinary retention, are technically easy to learn, and have less severe side effects. Patients who are coagulopathic or who have musculoskeletal deformities such as kyphosis or scoliosis should not be considered for a PVB.[5,6]
- Potential complications associated with a PVB are pneumothorax, vascular penetrance, sepsis, and hematoma. Pneumothoraces are more common with multiple-level injections in comparison to single-level injections. Patients can either be seated with the spine in a kyphotic curve or placed in a lateral decubitus position (**FIG 3**). The local anesthetic is injected in the paravertebral space where the thoracic spinal nerves emerge.
- Ultrasound can also help guide the correct placement of the local anesthetic. Patient comfort improves when an ultrasound is used, and the pneumothorax rate decreases due to the direct visualization of the pleura.
- Before patients enter the operating theater, they should be site marked in the preoperative area to ensure the correct side is being operated on. Radiologic imaging should be thoroughly reviewed prior to the procedure to ensure the location of the tumor and the proximity of it to the skin.
- Prophylactic antibiotics have been shown to reduce postoperative infections and should be administered prior to incision.[7] Most surgeons prefer to avoid the use of paralytics during an MRM in order to aid identification of important motor nerves, but excessive handling of these nerves is discouraged to prevent axonal injury.

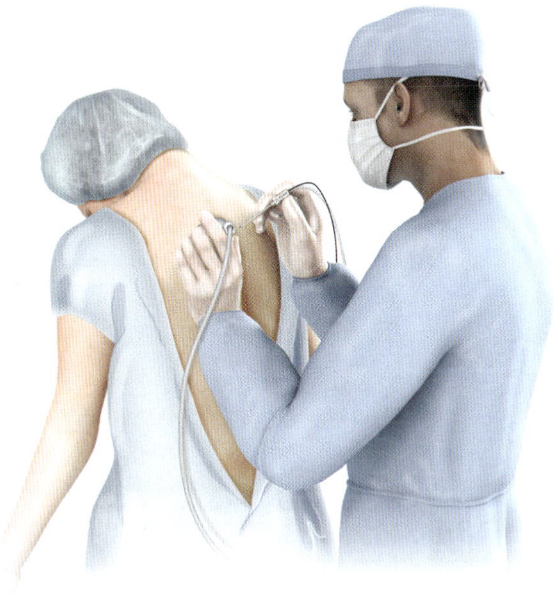

FIG 3 • When performing a PVB, the patient can be seated with the spine positioned in a kyphotic curve. (Modified from Hebl JR, Lennon RL. *Mayo Clinic Atlas of Regional Anesthesia and Ultrasound-Guided Nerve Blockade*. Rochester, MN and New York, NY: Mayo Clinic Scientific Press and Oxford University Press; 2010. Used with permission of Mayo Foundation for Medical Education and Research. All rights reserved.)

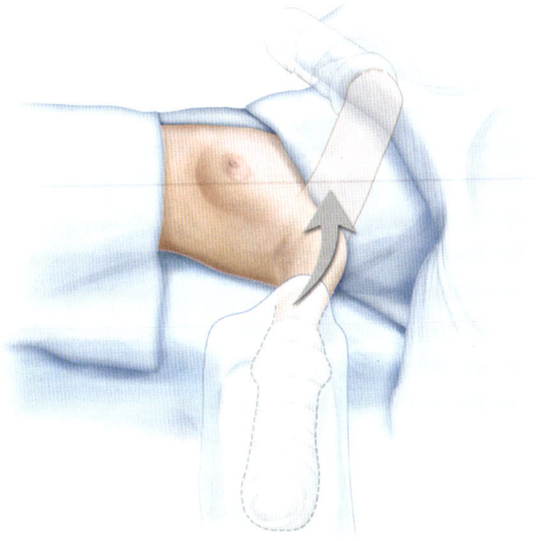

FIG 4 • Positioning and draping of a patient for an MRM. (Modified from Donohue JH, Van Heerden J, Monson JRT, eds. *Atlas of Surgical Oncology*. Cambridge, MA: Blackwell Science; 1995. Used with permission of Mayo Foundation for Medical Education and Research. All rights reserved.)

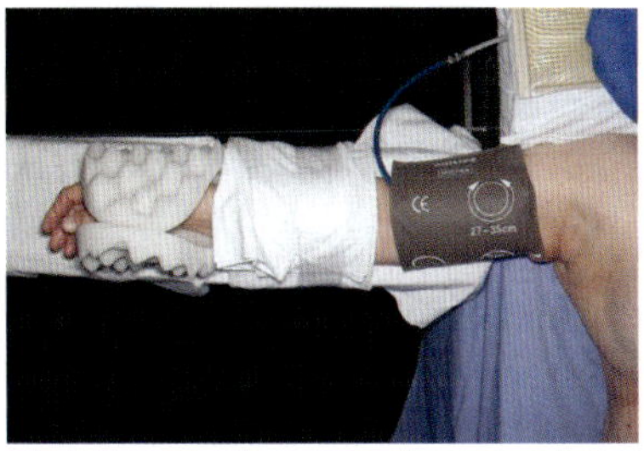

FIG 5 • The contralateral arm should contain the IV and blood pressure cuff.

- Prophylactic anticoagulants for prevention of venous thromboembolism (VTE), such as subcutaneous heparin, should be considered on a case-by-case basis. Sequential compression devices should be placed prior to initiation of general anesthesia for VTE prevention.

Positioning

- Correct positioning of patients undergoing an MRM is vitally important. Patients should be in a supine position with the side of the MRM close to the edge of the operating table. The endotracheal tube should be positioned toward the contralateral side of the mouth from the side of the MRM. Arms should not be abducted greater than 90 degrees to prevent injury to the brachial plexus. Arms should be placed on padded arm boards and positioned in a way that pressure points are alleviated. It is often helpful, particularly with bulky adenopathy, to prepare the ipsilateral arm into the field and wrap it with a sterile stockinette and Kerlix wrap (**FIG 4**). This allows for relaxation of the pectoralis muscles and easier access to the level II and III axillary nodes.
- The arm should be secured to the arm board. Blood pressure cuffs and intravenous (IV) lines should be placed in the contralateral upper extremity (**FIG 5**). Allow enough room between the operating table and anesthesiologist cart to allow an assistant to stand above the arm.
- Surgical preparation should include the breast and axilla and extend across the midline, inferiorly onto the abdomen, superiorly to the neck and the upper arm, and laterally to the level of the operating table. Draping should ensure preservation of a sterile field with exposure of the whole breast and axilla (**FIG 6**).

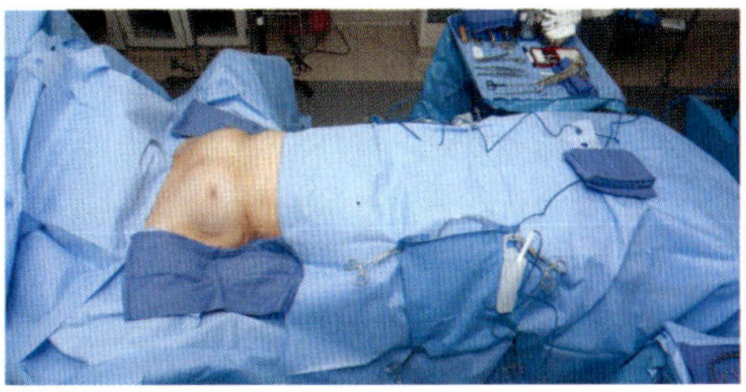

FIG 6 • Draping should ensure preservation of a sterile field with exposure of the whole breast and axilla.

INCISION PLACEMENT

- There are many options for incisions for a total mastectomy that are based on the tumor location. In an MRM, it is important to have an incision that provides good exposure to the axilla and reduces skin redundancy. The incision should include the skin overlying the tumor in cases where the tumor is close to the skin and a 1- to 2-cm margin around the tumor and include the previous biopsy site.
- The classic Stewart incision is a transverse elliptical incision, provides access to the axilla, and is the preferred incision of many plastic surgeons for patients seeking delayed reconstruction (**FIG 7**).
- When mapping the incision, it is important to make sure there will be adequate skin for a tension-free closure without excess skin for redundancy (**FIG 8A,B**). Most of these patients will be receiving postmastectomy radiation, which can lead to incision breakdown, and this is increased when incisions are under tension. The boundaries of the breast (clavicle superiorly, inframammary fold inferiorly, sternum medially, and midaxillary line laterally) define the extent of the flap dissection.
- Measuring the length of the planned superior incision and inferior incision to ensure that these are equal in length can help guide adjustments to allow equal length skin flaps.

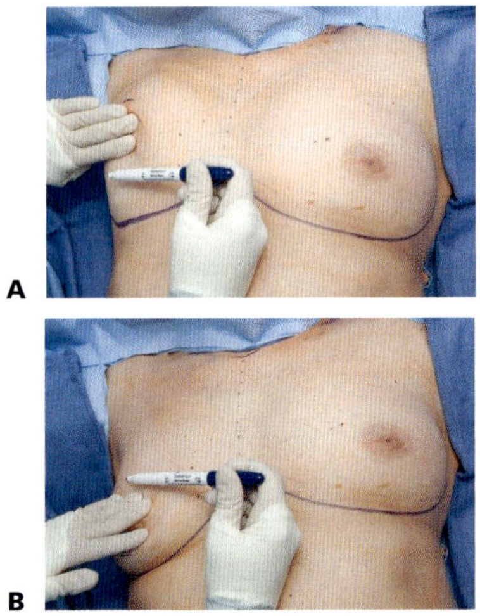

FIG 8 • **A,B.** Measuring the distance from the superior to the inferior incision with a marking pen will help provide a tension-free closure and reduce skin redundancy.

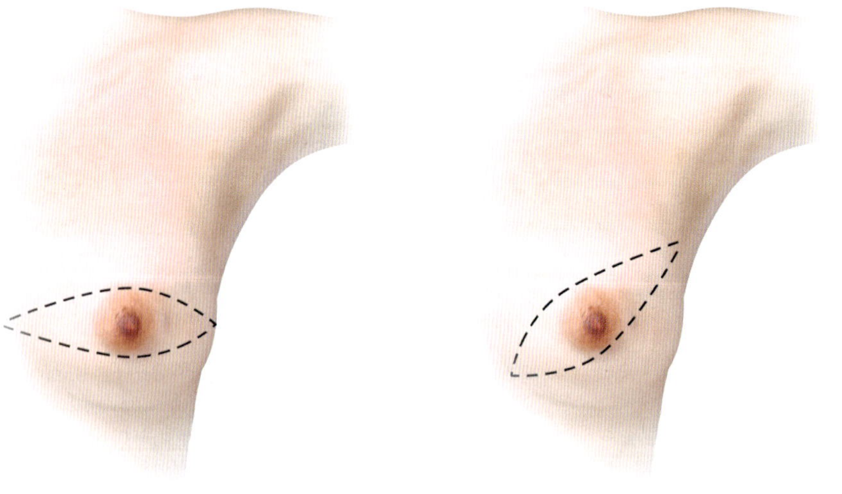

FIG 7 • The two most common and preferred incisions for an MRM, which provide good axillary exposure. **Left:** Stewart incision. **Right:** Modified Stewart incision. (Modified from Donohue JH, Van Heerden J, Monson JRT, eds. *Atlas of Surgical Oncology*. Cambridge, MA: Blackwell Science; 1995. Used with permission of Mayo Foundation for Medical Education and Research. All rights reserved.)

SKIN INCISION AND CREATION OF FLAPS

- Once the skin incision has been mapped out on the breast, a scalpel is used to cut through the skin and dermis. A small edge of tissue is raised below the dermal layer to develop the flap (**FIG 9**). Skin hooks are used to provide traction for flap elevation, and these should be replaced with deeper retractors or lighted retractors when the dissection flaps are extended (**FIG 10**). Traction of the contralateral hand of the surgeon with a sponge also provides necessary tension for appropriate plane dissection. Flap dissection can be done sharply or with electrocautery, but electrocautery will provide better hemostasis during the dissection.
- The goal of flap elevation is to remove all the breast tissue while maintaining vascular supply to the flaps. The dissection plane should be developed between the breast tissue and subcutaneous fat. Frequently, there will be an avascular plane that can help guide in the dissection. It is important to keep traction on the breast to assist in finding the correct plane, and intermittent flap palpation should be performed to determine the correct thickness of the flaps. Flap thickness will vary among patients and is dependent on the patient's body habitus.

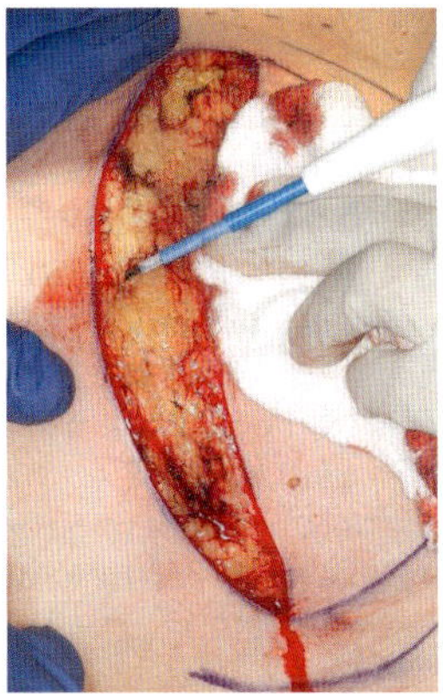

FIG 9 ● Raise an area of tissue under the dermis to begin the flap dissection. Using a sponge in the opposite hand can help provide traction, which will help in the flap creation.

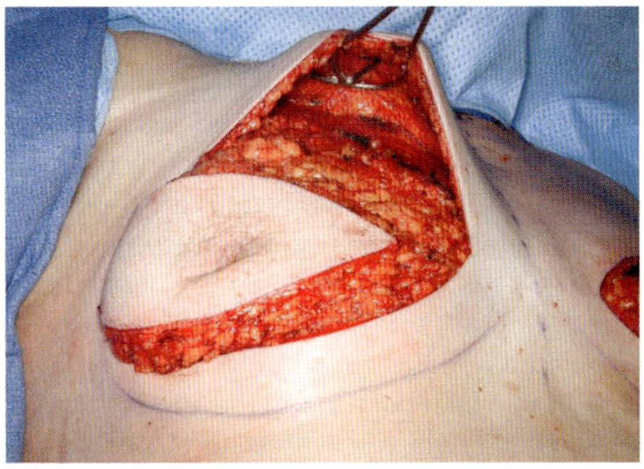

FIG 11 ● The superior flap dissection is extended up to the clavicle where the underlying muscle can then be exposed.

- The superior flap should be extended up to the inferior border of the clavicle, and the medial flap should be dissected to the sternal border (FIG 11). When creating the medial flap, careful attention should be directed to the medial perforators. These perforators should be preserved where feasible to maintain vascular supply to the flap. When these need to be sacrificed, clips or suture ligation should be used to assure hemostasis. The lateral flap should be extended to the latissimus dorsi and the inferior flap should be dissected to the inframammary fold (FIG 12). It is important to avoid excess traction as the dissection is extended to avoid flap ischemia.

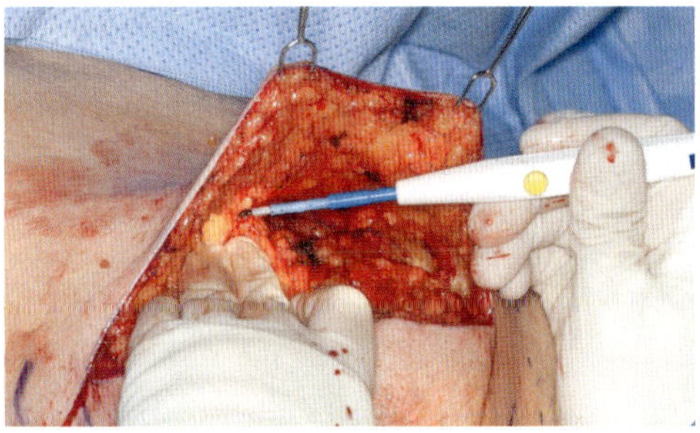

FIG 10 ● Joseph retractors or skin hooks are used at the beginning of the flap dissection. These should be switched out for deeper retractors as the dissection is extended.

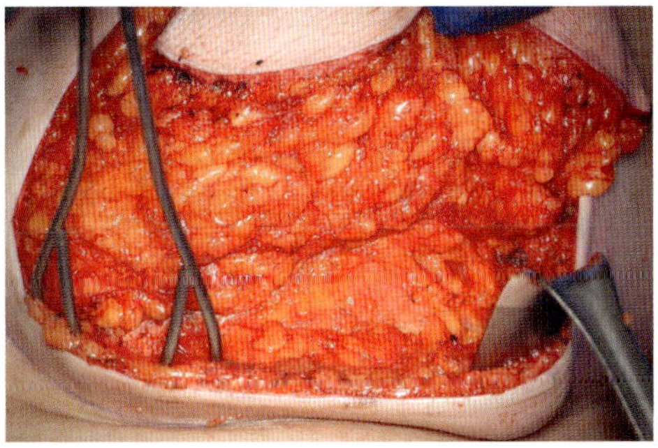

FIG 12 ● The inferior flap dissection is carried to the inframammary fold.

DISSECTION FROM THE PECTORAL MUSCLES

- When the flaps are completed to the appropriate landmarks, the breast tissue is dissected off the pectoralis muscle taking the pectoral fascia with the breast tissue using the electrocautery. The dissection should be started superiorly at the level of the clavicle. Traction should be applied with the contralateral hand to visualize the dissection plane (FIG 13).
- The dissection should continue inferiorly and in a medial to lateral fashion to follow the muscle fibers. The fascia surrounding the muscle should be dissected off with the breast in order to prevent local recurrence.[8,9] Careful attention should be provided to preserve the serratus anterior muscle fascia laterally and inferiorly and the rectus sheath fascia inferiorly. The axillary tail of the breast should remain attached in order to keep the breast and axillary contents as one pathologic specimen and also to guide the axillary dissection.

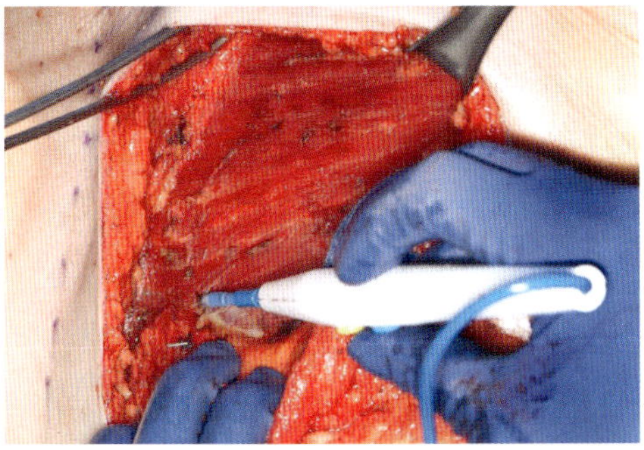

FIG 13 ● Dissection of the breast tissue off the pectoralis major muscle should be done with electrocautery in a medial to lateral fashion taking the pectoralis major muscle fascia with the specimen.

AXILLARY DISSECTION

- The axilla has a pyramidal shape and is located between the upper arm and thoracic chest wall. It is bounded superiorly by the axillary vein, anteriorly by the pectoralis muscle, medially by the serratus anterior muscle, and posterolaterally by the latissimus dorsi.
- The axilla can be reached when the breast tissue is positioned laterally and the dissection is continued under the pectoralis major muscle (**FIG 14**). The clavipectoral fascia should be incised along the edge of the pectoralis major muscle, which will free up the pectoralis major and minor muscle from the nodal tissue (**FIG 15**). Close attention should be paid to identify the medial pectoral neurovascular bundle. It sweeps laterally along the pectoralis minor, and care should be taken to preserve the bundle. The inferior border of the dissection should extend to the 4th or 5th rib to ensure that level I nodes are included in the specimen.[10]
- Once the axillary fat pad is encountered, the subcutaneous fat appears darker and is glistening. Once the axillary space is entered, it is vitally important to identify landmarks to guide your dissection and to prevent neurovascular injury. This ALND describes a lateral to medial approach to the axillary lymph node dissection. A medial to lateral approach is described in Chapter 28.
- The first vital structure to identify is the thoracodorsal bundle, and this is facilitated by visualizing the latissimus dorsi laterally (**FIG 16**). The thoracodorsal nerve inserts approximately 4 cm inferior to the axillary vein, and the bundle can be followed superiorly to its posterior insertion on the axillary vein (**FIG 17**).
- The next step is to identify the axillary vein. Richardson retractors should be used at this time to provide exposure to the vein by retracting the pectoral muscles (**FIG 18**). The axillary vein can be easily identified using

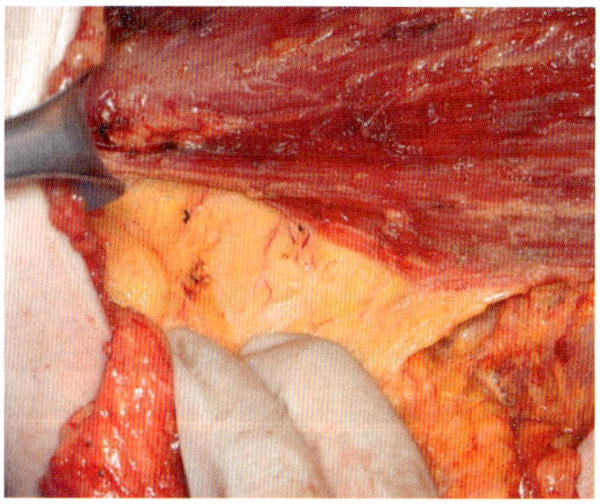

FIG 14 • The axilla can be reached when the breast tissue is positioned laterally and the dissection is continued under the pectoralis major muscle, where the clavipectoral fascia is exposed.

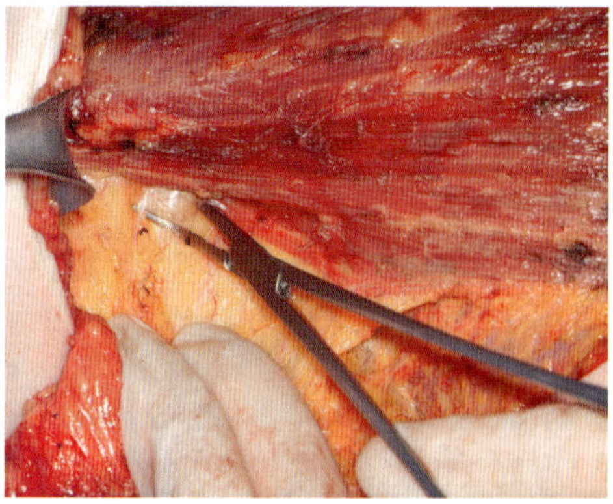

FIG 15 • The axillary fat pad is entered when the clavipectoral fascia is incised.

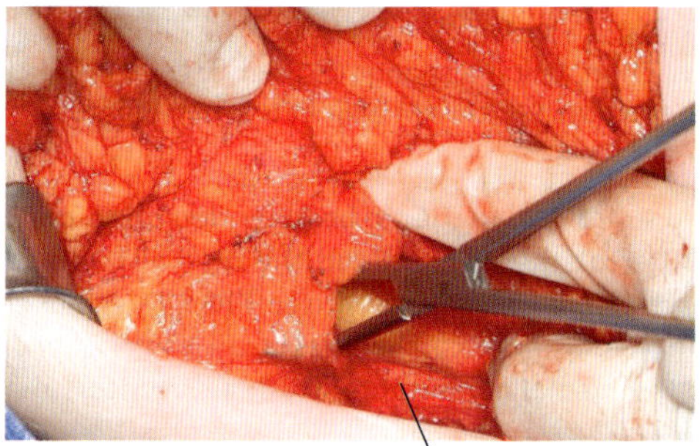

FIG 16 • Dissect laterally to identify the latissimus dorsi muscle and enter axilla just anterior to latissimus dorsi to find the thoracodorsal bundle.

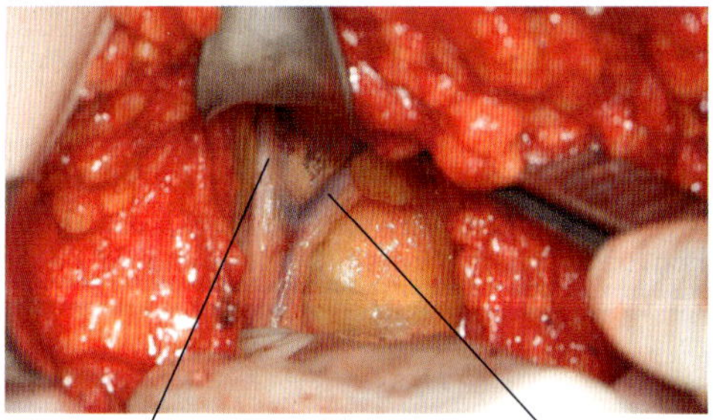

FIG 17 • The thoracodorsal bundle.

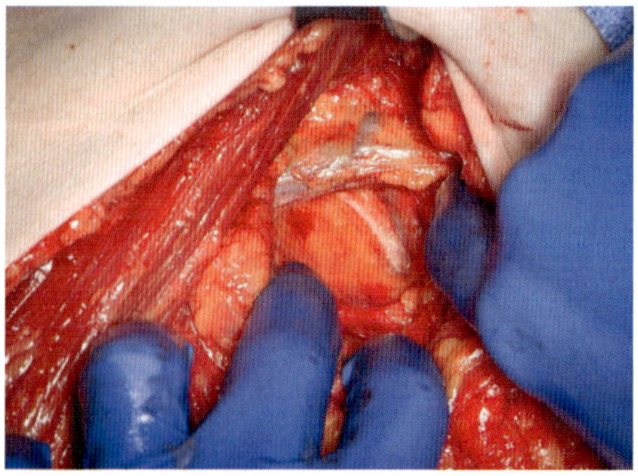

FIG 18 • The Richardson retractor is used to expose the axillary vein by retracting the pectoral muscles. The thoracodorsal bundle is seen posterior to the axillary vein.

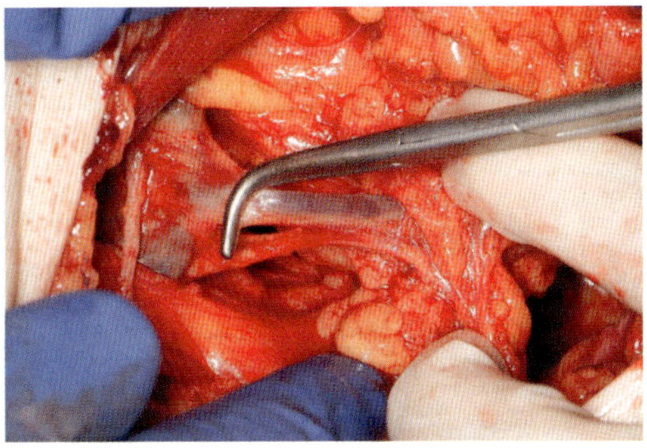

FIG 19 ● The thoracoepigastric vein is the only superficial tributary of the axillary vein and should be ligated with clips or ties.

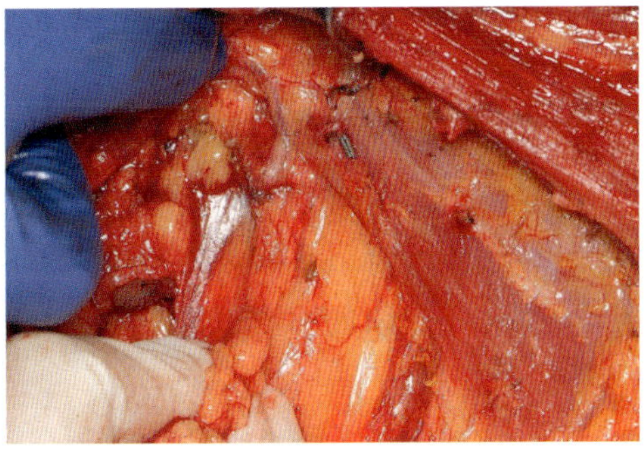

A

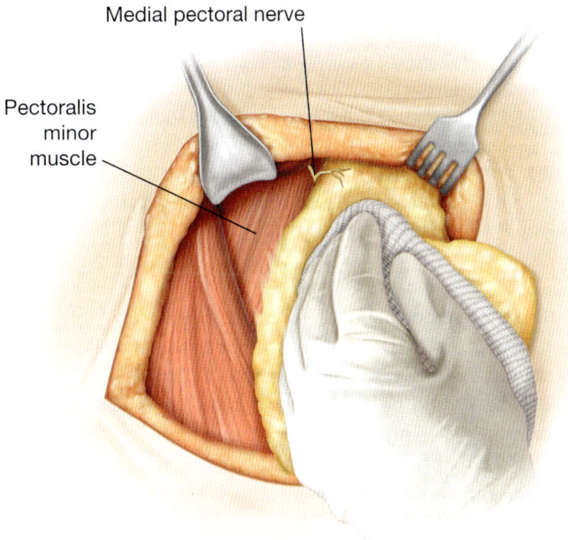

B

FIG 20 ● **A,B.** When placing the retractor deep under the muscles, pay careful attention to the medial pectoral bundle to prevent damage to these structures. The medial pectoral nerve wraps around the underside of the pectoralis minor muscle. (Part **B** modified from Donohue JH, Van Heerden J, Monson JRT, eds. *Atlas of Surgical Oncology*. Cambridge, MA: Blackwell Science; 1995. Used with permission of Mayo Foundation for Medical Education and Research. All rights reserved.)

blunt dissection of the axillary fat once the clavipectoral fascia has been divided. Once the vein is identified, the dissection should continue inferiorly to it. The nodal tissue superior to the axillary vein should be preserved to reduce lymphedema and brachial plexus injury. The thoracoepigastric vein is the only superficial tributary of the axillary vein and should be ligated with clips or ties (FIG 19). Before any ligation of this branch is performed, care must be taken to not mistake this vein for the thoracodorsal vein, which lies deep to it. All other lymphatic channels should be clipped and divided using scissors, and superficial branches of the axillary vein should be divided sharply between clips or sutures.

- Level II nodes are located underneath the pectoralis muscle, and level III nodes are located medial to the muscle. Level III nodes are rarely involved in most breast cancer metastasis and are not included in the traditional axillary lymph node dissection.[11] To gain access to the level II nodes, the Richardson retractor should retract the pectoral muscles medially. When placing the retractor deep under the muscles, pay careful attention to the medial pectoral bundle to prevent damage to these structures (FIG 20A,B). The dissection should continue to extend medially along the axillary vein, and the lymphatic tissue on the chest wall should be retracted inferolaterally. This tissue should be dissected off the chest wall with ties or clips to prevent lymphatic leaks.
- The long thoracic nerve lies along the chest wall and is superficial to the investing fascia of the serratus anterior muscle (FIG 21). This nerve can be difficult to identify, and palpation of this nerve can help to recognize it. The nerve feels like a string of spaghetti when running a finger along the serratus anterior muscle. Care should be taken to not retract the nerve off the chest wall with the specimen. If this nerve is inadvertently injured, it will cause patients to have a winged scapula. Dissection of the lymphatic tissue close to the nerve should be done with sharp dissection and not electrocautery.

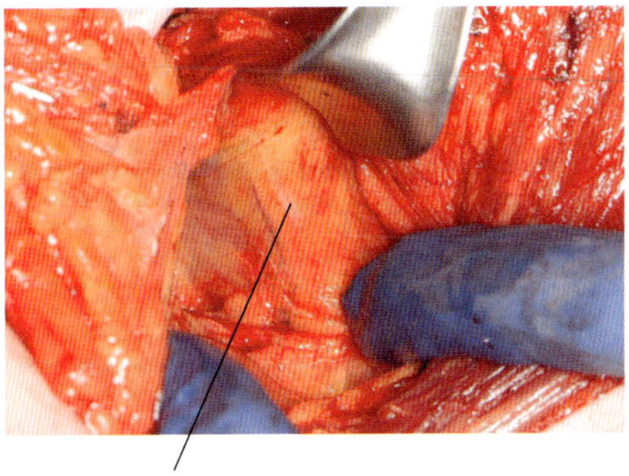

FIG 21 ● The long thoracic nerve lies along the chest wall and is superficial to the investing fascia of the serratus anterior muscle. Care should be taken to not pull the nerve laterally during the axillary dissection. The nerve can be difficult to identify and sometimes will only be felt on palpation. Running a finger along the lateral chest wall can aid in identifying the nerve.

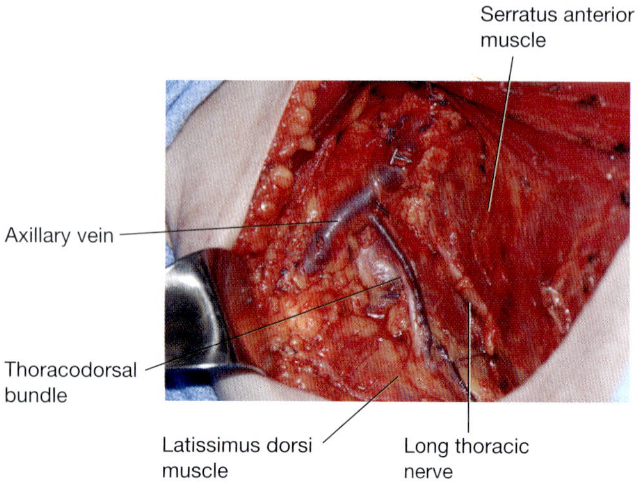

FIG 22 ● The axilla after removal of level I and II lymph nodes, with thoracodorsal bundle and long thoracic nerve and axillary vein intact.

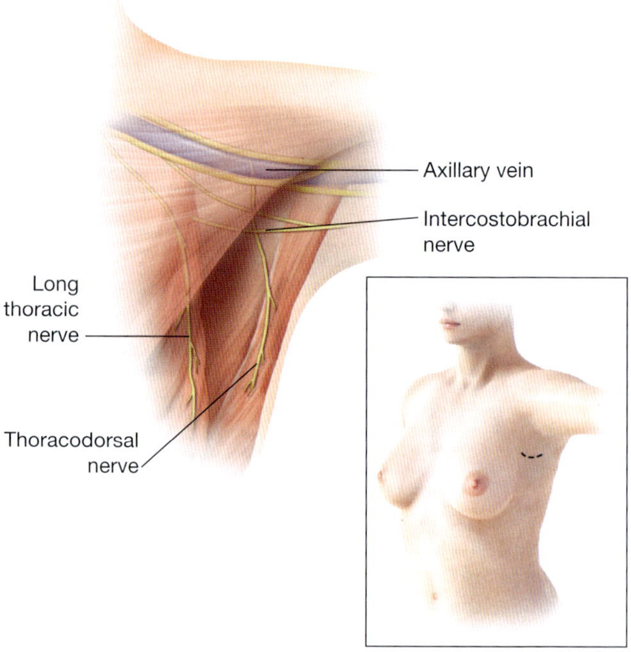

FIG 23 ● Schematic drawing of the relationship of the axillary nerves to each other. The intercostobrachial nerves should be preserved if possible. (Modified from and used with permission of Mayo Foundation for Medical Education Research. All rights reserved.)

- The thoracodorsal bundle is found lateral to the long thoracic nerve. The lymphatic tissue between the two nerves should be dissected and removed. The thoracodorsal bundle should be skeletonized. Any lymphatic channels or superficial branches should be clipped or suture ligated. The branches of the thoracodorsal vein and artery entering the chest medially should be preserved where possible (**FIG 22**).
- Attempts should also be made to try to preserve the intercostobrachial nerves, but if the path of the nerve is directly through the specimen, it can be ligated (**FIG 23**). Patients should know that the intercostobrachial nerves may need to be sacrificed preoperatively, and explain to them that ligating the nerve will cause loss of sensation to their upper inner arm.
- The breast and attached nodal tissue should be excised en bloc by dividing the remaining lateral pedicle. The specimen should be sent to pathology with sutures placed for orientation (**FIG 24**).

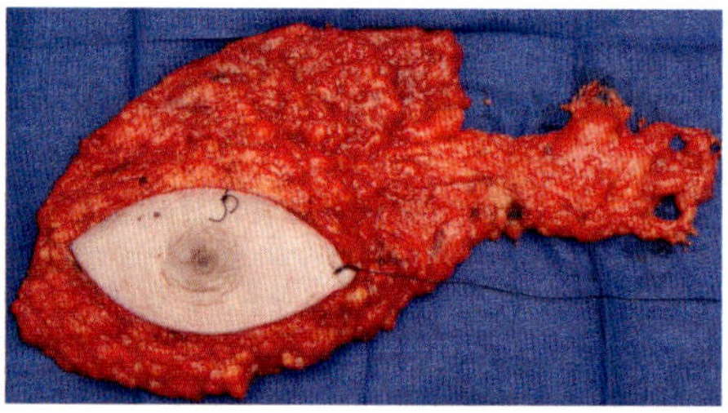

FIG 24 ● Suture orientation should be done before the specimen is passed off to pathology. A short stitch should be placed superiorly and a long stitch laterally.

DRAIN PLACEMENT

- Two closed suction drains should be placed to prevent seroma formation. Studies have shown two drains are superior in comparison to one drain placed.[12] One drain should be placed over the pectoralis major muscle and the other drain should be placed in the axillary space (**FIG 25A,B**). The drains should be sutured in place with a monofilament suture and dressed appropriately based on surgical preference.

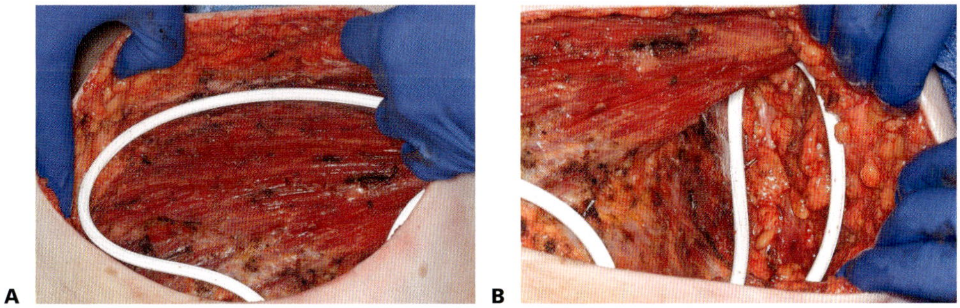

FIG 25 ● **A.** One drain should be placed over the pectoralis major muscle, **(B)** and the other should be placed in the axillary space. The drains should be secured to the skin.

CLOSURE

- A cosmetically pleasing closure is important for psychologic reasons. The goal is to provide a closure that will cause the chest to have a very flat appearance without excess skin redundancy.
- If the skin edges are traumatized, they should be excised with scissors or scalpel. Many times, dog ears appear at the medial and lateral edges of the incision. These should be excised to make the incision have a smoother and flatter appearance. The dermal layer should be closed with an inverted interrupted closure using absorbable suture. INSORB, an absorbable suture stapler, can also be used to close the dermal layer and is a faster alternative to traditional suture closure. The skin should be approximated with an absorbable 4-0 monofilament suture in a running subcuticular closure (**FIG 26**).

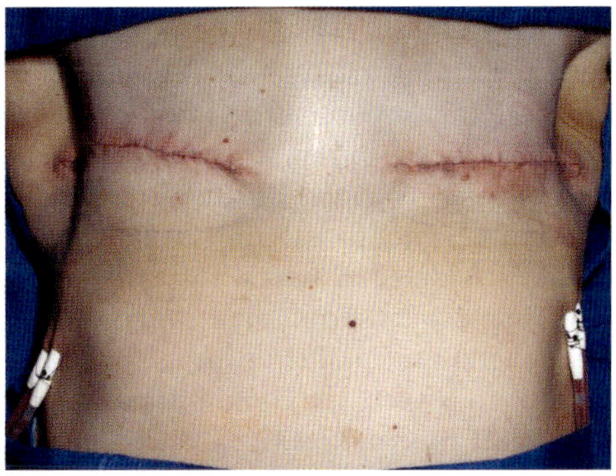

FIG 26 ● A cosmetic closure with a flat-appearing chest wall without skin redundancy is the goal.

PEARLS AND PITFALLS

Indications	■ A comprehensive history and physical examination should be undertaken, as well as review of the radiographic images of the breast and axilla and pathology from all biopsies. Patients with node-positive disease either not amenable to breast conservation or electing mastectomy are candidates for modified radical mastectomy, which encompasses a simple mastectomy together with an axillary lymph node dissection. ■ Once a cancer diagnosis is made, multidisciplinary coordination is essential for successful treatment planning.
Incision placement	■ When choosing an incision for a modified radical mastectomy, the goal is to provide great exposure to the axilla and a good cosmetic outcome. ■ The incision should include a 1- to 2-cm margin around the tumor (if close to the skin) and include the previous biopsy site. ■ The classic Stewart incision is the preferred incision for a modified radical mastectomy providing the necessary exposure and cosmetic outcome.
Flap dissection	■ Flaps should be extended to the borders of the breast tissue. Careful attention needs to be paid to ensure all the breast tissue is resected and the vascular supply to the remaining skin flaps is preserved to avoid flap ischemia.
Axillary lymph node dissection	■ Careful identification of vital structures and the axillary borders will define the dissection. ■ Close attention needs to be paid to the preservation of the axillary vein, thoracodorsal bundle, and long thoracic nerve during the dissection.

Closure	■ The goal is to reduce skin redundancy and create a smooth flat incision. Avoid medial and lateral dog ears. Two closed suction drains should be placed to avoid seroma.
Rehabilitation	■ Patients should have access to counseling or therapy to help in coping with issues of body image. Patients who do not desire reconstruction should also be set up to be fitted for a breast prosthesis. ■ All patients should meet with a lymphedema specialist to coordinate an exercise plan and be provided with compression garments if needed.

POSTOPERATIVE CARE

- Patients after an MRM should be placed in a breast binder or an Ace wrap following their surgery (**FIG 27**). This will provide good compression to prevent development of any hematoma. Steri-Strips or Xeroform dressing can be placed directly over the incisions. Fluffs or Kerlix gauze can be placed over the incision to act as a barrier between the incision and binder.
- Patients who have undergone an MRM will face a variety of rehabilitation issues pertaining to lymphedema, body image, and sexual dysfunction. It is important to have all these concerns addressed preoperatively, during their hospital stay, or at follow-up appointments. The most dreaded complication of having an axillary lymph node dissection is lymphedema. All patients should be scheduled to meet with a lymphedema therapist approximately 2 weeks from their surgery or after drain removal. The therapists can help educate patients on lymphedema and how to prevent the complication and provide them with exercises to avoid restricted shoulder range of motion.
- Patients who have undergone MRM without reconstruction should be referred to be fitted for a breast prosthesis after the drains are removed and the swelling has gone down.

OUTCOMES

- Patients who undergo an MRM are at risk for developing secondary lymphedema. This is one of the most dreaded fears of many breast cancer survivors, and many women are not educated on this complication preoperatively.
- Many patients undergoing an MRM will require postmastectomy radiation. The addition of radiation after a nodal dissection can substantially increase the risk of development of lymphedema to over 40%. Successful diagnosis and treatment of patients suffering from lymphedema should focus on risk-reducing therapies and lifelong self-directed care.[13,14]
- Survival outcomes in patients undergoing MRM are not based solely on the operative procedure but dependent on the tumor stage, nodal stage, and tumor biology. Studies have shown in node-positive patients that the number of positive lymph nodes, patient age, tumor grade, and race are significant variables to affect survival.[15]

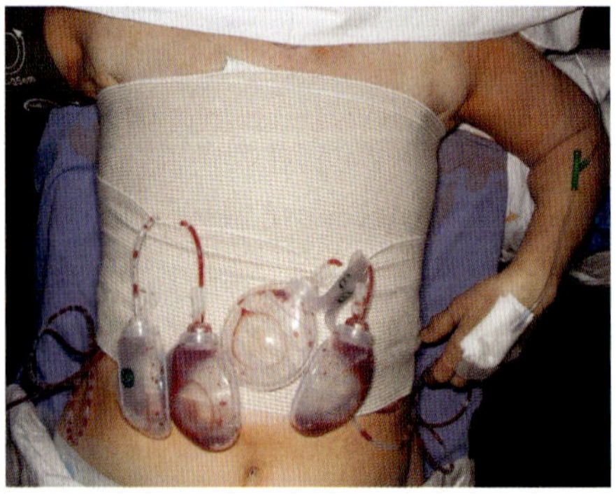

FIG 27 • Patients should be wrapped in an Ace binder or a breast binder to provide compression. The drains should be in view to monitor output and consistency.

COMPLICATIONS

- Seroma
- Wound infection
- Hematoma
- Wound dehiscence
- Flap necrosis
- Positive margins
- Brachial plexus injury
- Nerve injury
- Winged scapula
- Axillary vein thrombosis
- Lymphedema

REFERENCES

1. NCCN clinical practice guidelines in oncology: invasive breast cancer. National Comprehensive Cancer Network. Published 2012. http://www.nccn.org. Accessed January 8, 2013.
2. Kopans DB. The positive predictive value of mammography. *AJR Am J Roentgenol.* 1992;158(3):521–526.
3. Handel N, Silverstein MJ, Gamagami P, et al. Factors affecting mammographic visualization of the breast after augmentation mammaplasty. *JAMA.* 1992;268(14):1913–1917.
4. Exadaktylos AK, Buggy DJ, Moriarty DC, et al. Can anesthetic technique for primary breast cancer surgery affect recurrence or metastasis? *Anesthesiology.* 2006;105(4):660–664.
5. Coveney E, Weltz CR, Greengrass R, et al. Use of paravertebral block anesthesia in the surgical management of breast cancer: experience in 156 cases. *Ann Surg.* 1998;227(4):496–501.
6. Kairaluoma PM, Bachmann MS, Rosenberg PH, et al. Preincisional paravertebral block reduces the prevalence of chronic pain after breast surgery. *Anesth Analg.* 2006:103(3):703–708.
7. Tejirian T, DiFronzo LA, Haigh PI. Antibiotic prophylaxis for preventing wound infection after breast surgery: a systematic review and metaanalysis. *J Am Coll Surg.* 2006:203(5):729–734.
8. Dalberg K, Johansson H, Signomklao T, et al. A randomized study of axillary drainage and pectoral fascia preservation after mastectomy for breast cancer. *Eur J Surg Oncol.* 2004;30(6):602–609.
9. Dalberg K, Krawiec K, Sandelin K. Eleven-year follow-up of a randomized study of pectoral fascia preservation after mastectomy for early breast cancer. *World J Surg.* 2010;34(11):2539–2544.

10. Ung O, Tan M, Chua B, et al. Complete axillary dissection: a technique that still has relevance in contemporary management of breast cancer. *ANZ J Surg*. 2006;76(6):518–521.
11. Rosen PP, Lesser ML, Kinne DW, et al. Discontinuous or "skip" metastases in breast carcinoma. Analysis of 1228 axillary dissections. *Ann Surg*. 1983;197(3):276–283.
12. Terrell GS, Singer JA. Axillary versus combined axillary and pectoral drainage after modified radical mastectomy. *Surg Gynecol Obstet*. 1992;175(5):437–440.
13. Herd-Smith A, Russo A, Muraca MG, et al. Prognostic factors for lymphedema after primary treatment of breast carcinoma. *Cancer*. 2001;92(7):1783–1787.
14. Aitken RJ, Gaze MN, Rodger A, et al. Arm morbidity within a trial of mastectomy and either nodal sample with selective radiotherapy or axillary clearance. *Br J Surg*. 1989;76(6):568–571.
15. Fisher ER, Anderson S, Redmond C, et al. Pathologic findings from the National Surgical Adjuvant Breast Project protocol B-06. 10-year pathologic and clinical prognostic discriminants. *Cancer*. 1993;71(8):2507–2514.

Chapter 13

Techniques for Correcting Lumpectomy Defects

Julie E. Park Jonathan Bank David H. Song

DEFINITION

- Breast conservation therapy (BCT), the combination of lumpectomy and breast radiation, allows women with breast cancer to avoid mastectomy without compromising outcome. Although the majority of women will have an excellent cosmetic outcome, some women will develop asymmetry from volume loss and postradiation contour deformity and nipple–areolar complex (NAC) deviation. Several techniques exist for correcting lumpectomy defects to allow for oncologically sound and aesthetically acceptable BCT.

PATIENT HISTORY AND PHYSICAL FINDINGS

- In some situations, the plastic surgeon is asked to evaluate the patient prior to lumpectomy in order to plan for an immediate correction. In other situations, the patient is referred to plastic surgery after radiation therapy for correction of postradiation contour deformity and NAC deviation.
- It is important to discuss with the patient her expectations; specifically, whether she would accept a smaller breast.
- Does the patient have symptomatic macromastia and would she benefit from, or be interested in, breast reduction?
- Does the patient smoke? This might impact nipple perfusion.
- A thorough breast examination should take note of the breast size and any preexisting asymmetry. Any previous scars or contour deformities should be noted, especially in women who have already completed BCT.
- It is also important to document the position of the nipple, including any ptosis, and the distance from the sternal notch.
- For patients anticipated to have a significant deformity from BCT, a multidisciplinary approach is critical to achieving the optimal cosmetic outcome. Communication with the surgical oncologist is critical to both identifying appropriate patients, planning the site and expected volume of resection, and coordinating schedules. It is important to identify with the radiation oncologist if the patient will require a "boost," as this will limit how much tissue can be rearranged. In cases of wire-localized lumpectomy, marks should be placed prior to wire placement and this should be coordinated with the breast radiologist.

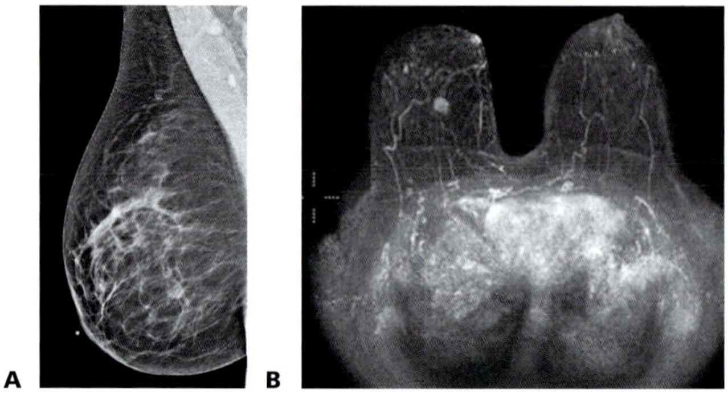

FIG 1 • Mammogram **(A)** and MRI **(B)** of patient with 1.1 × 1.0 × 0.8 cm right-sided breast cancer at 5 o'clock position.

IMAGING AND OTHER DIAGNOSTIC STUDIES

- Almost all patients who have undergone BCT should have had bilateral mammography as part of the workup (**FIG 1A**), and some women may have had magnetic resonance imaging (MRI) (**FIG 1B**).

SURGICAL MANAGEMENT

Preoperative Planning

- The goals of correcting lumpectomy defects include obliterating any dead space, supporting the NAC and maintaining adequate perfusion, and resecting any excess skin.
- There are two main options for reconstructing a lumpectomy defect. ***Volume displacement*** techniques use parenchymal remodeling (volume shrinkage). ***Volume replacement*** techniques use both local and distant tissue to preserve volume.
- After reviewing the preoperative imaging and discussing with the surgical oncologist, the next question is whether given the size and location of the tumor, will there be sufficient tissue in the breast to rearrange and obliterate dead space without losing too much volume?
  - Yes—volume displacement: reduction, mastopexy, or intrinsic breast flaps
  - No—volume replacement: local rotational flaps
    - Thoracodorsal artery perforator (TAP) or muscle-sparing latissimus dorsi (MSLD) flap
    - Lateral intercostal artery perforator (LICAP) flap

Positioning

- The patient is positioned supine with the arms secured to the arm boards at the side to allow for sitting the patient up during the surgery (**FIG 2**). The arms should be place on padded arm boards and positioned in a way that pressure points are alleviated.

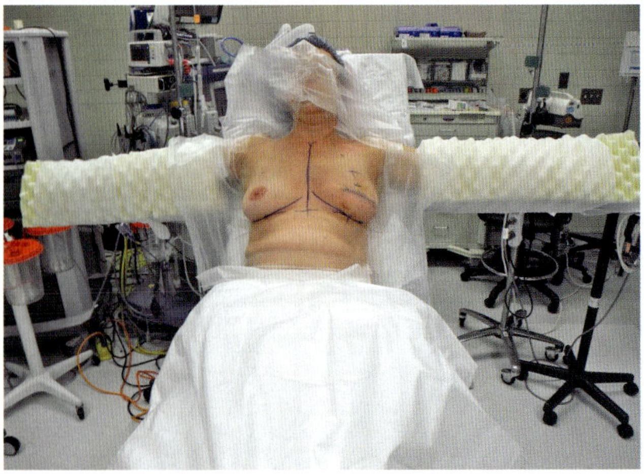

FIG 2 • Positioning of a patient with both arms abducted, padded, and secured, enabling seating the patient during surgery to assess for symmetry of reconstruction.

FREESTYLE INTRINSIC BREAST FLAPS

- For some defects, dermatoglandular flaps can be created to fill small defects. Depending on the location, even small defects can lead to unfavorable cosmetic results, particularly a significant concavity at the site of the lumpectomy after radiation. This can occur when there is minimal tissue between the skin and underlying muscle.
- The principle of intrinsic breast flaps is to focus on perfusion and support to the NAC and to obliterate the dead space.
- The lumpectomy cavity is examined to evaluate how much dead space there is and the remainder of the breast is assessed for where there is extra tissue (**FIG 4A**). An intrinsic breast flap is created by dissecting between the skin and breast parenchyma and between the breast parenchyma and pectoralis (**FIG 4B**). The flaps are based either on axial blood supply from perforators originating from the internal mammary artery or from the intercostal vessels. As these vessels are not typically identified in the dissection, the flaps should be created as random pattern flaps, adhering to the principles of creating broad-based flaps that are not too lengthy as to put the distal tip of the flap at risk of ischemia. The flap is then advanced and secured to fill the lumpectomy cavity and to maintain support to NAC (**FIG 4C**).
- Any excess skin is resected and the wound is closed.

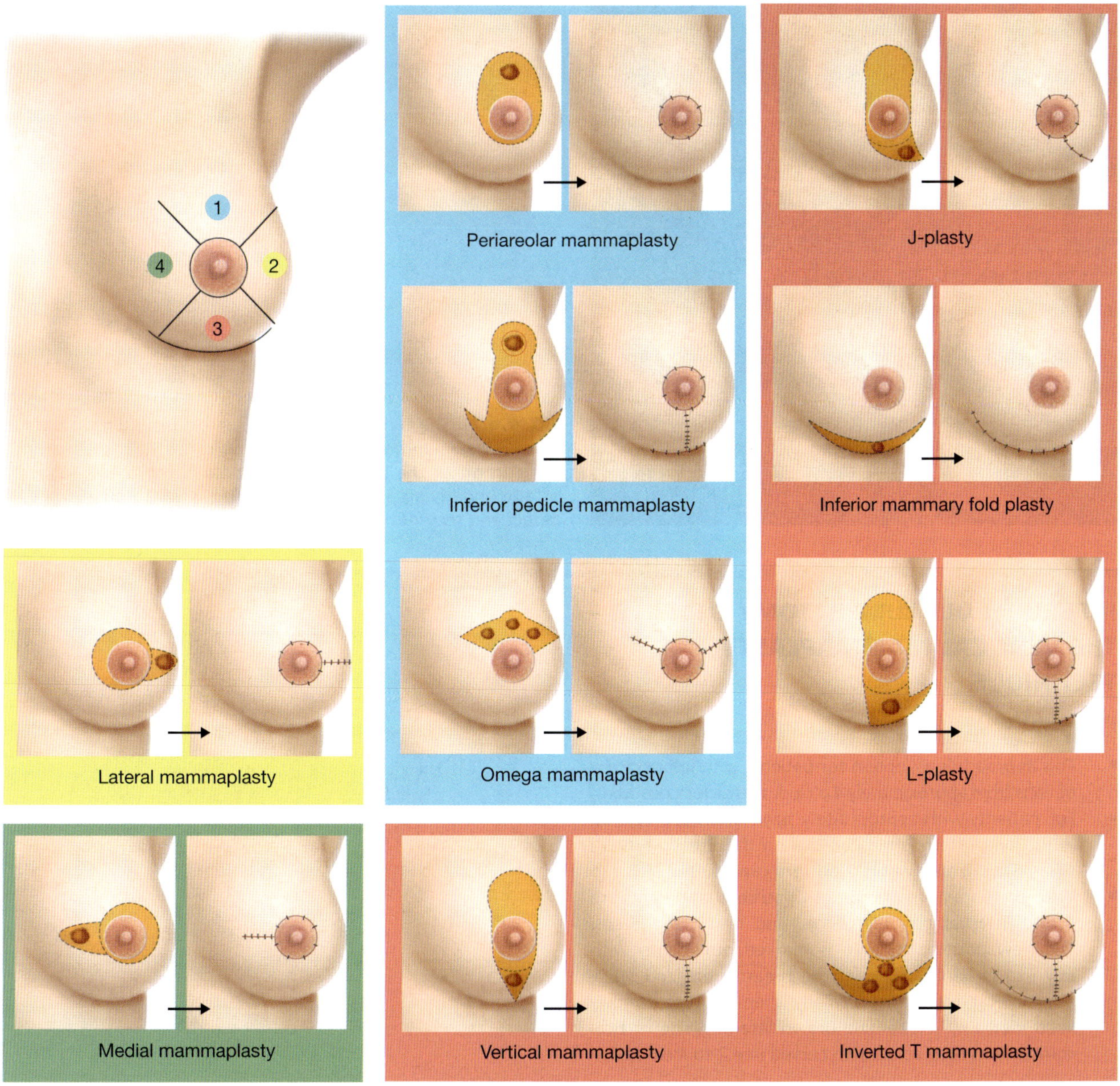

FIG 3 • There are multiple options for skin incisions for resections depending on the location of the defect, size of the defect, and size of the breast.

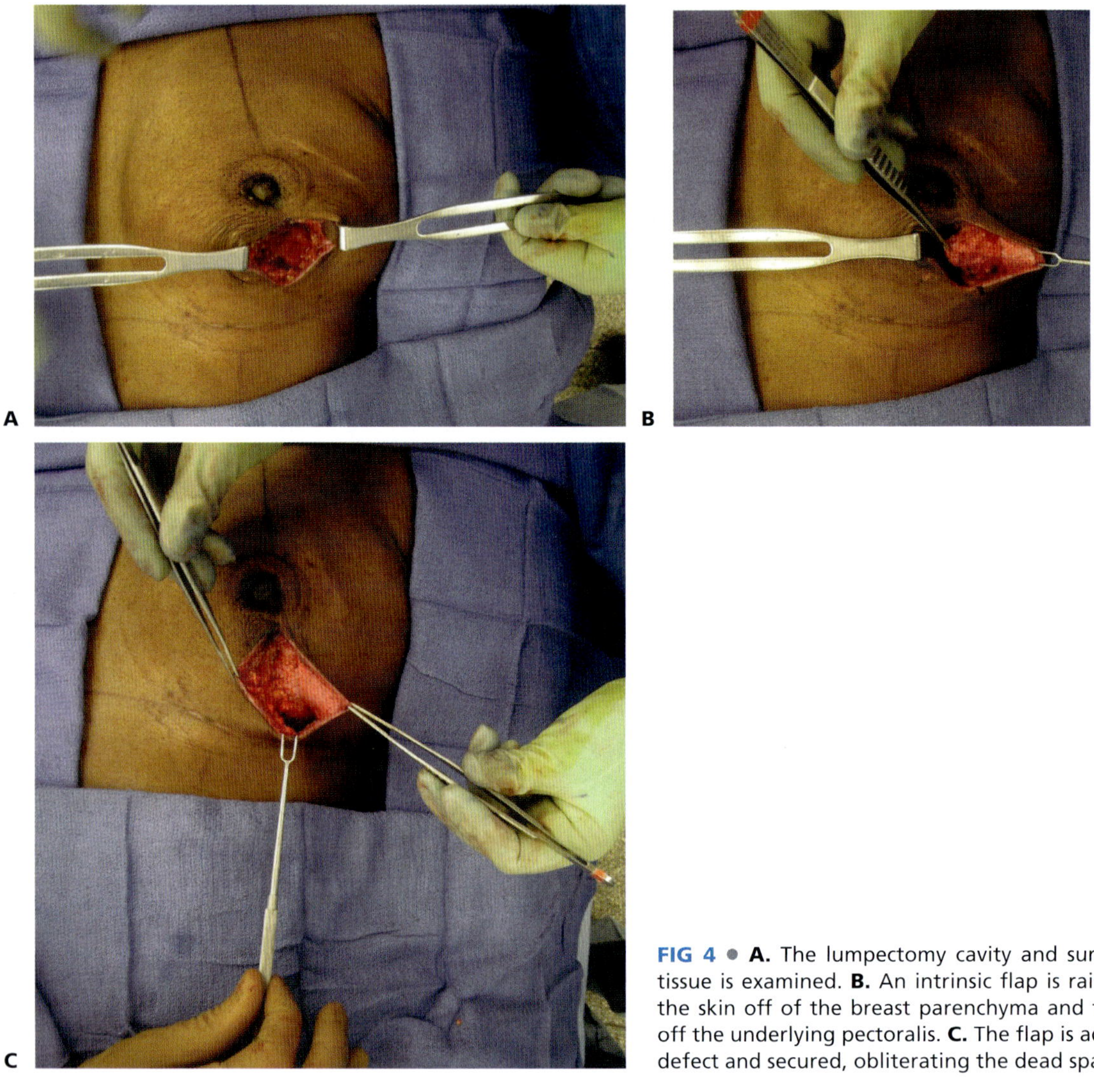

FIG 4 ● **A.** The lumpectomy cavity and surrounding breast tissue is examined. **B.** An intrinsic flap is raised by elevating the skin off of the breast parenchyma and the breast tissue off the underlying pectoralis. **C.** The flap is advanced into the defect and secured, obliterating the dead space.

INFERIOR POLE LUMPECTOMY DEFECTS—THE VERTICAL MAMMAPLASTY TECHNIQUE

Preoperative Marking

- This approach is an option for patients with lumpectomy defects from approximately 4 o'clock to 8 o'clock positions.
- For patients with appropriately sized breasts, a vertical reduction pattern is marked out on the breast (FIG 5). Alternatively, an inverted T pattern can be used.
- With the patient in the upright position, landmarks are drawn—sternal notch, midline, and breast meridians. The new position of NAC is marked out, along with any excess skin as follows: the breast mobilized laterally, vertical line drawn medially, then the breast mobilized medially, vertical line drawn laterally. The vertical components connected with curved line 2 to 4 cm above

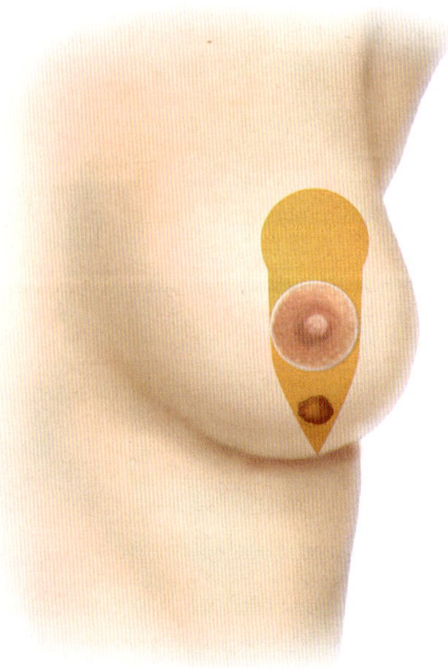

FIG 5 ● A vertical reduction pattern.

the inframammary fold (IMF). A mosque-shaped marking is drawn for inset of NAC.

Assess Lumpectomy Defect and Nipple–Areolar Complex

- In the operating room, the prior lumpectomy cavity is opened and the seroma evacuated. As there will no longer be a seroma to guide radiation, it is a good idea to place several small clips at the boundaries of the lumpectomy defect.
- Confirm perfusion and support to NAC and make sure that the lumpectomy cavity is not undermining the NAC. If it is, you need to plan on supporting it with intrinsic breast tissue. If this is not possible, a free nipple graft (FNG) will be needed: The NAC is excised as a full-thickness skin graft, defatted, replaced on a well-vascularized bed in the appropriate position on the breast mound, and secured in place with a bolster dressing.

Convert to Vertical Reduction

- Additional (i.e., more than the lumpectomy) breast tissue is resected as needed to allow for an acceptable final shape. Undermining of the breast off of the pectoralis is usually confined to inferior breast. Tissue is resected medial and lateral to vertical incision to allow "rounding off" of the breast. The parenchyma is approximated centrally (approximating the medial and lateral remaining portions of the breast—the medial and lateral "pillars").
- Skin closure—excessed gathered in subcuticular closure. A small horizontal excision is made along the IMF if needed to further reduce the skin.
- This approach will result in volume loss, so a contralateral reduction will be needed in the future, approximately 3 to 6 months after radiation therapy has been completed.

VOLUME REPLACEMENT PEDICLED FLAPS

- For patients with larger defects for which displacement techniques would not work, replacement techniques may be necessary. Pedicled flaps are recommended. Free tissue transfer is not initially recommended in this situation, as it eliminates the use of a flap in the future should the patient have a local recurrence or new tumor and require a mastectomy. Free flaps should only be considered if pedicled flaps are not feasible or fail.
- Flaps can be raised from the axillary and back region (thoracodorsal, intercostal) or from the upper abdomen (superior epigastric). The two most common types of pedicled flaps are (**FIG 6**) as follows:
  - Thoracodorsal artery perforator (TAP) flap, which is based on the perforators from the descending or the horizontal branches of the thoracodorsal vessels. This is most suitable for superior defects.
  - LICAP flap, which is based on perforators arising from the costal groove. This is a good alternative to the TAP flap for lateral and inferior breast defects.
  - Defects in the medial quadrant can be approached via an anterior intercostal artery perforator (AICAP) flap, which is supplied by perforators originating from the muscular segment, or the superior epigastric artery perforator (SEAP) flap, based on perforators from the superior epigastric. These are not described here.

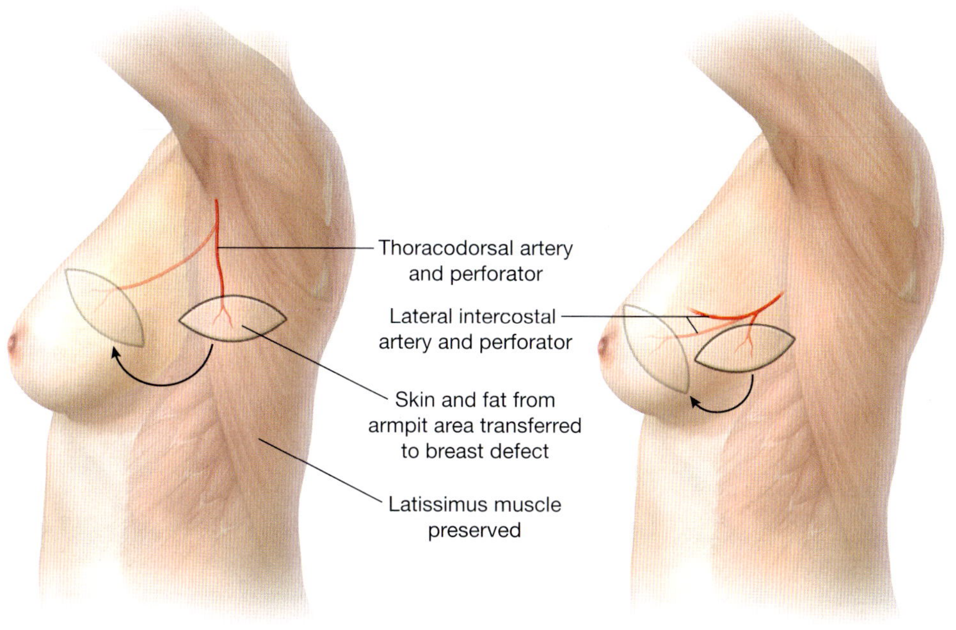

FIG 6 • The TAP and LICAP flaps.

SUPERIOR-LATERAL LUMPECTOMY DEFECTS—THE THORACODORSAL ARTERY PERFORATOR FLAP OR MUSCLE-SPARING LATISSIMUS DORSI FLAP

Preoperative Marking

- Preoperatively, the patient should be marked in the supine and upright position. Several anatomic landmarks should be identified and marked.
  - The borders of the breast, including the IMF, should be marked. The ideal position of the NAC should be drawn using the contralateral breast as a template. This will need to be adjusted accordingly if there is a plan to either lift or reduce the contralateral breast.
  - Identify and mark the tip of scapula and the anterior edge of the latissimus dorsi muscle.
  - A ***pinch test*** should then be performed to determine the amount of redundant skin in order to determine the size of flap.
- The perforator will determine the viability of the flap and knowing its location will reduce operating time and complications. The perforator emerges approximately 8 to 10 cm from the posterior axillary crease and 2 cm posterior to anterior border of the latissimus (**FIG 7**). This can be confirmed and the perforator marked in the preoperative area with a Doppler ultrasound device.
- Based on this exam, the surgeon should anticipate how to orient the flap.
  - Horizontal—"bra line"
  - Obliquely—line of relaxed skin tension
  - Vertically—along anterior edge of latissimus

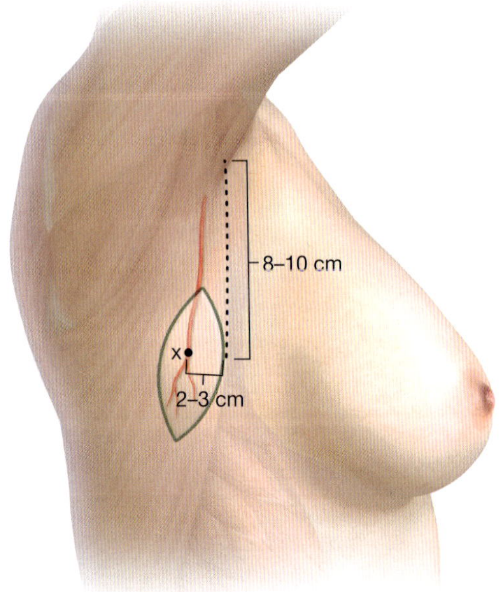

FIG 7 • The patient is placed in the lateral decubitus position to locate the perforators and design the flap. The *dotted line* is the anterior border of the latissimus dorsi muscle. "X" marks the main perforator artery for the flap, located 2 to 3 cm from the anterior margin of latissimus and 8 to 10 cm from the posterior axillary crease.

Intraoperative Assessment and Creation of Lateral Tunnel

- The patient should be placed on a beanbag. Initially, the patient will be supine. Both breasts are sterilely prepped into the field.
- The prior cavity should be opened and the seroma evacuated. At this point, multiple small clips are placed to mark all the boundaries of the lumpectomy defect. These are important for radiation oncology to know where the lumpectomy cavity was, as there will no longer be a seroma for guidance.
- The NAC should be examined to confirm perfusion and support. It is important to make sure the lumpectomy is not undermining the NAC. Otherwise, this will require support with intrinsic breast tissue. If there is insufficient tissue for perfusion, an FNG may be necessary.
- Assess the total volume of tissue that will be needed to fill the space.
- A tunnel is then created from the lumpectomy cavity to the anterior edge of the latissimus muscle.
- Once the latissimus muscle is identified, the skin edges are temporarily reapproximated with skin staples and the wound is covered with a large sterile occlusive dressing (i.e., Ioban).

Flap Creation

- The patient is repositioned in the lateral decubitus position. All pressure points are appropriately padded and the operative field is again sterilely prepped and draped.
- The perforating vessels are identified using a handheld pencil Doppler. Once the perforators have been identified, the flap position is adjusted as necessary.
- The skin of the flap is incised with a scalpel, beveling so as to capture as much sub–Scarpa's fat as needed. Dissection is then carried down to the muscle.
- Dissect from the midline anteriorly until the perforators are identified (**FIG 8**). The latissimus dorsi fascia should be included with the flap. Complete dissection from anterior to midline is necessary to isolate the perforators.

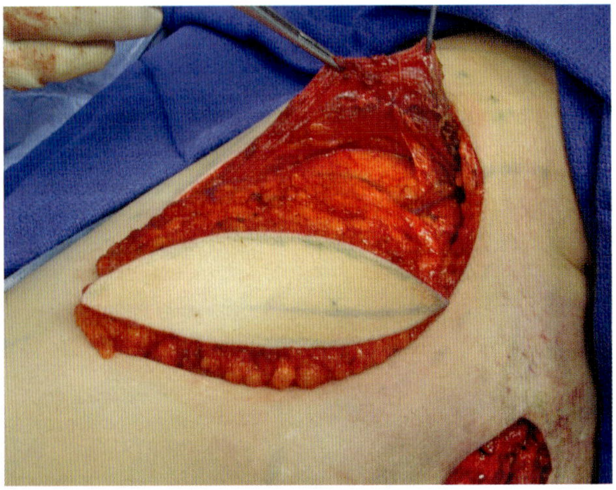

FIG 8 • The latissimus dorsi muscle is completely dissected from anterior to midline in order to identify the perforators.

- At this point, it becomes necessary to decide between a TAP flap and an MSLD flap based on the perfusion of the tissues, especially the venous drainage.
  - For a TAP flap, just one perforator is isolated. The muscle is then split and the descending branch of the thoracodorsal artery is dissected to the takeoff point of the transverse branch of the thoracodorsal.
  - For an MSLD flap, multiple perforators within 1 to 3 cm of the anterior edge of the latissimus need to be captured. Harvest the descending branch of the thoracodorsal artery at the takeoff point of the transverse branch.

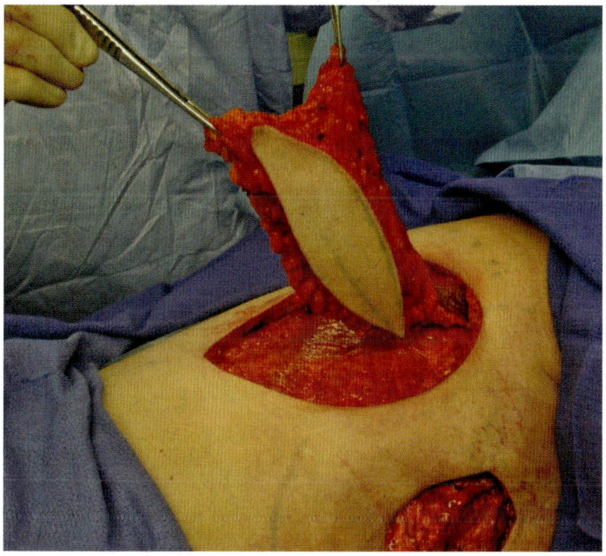

FIG 9 ● Once the flap has been elevated, a drain is placed and the skin is reapproximated. The patient is then repositioned supine.

- Once the flap has been created (**FIG 9**), a drain is placed and the skin is reapproximated. Sterile dressings are applied.

Flap Insertion

- The patient is repositioned supine, with the arms secured to the arm boards to that the table can be flexed and the two breasts compared with the patient in the upright position.
- The flap is inset in order to fill the volume defect. It is important that the NAC be supported.
- It is often necessary to de-epithelialize the skin, but a small skin island should be maintained in order to monitor the flap. The patient should be monitored in the hospital for 1 to 2 days postoperatively (**FIG 10**).

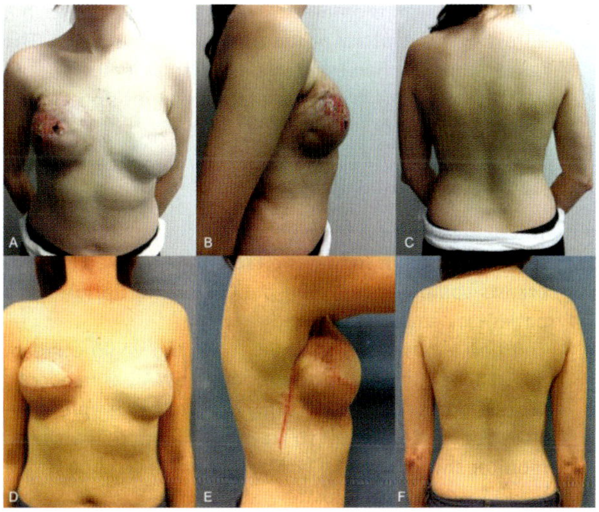

FIG 10 ● After a poor outcome with a superior lateral lumpectomy **(A–C)**, the defect was corrected using a TAP **(D–F)**.

LATERAL LUMPECTOMY DEFECTS—THE LATERAL INTERCOSTAL ARTERY PERFORATOR FLAP

Preoperative Markings

- The borders of the breast, including the IMF, should be marked. The ideal position of the NAC should be drawn, using the contralateral breast as a template. This will need to be adjusted accordingly if there is a plan to either lift or reduce the contralateral breast.
- Identify and mark at least 5 cm posterior to axillary line at the level of the future defect. (This marking is posterior to the LICAP and thus will ensure inclusion of the perforator in the flap.)
- Mark perforator with handheld pencil Doppler.

Intraoperative Assessment

- The patient is placed supine with a beanbag on the table. Both breasts are prepped and draped into the field.
- The prior lumpectomy cavity is opened and the seroma is evacuated. Multiple small clips are placed to mark all the boundaries of the lumpectomy defect. These are important for radiation oncology to know where the lumpectomy cavity was, as there will no longer be a seroma for guidance.
- Assess the total volume of tissue that will be needed to fill the space.
- The NAC should be examined to confirm perfusion and support. It is important to make sure the lumpectomy is not undermining the NAC. Otherwise, this will require support with intrinsic breast tissue.
- The skin is then temporarily closed with staples and covered with a large sterile occlusive dressing (i.e., Ioban).

Locate Perforators

- The patient is repositioned in the decubitus position. All pressure points are carefully padded and the patient is sterilely prepped and draped.
- A handheld pencil Doppler is used to locate the perforators. It may be necessary to adjust the flap position based on the location of the perforators.

Make Skin Incision

- An elliptical incision starting approximately 5 cm posterior to the axillary fold is created at the level of the defect.
- Bevel to capture as much of the sub–Scarpa's fat as needed, and then the incision is deepened to expose the latissimus dorsi muscle.

Identify Perforators

- The dissection is carried from the midline in the anterior direction until the perforators are found. The smaller posterior branch of the lateral cutaneous branch will be identified at the anterior border of the latissimus and this can be traced to find the larger anterior branch (**FIG 11**).
- The latissimus dorsi muscle belly is retracted and a pedicle of 3 to 5 cm is obtained. This is adequate to reach a defect over the lateral or superior part of the breast. The fascia should be harvested into the flap as well.
- A Jackson-Pratt (JP) drain is placed, the incision closed, and the donor site is dressed.

Rotate the Flap Anteriorly and Inset

- The patient is repositioned supine with the arms secured to the arm boards so that the table can be flexed and the breasts compared with the patient sitting upright. The patient is again prepped and draped.
- The flap is now inset in order to fill the volume defect (**FIG 12**). It is important to support the NAC as needed.
- A good portion of the skin may need to be de-epithelialized, but it is important to leave a skin island in order to monitor the flap (**FIG 13**). The patient should be monitored for 1 to 2 days postoperatively.

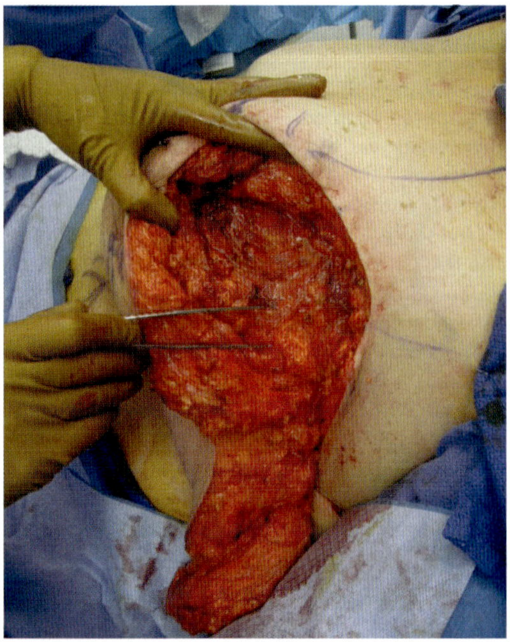

FIG 11 ● The smaller posterior branch of the lateral cutaneous branch will be identified at the anterior border of the latissimus and this can be traced to find the larger anterior branch.

A

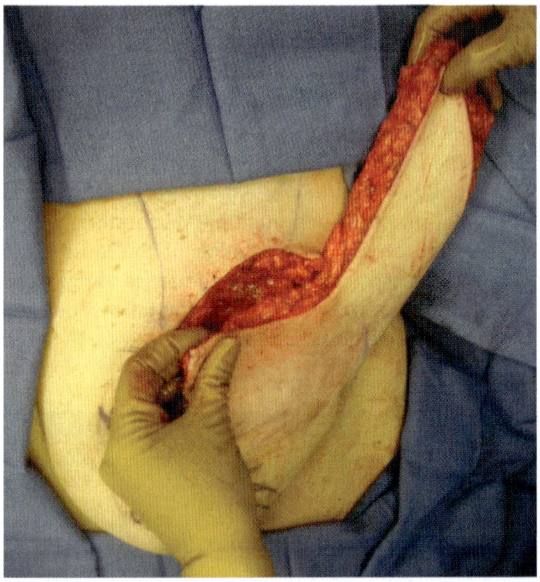

B

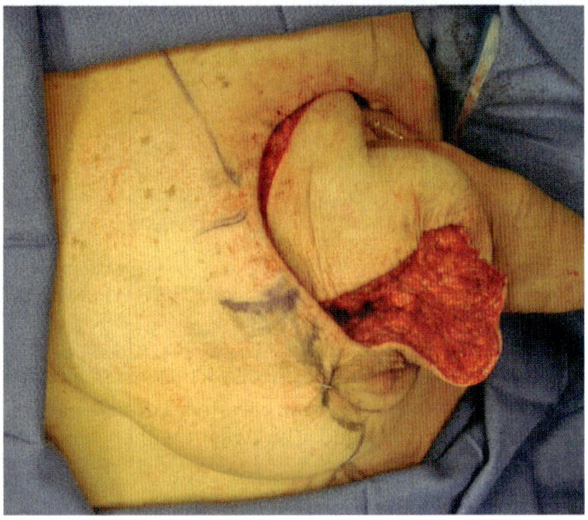

FIG 12 ● The LICAP flap is now inset in order to fill the volume defect.

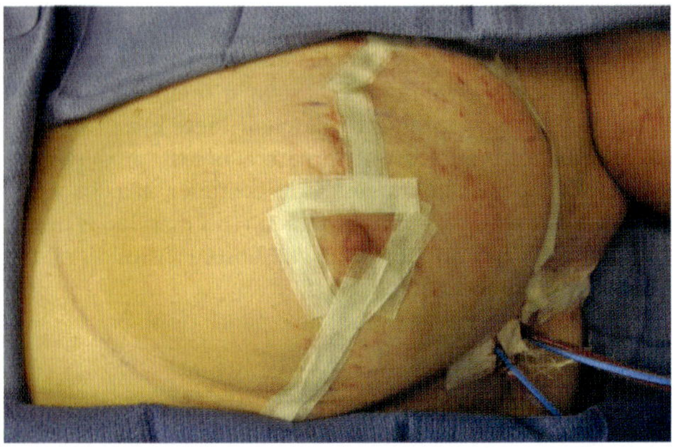

FIG 13 ● After the flap is inset, the skin is de-epithelialized except for a small skin island and the skin is then reapproximated.

CENTRAL LUMPECTOMY INCLUDING THE NIPPLE–AREOLAR COMPLEX

Preoperative Marking

- With the patient in the upright position, the new position of NAC is marked out, along with any excess skin.
- An inferior pedicle reduction pattern is marked out (**FIG 14**).

Assess Lumpectomy Defect and Nipple–Areolar Complex

- In the operating room, the prior lumpectomy cavity is opened and the seroma evacuated. As there will no longer be a seroma to guide radiation, it is a good idea to place several small clips at the boundaries of the lumpectomy defect.

Convert Reduction with Inferior Pedicle

- An inferior pedicle is designed to convert this to a reduction (**FIG 15**).
- A neoareola is created by leaving a skin paddle on the pedicle that will fill in the previous NAC when the pedicle is advanced superiorly.
- An inferior pedicle is created and advanced superiorly. Blood supply emanates from pectoral perforators from thoracoacromial artery. The pedicle design has a 3:1 ratio of length:width with a 30-cm maximal length.

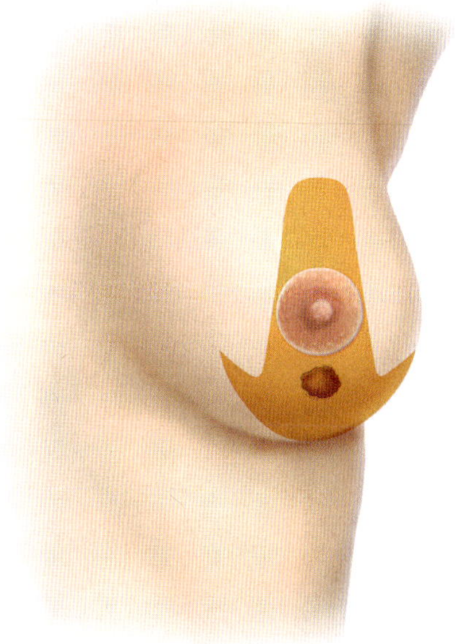

FIG 14 ● An inferior pedicle reduction pattern.

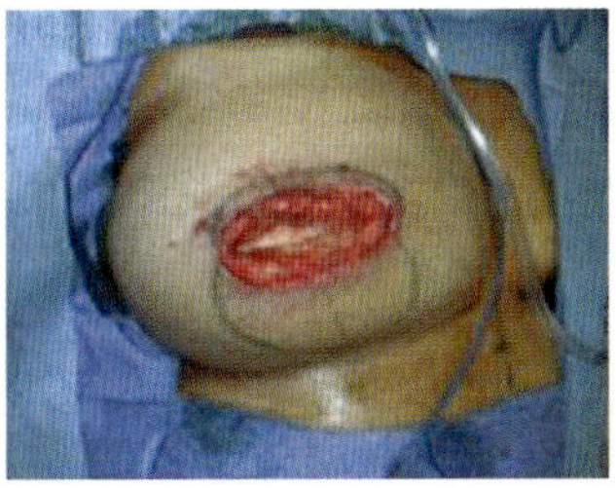

FIG 15 ● After the lumpectomy and NAC have been removed, an inferior pedicle reduction pattern is designed.

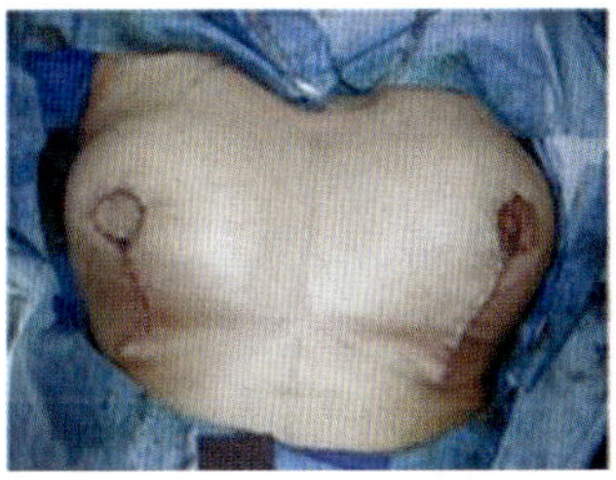

FIG 16 ● A neoareola has been created by leaving a skin paddle on the pedicle and brought out through the new NAC space.

- The skin paddle is brought out in the previous NAC space.
- The excess skin and tissue is excised and the remaining skin is reapproximated (**FIG 16**).

Creation of New Nipple–Areolar Complex

- Three to 6 months after radiation therapy is completed, the patient returns to the operating room for nipple reconstruction as per standard techniques for total breast reconstruction (see Chapter 20). They will also require a contralateral symmetry procedure at that time (**FIG 17**).

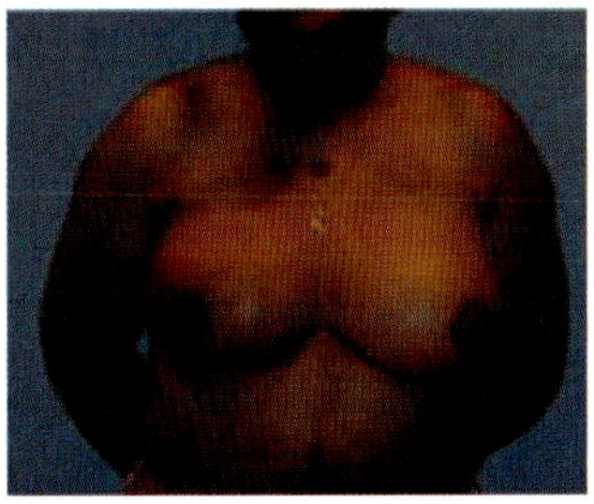

FIG 17 ● After the patient has undergone nipple–areolar reconstruction and contralateral reduction.

PEARLS AND PITFALLS

Timing 6 to 8 weeks to radiation therapy from lumpectomy	▪ Evaluate patient prior to lumpectomy. ▪ Schedule cases simultaneously. ▪ Discuss incision location with oncologic surgeon.
Adjust for postradiation contractures	▪ Likely will have a superior lift—do not err on placement of nipple being too high.
Not as much time for resolution of inferior dog ear	▪ Excise as needed.
Delay contralateral reduction if possible.	▪ Keeps healthy breast tissue out of the field of radiation
Postlumpectomy edema affecting venous perfusion, especially of NAC	▪ Good breast support after lumpectomy ▪ Convert to FNG as needed.
Will lumpectomy resection allow for NAC pedicle?	▪ FNG as needed
Unsure about volume?	▪ Evaluate the lumpectomy during first surgery.

POSTOPERATIVE CARE

- Monitor any flaps for at least 1 to 2 days in the hospital.
- Surgical support bra
- Immediate response to any wound dehiscence or breakdown to avoid delay to radiation therapy
- Consider drain placement to limit postoperative edema (limited time to get patient to radiation therapy)

COMPLICATIONS

- Fat necrosis
- Wound healing complications
- Potential delay to radiation therapy

SUGGESTED READINGS

1. Roughton MC, Shenaq D, Jaskowiak N, et al. Optimizing delivery of breast conservation therapy: a multidisciplinary approach to oncoplastic surgery. *Ann Plast Surg*. 2012;69(3):250–255.
2. Losken A, Styblo TM, Carlson GW, et al. Management algorithm and outcome evaluation of partial mastectomy defects treated using reduction or mastopexy techniques. *Ann Plast Surg*. 2007;59(3):235–242.
3. Hamdi M, Van Landuyt K, Hijjawi JB, et al. Surgical technique in pedicled thoracodorsal artery perforator flaps: a clinical experience with 99 patients. *Plast Reconstr Surg*. 2008;121(5):1632–1641.
4. Hamdi M, Van Landuyt K, de Frene B, et al. The versatility of the inter-costal artery perforator (ICAP) flaps. *J Plast Reconstr Aesthet Surg*. 2006;59(6):644–652.

Chapter **14** Direct-to-Implant Breast Reconstruction

Amy S. Colwell

DEFINITION

- Mastectomy is increasingly performed for breast cancer treatment or risk reduction in high-risk patients. The goal of breast reconstruction is to rebuild the breast and restore a sense of normalcy.

ANATOMY

- The breast glandular tissue extends to the clavicle superiorly, the inframammary fold (IMF) inferiorly, sternum medially, and latissimus dorsi laterally (**FIG 1**). With a skin-sparing or nipple-sparing mastectomy, the glandular tissue is removed and the skin is spared, thus making direct-to-implant breast reconstruction possible. In implant-based breast reconstruction, a space is created underneath the pectoralis muscle, and the serratus anterior is sometimes used to help define the lateral border of the reconstructed breast (**FIG 2**).

NATURAL HISTORY

- Mastectomy offers potential cure in breast cancer patients and prevention for those at high risk for cancer. Immediate breast reconstruction offers an improvement in health-related quality of life and patient satisfaction for women choosing mastectomy as part of their treatment plan.[1–3]

PATIENT HISTORY AND PHYSICAL FINDINGS

- Patient selection in immediate direct-to-implant breast reconstruction is one of the keys to success. A history is obtained to check for comorbidities that are known risk factors for increased complications including smoking, diabetes, body mass index (BMI), and previous breast radiation. On physical exam, the breast is assessed for skin quality, size, scars from previous procedures, symmetry, position of the IMF, and nipple position if a nipple-sparing mastectomy is being considered.

DIFFERENTIAL SURGICAL TREATMENT OPTIONS

- Two-stage tissue expander–implant reconstruction
- Autologous reconstruction using tissue from the body including the abdomen (TRAM, transverse rectus abdominis myocutaneous; DIEP, deep inferior epigastric perforator; SIEA [superficial inferior epigastric artery] flaps), buttocks (SGAP, superior gluteal artery perforator; IGAP [inferior gluteal artery perforator] flaps), thighs (TUG [transverse upper gracilis] flap), and back (latissimus dorsi)
- Fat transfer
- No, or delayed, reconstruction

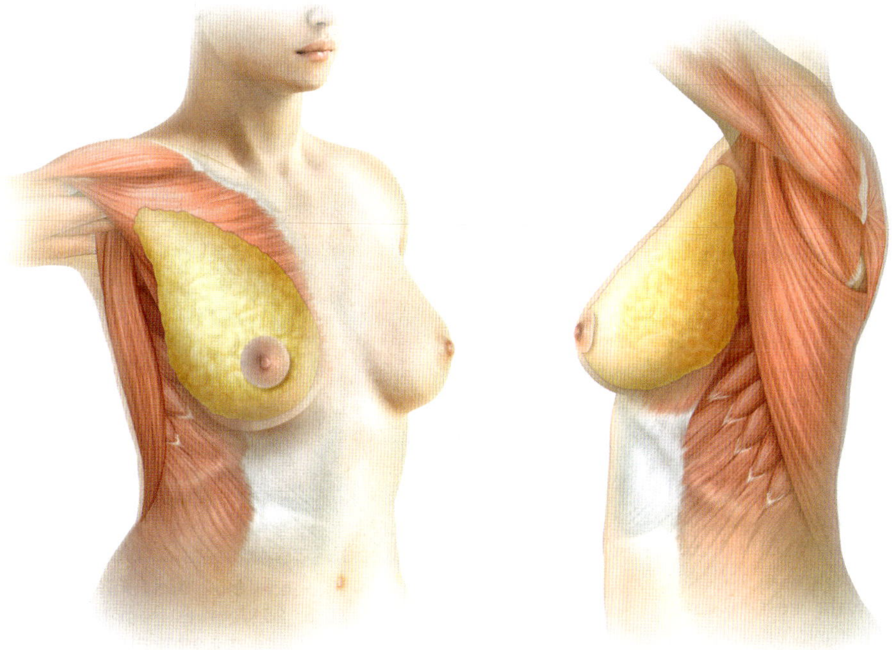

FIG 1 • The anatomic boundaries of the breast are the clavicle, sternum, inframammary fold, and latissimus dorsi.

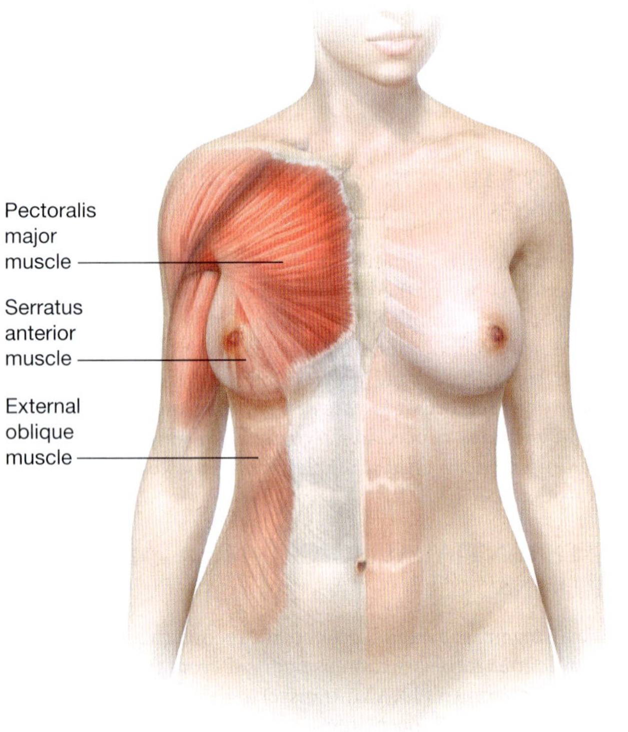

FIG 2 • A plane is created under the pectoralis muscle for implant placement. The pectoralis thus covers the implant superior and medially. The serratus muscle is sometimes elevated for lateral coverage or support.

NONOPERATIVE MANAGEMENT

- Breast reconstruction is a choice, and patients undergoing mastectomy may not elect to pursue reconstruction. If no reconstruction is planned, the breast skin is closed and the chest remains flat in contour. If desired, external breast prostheses are available for women to wear in their clothing to give the appearance of a breast.

SURGICAL MANAGEMENT

- The goals of reconstruction are considered in determining if the reconstruction is designed to augment, reduce, or maintain the current breast size. In general, if a woman wants a significant increase in breast size, this is more safely done in two stages using a tissue expander followed by exchange to implant in a second surgery (see Chapter 15). For single-stage implant reconstruction, the implant is placed directly in a partial subpectoral pocket in order to allow superior soft tissue coverage with muscle in the cleavage area of the breast and to help prevent contracture around the implant.[4] The implant is subcutaneous inferiorly, which allows a more natural teardrop shape, and is typically supported by a surgical acellular dermal matrix (ADM) or mesh. Currently, the most common ADM is AlloDerm (human dermis, LifeCell, Branchburg, NJ), but a variety of ADM or mesh material derived from human dermis, porcine dermis, bovine pericardium, fetal bovine dermis, silk, titanium, and Vicryl exist.

Preoperative Planning

- With immediate implant reconstruction, a foreign body (implant) is placed into a skin envelope that has been partially devascularized with the mastectomy. Therefore, sterility is an important component of preoperative planning and operative management. The patient sits upright and is marked prior to the procedure. Important landmarks include the IMF position, its relation to the IMF on the contralateral breast, and the lateral border of the breast. The mastectomy portion of the procedure is performed first followed by the reconstruction.

Positioning

- The patient is positioned supine with the arms secured on arm boards at the side, angled approximately 80 to 85 degrees from the operating table (**FIG 3**). This allows access to the axillary lymph nodes for sampling during the mastectomy. Both breasts are prepped and draped into the field.

Approach

- The mastectomy and reconstruction may be performed using various incisions. If a nipple-sparing approach is chosen, the safest option is to use a radial lateral incision extending from the areola toward the axilla without a full-thickness incision around the nipple. The incision that maximizes cosmesis is an inferolateral or standard IMF incision under the breast.[5] For skin-sparing mastectomies, the incision is made around the areola and extended laterally if needed for access. For larger breasts, a skin-reducing pattern is designed to remove excess skin in a vertical or horizontal direction. The inverted T/Wise/anchor skin pattern is typically avoided (secondary to higher risk of skin necrosis and complications). The pectoralis muscle is partially released inferiorly to accommodate the implant size and allow more natural breast shape. The challenge of direct-to-implant breast reconstruction is in replacement of the breast volume with an implant that closely matches the breast base diameter but without placing undue stress on the breast skin envelope. If this cannot be achieved in one stage, a two-stage approach is used with a tissue expander intermediary step.

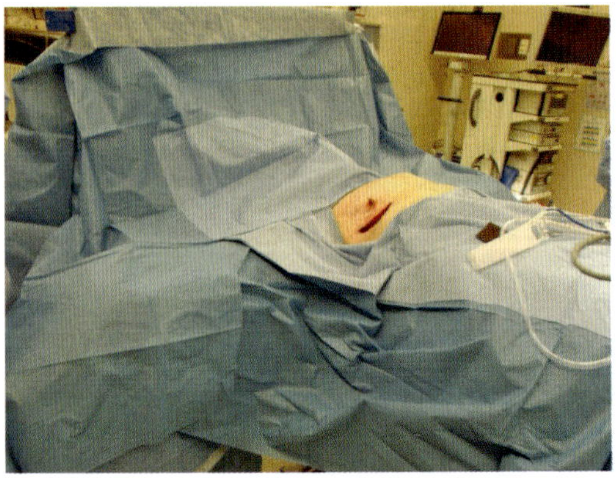

FIG 3 • The patient is positioned supine with arms out on arm boards at approximately 80 to 85 degrees from the operating room table. Care is taken to secure the arms firmly as the back of the operating room table will be raised to a sitting position to check implant placement in the breast pocket while the patient is under anesthesia.

DIRECT-TO-IMPLANT BREAST RECONSTRUCTION WITH PARTIAL PECTORALIS MUSCLE COVERAGE AND ACELLULAR DERMAL MATRIX

- Following mastectomy, the skin is reprepped using a chlorhexidine scrub, and new sterile drapes are placed over the mastectomy drapes. The patient is paralyzed in order to allow easier dissection and pocket creation under the pectoralis muscle. The color of the skin and thickness of the skin flaps are observed to determine if the patient is a candidate for direct-to-implant reconstruction. If there are ischemic changes to the skin marked by pink or blue discoloration, or if the skin flaps are very thin with areas of dermis exposed on the undersurface, it is unlikely that the skin will be able to support the additional stress and weight of a full-size implant at the time of mastectomy. If the skin color is good and the skin flaps have a uniform marbling of subcutaneous fat on the undersurface, then the patient is a candidate for direct-to-implant reconstruction.

Pectoralis Muscle Release

- Using the same access incision used for the mastectomy, the pectoralis muscle is raised from lateral to medial in the loose areolar tissue plane underneath the muscle until the medial origin on the sternum is reached. The pectoralis muscle is then detached from its origin on the external oblique aponeurosis and rectus sheath inferiorly. Dissection continues to the medial muscle origin on the sternum at approximately the 4 o'clock or 8 o'clock position on the chest wall (**FIG 4**) using electrocautery. Inadequate medial release will lead to lateral malposition of the implant. The remaining pectoralis attachment to the sternum is preserved. If necessary, the muscle may be released further to the 3 o'clock or 9 o'clock position on the chest wall to facilitate medial positioning, but this also results in greater pectoralis muscle retraction and thus less muscle coverage over the implant. The pectoralis muscle becomes the superior and medial border of the implant pocket.

Pocket Creation

- Although the pectoralis muscle serves as the superior and medial pocket borders, the inferior and lateral pocket borders are formed by the ADM. The ADM is washed and rehydrated according to the manufacturer. The ADM is then first stitched to the medial border of the released pectoralis muscle (**FIG 5**). If the IMF is intact inferiorly, the ADM is sewn to the IMF using simple buried interrupted sutures. If the IMF is not intact, the ADM is sewn to the chest wall at the desired location for the IMF using a permanent suture (0 Ethibond). Care is taken to leave the ADM loose medially in preparation for accommodating an implant. Laterally, the ADM is sewn to the chest wall at the lateral border of the breast as marked preoperatively or to a raised edge of serratus muscle if the ADM is insufficient in horizontal length. Once the pocket has been created, the base diameter is measured with a ruler to help determine implant choice. A sizer is then placed into the subpectoral, sub-ADM pocket and one or two sutures are placed from the pectoralis muscle to the ADM to keep the sizer in place in the pocket. The skin is stapled shut and the patient is sat upright on the operating room table. The breast reconstruction is observed with different sizer volumes to help determine if it is safe to place an implant, to determine volume, and to assess pocket dimensions.
- The pocket is copiously irrigated with a triple-antibiotic solution of cefazolin, gentamicin, and bacitracin. The surgeon's gloves are changed and the implant is inserted

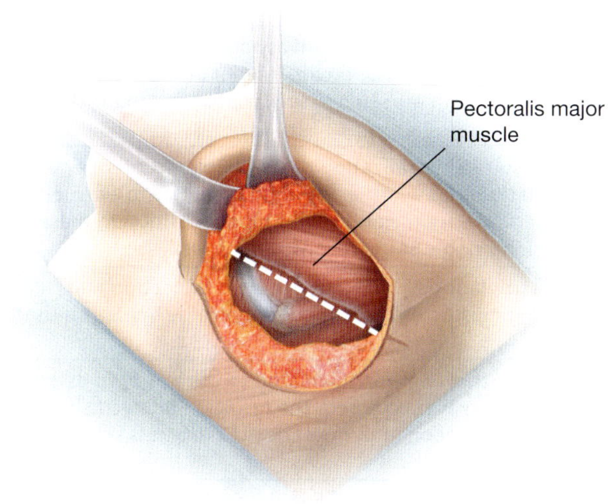

FIG 4 • The pectoralis muscle is released from its insertion inferiorly to the 4 o'clock or 8 o'clock position on the chest wall to allow medial placement of the implant.

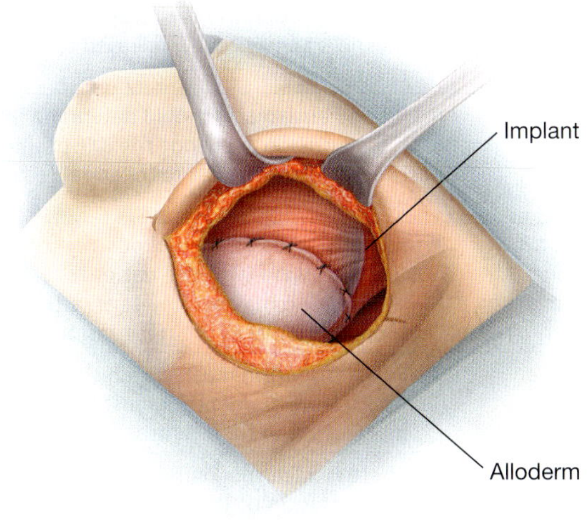

FIG 5 • To create the inferior and lateral portions of the implant pocket, an ADM or scaffold is sewn to the IMF or chest wall inferiorly and laterally. The implant is placed inside the pocket and then the pectoralis-ADM pocket is closed using absorbable sutures.

into the newly created pectoralis-ADM pocket. The pocket is closed using figure-of-eight or horizontal mattress absorbable sutures (2-0 Vicryl) (**FIG 6A,B**). Two closed suction drains are placed with one inside the ADM pocket along the IMF and the other outside the pocket in the axilla. The skin edges are trimmed and closed in two layers. Incisions are sealed with surgical glue (Dermabond) and covered with a clear semipermeable dressing (Tegaderm). A chlorhexidine-impregnated sponge (Biopatch) can be used around the drains. If desired, Microfoam tape can be placed laterally and inferiorly to help support the implant position.

A 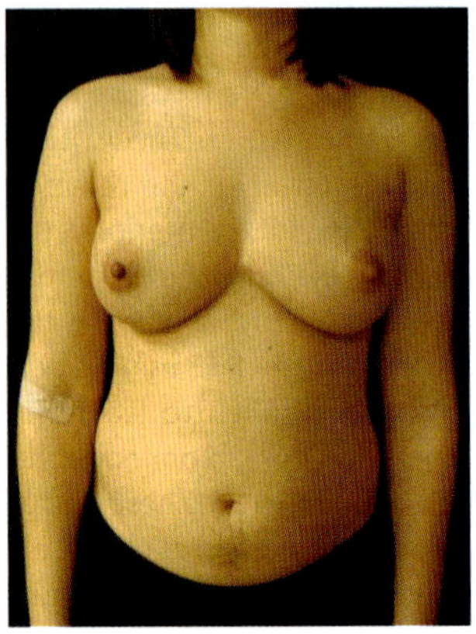

B 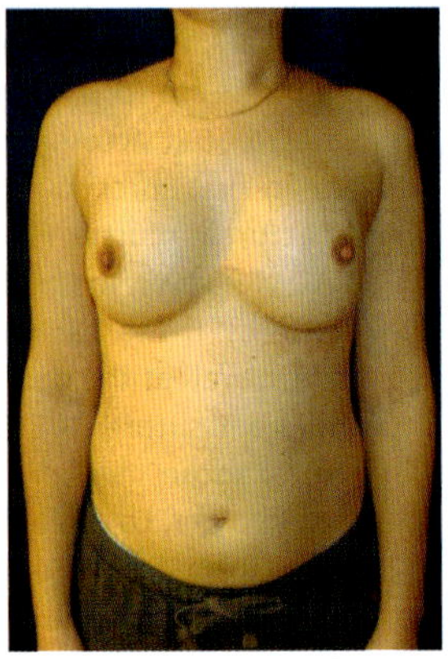

FIG 6 • This 34-year-old female developed breast cancer and had bilateral nipple-sparing mastectomy procedures through inferolateral IMF incisions with single-stage direct-to-implant reconstructions. **A.** Preoperative photo, **(B)** postoperative photo.

DIRECT-TO-IMPLANT BREAST RECONSTRUCTION WITH TOTAL MUSCLE COVERAGE

- Direct-to-implant breast reconstruction with total muscle coverage of the implant is uncommonly performed due to limitations in achievable volume and less desirable implant shape and position. In select patients with small breast volumes, it can be performed by elevating the pectoralis muscle from lateral to the medial sternal origin. The pectoralis may be partially released inferiorly by dissecting through the rectus abdominis fascia centrally to help avoid superior malposition. A serratus flap is raised laterally to form the lateral borders of the implant pocket. Once the implant is placed, the pectoralis-serratus pocket is closed using absorbable sutures.

PEARLS AND PITFALLS

Lateral malposition of implant	▪ Check placement of lateral sutures and determine if lateral border should be medialized to shift implant position. If appropriate, check base diameter of implant to ensure proper fit into pocket. Make sure pectoralis muscle is appropriately released to sternal origin medially and to the 4 o'clock or 8 o'clock position on the chest wall.
Asymmetry of IMF positions	▪ Preoperative marks should determine if the IMF position is similar on the breasts. If asymmetric, a decision is typically made to change the IMF position on one breast to match the other breast. Inferior suture placement is checked on both sides for bilateral reconstruction to make sure both are sewn to similar positions on the chest wall or IMF.
Lateralization of nipples on nipple-sparing mastectomy	▪ For large breasts, medial positioning of implants may result in lateralization of the nipples. A preoperative discussion with the patient sets expectations and determines whether it would be better to pursue a skin-sparing mastectomy as an alternative. A radial inferior incision yields better nipple position in these breasts but places greater tension on the skin, thus making single-stage reconstruction less likely.
Implant choice	▪ For skin-sparing mastectomies, a moderate plus profile implant best matches goals for projection and breast base diameter in most patients. For nipple-sparing mastectomies, a moderate profile implant is used more often to help centralize the nipple.
Learning curve	▪ There is a learning curve for surgeons using this technique that is primarily related to the ability to assess the perfusion of the breast skin flap. If the limits of perfusion are surpassed, the result is skin necrosis. Experience with the technique, experience with the breast surgeon, and novel devices to assess skin perfusion decrease the complication rate for this technique.
Fat transfer	▪ Fat transfer is increasingly used in implant-based breast reconstruction to fill in defects around the implant. This is not recommended at the time of immediate breast reconstruction with implants, but may be safely done in a second procedure.

POSTOPERATIVE CARE

- The patient stays in the hospital for one or two nights. Prior to discharge, a loose-fitting surgical bra is placed. Care is taken to avoid a tight or constricting dressing or bra that may compromise the blood flow of the mastectomy skin flaps. Patients are seen weekly until drains are removed. Criteria for drain removal is less than 30 mL per day. If skin necrosis develops, it is treated aggressively with sharp debridement and closure. For smooth round implants, gentle medial massage of the implants is started 4 weeks postoperatively to help prevent implant contracture.

OUTCOMES

- Immediate breast reconstruction following mastectomy leads to improved psychosocial outcomes and patient satisfaction compared to patients who decide not to have reconstruction.

COMPLICATIONS

- Total complications following direct-to-implant reconstruction are 3% to 15%.[6,7] The explant rate ranges from 1% to 4%. The most common complication is skin necrosis. Other complications include infection, seroma, hematoma, nipple necrosis, implant malposition, and deep venous thrombosis. The most common late complication is capsular contracture.

REFERENCES

1. Alderman AK, Wilkins EG, Lowery JC, et al. Determinants of patient satisfaction in post-mastectomy breast reconstruction. *Plast Reconstr Surg*. 2000;106:769–776.
2. Alderman AK, Kuhn LE, Lowery JC, et al. Does patient satisfaction with breast reconstruction change over time? Two-year results of the Michigan Breast Reconstruction Outcomes Study. *J Am Coll Surg*. 2007;204:7–12.
3. Christensen BO, Overgaard J, Kettner LO, et al. Long-term evaluation of postmastectomy breast reconstruction. *Acta Oncol*. 2011;50(7): 1053–1061.
4. Breuing KH, Colwell AS. Inferolateral AlloDerm hammock for implant coverage in breast reconstruction. *Ann Plast Surg*. 2007;59(3):250–255.
5. Colwell AS, Gadd M, Smith BL, et al. An inferolateral approach to nipple-sparing mastectomy: optimizing mastectomy and reconstruction. *Ann Plast Surg*. 2010;65(2):140–143.
6. Colwell AS, Damjanovic B, Zahedi B, et al. Retrospective review of 331 consecutive immediate single-stage implant reconstructions: indications, complications, trends, and costs. *Plast Reconstr Surg*. 2011; 128:1170–1178.
7. Salzberg CA, Ashikari AY, Koch RM, et al. An 8 year experience of direct-to-implant immediate breast reconstruction using human acellular dermal matrix (AlloDerm). *Plast Reconstr Surg*. 2011;127(2):514–524.

Chapter **15**

Two-Stage Implant Breast Reconstruction

Eric G. Halvorson

DEFINITION

- Two-stage implant breast reconstruction is performed in either the immediate or delayed setting following mastectomy.
- The advantages of two-stage implant reconstruction (compared to autologous reconstruction) include shorter operation, lack of donor site, shorter hospital stay, shorter recovery, patient control over final volume, and a "perkier" result.
- The disadvantages of two-stage implant reconstruction include multiple postoperative office visits for expansions, discomfort associated with the expansion process, a second (albeit outpatient) surgery, and the permanent risks of implants (capsular contracture, rupture, rippling, infection, malposition, and exposure).

PATIENT HISTORY AND PHYSICAL FINDINGS

- It may be beneficial for the initial consultation to occur separate from multidisciplinary clinic visits focused on cancer care. Patients presenting to the plastic surgeon after such visits are often overloaded with information and overwhelmed by all the options and information related to reconstruction. It is critical to determine the patient's goals for reconstruction and to ascertain their preferences with respect to breast size, breast shape, willingness to accept surgical risk, willingness to accept donor site morbidity, operative length, hospital stay, recovery process, postoperative follow-up protocol, secondary surgeries, and long-term complications.
- Having a clinic nurse well versed in reconstructive options to meet with patients and show them patient photographs is an incredibly helpful prelude to the physician–patient consultation.
- Physical examination of the breasts is performed to evaluate any masses and whether or not skin involvement or peau d'orange is present. The overall size and degree of ptosis is noted. Patients with significant ptosis will typically require skin excision. If performed as an inverted "T" or Wise pattern, there is significant risk for mastectomy flap necrosis. Alternatively, one can perform a generous horizontal ellipse, vertical ellipse, or two-stage Wise pattern excision with the vertical closure first and a horizontal excision at the inframammary fold (IMF) 3 to 6 months later.
- The breast width, height, and projection is measured in centimeters. These measurements are used for selecting a tissue expander (as described in the following text).

SURGICAL MANAGEMENT

- Ideal candidates for two-stage implant reconstruction are thin, nonsmokers undergoing bilateral mastectomy who have not, and will not, receive radiotherapy. Smokers are prone to mastectomy flap necrosis and infection. Radiotherapy increases the risk of infection, implant exposure, and capsular contracture. Previously radiated skin will not expand well.
- Although obesity increases the risk of complication for any type of reconstruction, heavier patients tend to have better cosmetic results with autologous reconstruction than with implants, as it can be difficult to match the opposite breast after a unilateral mastectomy or give adequate volume/ptosis after a bilateral mastectomy.
- Patients with very large breasts who require skin removal during mastectomy are at risk for mastectomy flap necrosis and tend to require secondary procedures to address residual excess skin. These patients often have ample donor sites for autologous reconstruction, which may be a better option. Patients with small breasts who want them to be larger can achieve that goal through expansion. Patients who have minimal ptosis and want their breasts to be slightly smaller are candidates for single-stage implant reconstruction.

Preoperative Planning and Implant Selection

- Good communication with the breast surgeon is important to ensure oncologic goals are maintained and that reconstruction is appropriately staged. Patients with advanced disease, requirement for immediate postoperative adjuvant therapy, unstable social environment, and/or uncertainty regarding goals for reconstruction may be better served by delayed reconstruction.
- Prior to mastectomy, the patient must be marked in the standing position. The IMF is marked on each side and the midline is drawn between the sternal notch and xiphoid process. The overall outline of the breasts is marked. Although a transverse ellipse around the nipple–areolar complex (NAC) is commonly used for the mastectomy incision, the author's preference is an oblique ellipse parallel to the pectoralis major fibers (**FIG 1**). This renders the medial scar less visible

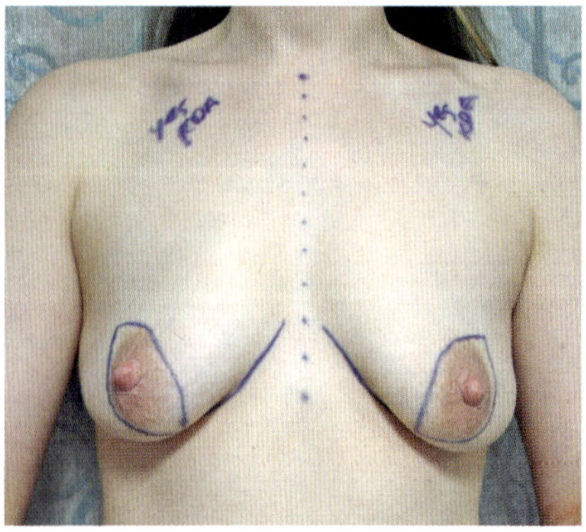

FIG 1 • This patient will be used for the majority of photographs in this chapter. She is a woman in her late 20s with genetic predisposition (*BRCA* gene) undergoing bilateral prophylactic mastectomy and two-stage implant reconstruction. Preoperative markings for the mastectomy are shown, demonstrating the oblique ellipses for incision preferred by the author.

in clothing, allows for better subincisional muscular coverage, and facilitates a stair-step approach during the exchange procedure (as described in the following text).

- Tissue expanders are selected preoperatively based on the width of the patient's breast. There are many different tissue expanders to choose from, but most are textured and anatomic, providing lower pole projection. Some are taller than they are wide, some are wider than they are tall, and some are semicircular or crescentic and focus on lower pole expansion. Most have integrated metal ports that are located with magnets, although a remote port is useful when placing the expander under a thick flap (such as a latissimus dorsi flap in an obese patient). In such patients, finding the port with a magnet can be difficult and a long needle is required, placing the expander at risk for rupture.
- Intraoperatively, a ruler is used to measure the width of the surgically created implant pocket, which ultimately determines the expander to be used. Alternatively, one can create a pocket wide enough to accommodate the desired expander. The author's preference is to measure the surgically created pocket based on native patient anatomy and choose an expander that is 1 cm narrower in width.
- Prior to the exchange procedure, the patient is again marked in the standing position. The midline is marked and asymmetries in implant position are noted. The ideal contour for the final implants is marked.
- Final implants are selected primarily based on volume, although width should be taken into consideration. A full discussion of implant types is beyond the scope of this chapter. The majority of surgeons use smooth, round, high-profile implants for reconstructive purposes, although textured anatomic silicone implants may gain popularity if or when they gain U.S. Food and Drug Administration (FDA) approval. Patients with very wide chests may require a moderate-profile implant that will have a larger base diameter for a given volume (although less projection). A comparison of saline versus silicone implants is also beyond the scope of this chapter, but suffice it to say that the issue is controversial. The author's preference is to offer both types to patients noting the following advantages and disadvantages for each implant type:
  - Saline
    - Advantages: Implant rupture is immediately detected; removal of a ruptured implant is simple and quick.
    - Disadvantages: Reexpansion may be required if implant ruptures and is not replaced expeditiously; firmer than silicone, although this difference is diminished when good soft tissue coverage is present; higher potential for rippling if underfilled.
  - Silicone
    - Advantages: Softer, more "natural" feel
    - Disadvantages: Rupture is often clinically silent until extracapsular rupture and silicone granuloma formation is present, removal of a ruptured implant is a difficult operation that often involves removal of native tissue thus compromising subsequent reconstruction, and monitoring for silent implant rupture using magnetic resonance imaging (MRI) is not proven and has a definite risk of false positives and unnecessary surgeries.

Positioning

- Patients are placed in the supine position under a general anesthetic with arms padded circumferentially and abducted at 80 degrees. Following mastectomy, the patient is positioned such that the sternum is parallel to the floor.

TISSUE EXPANDER PLACEMENT

First Step—Wound Assessment

- Following mastectomy, the wounds are irrigated and hemostasis is obtained. The mastectomy flaps are evaluated by examining their thickness and assessing color and capillary refill. Areas where dermis is exposed internally should be carefully evaluated externally. Areas where the external skin is pale without capillary refill should be considered for debridement. Laser-assisted indocyanine-green fluoroscopy has been promoted to assess mastectomy flap perfusion; however, guidelines for its use and interpretation have not been firmly established.[1]
- Use of tumescent solution by the extirpative surgeon makes assessment of mastectomy flaps difficult and has been shown in some studies to be associated with a higher rate of mastectomy flap necrosis.[2–4]
- When there is significant concern for mastectomy flap necrosis, or if debridement of questionable tissue will lead to closure under tension or an open wound, then aborting reconstruction is strongly advised.
- If necessary, the IMF can be recreated with interrupted suture; however, the position of the inferior edge of the expander will ultimately determine the IMF, which can be adjusted further during an exchange procedure if desired. Some surgeons try to establish the native IMF during this initial procedure (which may make the exchange procedure simpler), whereas others intentionally place the expander lower than the IMF to increase lower pole expansion and projection (which requires recreation of the IMF with suture during the exchange procedure). The author's preference is to preserve the native IMF when performing single-stage implant reconstruction, when placing a significant initial fill volume in the expander, or when the IMF is already low. When performing delayed two-stage implant reconstruction or when placing minimal initial fill volume in the expander, placing the implant below the IMF will preferentially expand the lower pole and permit the surgeon to create minimal ptosis at the exchange procedure (as described in the following text).

Second Step—Creation of Implant Pocket

- The tissue expander cannot be covered by the mastectomy flaps alone, which are thin and offer poor soft tissue coverage. Ideally, the surgeon should provide complete musculofascial coverage with the pectoralis major and serratus anterior muscles (**FIG 2**), or use an acellular dermal allograft (ADA) or other product in addition to the pectoralis major muscle.

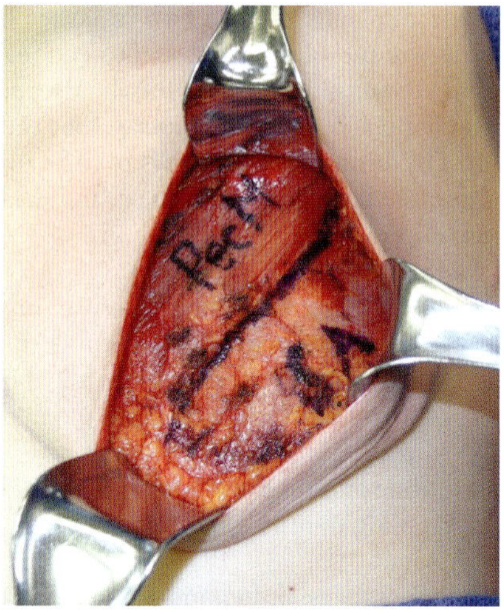

FIG 2 ● Following mastectomy, the pectoralis major and serratus anterior muscles are visualized as these are the muscles used for expander coverage. If these muscles have been affected by mastectomy, using an ADA in their place is considered.

- The lateral edge of the pectoralis major muscle is pinched between the surgeon's index finger and thumb and pulled away from the chest, revealing a loose areolar plane between the pectoralis major and minor muscles. Dissection in this plane commences with Bovie cautery, but once the subpectoral space is entered, much of the superior and medial implant pocket can be created via blunt digital dissection before using lighted retractors for direct visualization. A lighted retractor is quite helpful to finish medial dissection, as great care must be taken to ligate or cauterize the intercostal perforators of the internal mammary vessels (**FIG 3**).
- The medial boundary is defined externally by the preoperative markings that define the patient's native breast form. Internally, it is quite common to release the medial and inferomedial origins of the pectoralis major muscle. It is important not to release this area excessively, as symmastia can result and is difficult to correct.
- After the subpectoral plane is developed, the inferior insertion of the pectoralis major muscle is examined (**FIG 4**). If the patient's muscle reaches the IMF, then a submuscular pocket can be created down to the IMF with supple and adequate soft tissue coverage that will respond well to expansion (**FIG 5**). More commonly, however, the pectoralis major inserts above the IMF. In this scenario, to provide autologous implant coverage inferiorly, one must continue dissection past the pectoralis major insertion and under the anterior rectus sheath until just below the IMF. Transitioning from the subpectoral plane to underneath the anterior rectus sheath is sometimes technically difficult and may result in a few gaps in coverage that can be closed after the pocket is fully created. A lighted retractor is necessary for this portion of the procedure. The anterior rectus sheath is quite stiff and will not expand well unless an incision is made transversely across the sheath just below the IMF, entering the subcutaneous

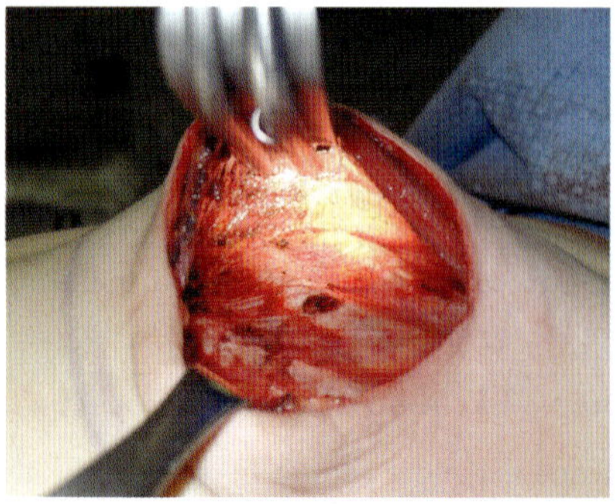

FIG 3 ● A lighted retractor is very helpful for both expander placement and the implant exchange procedure. Here, the lighted retractor is shown during creation of the subpectoral pocket superomedially, where dissection proceeds carefully so intercostal perforators can be visualized and carefully ligated if necessary.

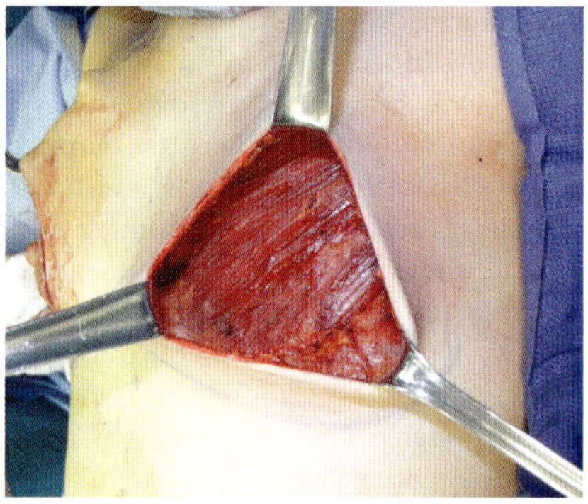

FIG 4 ● The relationship between the most caudal extent of the pectoralis major muscle and the IMF determines whether or not the anterior rectus sheath will be necessary to provide complete submusculofascial coverage of the expander. If the muscle originates at or below the IMF, as shown in this figure, then there is no need to elevate the anterior rectus sheath.

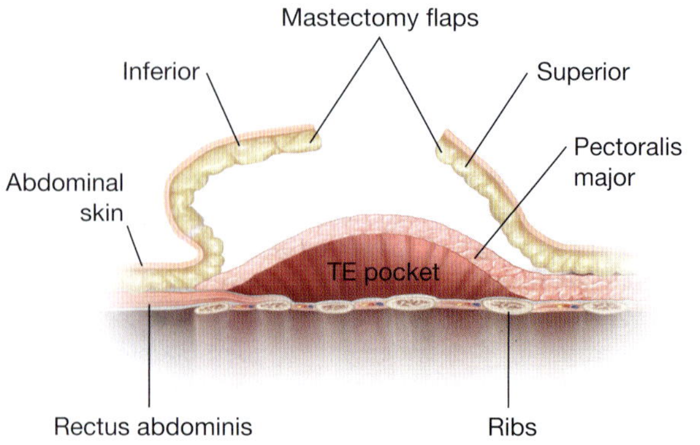

FIG 5 ● Schematic diagram patient anatomy when the pectoralis major originates at or below the IMF. In this case, a submuscular pocket can be created down to the IMF that will be supple and respond well to expansion. TE, tissue expander.

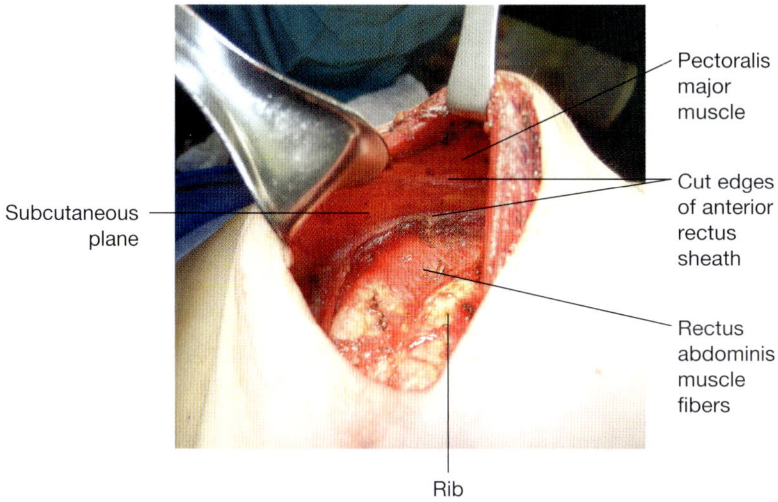

FIG 6 ● At or just below the IMF, the anterior rectus sheath is divided horizontally to enter the subcutaneous plane. If this is not performed, lower pole expansion will be limited by the stiff anterior rectus sheath.

plane (**FIGS 6** and **7**). If the anterior rectus sheath is released above the IMF, one would obviously enter the implant pocket. The goal is to provide complete and supple submusculofascial coverage without gap between the pectoralis major and the IMF. Alternatively, the pectoralis major can be released from the chest wall and a piece of ADA (or other product) can be sewn to the IMF inferiorly and the cut edge of the muscle superiorly.

- Following creation of a subpectoral pocket with or without elevation of the anterior rectus sheath, inferolateral coverage must be provided. Autologous coverage is provided by elevating the serratus anterior fascia if robust, or a partial thickness muscle flap if the fascia is thin or traumatized from the mastectomy. An incision in the serratus anterior is made at the level of, and parallel to, the inferolateral edge of the pectoralis major muscle and a fascial or musculofascial flap is elevated to the anterior axillary line (**FIG 8**). Alternatively, one can determine the width of the implant pocket based on the width of the desired tissue expander and stop lateral dissection when a sufficient pocket width is achieved (usually 1 cm wider than tissue expander). At this point, the inferior and lateral dissections will be complete, but the inferior serratus and superolateral external oblique muscles will still be attached to the chest wall. By retracting inferiorly and laterally, this plane is exposed and the muscles can be elevated off the chest wall to open the inferolateral pocket (**FIG 9**).

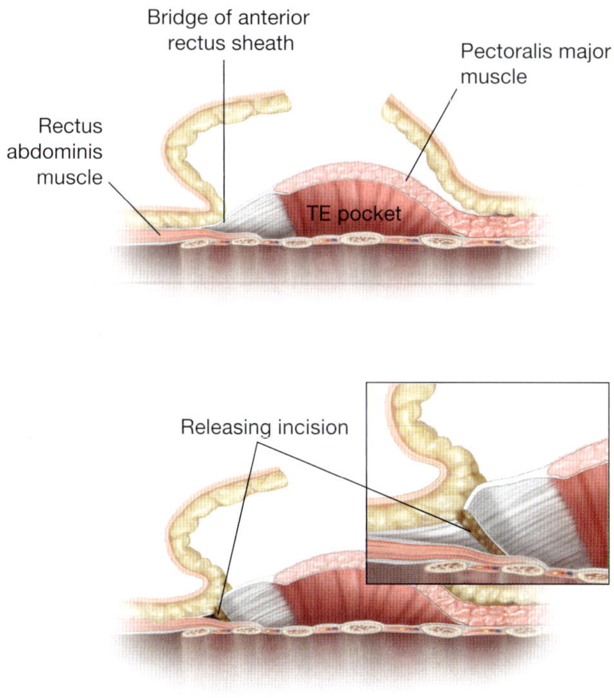

FIG 7 ● Schematic diagram patient anatomy when the pectoralis major muscle originates above the IMF. In this case, the gap between the caudal border of the pectoralis and IMF must be bridged by elevating the anterior rectus sheath. At or just below the IMF, the sheath must be incised horizontally to enter the subcutaneous space; otherwise, the inferior pocket will not expand well. Alternatively, an ADA can be used to bridge this gap. TE, tissue expander.

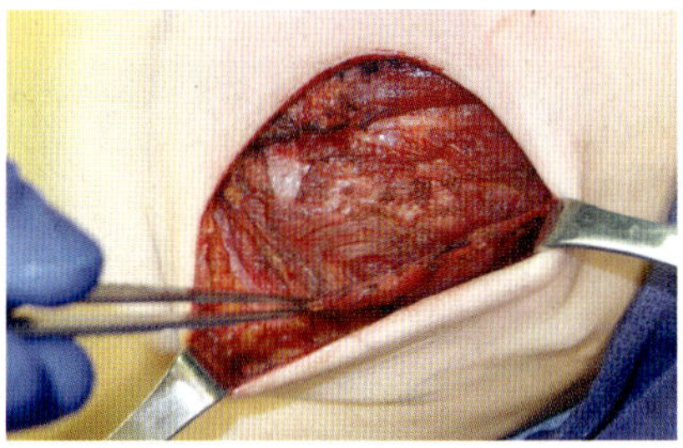

FIG 8 ● For lateral and inferolateral coverage, a partial-thickness serratus anterior muscle flap is elevated and shown in this photograph. If the fascia is robust and intact, that can be used alone; however, this is seldom the case. An incision in the muscle parallel to the inferolateral edge of the pectoralis major muscle is made and the flap is elevated laterally until the anterior axillary line or sufficiently to create the desired pocket width for the chosen expander.

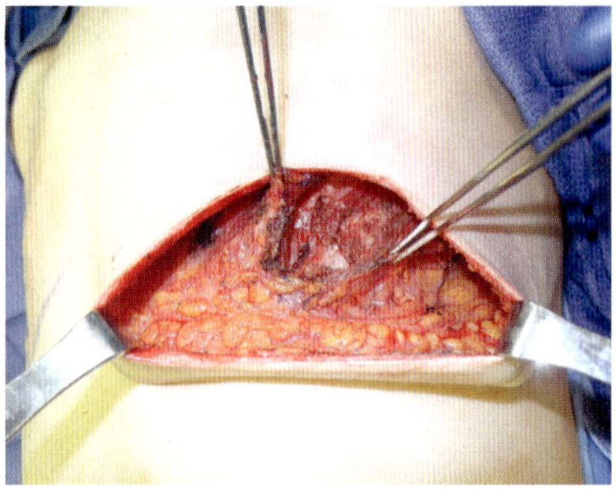

FIG 9 • Following elevation of the serratus anterior muscle, the inferolateral aspect of the implant pocket will still be adherent to the chest wall. If retractors are placed under the pectoralis major and serratus anterior muscles, this area of adhesion will be exposed and inferolateral dissection will elevate the serratus anterior and external oblique muscles off the chest wall to complete implant pocket dissection.

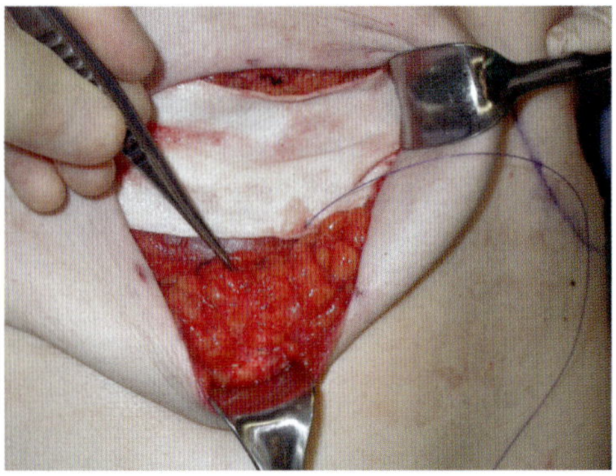

FIG 11 • A piece of ADA is prepared appropriately, according to the manufacturer's recommendations, and is sewn in with the epidermis side facing the implant. A 6 × 16 cm piece is usually sufficient. The inferomedial and inferolateral corners of the ADA are trimmed to create a curved inferior border and it is secured to the IMF and lateral pocket using a running 2-0 monofilament slowly absorbing suture. The transition from the IMF to the lateral pocket must be a gentle arc that mimics the opposite side.

- If an ADA is used, the origin of the pectoralis major is taken down starting inferolaterally and extending medially and then superiorly along the sternal origin to approximately the 3rd or 4th rib (**FIG 10**). The ADA will provide inferolateral implant coverage and there is no need to elevate the serratus anterior. In this case, the IMF and anterior axillary line are marked internally and the ADA is sutured along a line that transitions in an arc from the IMF to the anterior axillary line (**FIG 11**). Alternatively, one can mark the lateral mammary fold based on the width of the desired tissue expander and suture the ADA to this line (**FIG 12**). One can tailor the surgically created IMF to match the contralateral native IMF during unilateral reconstruction. If performing bilateral reconstruction, then it is imperative to create symmetric IMFs.
- The advantages of using an ADA are that it avoids any morbidity associated with elevation of the rectus sheath and serratus anterior, it allows for a greater initial fill volume (and thus fewer postoperative expansions), it allows precise control of the IMF, it may reduce operative time, and it may preserve lower pole fullness. Disadvantages include cost and an increased incidence of seroma, infection, and reconstructive failure in patients with risk factors such as obesity, smoking, and/or radiation.[5] Although some surgeons use an ADA routinely and others do not, the author's preference is to use ADA selectively (**FIG 13**). If the anterior rectus sheath or serratus anterior have been affected by the mastectomy and will not provide adequate coverage, ADA is an option, provided the patient does not have risk factors such as prior radiation, obesity, or smoking. In patients who have excess skin, it is advantageous to take advantage of this by placing a higher initial fill volume and an ADA will allow the surgeon to do this (again, provided the patient does not have the risk factors mentioned earlier). When the pectoralis major does not extend down to the IMF in a patient with some excess skin and no risk factors, ADA is a good option. However, in a patient without skin excess, who desires small breasts, and in whom very little initial fill volume will be placed, submusculofascial coverage is provided without ADA.

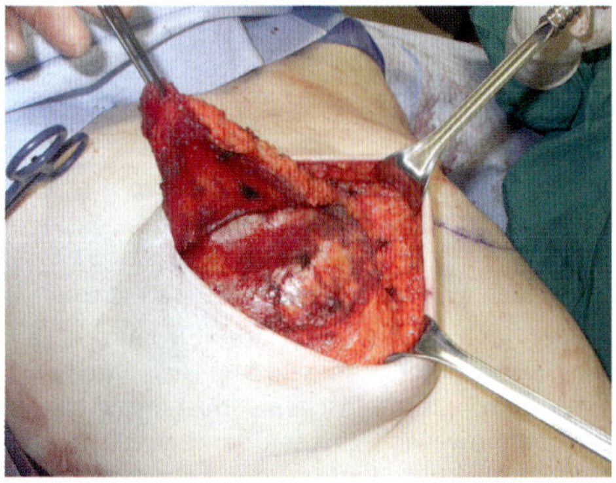

FIG 10 • If an ADA is used, the pectoralis major muscle is elevated from the chest wall by dividing its inferior and inferomedial origin.

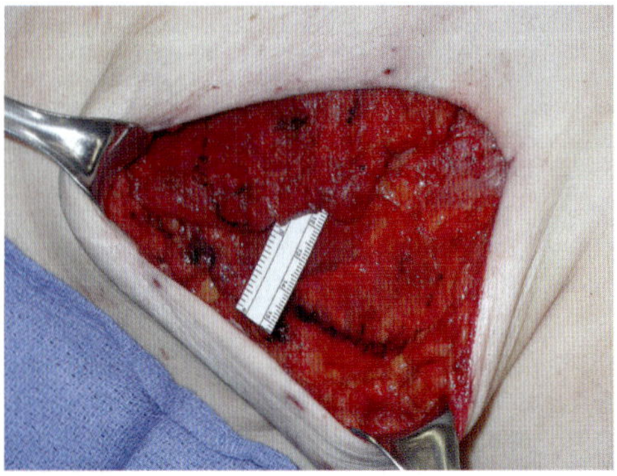

FIG 12 • A ruler is used to measure the width of the surgically created pocket. The proper pocket width can be determined either by patient anatomy (e.g., the anterior axillary line) or the dimensions of the expander desired.

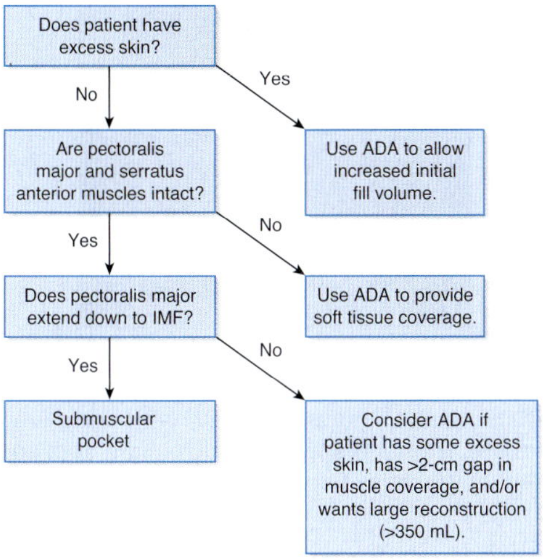

FIG 13 ● Algorithm to determine when to use ADA. IMF, inframammary fold.

Third Step—Preparation of Tissue Expander

- Tissue expanders come with air in them to prevent the inner shell from sticking to itself. There are usually markings for orientation, but it is helpful to draw a vertical line on the expander with a marking pen to assist with positioning the expander in the pocket. A needle (usually 23 gauge) is inserted into the port and all air is removed. The most commonly used tissue expanders are anatomic (creating lower pole expansion) and thus they are textured (to prevent rotation). There is typically more shell inferiorly, and while deflating the expander, it is important to fold excess shell inward as opposed to folding it upward and on to itself, where it might cover the port and get punctured (**FIG 14**).
- The author's preference is to place 60 to 180 mL of sterile saline in the tissue expander prior to placement, which allows the anterior shell to move away from the rigid backing. It is important to control positioning of this backing as it is what determines final expander position.

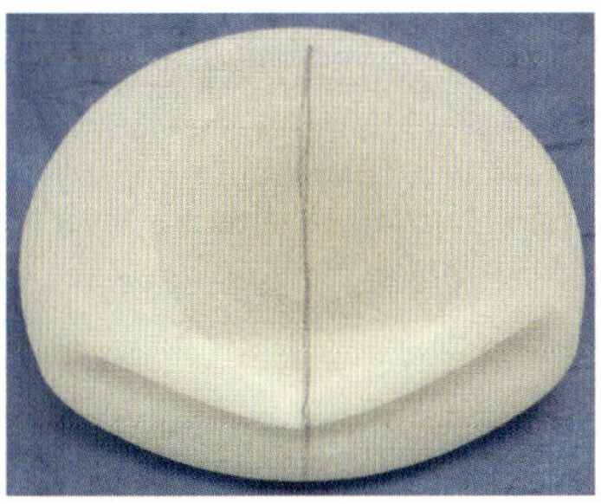

FIG 14 ● The tissue expander is marked with a vertical line for orientation. All air is removed with the excess inferior implant folded inward as shown to avoid puncturing the inferior implant while placing needles for expansion in clinic postoperatively. A minimum of 60 mL of saline is instilled, dyed with methylene blue. This allows for quick identification of inadvertent implant rupture during wound closure and also allows the clinic staff to confirm placement of the filling needle during subsequent expansions.

- It is extremely helpful to put 1 mL of methylene blue in 1 L of injectable saline and use this for the initial expander fluid. If the expander is punctured during closure, it will be evident due to the dye. Additionally, during expansions in clinic, the blue dye will confirm when the port is accessed.

Fourth Step—Placement of Tissue Expander and Closure

- The pectoralis is retracted away from the chest wall and the expander is placed into the pocket taking great care to orient it correctly. It is important to note the rigid backing of the expander and place the caudal edge at the IMF or below if desired. Be sure to unfold all edges of the expander. If performing bilateral reconstruction, symmetry in expander placement should be confirmed by palpating the expander ports on each side and ensuring symmetric horizontal and vertical positioning. If an expander requires adjustment in positioning, it is critical to grasp the rigid backing of the implant and then adjust the position. If only the ports or anterior shell are adjusted, this usually has no effect on the position of the backing, which determines implant position once fully inflated.
- The inferolateral edge of the pectoralis major muscle is sutured to the anteromedial edge of the serratus anterior muscle with running absorbable 2-0 braided suture, closing the pocket. A small opening is left superolaterally to allow egress of fluid. Alternatively, if an ADA is used, the pectoralis major muscle is sewn to the ADA with interrupted figure-of-eight braided absorbable 2-0 suture (**FIG 15**).
- The author's preference is to inflate the tissue expander with sterile saline as much as the soft tissue (muscle/skin) will allow without undue tension. This is typically 180 to 240 mL. It is important to do this prior to skin closure, as placing the needle through the muscle will occasionally cause bleeding, which can be controlled directly. Otherwise, a hematoma could expand in the subcutaneous space without notice until the patient is

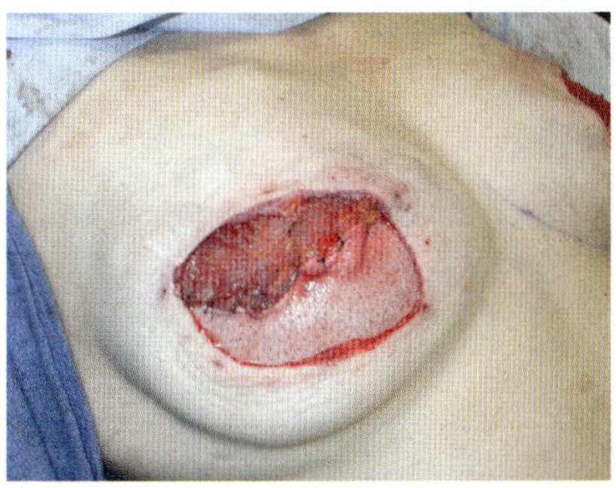

FIG 15 ● The inferolateral edge of the pectoralis major is sewn to the superomedial edge of the serratus anterior with a running 2-0 absorbable polyfilament suture to cover the implant. If an ADA is used, the pectoralis major is sewn to the edge of the ADA with interrupted figure-of-eight 2-0 absorbable polyfilament suture, as shown.

out of surgery. In cases where there is significant concern regarding the cutaneous circulation, then only 0 to 60 mL of inflation is advisable.

- Two closed suction drains are placed in the subcutaneous space. One is oriented superiorly and the other inferiorly. The skin is closed with interrupted 3-0 absorbable monofilament suture for the dermis and a running 4-0 absorbable monofilament suture for subcuticular closure (**FIG 16**). The author's preference is to use skin glue alone as a dressing, without placement of a surgical bra, which applies pressure to the tenuous mastectomy flaps and is an impediment to physical examination.
- Antibiotics are continued parenterally for at least 24 hours postoperatively and transitioned to oral antibiotics for a week, as withholding postoperative antibiotics has been shown to be associated with an unacceptable rate of implant infection.[6] Drains are removed when output is less than 30 mL per 24 hours and expansion is begun typically 2 weeks postoperatively. Expansion can continue on a weekly basis, adding as much fluid as the patient will tolerate without discomfort (usually 60 to 120 mL). Once expansion is complete according to patient preference and surgeon's satisfaction, the author's preference is to perform one additional overexpansion, which can provide some additional tissue to create minimal ptosis at the exchange procedure at least 1 month later (as described in the following text).

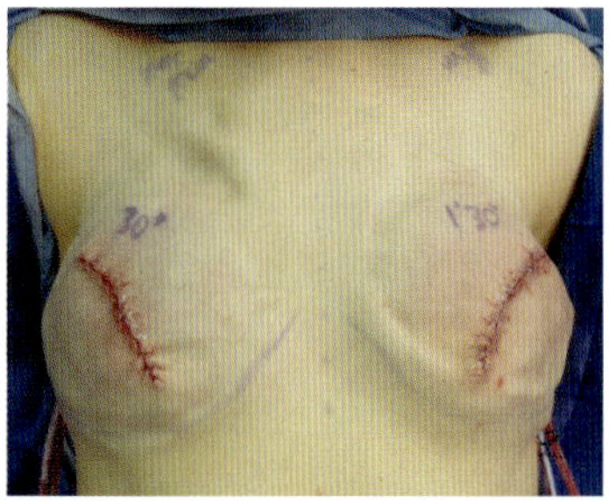

FIG 16 • The patient is shown following placement of tissue expanders and closure over two closed suction drains. Internal absorbable sutures are used, with skin glue as the only dressing. No bra is applied, which might apply pressure to tenuous mastectomy flaps.

IMPLANT EXCHANGE

First Step—Removal of Tissue Expander

- As noted earlier, the patient is marked in the standing position. Asymmetries are noted and the ideal contour for the final implants is marked.
- The mastectomy scars have often widened during expansion and these can be excised. A stair-step approach to the implant pocket is usually performed, so any wound breakdown in one layer does not expose the suture line of the other layer. If the scar is oriented obliquely (**FIG 17**), 2 to 4 cm of superomedial skin elevation will expose the pectoralis major, which can be incised parallel to the muscle fibers (**FIGS 18** and **19**). If a transverse approach was used, then superolateral and inferomedial skin elevation is required to expose the pectoralis major and allow for an incision parallel to the muscle fibers.
- The implant pocket is entered and the capsule is bluntly separated from the expander, which is removed. If the expander is too large, it can be ruptured with a needle or scalpel to assist in removal. If there was any doubt about the final expander volume, it can be measured at this point.

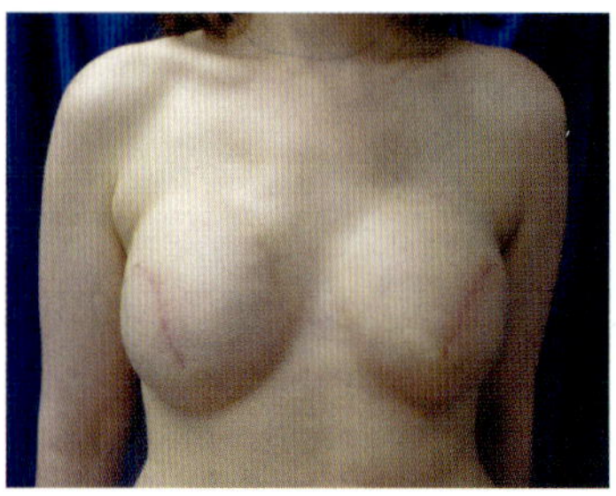

FIG 17 • The patient is shown prior to the exchange procedure, 1 month following the last expansion in clinic. She has been expanded to 600 mL and desires 550 mL implants.

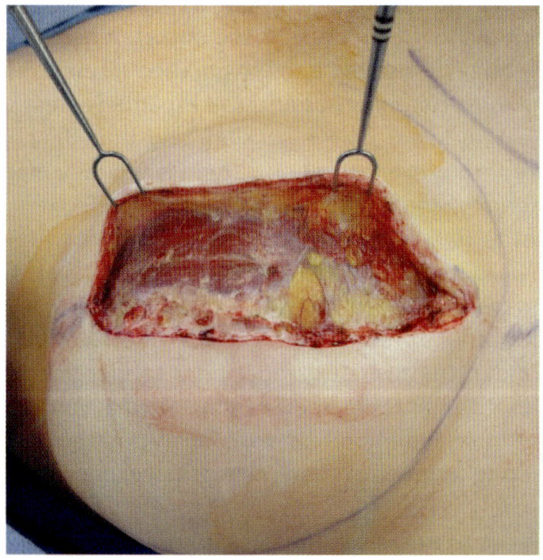

FIG 18 • If the oblique incision is used for mastectomy, it is easy at the exchange procedure to elevate a superomedial flap exposing the pectoralis major muscle where it tends to be thicker. This will allow a "stair-step" approach to the implant pocket. Any wound healing issue at one level will not expose the suture line at the other level.

Second Step—Creation of Implant Pocket

- Ideally, the expanders can be removed and the permanent implants placed without further intervention; however, this is almost never the case. Superior and superomedial capsulotomy is often required to soften the transition from the chest wall to the implant (**FIG 20**). The pocket may need to be medialized, lateralized, elevated, or displaced inferiorly.

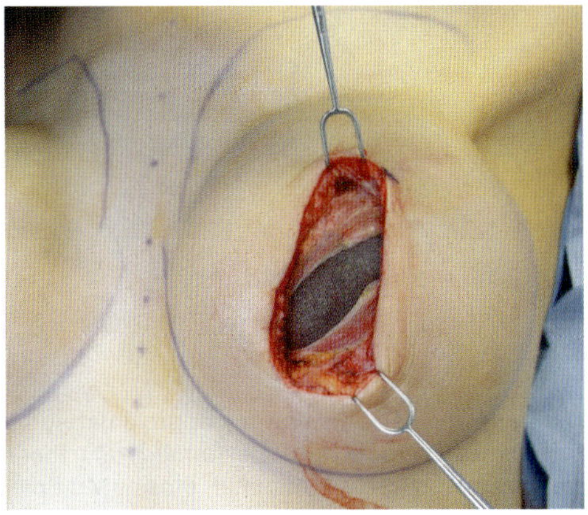

FIG 19 ● A muscular incision is made parallel to the pectoralis major muscle fibers to access the implant pocket. The capsule is also incised with cautery and the expander is bluntly separated from the capsule.

These can all be accomplished through capsulotomy. If the final implant is roughly the same width as the expander, then a corresponding capsulorrhaphy at the opposite side of the pocket is necessary using figure-of-eight interrupted 0 absorbable suture. If the implant is wider than the expander, this may not be necessary as the capsulotomy will increase pocket diameter.

- If the expander was placed below the IMF, or if the IMF needs to be elevated, this is accomplished with figure-of-eight interrupted 0 absorbable suture. The patient is sat upright (**FIG 21**) and the inferior mastectomy flap is lifted away from the chest wall. Usually, the old IMF can be visualized and marked (**FIG 22**); otherwise, the desired IMF can be marked. The needle is passed through the capsule and the IMF marking externally is visualized. The needle tip should just catch the deep dermis, resulting in a small indentation when tied. These indentations will resolve in several weeks. After passing the needle through the capsule/dermis, tension can be adjusted by examining the fold externally (**FIG 23**) and elevating it

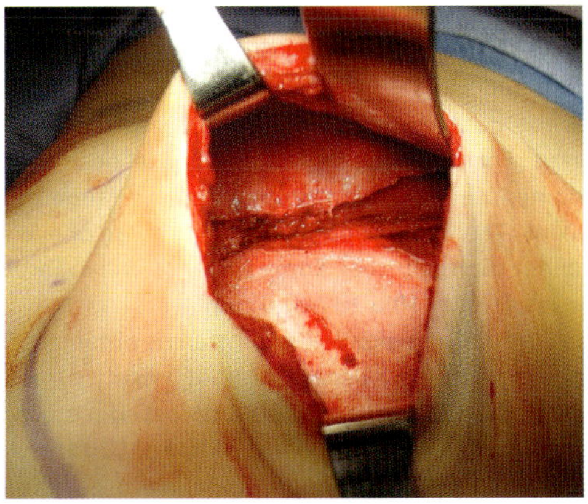

FIG 20 ● A superomedial and superior capsulotomy is made just above the chest wall using a lighted retractor. This will soften the transition from chest wall to implant and allow for more implant mobility within the pocket.

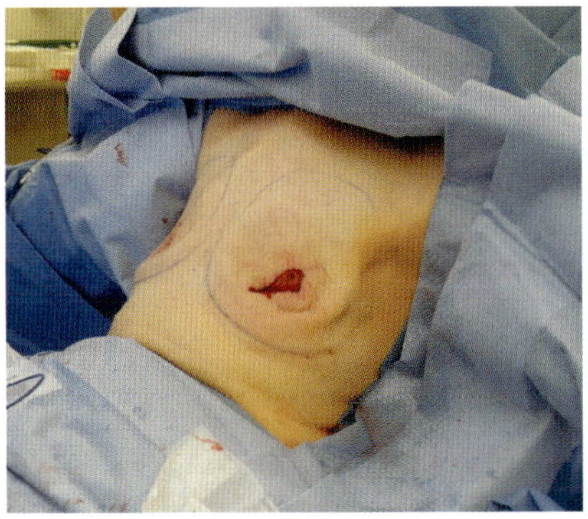

FIG 21 ● The patient is positioned upright with both upper extremities well padded and secured to arm boards abducted less than 90 degrees.

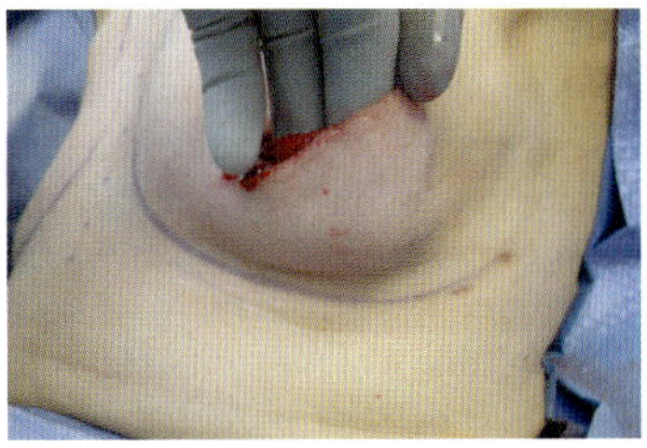

FIG 22 ● When the inferior mastectomy flap is elevated gently from the chest wall, the patient's original IMF is still visible and can be marked for recreation of the native IMF. A higher or lower IMF can also be created.

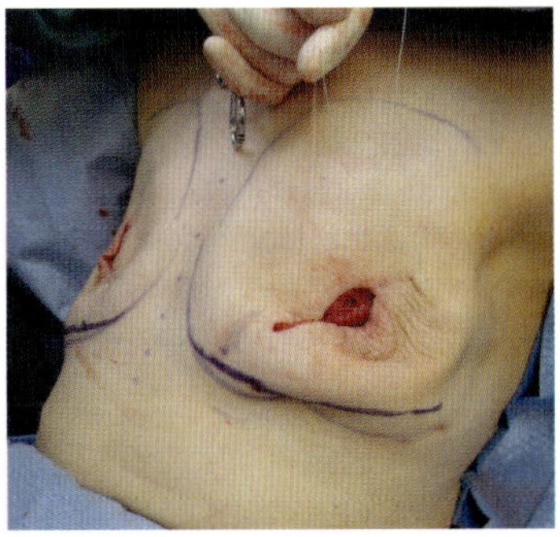

FIG 23 ● A suture is placed in the center of the IMF, through the capsule and just catching the deep dermis. The suture is pulled upward and the level of the IMF adjusted as desired to recreate a sharp and well-defined IMF. Once held in appropriate position, internal inspection will reveal where a suture should be placed on the chest wall. To minimize pain, suturing to the ribs should be avoided if possible. If the lower portion of the expander was placed at the IMF and good lower pole expansion and a crisp IMF in good position has resulted, then this maneuver is unnecessary.

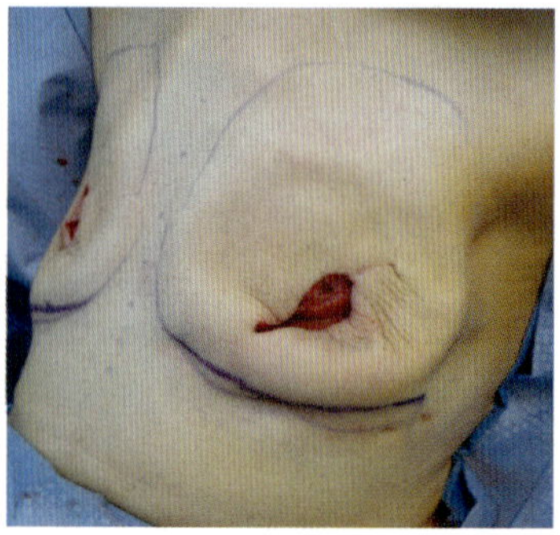

FIG 24 ● The IMF has been reestablished with multiple figure-of-eight capsulorrhaphy sutures, starting in the center of the IMF and proceeding medially and laterally until an adequate IMF is recreated. A temporary implant sizer is helpful to assess the reconstructed IMF during this process.

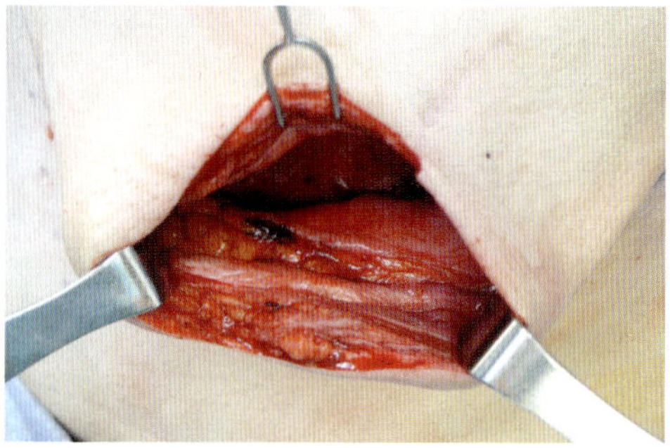

FIG 26 ● A horizontal capsulotomy approximately half way up the inferior mastectomy flap is performed to further expand the lower pole and create minimal ptosis. Multiple radial capsulotomies (perpendicular to the horizontal capsulotomy and extending from the IMF to the incision) will further expand the lower pole.

as desired. Internal inspection with the suture still under tension will indicate where the corresponding suture throw in the chest wall must be made. Suturing into the rib should be avoided, as this results in pain. The first suture is placed at the center of the IMF and then one to two sutures are placed medially and laterally until an adequate fold is created (FIGS 24 and 25).

- Some surgeons prefer to establish the IMF at the initial operation, potentially with an ADA, which has the added benefit of permitting a higher initial fill volume. A higher initial fill volume has the potential to better preserve lower pole fullness. No time is spent reconstructing the IMF at the exchange procedure. Although this may be a simpler approach, it may result in a blunted IMF. The author's preference is to treat each case individually and surgically create a crisp IMF at the exchange procedure if necessary. For example, patients undergoing delayed reconstruction will benefit from significant lower pole expansion and thus the expander is placed inferior to the desired IMF and the IMF is reconstructed at the exchange procedure. A patient with minimal excess skin and ptosis undergoing immediate reconstruction will benefit from an ADA to maximize the initial fill volume (preserve lower pole fullness), establish the IMF, and avoid inferior capsulorrhaphy at the exchange procedure.
- To further expand the lower pole and create minimal ptosis, capsulotomy of the inferior pocket is then performed. A horizontal capsulotomy half way up the inferior mastectomy flap, at least 4 cm off the chest wall, will expand the lower pole of the pocket (FIG 26). Additional radial capsulotomies can be added for further lower pole expansion or elsewhere to create symmetric pockets.

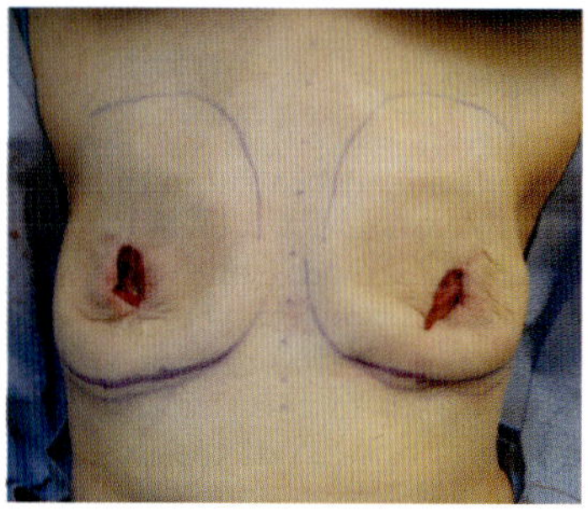

FIG 25 ● Comparison of the left side, where the IMF has been recreated, and the right side, where it has not.

- During pocket creation, it is helpful to have a temporary sizer inflated (with air or saline) to roughly the desired implant volume, which can be placed into the implant pocket to assess position, shape, and volume. This is particularly important in bilateral reconstructions, where two sizers are required to confirm pocket symmetry.

Third Step—Implant Selection and Closure

- When ordering implants for the exchange procedure, it is wise to order implants that are one size smaller and one size larger than the implant size determined by the patient's final expansion volume (prior to final overexpansion). As mentioned earlier, temporary sizers are usually used and can be adjusted to determine an acceptable final implant volume. Inflating the sizer beyond the final expander volume usually results in excessive upper pole fullness, a noticeable step-off between the chest and implant, and tight closure. The chest should transition to the implant smoothly and the breast mound should have slight ptosis.
- When placing saline implants, choose an implant that has the desired volume as the upper end of its volume range. For example, if 380 mL is the desired implant volume, use an implant with a volume range of 360 to 390 mL. This avoids rippling at the expense of making the implant slightly firmer. Some surgeons will in fact overfill the implant by 10% to avoid rippling.
- The pockets are irrigated, hemostasis is obtained, and the final implants are opened. Although many surgeons will reprep the patient, place new drapes, dip retractors in prep solution, and handle the implants with fresh gloves, there is no data to support these practices. The author does not take any special precautions, as the procedure is a clean, sterile procedure. The implants are placed and the muscular closure is performed with a running 2-0 braided absorbable suture. The capsule is not included

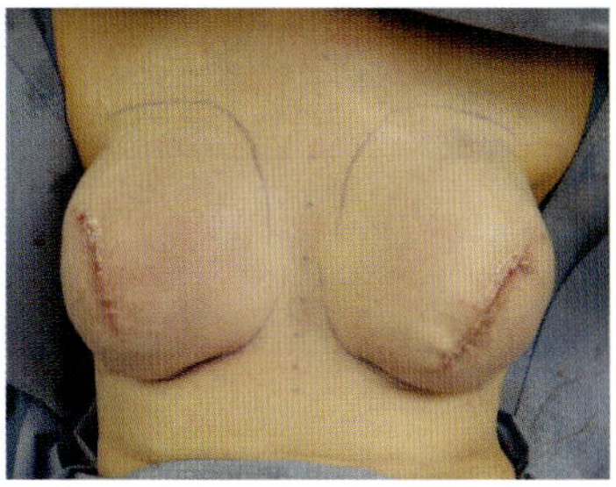

FIG 27 ● The implants have been placed and the wounds closed without drains. Skin glue has been applied. The dimpling observed at the IMFs will resolve in several weeks.

in this closure if possible, thus creating an anterior capsulotomy (made upon initial approach to the implant pocket). No drains are placed. The skin is closed with interrupted deep dermal 3-0 monofilament absorbable suture and a running 4-0 subcuticular absorbable suture (**FIG 27**). A skin glue is applied, and a bra is only used if supporting the implant in a particular position is desired.

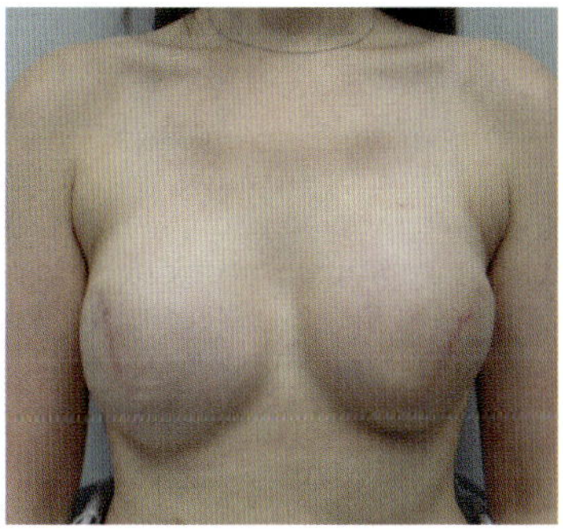

FIG 28 ● Three months following the exchange procedure, the patient is very happy and interested in nipple reconstruction. The right IMF is 2 cm lower than the left IMF, but the patient does not desire correction. It is important to establish the final implant position prior to nipple reconstruction; otherwise, later implant repositioning will affect how the nipple is positioned on the breast mound. There is minimal step-off from the chest wall to the implants, which is the result of mastectomy and commonly seen in implant reconstruction. This can be corrected with fat grafting—an effective and popular but controversial procedure at this time. The patient did not desire fat grafting.

Additional Procedure—Nipple Reconstruction and Revisions

- When examined with a critical eye, almost all patients have some degree of asymmetry following reconstruction (**FIG 28**). Approximately 30% will request a third procedure to address this asymmetry. Correcting the unfavorable result in implant breast reconstruction is a complex subject, involving techniques to alter implant position, breast shape, implant type, and soft tissue characteristics. Many patients ultimately opt for NAC reconstruction (**FIG 29**) (see Chapter 20). In many cases, minor revisions can be performed at the time of NAC reconstruction; however, the nipple should only be created once the breast mound is in its final position, and thus it is not advisable to adjust the implant pocket and create the nipple during the same operation.

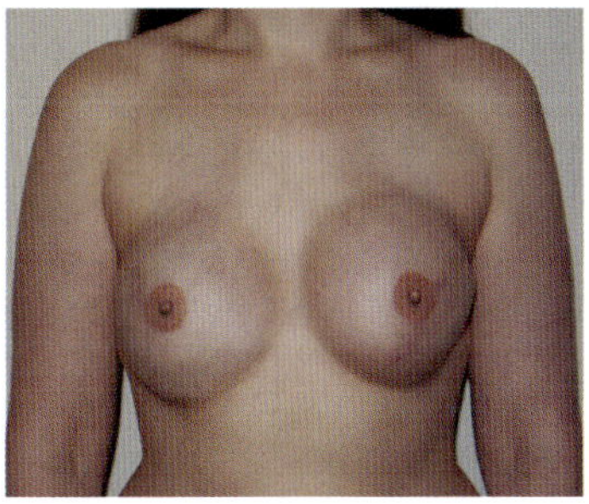

FIG 29 ● Options for nipple–areolar complex (NAC) reconstruction include tattoo only, nipple reconstruction with areola tattoo, and nipple reconstruction with areola graft. This patient opted for a "3-D" tattoo performed by a professional tattoo artist that specializes in NAC tattoo (Vinnie Myers in Finksburg, MD—http://www.vinniemyers.com). She is very happy with the aesthetic result, although she has some chronic discomfort lateral to the right breast. It is very common for patients to have some degree of chronic sensory dysfunction following mastectomy. Much of this resolves with time and can improve with therapy and massage; however, every patient should be counseled of this risk. It is also very common for patients with implants to be aware of their presence permanently. No patients think the implants feel just like their native breasts. The implants have dropped slightly, resulting in a more obvious step-off from the chest wall to the implants, and could be corrected with elevation of the implants (which would affect NAC position on the breast mound) or fat grafting.

PEARLS AND PITFALLS

Indications	■ Patients with a history of radiation are poor candidates for implant reconstruction. ■ Risk factors for infection and wound healing complications include smoking, radiation, and obesity.
Incision placement	■ An oblique incision parallel to the pectoralis muscle fibers provides the best cosmesis and easiest approach for the exchange procedure. ■ Excess skin can be excised through a linear incision only, as additional incisions will compromise circulation and risk mastectomy flap necrosis. Secondary procedures are frequently necessary in patients with excess skin.
Expander selection	■ Expanders are selected based on breast width, not volume.

Expander placement	■ Marking the expander assists in correct orientation. ■ Remove all air and place saline dyed with methylene blue to allow detection of implant rupture as well as confirmation of port access for staff performing expansions. ■ Provide at least 24 hours of postoperative antibiotics.
Implant selection	■ Implants are selected based on volume primarily, taking breast width into consideration. High-profile implants are typically used, except in patients with wide chests who benefit from moderate profile, wider implants.
Patient expectation	■ Two-stage implant breast reconstruction is typically a year-long process. ■ Symmetry in the nude is always the goal but is seldom achieved. Symmetry in clothing is the most reasonable expectation.

POSTOPERATIVE CARE

- Following the mastectomy and tissue expander placement, the patient is maintained on antibiotics for at least 24 hours and more commonly for 1 week or until drains are removed. Drains remain in place at least 3 days and then are removed when output is less than 30 mL per day. Only one drain from each side should be removed at a time, as sometimes the output of the second drain will increase after the first drain is removed. The author's preference is to allow patients to shower with drains in place. The patient should be seen within 1 week to evaluate for postoperative infection and/or mastectomy flap necrosis and to remove drains if appropriate. Expansion is begun 2 weeks after surgery and continued on a weekly basis thereafter until the patient and surgeon are happy with the final volume. One additional "overexpansion" is performed and the exchange procedure is scheduled at least 1 month later to allow the tissues to soften.
- Following the exchange procedure, patients may shower after 48 hours. Although the author feels very strongly about giving patients extended postoperative prophylactic antibiotics after mastectomy and expander placement, the exchange procedure is a clean procedure and the mastectomy flaps have been delayed and have robust perfusion. Thus, no postoperative antibiotics are usually given. Although there is little data to support practices such as repreping the patient, changing drapes, changing gloves, or dipping retractors in prep solution, this is commonly performed by surgeons placing implants.

OUTCOMES

- Patient satisfaction with implant breast reconstruction is high, provided the preoperative consultation appropriately identified the patient's priorities, goals, and preferences with respect to reconstructive options, and realistic expectations were discussed (**FIGS 30** to **32**). Although some studies have indicated that patients undergoing prosthetic reconstruction are less satisfied than those undergoing autologous tissue reconstruction,[7,8] other studies have shown significant improvements in psychosocial outcomes regardless of the type of reconstruction.[9]
- It is common to tell patients undergoing implant reconstruction that, on average, they will require some form of surgery every 10 years. These could be procedures for symmetry, infection, rupture, or capsular contracture. Although some surgeons exchange silicone implants every 10 years to avoid extracapsular ruptures, most only offer surgery if a problem is identified. One study evaluated long-term outcomes of autologous versus implant reconstruction and noted stable survival of 90% of autologous reconstructions

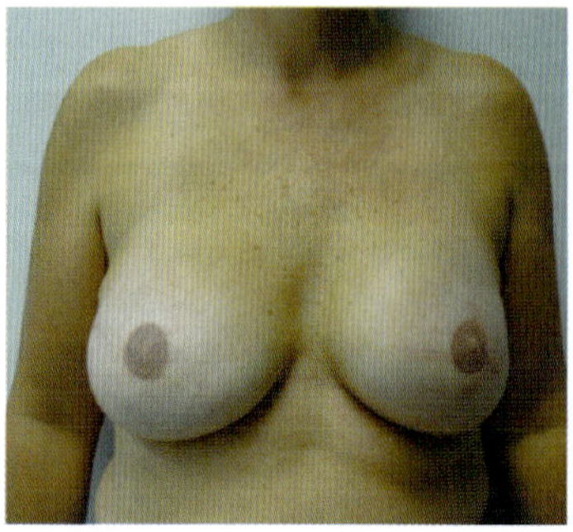

FIG 30 • This patient is 1 year out from the exchange procedure and 6 months out from NAC reconstruction with local flaps to reconstruct the nipple and areola tattoo. She has a higher body mass index (BMI) and more subcutaneous fat, and the mastectomy did not extend very far superiorly. Thus, she has a smooth transition from the chest wall to the implants.

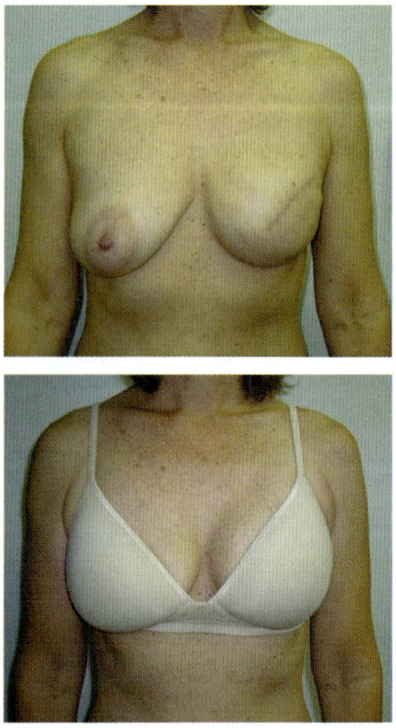

A

B

FIG 31 • **A,B.** This patient is 6 months out from unilateral reconstruction. She did not desire NAC reconstruction or a contralateral mastopexy for symmetry. She has a very acceptable appearance in a bra.

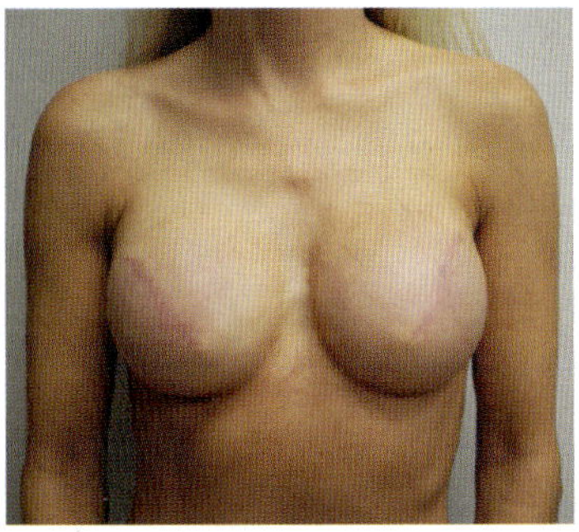

FIG 32 • This patient is 9 months out from her exchange procedure. She had prior augmentation mammaplasty and thin soft tissue coverage inferiorly; therefore, an ADA was used to augment soft tissue coverage of the expanders.

versus a gradual decline to 70% survival of implant reconstructions.[10] In general, autologous reconstructions improve or remain stable with time, whereas implant reconstructions tend to worsen slightly over time.

- There is no increased risk of breast cancer recurrence in patients undergoing therapeutic mastectomy and implant reconstruction. Detection of recurrence and outcome when recurrence is detected are not affected by the presence of an implant reconstruction.[11]

COMPLICATIONS

- Bleeding
- Infection
- Injury to surrounding structures (e.g., cutaneous nerves)
- Mastectomy flap necrosis
- Long-term risks of implants: capsular contracture, rupture, rippling, infection, malposition, and exposure
- Asymmetry, imperfect cosmetic result

REFERENCES

1. Moyer HR, Losken A. Predicting mastectomy skin flap necrosis with indocyanine green angiography: the gray area defined. *Plast Reconstr Surg*. 2012;129(5):1043–1048.
2. Abbott AM, Miller BT, Tuttle TM. Outcomes after tumescence technique versus electrocautery mastectomy. *Ann Surg Oncol*. 2012;19(8):2607–2611.
3. Seth AK, Hirsch EM, Fine NA, et al. Additive risk of tumescent technique in patients undergoing mastectomy with immediate reconstruction. *Ann Surg Oncol*. 2011;18(11):3041–3046.
4. Chun YS, Verma K, Rosen H, et al. Use of tumescent mastectomy technique as a risk factor for native breast skin flap necrosis following immediate breast reconstruction. *Am J Surg*. 2011;201(2):160–165.
5. Ho G, Nguyen TJ, Shahabi A, et al. A systematic review and meta-analysis of complications associated with acellular dermal matrix-assisted breast reconstruction. *Ann Plast Surg*. 2012;68(4):346–356.
6. Clayton JL, Bazakas A, Lee CN, et al. Once is not enough: withholding postoperative prophylactic antibiotics in prosthetic breast reconstruction is associated with an increased risk of infection. *Plast Reconstr Surg*. 2012;130(3):495–502.
7. Alderman AK, Wilkins EG, Lowery JC, et al. Determinants of patient satisfaction in postmastectomy breast reconstruction. *Plast Reconstr Surg*. 2000;106:769–776.
8. Christensen BO, Overgaard J, Kettner LO, et al. Long-term evaluation of postmastectomy breast reconstruction. *Acta Oncol*. 2011;50(7):1053–1061.
9. Wilkins EG, Cederna PS, Lowery JC, et al. Prospective analysis of psychosocial outcomes in breast reconstruction: one-year postoperative results from the Michigan Breast Reconstruction Outcome Study. *Plast Reconstr Surg*. 2000;106(5):1014–1025; discussion 1026–1027.
10. Rusby JE, Waters RA, Nightingale PG, et al. Immediate breast reconstruction after mastectomy: what are the long-term prospects? *Ann R Coll Surg Engl*. 2010;92(3):193–197.
11. McCarthy CM, Pusic AL, Sclafani L, et al. Breast cancer recurrence following prosthetic, postmastectomy reconstruction: incidence, detection, and treatment. *Plast Reconstr Surg*. 2008;121(2):381–388.

Chapter 16 Pedicled Latissimus Dorsi Flap Breast Reconstruction after Mastectomy

Frank Fang   Adeyiza O. Momoh

DEFINITION

- The latissimus dorsi myocutaneous flap was originally performed for chest wall reconstruction after radical mastectomy by Iginio Tansini in 1906 but fell out of favor when mastectomies were primarily closed or skin grafted.[1] Although the latissimus flap remained a dependable option for anterior chest wall reconstruction,[2–4] it was not until 1977 when it was first described to reconstruct a true breast mound in combination with a prosthetic implant.[5]
- The latissimus dorsi myocutaneous flap currently remains a viable and frequently used option for breast reconstruction. Typically, patients who required chest wall irradiation and are either unwilling or unable (lack of donor site tissue volume) to undergo one of the other autologous flap options for breast reconstruction will proceed with this option. Furthermore, this flap has found use in the reconstruction of congenital defects such as Poland syndrome in the younger patient population.[6] For the purpose of breast reconstruction, this technique usually requires flap transfer combined with an initial tissue expansion process followed by a subsequent saline- or silicone-filled prosthetic implant placement. Breast reconstruction with a latissimus dorsi myocuataneous flap without an implant is also possible but less commonly used due to flap volume limitations.[7]

ANATOMY

- The latissimus dorsi is a large, flat, triangle-shaped muscle on the back measuring approximately 25 × 35 cm; it mirrors the pectoralis major posteriorly.
- The muscle origin is a broad aponeurosis that spans the lower six thoracic vertebrae (superomedially), supraspinous ligament (central medial region), thoracolumbar fascia (inferomedially), and posterior iliac crest (inferiorly).
- The lateral border of the muscle separates from the serratus anterior as a free potential space until one encounters the small slips of origin from the 10th to 12th ribs, where the latissimus interdigitates with the slips of origin of the external oblique and serratus anterior muscles.
- The superior border of the muscle has an area of adhesion to the region of the inferior angle of the scapula but otherwise contains free potential space with the underlying layer.
- The muscle converges in the axilla to insert on the crest of the lesser tuberosity of the humerus.
- The latissimus dorsi adducts, extends, and rotates the humerus medially ("pull-up," rowing, or free-style swimming motions).
- The latissimus dorsi flap is a Nahai-Mathes type V myocutaneous flap, meaning that it may survive based solely on either the thoracodorsal artery or the segmental perforators from the intercostal and lumbar arteries.
- The thoracodorsal artery (arising from the subscapular branch off the axillary artery) enters the deep surface of the latissimus dorsi muscle in the posterior axilla approximately 10 cm inferior to the muscle insertion into the humerus and 2.6 cm medial to the lateral border of the muscle (**FIG 1**).
- The artery then divides into the medial (also known as transverse) and the lateral (also known as vertical or descending) branches. The medial branch is located approximately 3.5 cm below and parallel to the superior border. The lateral branch

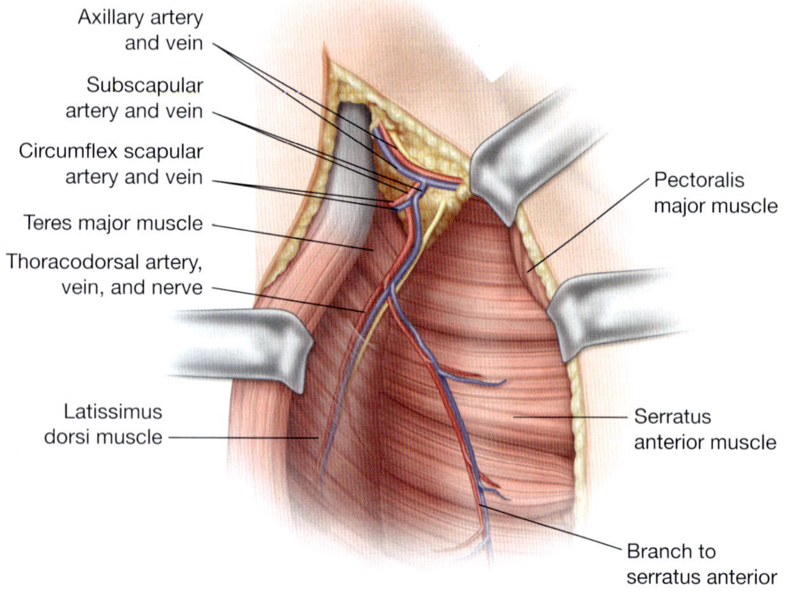

FIG 1 • Vascular anatomy of the thoracodorsal artery and vein.

is located approximately 2.6 cm medial and parallel to the lateral border. The serratus branch (artery to the serratus anterior), which joins the thoracodorsal artery just before its entrance to the latissimus muscle, is a useful landmark as it guides one directly to the thoracodorsal pedicle. There is usually a single vena comitans of the thoracodorsal artery.[8,9]

- The thoracodorsal motor nerve enters the muscle with the vascular pedicle. Cutaneous sensory nerves arise from the intercostal nerves at the midaxillary line and also in the paraspinal region.

PATIENT HISTORY AND PHYSICAL FINDINGS

- A thorough history and physical examination are critical in preparing for reconstruction.
- Pertinent aspects of the history include previous axillary operations (e.g., lymph node dissections or biopsies) and medical conditions that would preclude patients from an operation of moderate length under general anesthesia.
- Certain patients (e.g., paraplegic or wheelchair-dependent individuals who cannot afford even a minimal weakening of shoulder strength) probably should not undergo latissimus dorsi breast reconstruction. The average patient, however, will likely not notice a difference in shoulder function after a period of full recovery.
- A focused exam of the axilla and back for scars that may preclude use of the muscle flap or affect placement of the skin paddle is necessary.
- The presence of a viable and innervated muscle may be confirmed by having the patient activate the muscle by placing the hands on the hips and pushing firmly. However, a vigorous muscle contraction does not necessarily indicate an intact thoracodorsal arterial pedicle, as the nerve is quite separated from the thoracodorsal artery proximal to the branch point from the subscapular artery and could be potentially preserved despite ligation of the thoracodorsal artery.
- A team-based approach involving surgeons, anesthesiologists, primary care physicians, and other specialists such as cardiologists when needed ensures that patients are evaluated as a whole and all key concerns are addressed.

IMAGING AND OTHER DIAGNOSTIC STUDIES

- Preoperative computed tomography (CT) angiography of the donor site (**FIG 2**) is recommended in patients with previous surgical procedures during which the thoracodorsal arterial pedicle may have been sacrificed (e.g., axillary lymph node dissection or modified radical mastectomy).

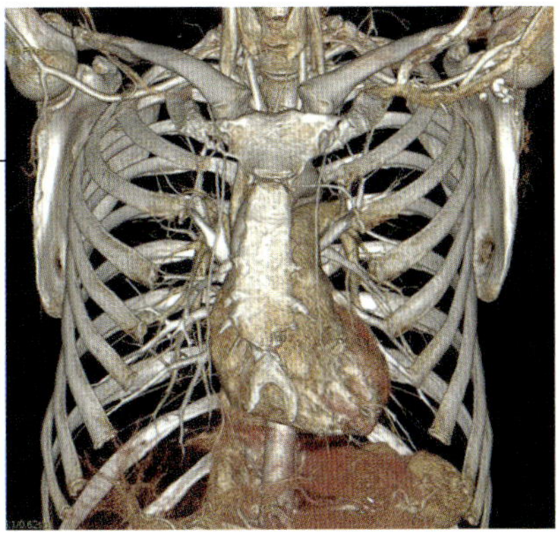

FIG 2 ● Preoperative CT angiography of the thoracodorsal vessels.

SURGICAL MANAGEMENT

- In consulting with patients, decisions about the timing of reconstruction (immediately after mastectomy or delayed) and the type of reconstruction are made taking patient factors and tumor characteristics into consideration.
  - Patient factors of significance include the following:
    - Patient preference
    - Smoking history
    - History of previous axillary operations that compromise the vascular pedicle of the donor site
    - Medical comorbidities that would preclude patients from undergoing an operation of moderate length.
  - Tumor characteristics as they relate to the following:
    - The need for postmastectomy radiation therapy
    - The need for close postmastectomy surveillance prior to reconstruction
    - In general, patients known to require postmastectomy radiation therapy are reconstructed in a delayed fashion to avoid the detrimental effects of radiation on flaps. A history of radiation therapy also serves as a relative indication for use of an autologous form of reconstruction, as implant-only reconstructions in the setting of radiation are prone to higher rates of complications and failure.

Preoperative Planning

- Basic labs (chemistry and blood counts)
- All anticoagulant and antiplatelet medications should be stopped a week prior to the operation. Warfarin can be bridged with enoxaparin a week prior.
- Smokers are required to quit for a minimum of 4 weeks prior.
- Patients receive preoperative antibiotics with intraoperative redosing.
- Patients receive deep vein thrombosis (DVT) prophylaxis with use of a pneumatic compression device at the beginning of the case; preoperative subcutaneous heparin is not typically used in our practice.
- A Foley catheter will be needed, given the length of the case.
- A headlight may be helpful in the harvest of the latissimus dorsi muscle.
- A beanbag is needed for lateral decubitus positioning.
- A sterile Doppler probe is helpful to have available in case there is any concern for the location or integrity of the thoracodorsal pedicle during the case.

Positioning

Marking/positioning

- The inframammary fold (IMF), medial limit, and lateral limit of the breast should be marked with the patient upright.
- With the patient in the sitting position, have the patient activate the latissimus muscle (by placing hands on the hips and coughing) and mark anterolateral margin of the muscle.

- Other key landmarks for the limits of the latissimus muscle are the tip of scapula, vertebral column, and posterior iliac crest. They should be marked for additional orientation.
- The pivot point for the flap is the approximate pedicle location: It should be marked 2 to 3 cm medial to lateral border and 9 cm below the apex of the axilla.
- Eight to 10-cm–wide skin paddles can generally be closed primarily (verify adequate skin laxity by pinching). The skin paddle must be placed over the muscular portion of the latissimus, as the vascularity of the skin over the thoracolumbar fascia is notoriously poor. In most patients, it is necessary to stay at least 8 cm superior to the posterior iliac crest to avoid the thoracolumbar fascia (**FIG 3**).
- Verify that the skin paddle has been designed correctly for rotating to the planned anterior position by measuring from the estimated pedicle pivot point to the inferolateral tip of the skin paddle. This distance must equal the distance from the pivot point to the medial limit of your planned mastectomy incision.
- The orientation of the axis of the skin paddle can be varied (**FIG 4**). A horizontally oriented skin paddle allows the scar to be hidden by a bra strap but may limit the size of the paddle harvested.

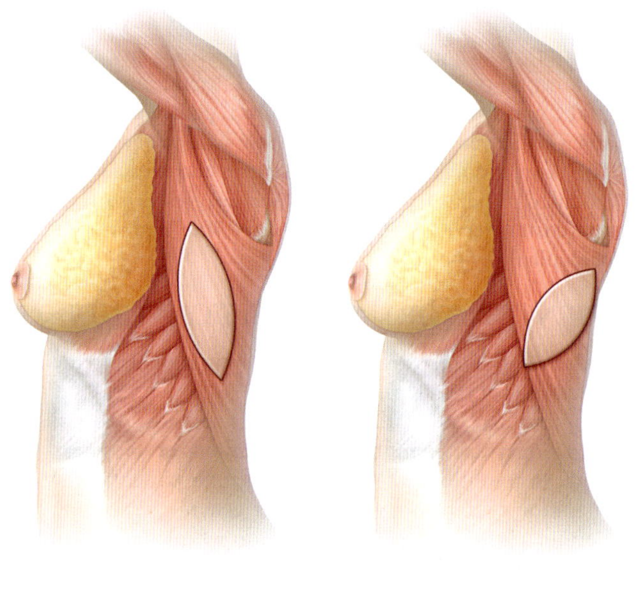

FIG 4 • Possible orientations of the latissimus dorsi flap skin paddles.

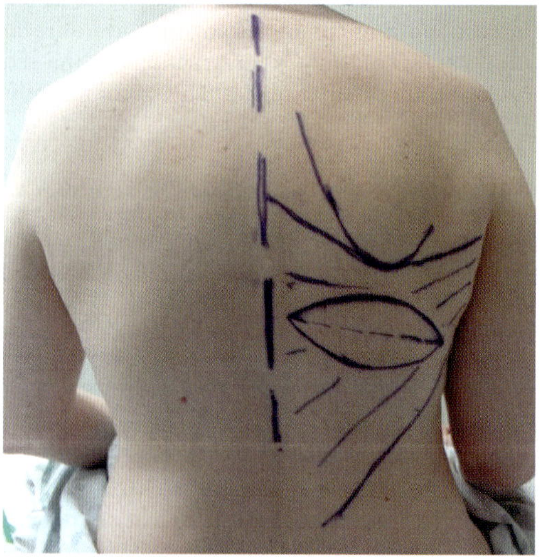

FIG 3 • Flap markings.

- Measure the breast base width to guide your choice of tissue expander size.
- Patient positioning varies by surgeon. Harvesting a full latissimus dorsi flap requires a lateral decubitus position with a special arm support for the ipsilateral arm and an axillary roll under the contralateral axilla to prevent brachial plexopathy. The lower extremities will also require adequate padding.
- Placing patients in the supine position during the earlier or latter parts of the case is based on surgeon preference and laterality of reconstruction (unilateral vs. bilateral). Bilateral procedures absolutely require position changes.
- The description in the following text will include multiple position changes to make clear the sequence of events for the procedure. This sequence can then be modified.

TECHNIQUES

RECIPIENT SITE PREPARATION (IN EITHER SUPINE OR LATERAL POSITION)

- Develop the recipient site with the patient in supine position: Elevate the skin and subcutaneous flaps off the pectoralis major to recreate the mastectomy defect in cases of delayed reconstruction; for immediate reconstruction, the mastectomy skin flaps are already developed by the breast surgeon.
- Natural borders of the breast should be preserved, including the IMF and skin adherence to the sternum along the midline. A possible exception would be in delayed reconstruction where the inferior dissection can extend approximately 0.5 to 1.0 cm inferior to the IMF to allow the expander to sit at the IMF after the latissimus is inset.
- Limit the lateral dissection, when possible, to the anterior axillary line with the exception of a three to four fingerbreadths tunnel created to allow for transfer of the flap. This tunnel should not violate the IMF.
- The lateral dissection is performed in a suprafascial plane within the tunnel and extends to the lateral border of the latissimus.
- Dissect 2 to 3 cm past the border of the latissimus, on its deep surface, to facilitate flap elevation when the patient is repositioned (**FIG 5**).
- Elevation of the pectoralis major muscle is then performed, disinserting the muscle from its attachments to ribs at the IMF. This disinsertion is terminated at lateral border of the sternum.

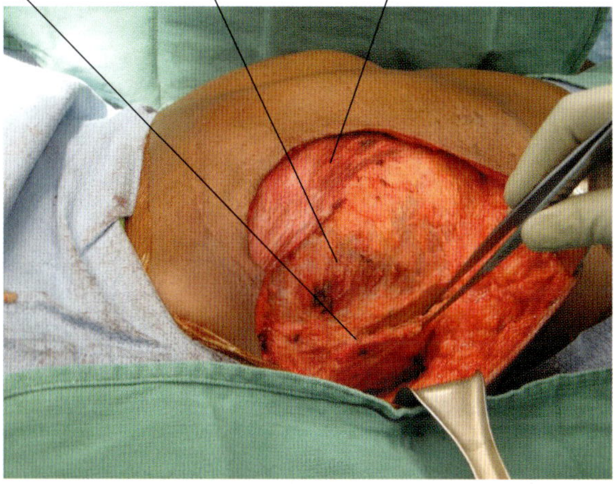

FIG 5 ● View of the chest wall with exposure of the pectoralis major, serratus anterior, and lateral border of the latissimus dorsi muscle.

- The anterior chest surgical site is then packed with moist laparotomy sponges, tucking a sponge laterally under the lateral border of the latissimus. This also helps identify this border of the flap during harvest in the lateral decubitus position. An Ioban sheet is then used to seal the mastectomy defects.

FLAP HARVEST

- The patient is either placed in a lateral decubitus position (**FIG 6**) for a unilateral flap harvest or in a prone position for bilateral flap harvests.
- All position changes require reprepping and redraping of the operative fields.
- The incision is made on the lines of the designed skin paddle. As soon as subcutaneous fat is visualized, the plane of dissection should be beveled outward in a fashion to preserve as many vascular perforators as possible.
- The skin and subcutaneous tissue are elevated off the latissimus muscle until the superior, medial, and inferior limits of the muscle are visualized.

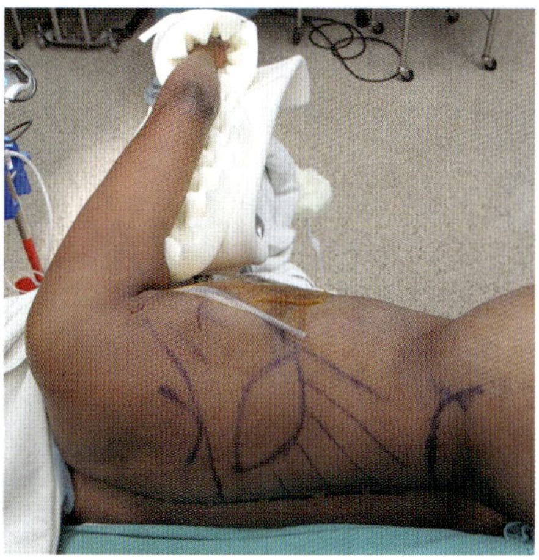

FIG 6 ● Patient positioning (lateral decubitus) for flap harvest.

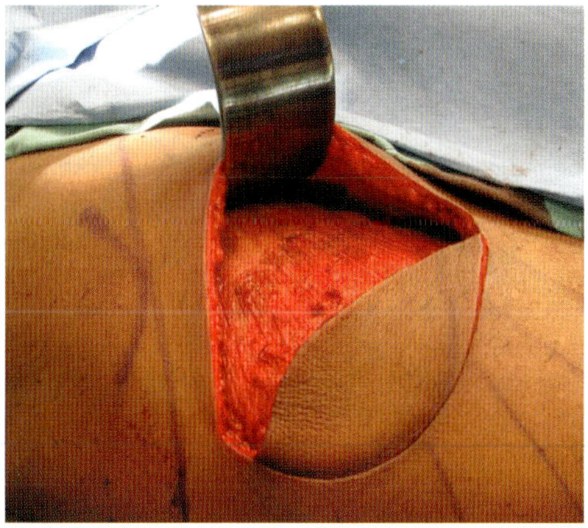

FIG 7 ● Exposure of superficial surface of the muscle during flap harvest.

- Retraction can be a challenging aspect of this step. A Deaver or Harrington retractor and Bovie electrocautery extension are helpful (**FIG 7**).
- Dissection under the lateral edge of the latissimus is now initiated, starting in the area inferolaterally. Note that the anterior edge of the muscle often approaches the midaxillary line.
- Identification of the lateral border of the muscle is easy if elevation is begun while the patient is supine, with placement of a laparotomy sponge under the muscle edge as outlined previously.
- Dissection deep to the latissimus near the pedicle should be done cautiously with electrocautery to minimize the chance for pedicle damage.
- Visualization of the pedicle is not necessary for most pedicled flaps with the exception of flaps requiring

a division of the muscle insertion or flaps requiring denervation.

- Note that the serratus branch artery (FIG 1) can guide you from the serratus anterior muscle to the superiorly located thoracodorsal vessels.
- Lateral and medial row segmental pattern perforators to the skin will be encountered in the paraspinal region and should be meticulously cauterized.
- The latissimus muscle is divided medially and inferiorly at the point where the muscle fibers transition into the thoracolumbar fascia.
- Deep to the latissimus muscle, the dissection should be limited to muscle only, leaving behind adipose tissue, as this contains many lymphatic channels; preserving this lymphatic circulation is thought to reduce the risk for seroma.
- The fully elevated flap (FIG 8) is then rotated into the previously created lateral chest wall tunnel for passage to the mastectomy defect.
- Placing a large silk stitch on the medial edge of the flap skin paddle is helpful for locating the flap within the tunnel and subsequently for traction to slide the flap through the subcutaneous tunnel.
- A drain tube is placed in back donor site.

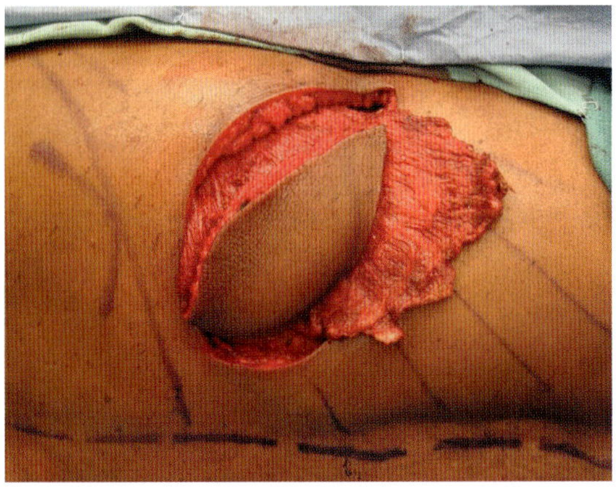

FIG 8 • Elevated latissimus dorsi myocutaneous flap.

- The back donor site is then closed in layers.
- Prior to closure, fibrin sealant such as Tisseel or Evicel can be instilled into the donor site. Although not absolutely necessary, this maneuver is thought to reduce the risk for seroma.
- Dressings in the form of a skin glue product, Steri-Strips, or an ointment are then applied to the suture line.

INSETTING OF THE FLAP

- The patient is repositioned to the supine position.
- The latissimus muscle is advanced into the recipient site. Any restricting bands of tissue near the pedicle pivot point can be carefully lysed to yield better flap rotation and an ideal position of the pedicle.
- Complete skeletonization of the pedicle is not necessary. Disinsertion of the muscle attachments to the humerus can be performed to gain a few additional centimeters of reach.
- Ligation of the thoracodorsal nerve eliminates contraction of the muscle, which can be bothersome to some patients. Most patients, however, do not complain about persistent muscle contractions after transposition of this muscle without sacrificing the motor nerve.
- The latissimus muscle is then inset to the IMF with interrupted absorbable sutures.
- A tissue expander selected based on the patient's chest wall dimensions (primarily breast base width) is then placed in the pocket flanked superiorly by the pectoralis major muscle flap and inferiorly by the latissimus dorsi myocutaneous flap (FIG 9).
- Tissue expanders with suture tabs can be used, as they allow the expander to be secured to the chest wall temporarily, preventing migration and optimizing expansion of desired areas of the breast mound.
- The pectoralis major muscle is then approximated to the latissimus with interrupted or running absorbable sutures.
- If there are concerns for tension on the flap, filling of the tissue expander (FIG 10) should be delayed.

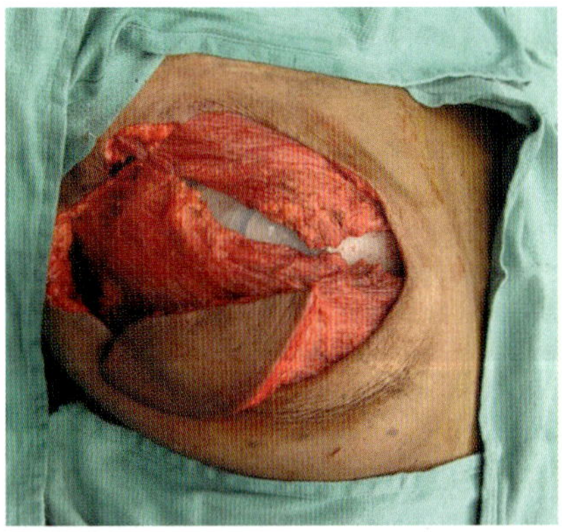

FIG 9 • Tissue expander placed behind the pectoralis major (superior) and latissimus dorsi (inferior) muscle flaps within the mastectomy defect.

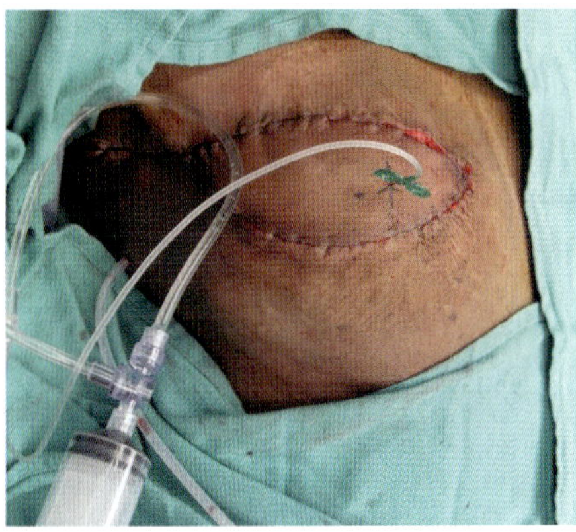

FIG 10 • Intraoperative fill of the tissue expander.

- The subcutaneous tunnel opening to the lateral tissue expander pocket can be closed to prevent lateral migration of the implant.
- A drain tube is placed deep to the skin flaps but superficial to the muscle flaps at the inferior pole of the breast, exiting at the lateral chest wall.
- Skin closure is performed in layers with absorbable interrupted deep dermal sutures and a running subcuticular suture (**FIG 11**).
- Dressings in the form of a skin glue product, Steri-Strips, or an ointment are then applied to the suture line.

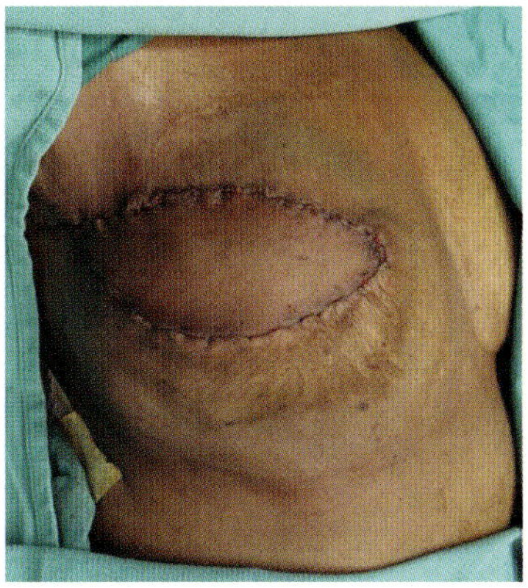

FIG 11 ● Inset flap skin paddle.

PEARLS AND PITFALLS

Preoperative planning	■ Preoperative CT angiography is worthwhile when axillary lymph node dissection has been performed previously. The thoracodorsal vessels are occasionally ligated during axillary dissections.
Positioning	■ Minimizing the position changes will reduce surgical duration. For instance, a lateral position for both recipient site preparation and donor site harvest followed by supine positioning for the inset and expander placement takes advantage of a single position change.
Freeing the latissimus dorsi	■ Identifying and beginning the dissection underneath the lateral border of the latissimus while the patient is supine allows for an easier flap elevation once the patient is in a lateral position. ■ Disinserting the muscle attachments to the humerus improves the reach of the muscle.
Postoperative seroma	■ Avoid taking out donor site drains too early as seromas are common with this flap elevation.

POSTOPERATIVE CARE

- Patients can be transferred from the operating room (OR) to a postanesthesia care unit (PACU) or directly to a unit with nursing capabilities for flap monitoring.
- Flaps are monitored by physical exams (color, temperature, capillary refill) performed every hour for the first 4 hours and then checks can be spaced out to every 2 hours and 4 hours over subsequent hospital days.
- DVT prophylaxis is the only form of anticoagulation used routinely.
- Diet is advanced from clear liquids to regular on postoperative day 1; there are no restrictions on caffeine.
- Patients are assisted to ambulate beginning on postoperative day 1.
- Foley catheters and intravenous (IV) fluids are discontinued; IV medications/patient-controlled analgesias (PCAs) are converted to orals on postoperative day 1.
- Patients are typically ready for discharge home from postoperative days 2 to 4.
- Surgical drains are discontinued once the output is less than 30 mL for 2 consecutive days.
- Activities are limited and weight-lifting restrictions are in place for 6 weeks postoperative.
- The first postoperative visit is at 1 week following discharge.
- Postoperative results for a left delayed breast reconstruction in an irradiated patient (**FIG 12**).

OUTCOMES

- Breast reconstruction outcomes may be assessed in several ways. Patient satisfaction, shoulder girdle function and reoperation rates are all parameters that have been analyzed in recent literature. An evaluation of patient satisfaction showed that latissimus dorsi breast reconstruction patients are generally satisfied with their decision, with 80% of surveyed patients indicating that they would both recommend the surgery to another person and undergo the surgery again if given the choice. Over 70% of surveyed patients found the size, shape, and scars associated with their reconstructions to be "good" or "excellent." However, contrary to what is previously believed, over one-third of patients questioned reported moderate to severe loss of shoulder force and function. By strict physiometric measurements, there is comparable shoulder range of motion and slight decrease in shoulder strength when compared to preoperative measurements at 1 year postoperatively. This amount of change does not substantially affect the ability to perform daily activities for most patients.[10] Also, reoperation rate was 50% for prosthesis-related problems at a mean follow-up time of 14.9 years.[11]

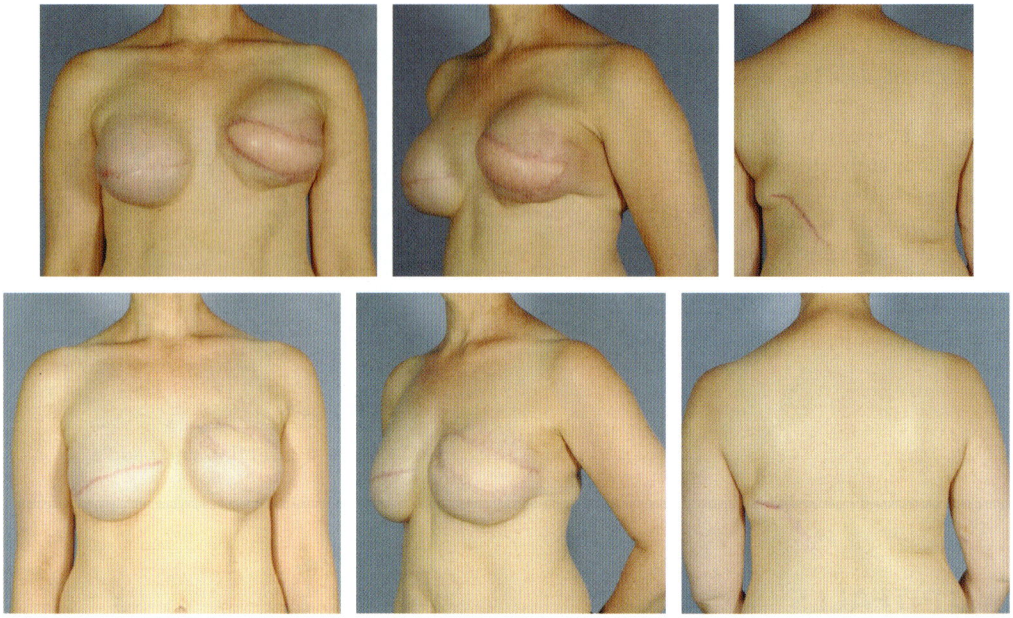

FIG 12 • A patient with left breast invasive ductal carcinoma who underwent bilateral mastectomies, adjuvant chemotherapy, and left chest wall radiation. *Above*, 4-month postoperative result after completion of tissue expansion. *Below*, 9 months after exchange of the tissue expanders for silicone implants.

- Breast reconstruction patients are typically satisfied in the short term (<5 years) with their choice of reconstruction across implant-based to autologous forms of reconstruction.[12]
- Over the long term (>8 years), satisfaction with abdominal-based flap reconstruction is maintained, whereas satisfaction with implant-based techniques tends to depreciate.[12]
- Studies have also shown greater satisfaction with autologous reconstruction in patients requiring unilateral reconstructions. This is likely the result of better symmetry with the natural contralateral breast.[12]
- Patient satisfaction in bilateral reconstructions has been found to be similar across all techniques provided that the same technique is used on both sides,[12] highlighting again the importance of symmetry.

COMPLICATIONS

Flap-Related Complications

- Infections/implant extrusions—risks for these complications are elevated for implant-only reconstruction of irradiated sites. Autologous tissue transferred to the chest over a prosthesis offers greater resistance to infection or implant extrusion than do prostheses alone on irradiated sites.[13,14]
- Delayed wound healing—this complication typically occurs at the interface between the mastectomy flap and latissimus flap skin paddle. It often is a result of marginal mastectomy flap necrosis from poor skin perfusion, which is more likely in smokers and in the previously radiated breast skin.
- Partial flap loss—an uncommon complication (~3% or less) that is also related to poor perfusion.[15,16] It can be the result of poor skin paddle design. An excision of the necrotic segment is usually required.
- Total flap loss—this is one of the most devastating complications encountered and it occurs in less than 1% of reconstructions.[15,16]
- Capsular contracture—recent studies based on the newest generation implants report approximately 16%.[17]

Donor Site Complications

- Seroma—approximately 9% of latissimus dorsi flap donor sites encounter a seroma.[15,16] Some studies report as high as 34%.[17]
- Delayed wound healing—wound healing problems are encountered often in morbidly obese patients, diabetics, and smokers. These wounds are managed by debridement and dressing changes with healing by secondary intention.

REFERENCES

1. Maxwell GP. Iginio Tansini and the origin of the latissimus dorsi musculocutaneous flap. *Plast Reconstr Surg*. 1980;65(5):686–692.
2. Davis HH, Tollman JP, Brush JH. Huge chondrosarcoma of rib. *Surgery*. 1949;26:699.
3. Campbell D. Reconstruction of the anterior thoracic wall. *J Thorac Surg*. 1950;19(3):456.
4. Olivari N. The latissimus flap. *Br J Plast Surg*. 1976;29(2):126–128.
5. Schneider WJ, Hill HL Jr, Brown RG. Latissimus dorsi myocutaneous flap for breast reconstruction. *Br J Plastic Surg*. 1977;30(4):277–281.
6. Hester TR Jr, Bostwick J III. Poland's syndrome: correction with latissimus muscle transposition. *Plast Reconstr Surg*. 1982;69(2):226–233.
7. Chang DW, Youssef A, Cha S, et al. Autologous breast reconstruction with the extended latissimus dorsi flap. *Plast Reconstr Surg*. 2002; 110(3):751–759.
8. Zenn MR, Jones GE. *Reconstructive Surgery: Anatomy, Technique, and Clinical Applications*. St. Louis, MO: Quality Medical; 2012.
9. Strauch B, Yu H-L. *Atlas of Microvascular Surgery: Anatomy and Operative Techniques*. 2nd ed. New York, NY: Thieme; 2006.
10. Glassey N, Perks GB, McCulley SJ. A prospective assessment of shoulder morbidity and recovery time scales following latissimus dorsi breast reconstruction. *Plast Reconstr Surg*. 2008;122(5):1334–1340.
11. Tarantino I, Banic A, Fischer T. Evaluation of late results in breast reconstruction by latissimus dorsi flap and prosthesis implantation. *Plast Reconstr Surg*. 2006;117(5):1387–1394.

12. Hu ES, Pusic AL, Waljee JF, et al. Patient-reported aesthetic satisfaction with breast reconstruction during the long-term survivorship period. *Plast Reconstr Surg*. 2009;124(1):1–8.
13. Kroll SS, Schusterman MA, Reece GP, et al. Breast reconstruction with myocutaneous flaps in previously irradiated patients. *Plast Reconstr Surg*. 1994;93(3):460–469.
14. Spear SL, Boehmler JH, Taylor NS, et al. The role of the latissimus dorsi flap in reconstruction of the irradiated breast. *Plast Reconstr Surg*. 2007;119(1):1–9.
15. De Mey A, Lejour M, Declety A, et al. Late results and current indications of latissimus dorsi breast reconstructions. *Br J Plast Surg*. 1991;44(1):1–4.
16. Moore TS, Farrell LD. Latissimus dorsi myocutaneous flap for breast reconstruction: long-term results. *Plast Reconstr Surg*. 1992;89(4): 666–672.
17. Sternberg EG, Perdikis G, McLaughlin SA, et al. Latissimus dorsi flap remains an excellent choice for breast reconstruction. *Ann Plast Surg*. 2006;56(1):31–35.

Chapter 17

Pedicled Transverse Rectus Abdominis Myocutaneous Flap Breast Reconstruction

Dale Collins Vidal Emily B. Ridgway

DEFINITION

- All patients undergoing mastectomy, or those who have undergone a prior mastectomy, are potential candidates for breast reconstruction. The choice to have breast reconstruction is personal, and the options available for breast reconstruction are affected by an individual's anatomy, weight, prior surgical procedures and radiation, and personal preferences. Each patient is unique and consideration must be made of their current breast size, goal breast size, and anatomic limitations.
- The pedicled transverse rectus abdominis myocutaneous (TRAM) flap was first described by Hartrampf in the 1980s and remains the autologous "workhorse" of breast reconstruction. Diabetic patients, smokers, and patients with an elevated BMI or a pendulous panniculus have higher risk for flap failure.

PATIENT HISTORY AND PHYSICAL FINDINGS

- A complete medical and surgical history is essential.
- Prior comorbidities should be identified and the decision for preoperative anesthesia evaluation should be made.
- Current related history must include cancer stage; *BRCA* status; and prior treatments including lumpectomy, biopsy, neoadjuvant chemotherapy, and radiation.
- Accurate documentation of any prior abdominal, pelvic, cardiac, and groin surgery is necessary in order to evaluate the candidacy for a TRAM flap.
- Current breast size, the patient's goal for breast size, and the amount of abdominal tissue will also guide surgical planning and the need for a contralateral symmetry surgery.
- Risks, benefits, and alternate therapies must also be reviewed with the patient including other autologous options (free and pedicled) and implant-based reconstruction options.

Anatomy

- As with any surgical technique, a thorough working knowledge of the anatomy of the chest and abdominal wall and any variants is essential. The primary blood supply of the breast originates from internal mammary perforating branches. Secondary blood supply is received via perforating arteries from the lateral thoracic, pectoral, thoracic, and lateral intercostal arteries. Many of these vessels are injured during mastectomy and much of the mastectomy flap blood supply is compromised and relies on dermal and subcutaneous vessels running just deep to the dermis.
- The abdominal wall is made of skin, varying thickness of subcutaneous adipose tissue, and an anterior rectus fascia overlying the paired rectus abdominis muscles (**FIG 1**).
- Deep to the muscles is the posterior rectus fascia made up of the transversus fascia and internal oblique muscle fascia above the arcuate line and the transversus fascia below the arcuate line.
- The paired rectus muscles originate from the pubic bone and extend to the cartilage of the 6th, 7th and 8th ribs. The blood supply comes from the dominant deep inferior epigastric artery and the superior epigastric artery (**FIG 2**).

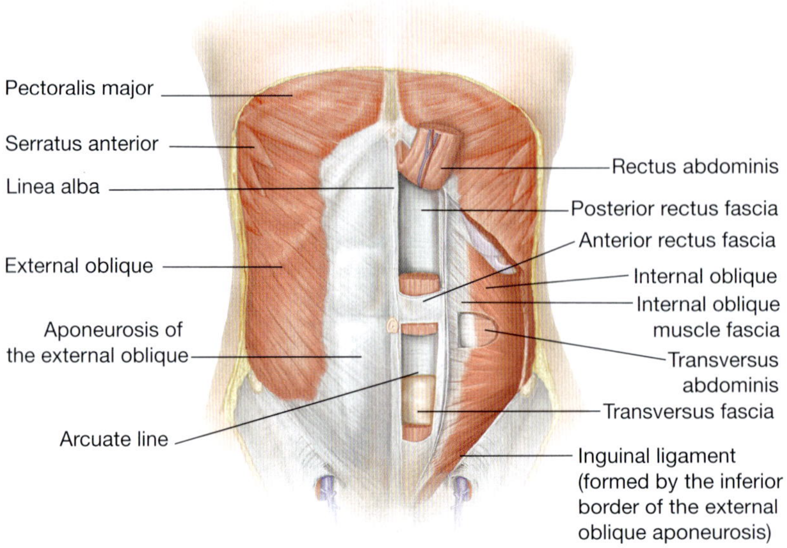

FIG 1 • Abdominal wall musculature.

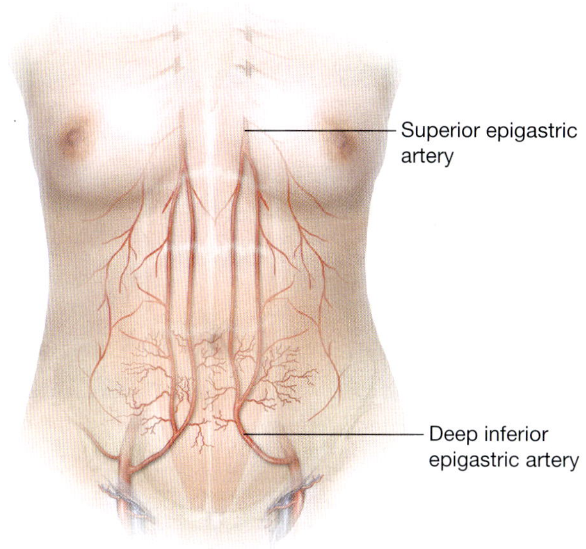

FIG 2 ● Abdominal wall blood supply.

Additional blood supply comes from the posterior perforating vessels accompanying the 8th through 12th intercostal neurovascular bundles.

- Within the muscle, the superior and inferior epigastric arteries may not have direct anastomoses under normal conditions. These connections are made or increased with surgical delay of the deep inferior epigastric artery.
- Musculocutaneous perforators pass through the muscle and anterior rectus fascia (**FIG 3**). They are often gathered in the periumbilical area and in mirrored medial and lateral rows of perforators. The medial and lateral row of perforators on a given side is separated by approximately 1.5 to 2 cm.

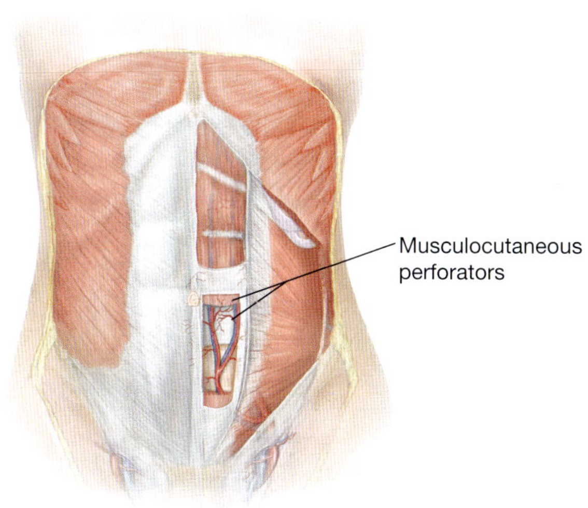

FIG 3 ● Surgical delay is performed to ligate the deep inferior epigastric artery and vein.

In the case of the pedicled TRAM flap, the flap is based on the superior epigastric vessels.

SURGICAL MANAGEMENT

Preoperative Planning

- For high-risk patients, ligation of the inferior epigastric artery (surgical delay) should be considered. Surgical delay of the inferior epigastric artery is performed 10 to 14 days prior to the mastectomy. This is often performed at the time of sentinel lymph node biopsy in order to limit events requiring anesthesia.
- On the day of reconstruction, the patient is marked first in the standing position. At the breast, the inframammary fold (IMF), midline and a line 1 cm off the midline on either side, the lateral breast extension, and proposed or prior mastectomy skin incision approach are marked. The width of the proposed breast reconstruction is measured as this will guide the ideal width of the abdominal flap, which is particularly important in delayed breast reconstruction where there is often a paucity of breast skin (**FIG 4**).
- On the abdomen, the midline is marked and an ellipse of skin including the umbilicus is marked. In our experience, all patients offer at least 13 cm in width of the ellipse and this can be assessed with a pinch test (**FIG 4**).
- The patient is then seated and any further extensions of the incisions are laterally marked to remove any "dog ear."

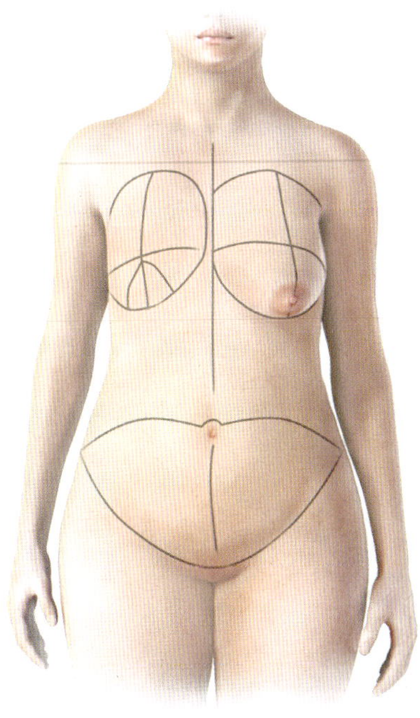

FIG 4 ● Preoperative marking of chest and abdomen in the standing position. Note the lateral dimension of the planned breast should correlate to the height of the planned TRAM flap. The TRAM flap is centered around the site of largest perforators at the periumbilical region.

- Perioperative antibiotics are provided and a Foley catheter and sequential compression device (SCD) boots are placed.
- The flap can be raised while the mastectomy is being performed. No tumescence is used. The superior incision is made first, and the upper abdominal wall is raised to the level of the costochondral cartilages. On the side of the planned reconstruction, a tunnel is made through the IMF into the mastectomy pocket that fits a fist and the planned flap.
- The patient is then flexed and the superior abdominal flap brought down to verify its pending closure and the possible height of the flap to be created. The inferior incision is then made. Beginning laterally on each side, the flap is then elevated with electrocautery above the level of the fascia until the lateral border of the rectus abdominis is seen. At this point, either bipolar or very low cautery is recommended for continuing to complete the identification of both the medial and lateral rows of perforators (**FIG 5**). If a bilateral reconstruction is planned, the midline incision may also be made to help in exposure for dissection (**FIG 6**). No perforators should be sacrificed at this time.
- Once all perforators have been identified, the flap vascularity is assessed. In unilateral reconstruction cases, if one flap has a heartier blood supply, this flap is chosen.
- Methylene blue is then used to mark the planned fascia incisions including each row of perforators and only the intervening fascia. A no.10 blade is used to incise the fascia and sharp dissection around the outside of each medial and lateral perforator under loupe magnification (**FIGS 7** and **8**). The width of this fascia (approximately 2 cm) is also included in the flap superiorly to the level of the costochondral cartilage (**FIG 8**). The underlying rectus muscle is then secured to the anterior rectus fascia and overlying Scarpa's fascia with several 3-0 Vicryl sutures on either side to prevent the flap from being avulsed from the muscle.

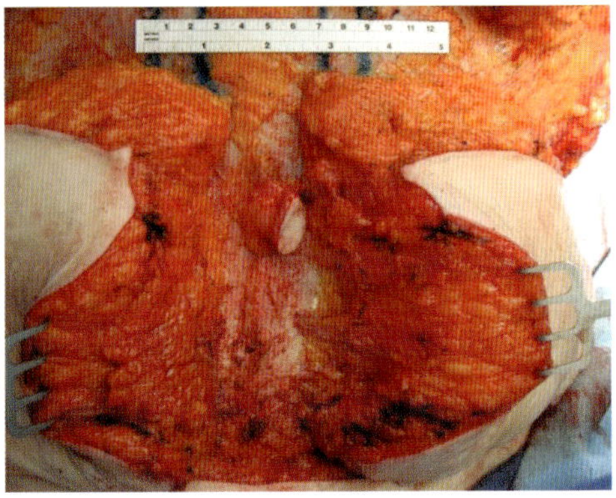

FIG 6 • If a bilateral reconstruction is planned, the midline incision may also be made to help in exposure for dissection.

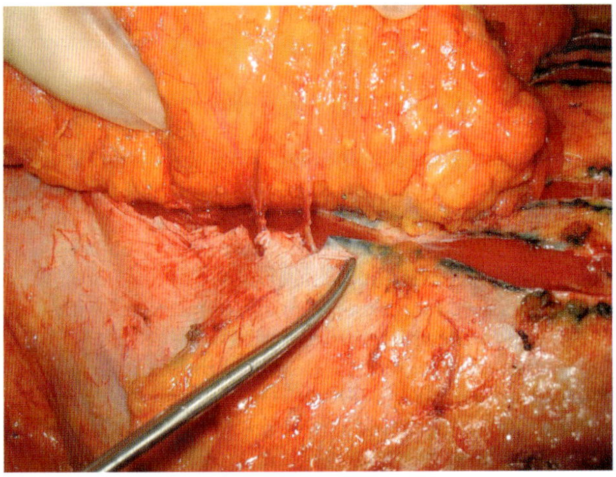

FIG 7 • Methylene blue is then used to mark the planned fascia incisions including each row of perforators and only the intervening fascia.

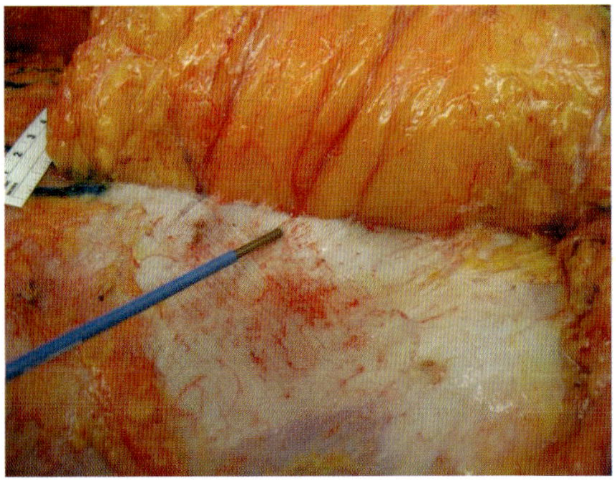

FIG 5 • Lateral flap elevation: Beginning laterally on each side, the flap is elevated with Bovie cautery above the level of the fascia until the lateral border of the rectus abdominis is seen. At this point, either bipolar or very low cautery is recommended for continuing to complete the identification of both the medial and lateral rows of perforators.

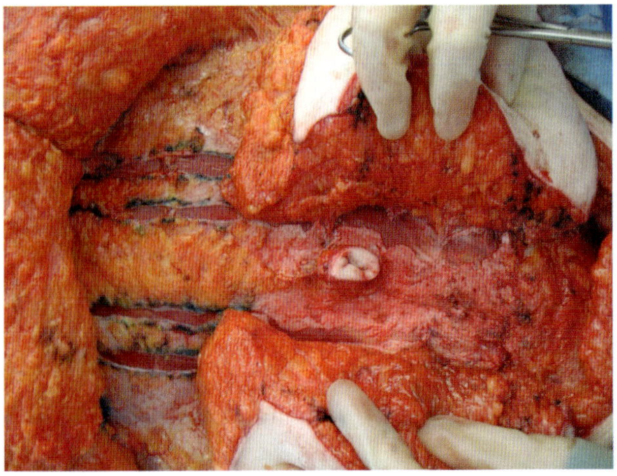

FIG 8 • Perforator dissection. A no. 10 blade is used to incise the fascia and sharp dissection around the outside of each medial and lateral perforator under loupes magnification.

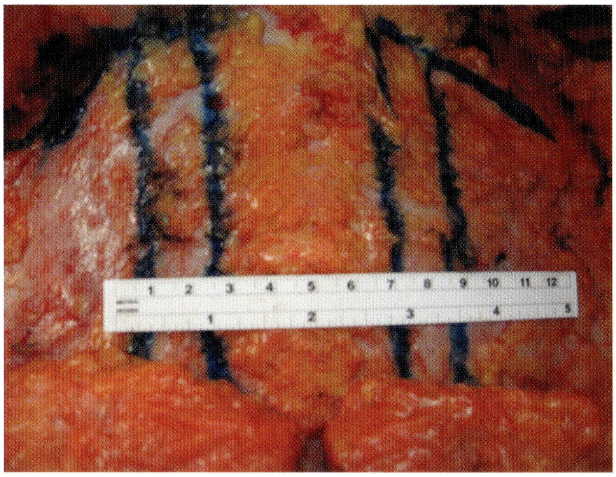

FIG 9 • Flap elevation: The width of the fascia within the TRAM (approximately 2 cm) is also included in the flap superiorly to the level of the costochondral cartilage.

- Circumferential muscle dissection is then completed, the deep inferior epigastric artery identified and clipped, and the inferior portion of the muscle divided. The flap is then raised and any posterior perforators and intercostal nerves clipped such that there is no tethering of the flap (FIG 9. At the superior border of the fascial dissection, a back cut is made to allow the flap to rotate superiorly without tension or kinking of the blood supply. The flap is then placed within the mastectomy pocket.
- The donor site is then verified for hemostasis particularly at the site of the deep inferior epigastric artery ligation and the narrow gap in the anterior rectus fascia closed with 0-Vicryl and 0-polydioxanone (PDS) sutures (FIG 10).

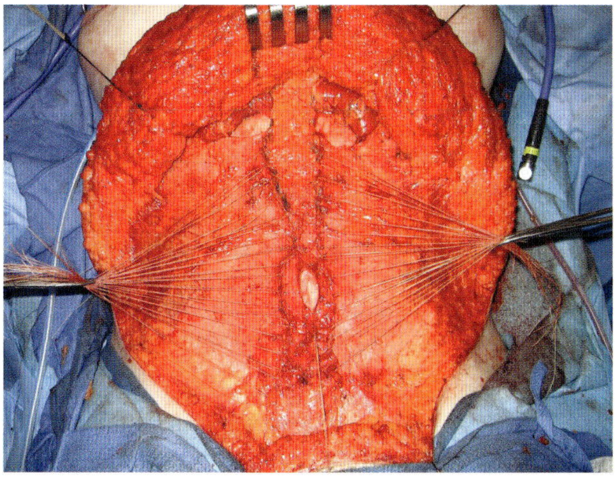

FIG 10 • Fascia closure: The anterior rectus fascia is closed with interrupted 0-Vicryl and a running 0-PDS suture. The posterior sheath has not been violated. Hemostasis is crucial prior to closure of the fascia.

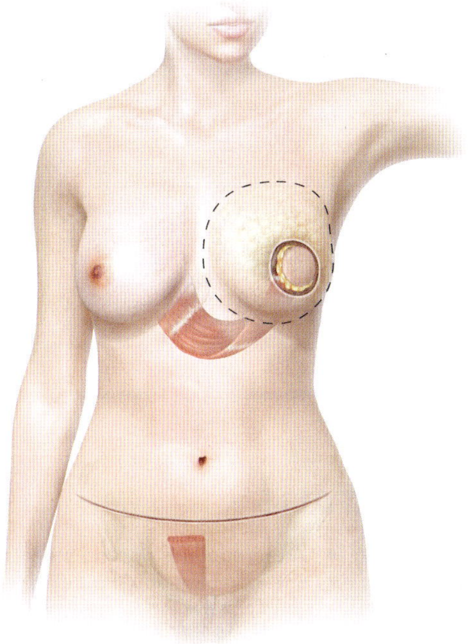

FIG 11 • Flap placement: The flap is then rotated into the ipsilateral or contralateral mastectomy defect via the prepared tunnel.

In unilateral cases, a plication may be performed on the contralateral side to restore the umbilicus to the midline. This plication and closure should extend from the costochondral margin to the pubic bone to create a smooth desirable abdominal contour. The bed is then flexed and two drains are placed exiting through inferolateral stab incisions. The Scarpa's fascia is then approximated with 0-Vicryl sutures and the dermis closed with buried deep dermal 3-0 Vicryl followed by a subcuticular 4-0 Monocryl and dermal glue.

- By this time, the mastectomy flap can be either clinically assessed or studies used to assess the viability of the mastectomy flaps. The lateral border of the breast can be recreated using dermal to fascia 3-0 Vicryl sutures. Puckering at this time is expected and will resolve. In cases of questionable flap viability, these areas may be excised or the flap inset delayed to allow further debridement of the flaps 3 to 5 days later. In cases where the mastectomy flap is viable, the TRAM flap is de-epithelialized in non–nipple-sparing cases except for the site of the nipple–areolar complex (NAC) or entirely in cases of nipple-sparing mastectomies (FIG 11). The flap is then secured medially and superiorly with Vicryl sutures to the pectoralis fascia. A drain is placed running along the IMF and exiting through a lateral stab incision (two drains are placed if axillary lymph node dissection has been performed) and the wound is closed with deep dermal 3-0 Vicryl sutures and a 4-0 Monocryl subcuticular suture followed by dermal glue (FIG 12).

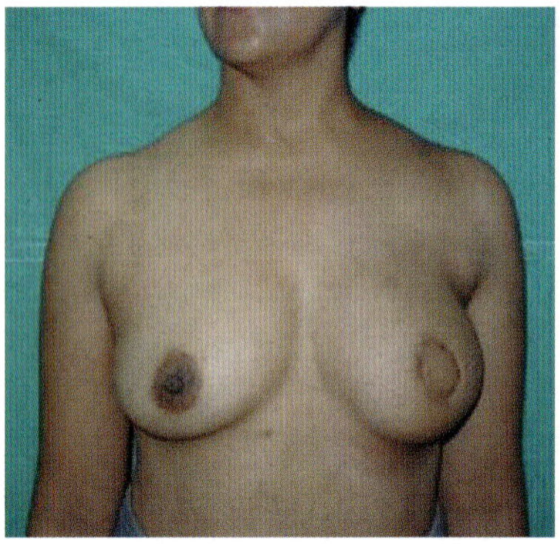

FIG 12 ● Immediate tram reconstruction for left skin sparing mastectomy.

PEARLS AND PITFALLS

Preoperative planning	▪ A thorough history and physical will identify high-risk factors. ▪ Smoking cessation should be strongly encouraged. ▪ High-risk patients should be considered for surgical delay. ▪ A thorough discussion with the patient regarding goals and reasonable expectations is essential.
Patient marking	▪ Careful marking of the patient in the standing and seating positions is essential to a successful TRAM flap.
Intraoperative technique	▪ Use either bipolar or very low cautery to avoid injury to the medial and lateral rows of perforators. ▪ Carefully assess the mastectomy flap viability. Excise any questionable areas or consider delaying the flap inset.

POSTOPERATIVE CARE

- Awaiting extubation and during transfer of the patient, the bed is kept in the flexed position.
- Routine postoperative care includes removal of the Foley catheter on the night of surgery, SCD boots, and subcutaneous deep vein thrombosis (DVT) prophylaxis beginning 6 hours after the procedure is completed and per the Caprini scale.
- Patients are moved to the chair and ambulated the afternoon of surgery or next morning.
- Incentive spirometry is encouraged hourly.
- No bra is initially placed to prevent compression of the pedicle, and a binder is placed when patient is ambulating but not while in the chair or sitting up in bed again to avoid compression of the pedicle. The binder is recommended for 6 to 8 weeks followed by use of compression undergarments for comfort. A surgical bra without underwire is placed in clinic on the first visit once the mastectomy flap has matured.
- No postoperative antibiotics are given after inset of the flap.
- Patients are discharged between 1 and 3 days after the procedure or on the day of inset if inset has been delayed.

COMPLICATIONS

- The most common complications related to breast reconstruction is mastectomy flap necrosis. Careful inspection and experience with your breast surgeon is critical.
- Partial flap loss or fat necrosis are also possible but have been limited by our requirements of smoking cessation and experience with surgical delay prior to TRAM. Complete flap loss is very unusual.
- Abdominal bulge, hernia, and back pain are also reported complications of TRAM patients.
- DVT and pulmonary embolus are life-threatening complications.

OUTCOMES

- In immediate breast reconstruction cases, common revisions include lateral abdominal dog ear scar revision. If the case was not nipple sparing, this can be performed under local anesthesia at the time of nipple reconstruction.
- Asymmetry can be improved also based on the patient's breast size goal and preoperative size, with contralateral breast reduction or mastopexy.
- Secondary revisions are more common in cases of delayed reconstruction. These can be performed to improve symmetry at the time of nipple reconstruction.
- In all cases, the superior pole may have a paucity of tissue and can be improved with autologous fat grafting. A common secondary procedure includes NAC reconstruction, dog ear revisions, and fat grafting to the superior pole.
- With these revisions, we have found patients to be very satisfied with their outcomes, with a few number of interventions (**FIG 13**).

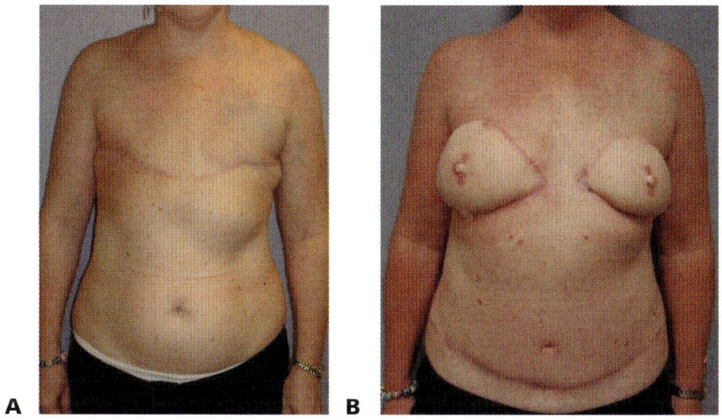

FIG 13 • **A,B.** Pre- and postoperative images of delayed TRAM flap breast reconstruction.

SUGGESTED READINGS

1. Hartrampf CR, Scheflan M, Black PW. Breast reconstruction with a transverse abdominal island flap. *Plast Reconstr Surg.* 1982;69(2): 216–225.
2. Kanchwala SK, Bucky LP. Optimizing pedicled transverse rectus abdominis muscle flap breast reconstruction. *Cancer J.* 2008;14(4): 236–240.
2. Serletti JM. Breast reconstruction with the TRAM flap: pedicled and free. *J Surg Oncol.* 2006;94(6):532–537.
3. Shestak KC. Breast reconstruction with a pedicled TRAM flap. *Clin Plast Surg.* 1998;25(2):167–182.
4. Mizgala CL, Hartrampf CR Jr, Bennett GK. Assessment of the abdominal wall after pedicled TRAM flap surgery: 5- to 7-year follow-up of 150 consecutive patients. *Plast Reconstr Surg.* 1994;93(5):988–1002.
5. Atisha DM, Comizio RC, Telischak KM, et al. Interval inset of TRAM flaps in immediate breast reconstruction: a technical refinement. *Ann Plast Surg.* 2010;65(6):524–527.
6. Nair N, Atisha DM, Streu R, et al. An innovative approach to the primary surgical delay procedure for pedicle TRAM flap breast reconstruction. *Plast Reconstr Surg.* 2010;125(4):173e–174e.
7. Kerrigan CL, Collins ED. Are perforator flaps truly more cost-effective than TRAM flaps? How good is the evidence. *Plast Reconstr Surg.* 2001;107(3):881–883.

Chapter **18**

Free Transverse Rectus Abdominis Musculocutaneous Flap Reconstruction after Mastectomy

Maurice Y. Nahabedian Ketan M. Patel

DEFINITION

- Breast reconstruction using free tissue transfer techniques have become routine procedures following mastectomy.
- The most common free flaps for breast reconstruction include the free transverse rectus abdominis musculocutaneous (TRAM) flap and the deep inferior epigastric perforator (DIEP) flap. Indications for these flaps are primarily based on the availability of sufficient skin and fat at the abdominal donor site.
- There are several decision points to be considered when determining candidacy for a free TRAM or DIEP flap. Many patients are now choosing to have bilateral mastectomy and reconstruction in the setting of unilateral breast cancer or for prevention of breast cancer.
- Once the decision to proceed with an abdominal free flap for breast reconstruction has been made, decisions relating to the type of abdominal flaps are considered and based on patient anatomy and surgical experience.
- Non–muscle-sparing free TRAM flaps are technically easier but are associated with increased donor site morbidity that includes contour abnormalities and weakness. These morbidities are increased when the continuity of the rectus abdominis muscle has been disrupted, such as with the traditional pedicle TRAM and the MS-0 (full width) free TRAM. For these reasons, the full-width free TRAM flap is rarely performed and will not be included in this review.
- Muscle-sparing free TRAM flaps and DIEP flaps are technically more challenging and require a better understanding and appreciation of perforator anatomy and dissection techniques. This chapter will focus on the free TRAM flap, whereas the DIEP flap is covered in Chapter 19.
- Muscle-sparing TRAM flap classification[1] (**FIG 1** [top])
  - MS-0: no muscle preservation (traditional TRAM flap)
  - MS-1: medial *or* lateral muscle preservation
  - MS-2: medial *and* lateral muscle preservation (central muscle sacrificed)
  - MS-3: total muscle preservation (DIEP flap)

PATIENT HISTORY AND PHYSICAL FINDINGS

- Many women with moderate to excessive volume are interested in these options because of the abdominoplasty appearance of the abdomen that is usually obtained.
- In women that lack a suitable quantity of abdominal soft tissue, alternative donor site options such as the gluteal or medial thigh region are considered.
- Sufficient donor site volume must be assessed to deliver appropriate breast volume. In some cases of bilateral free flap reconstruction, a hemiabdominal flap may not provide adequate volume and adjuncts such as combining flaps with implants or autologous fat grafting may warrant consideration.
- Prior abdominal surgery or body habitus may necessitate the use of computerized tomographic angiography (CTA) or magnetic resonance angiography (MRA) to assess the patency and location of the perforators and deep inferior epigastric artery and vein.

SURGICAL MANAGEMENT

Preoperative Planning

- A thorough history should focus on comorbidities, smoking history, previous surgeries, and medications that can alter surgical management and affect microvascular reconstruction. (Examples include coagulopathies, previous cardiac bypass surgery, previous abdominal surgery, and antiplatelet medications.)
- Physical exam will uncover hernias and previous abdominal scars. In addition, an assessment of the anterior abdomen for thickness and dimensions will aid in estimating a reconstructed breast volume.
- General complications include bleeding, hematoma, seroma, infection, delayed healing, and injury to surrounding structures.
- Specific complications include a 1% to 3% total flap failure rate,[2] early revisional surgery for microsurgical anastomotic thrombosis, late revisional surgery for contour irregularities, breast asymmetry, poor cosmetic result, and donor site complications that include an abdominal bulge/hernia (3% to 5%),[3] complex scarring, lateral "dog ears," and prolonged pain.
- Average length of surgery can range from 4 to 8 hours for a unilateral reconstruction and 6 to 12 hours for a bilateral reconstruction. Appropriate deep vein thrombosis (DVT) prophylaxis and perioperative antibiotics are routinely used due to the length and extent of surgery.
- The decision to proceed with a free TRAM or DIEP flap is sometimes made preoperatively and other times intraoperatively. Patients with a high body mass index (BMI) (>35) who have an overriding pannus are usually scheduled preoperatively for a muscle-sparing free TRAM flap. In other patients, who are found to lack a dominant perforator intraoperatively, the decision to convert from a DIEP to a free TRAM is made. If one or two dominant perforators are found, a DIEP flap is performed.

Anatomy

- The lower abdominal skin is supplied by perforating vessels from the primary source vessels that include the superior and deep inferior epigastric system.

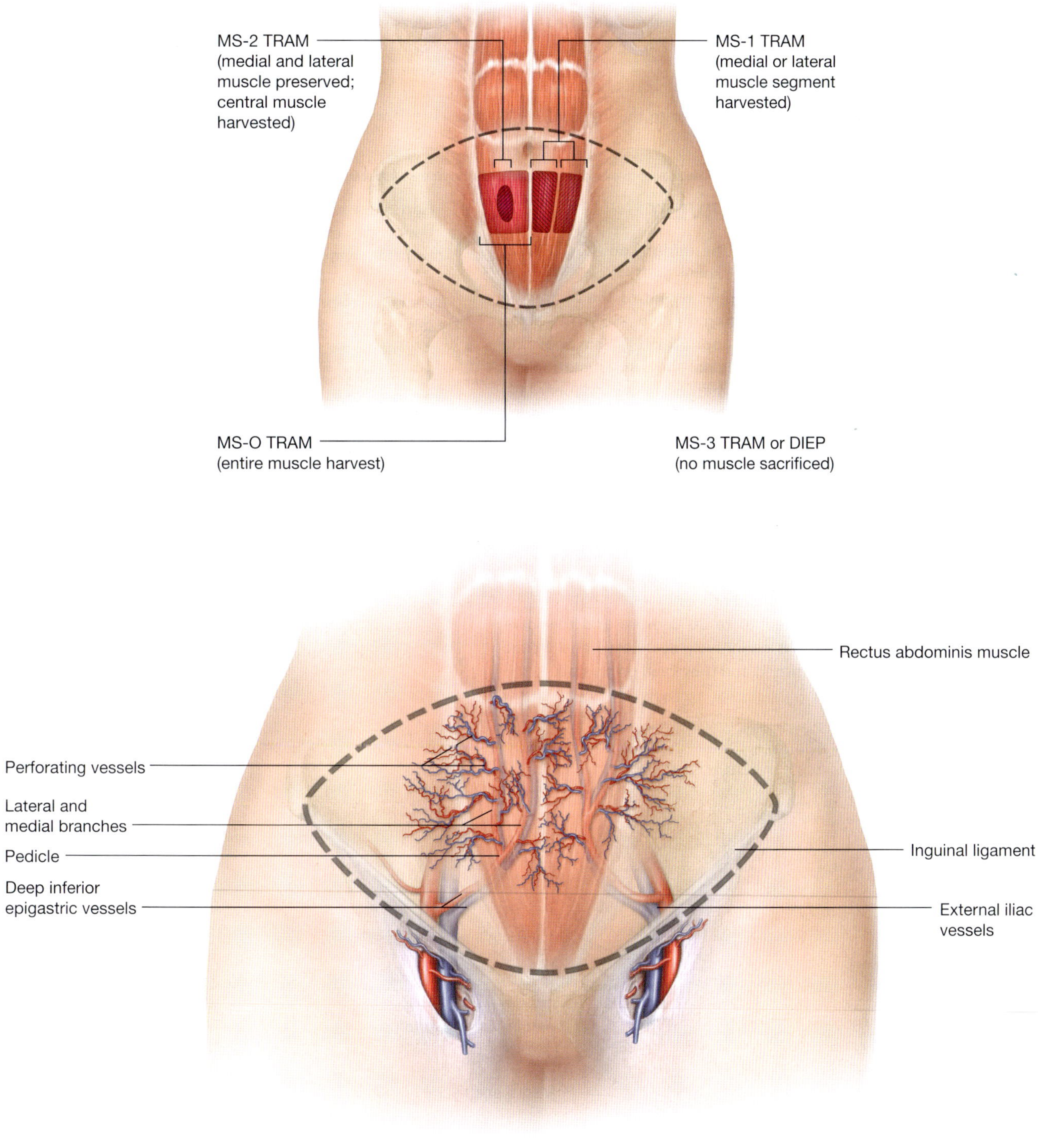

FIG 1 • The variations of muscle preservation during abdominal flap harvest are shown. A traditional MS-0 represents the entire horizontal segment of rectus harvest. An MS-1 harvest can either spare the medial *or* lateral segments of rectus abdominis muscle as shown. Sparing of the lateral segment of muscle may result in an improved functional benefit as motor innervation to this segment is spared. MS-2 flap harvest spares the medial *and* lateral muscle segments with harvest of a central portion of the muscle. An MS-3 or DIEP flap spares the entire muscle and requires intramuscular perforator dissection.

- Source vessels travel vertically along the fibers of the rectus abdominis muscle on each side of the abdomen and send vertical perforating vessels to the overlying skin and subcutaneous tissue.
- The inferior epigastric system originates from the medial aspect of the external iliac system just superior to the inguinal ligament. The pedicle enters the rectus abdominis muscle on the undersurface from the inferolateral aspect of the muscle at the junction of the lateral and central third of the muscle.
- Two main intramuscular branches are identified: a lateral and medial branch. These branches then send perforating vessels to the overlying skin (**FIG 1** [bottom]).

ABDOMINAL FLAP HARVEST

- The patient is marked in the upright position (**FIG 2**). The anterior superior iliac spine (ASIS) is palpated and marked bilaterally. The upper extent of the abdominal flap is delineated, connecting the two ASIS marks across the abdomen and staying approximately 1 cm above the umbilicus. The lower abdominal line is an estimation that extends from the two ASIS markings in a curvilinear fashion. The inferior limit of this line is the pubic symphysis. The final inferior line is determined in the operating room after the upper skin flap is redraped. The markings for a free TRAM flap and a DIEP flap are identical (**FIG 3**).
- The initial incision is the upper abdominal ellipse. The incision extends to the anterior rectus sheath using electrocautery (**FIG 4**). The upper abdominal adipocutaneous flap is typically undermined to the midpoint between the umbilicus and the xiphoid process.
- The patient is flexed 10 to 30 degrees and the lower abdominal ellipse is definitively delineated and incised. The umbilicus is incised and preserved on its stalk.
- Flap elevation begins from a lateral to medial direction at the level of the anterior rectus sheath. The "safe zone" extends to the lateral edge of the linea semilunaris. Medial to the linea semilunaris, extreme precautions are taken to preserve and avoid injury to perforating vessels from the deep inferior epigastric system (**FIG 5**).
- A decision at this stage must be made to determine if a muscle-sparing free TRAM flap or DIEP flap will be performed. In either case, the lateral innervation to the rectus abdominis muscle is preserved.
- If bilateral free DIEP flaps are to be performed, medial to lateral and lateral to medial perforator dissection is performed (**FIG 6**). This is facilitated using bipolar cautery or monopolar cautery at very low current. Mosquito clamps are used to elevate and divide strands of muscle fibers without injury to the perforators or underlying vasculature.
- With the muscle-sparing free TRAM technique, an island of perforators is defined and the anterior rectus sheath surrounding the island of perforators is incised (**FIG 7**).

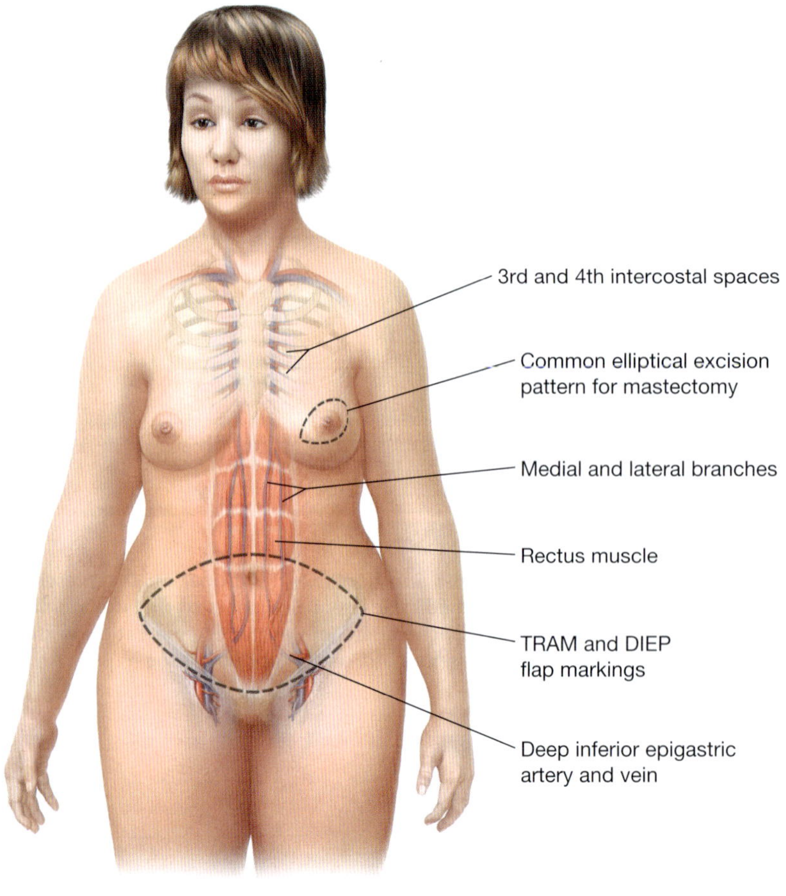

FIG 2 • An oblique or horizontal ellipse is traditionally performed during a non–nipple-sparing mastectomy. Other configurations that can be used include a periareolar circular pattern or a vertically oriented pattern. Knowledge of the rib anatomy and intercostal spaces will aid in selecting a recipient site for microsurgical anastomosis. A large interspace, usually the 3rd or 4th intercostal space, is usually selected. The internal mammary vessels are located close to the sternocostal junction.

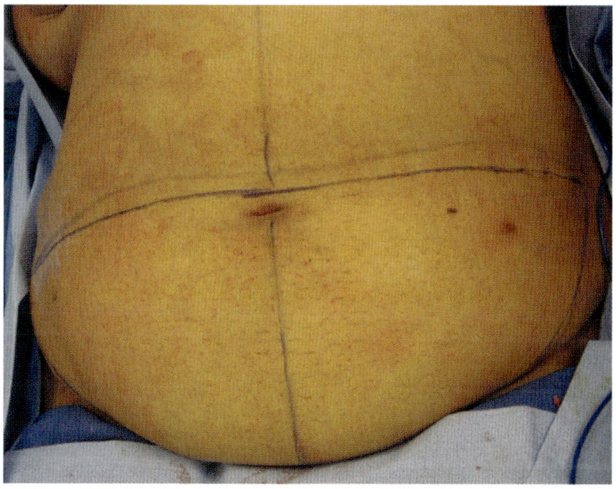

FIG 3 ● The abdomen in supine position is shown. The upper incision is usually located just above the umbilicus. The lower incision is placed in the lower abdominal crease or in a position to allow for donor site closure.

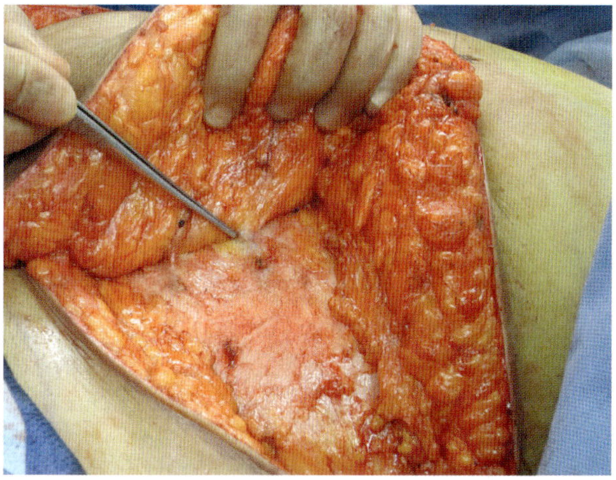

FIG 5 ● Flap elevation begins from the lateral edge. As the rectus sheath is encountered, lateral row perforators can be found piercing the fascia to perfuse the overlying skin and fat.

The medial and lateral sheath is elevated off the muscle and the retrorectus space is defined. The surrounding muscle is divided using monopolar or bipolar cautery.

- The superior portion of the rectus muscle is cauterized and the distal extent of the vascular pedicle is clipped. Palpation beneath the muscle will help identify the pulse and location of the pedicle to ensure that the pedicle is within the muscle segment (**FIG 8**).
- Once this is performed, the flap is solely based on the deep inferior epigastric system and elevated from distal to proximal. Cautery dissection proceeds at low current (**FIG 9**).
- The proximal portion of the pedicle can be visualized travelling toward the lateral edge of the rectus muscle and is dissected using sharp instruments. All side branches are clipped or ligated. Care must be taken to avoid injury to the vessels and intercostal nerves at this stage as diathermic injury may result in vessel thrombosis or neural injury (**FIG 10**).
- Pedicle dissection is continued proximally as deemed necessary for adequate pedicle length. Slightly increased caliber of the deep inferior epigastric artery (DIEA)/deep inferior epigastric vein (DIEV) is seen with more proximal dissection. Approximately 10 to 12 cm may be obtained if dissection is continued to the external iliac vessels.

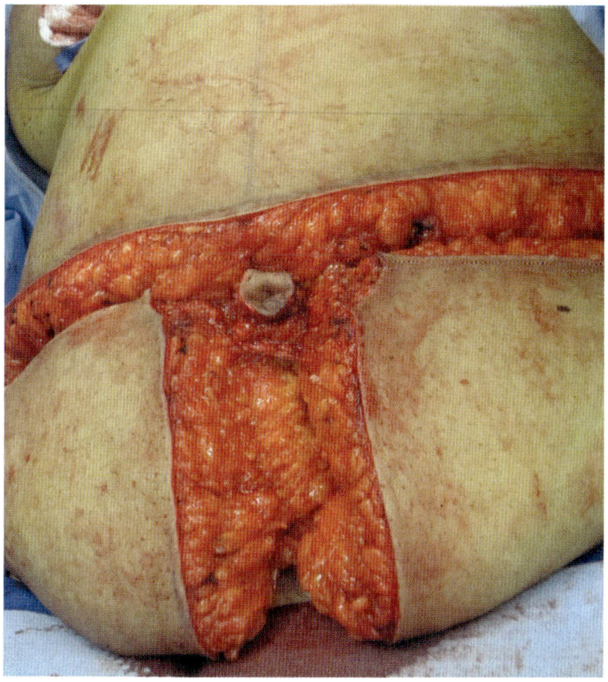

FIG 4 ● The upper incision is performed first. If bilateral reconstruction is being performed, the abdominal flap can be divided down the midline.

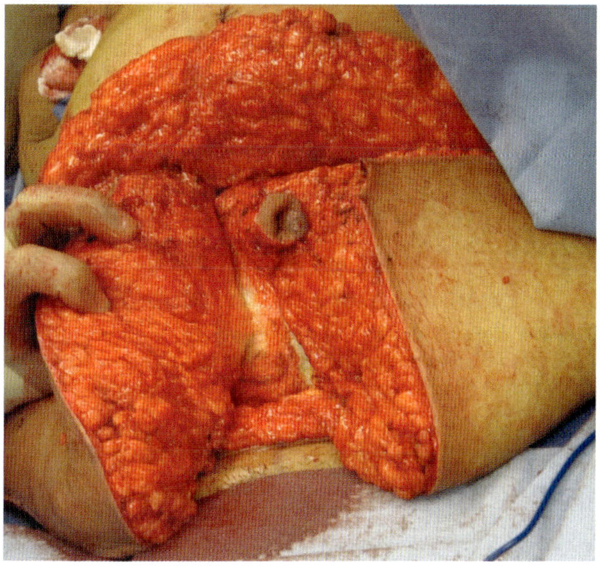

FIG 6 ● Dissection from the medial aspect of the flap is performed until medial row perforators are encountered and/or until safely over the rectus muscle.

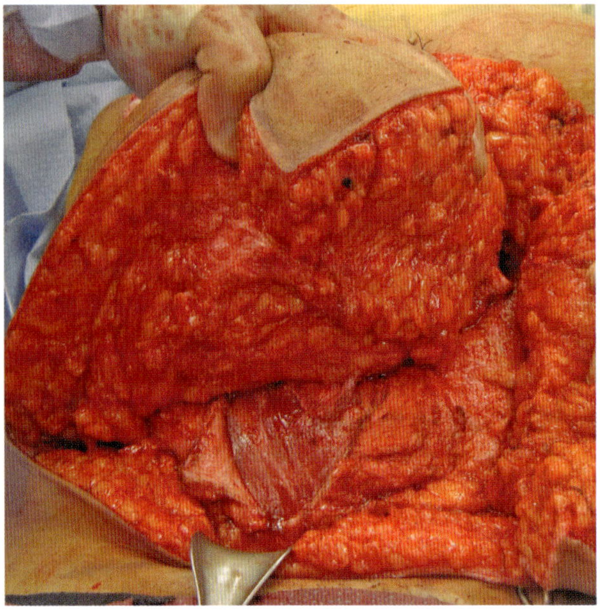

FIG 7 ● When harvesting a muscle-sparing TRAM flap, a fascial island is created around the perforators. The remaining fascia is elevated off of the surrounding muscle for better visualization and dissection.

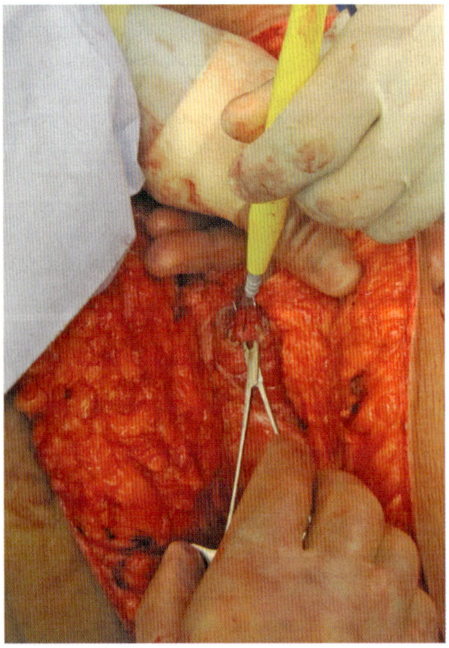

FIG 8 ● Careful dissection of the superior extent of the flap will allow for ligation of the distal pedicle to allow for distal to proximal flap harvest.

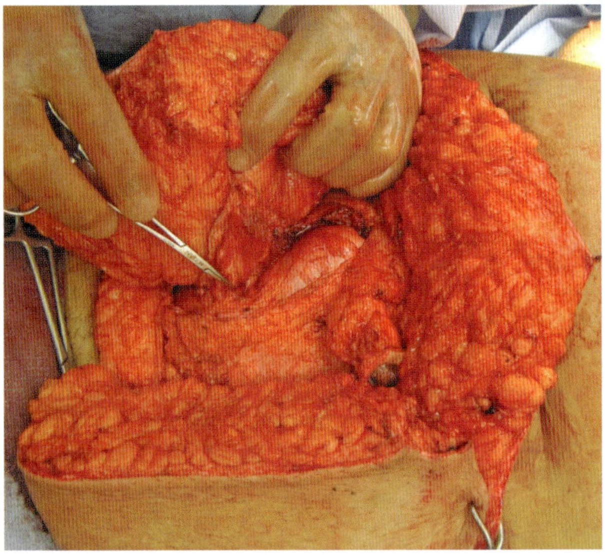

FIG 9 ● Once the muscle cuff is harvested, proximal dissection will reveal the pedicle vessels.

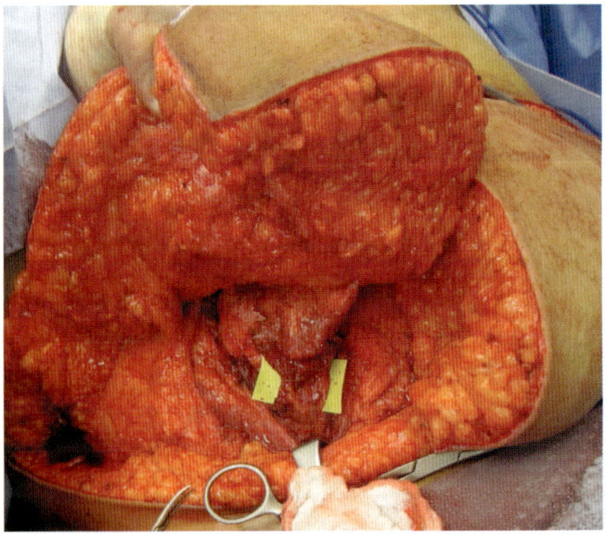

FIG 10 ● Care is taken to avoid injury to the pedicle during retrograde pedicle dissection.

RECIPIENT VESSEL DISSECTION

- The two sets of recipient vessels for free flap breast reconstruction include the internal mammary and thoracodorsal artery and vein. The most commonly used recipient vessels are the internal mammary system.
- The internal mammary vessels run paramedian to the sternum directly beneath the costal cartilage on the left and the right side. The thoracodorsal vessels are posterior in the axillary space and traverse along the anterior surface of the latissimus dorsi muscle.

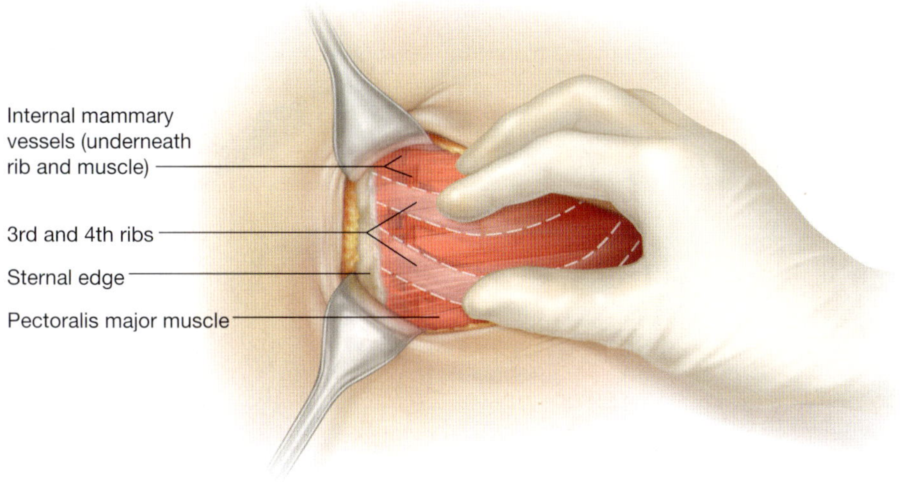

FIG 11 ● Selection of the interspace is usually performed intraoperatively with palpation of the intervening rib segments. Selection of a rib too low can result in a smaller caliber vein and a narrow interspace.

- The exposure technique described is for the internal mammary system. An appropriate intercostal space is chosen that will allow for adequate access for performing microsurgery. This is usually the 3rd or 4th interspace (**FIG 11**).
- The pectoralis major muscle overlying the desired rib is divided along the direction of the fibers using electrocautery. An adequate window is made, allowing for further rib and vessel dissection (**FIG 12**).
- The perichondrium is then removed overlying the costal portion of the rib and dissection proceeds in a subperichondrial fashion (**FIG 13**).
- Doyen surgical instruments are used to release the posterior perichondrium. Caution is taken in this dissection, as inadvertent passage through the posterior perichondrium can result in internal mammary artery and internal mammary vein (IMA/IMV) vessel injury or entry into the pleural space. A rib cutter is then used to isolate and remove a lateral segment of costal cartilage (**FIG 14**).
- Rib removal with a bone rongeur then proceeds from lateral to medial, again avoiding injury to the posterior perichondrium (**FIG 15**).
- Following complete removal of the costal cartilage segment, the posterior perichondrium is divided, elevated, and carefully excised using bipolar cautery and microdissection (**FIG 16**).
- The internal mammary artery and vein are visualized. The vein is usually the medial structure. Occasionally, a vena comitans is present. The recipient vessels are further dissected to clear the perivascular tissue using loupe magnification (**FIG 17**).

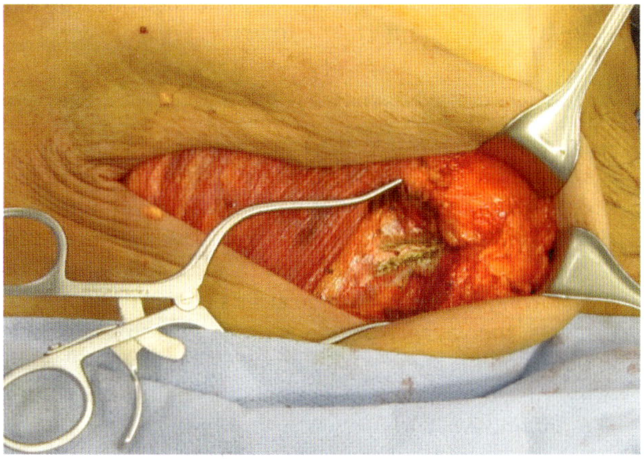

FIG 12 ● Division along the pectoralis major fibers will reveal the desired cartilaginous rib for resection.

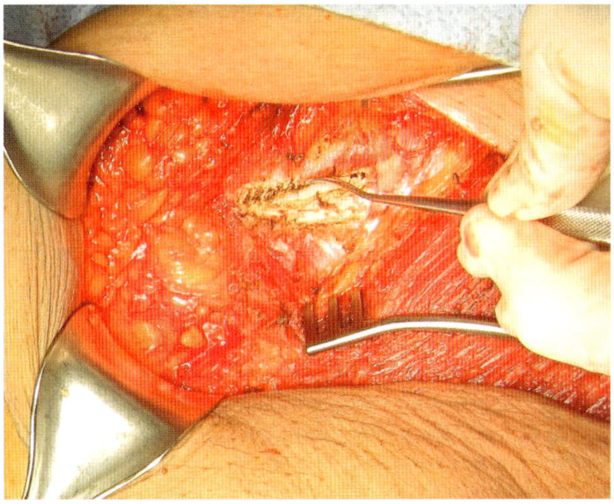

FIG 13 ● The perichondrium is incised and an elevator is used to circumferentially dissect around the rib segment.

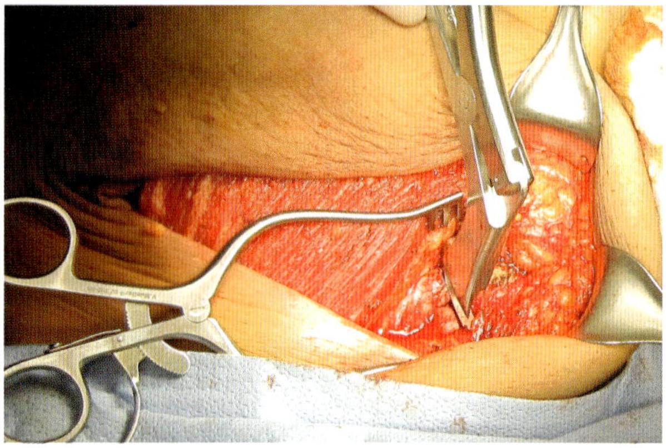

FIG 14 • A rib cutter is used to remove the cartilaginous segment of rib.

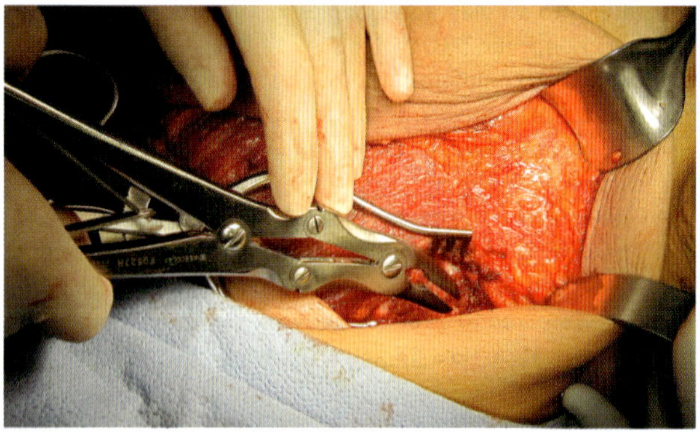

FIG 15 • A rongeur is used to finish the removal of the cartilaginous portion of rib. Care is taken to avoid injury to the posterior perichondrium as the internal mammary vessels lie deep to this structure.

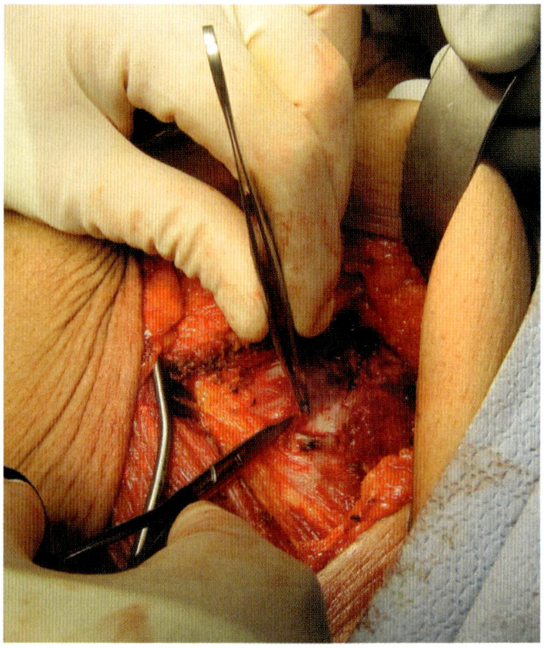

FIG 16 • Careful dissection is performed to separate the posterior perichondrium from the underlying vessels.

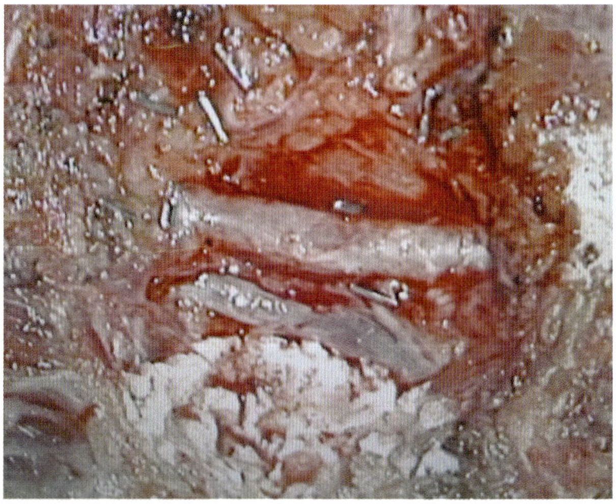

FIG 17 • Perivascular dissection is performed in order to prepare the vessels for microanastomosis.

MICROSURGICAL ANASTOMOSIS

- Intravenous heparin is usually administered prior to division of the inferior epigastric vessels.
- The harvested flap is positioned over the chest wall such that the inferior epigastric artery and vein are aligned with the internal mammary artery and vein.
- The medial anastomosis is usually performed first, which is typically the venous anastomosis. This is followed by the lateral or arterial anastomosis.
- The decision to use the vascular coupler (FIG 18) or to perform a hand-sewn anastomosis is based on surgeon preference. If a coupler is chosen, 2.0- to 3.0-mm ring is usually recommended. If a hand-sewn venous anastomosis is chosen, 8-0 or 9-0 sutures are used in an interrupted or continuous fashion. Avoidance of back-wall sutures is critical (FIG 19). Usually 8 to 10 sutures are needed to complete the artery (FIG 20).
- Following completion of the arterial and venous anastomoses, the vascular pedicle must be appropriately positioned on the chest wall to prevent twisting and kinking in order to minimize pedicle-related complications such as thrombosis.
- Positioning of the flap on the chest wall is an important step to recreate the breast contour and shape. Fortunately

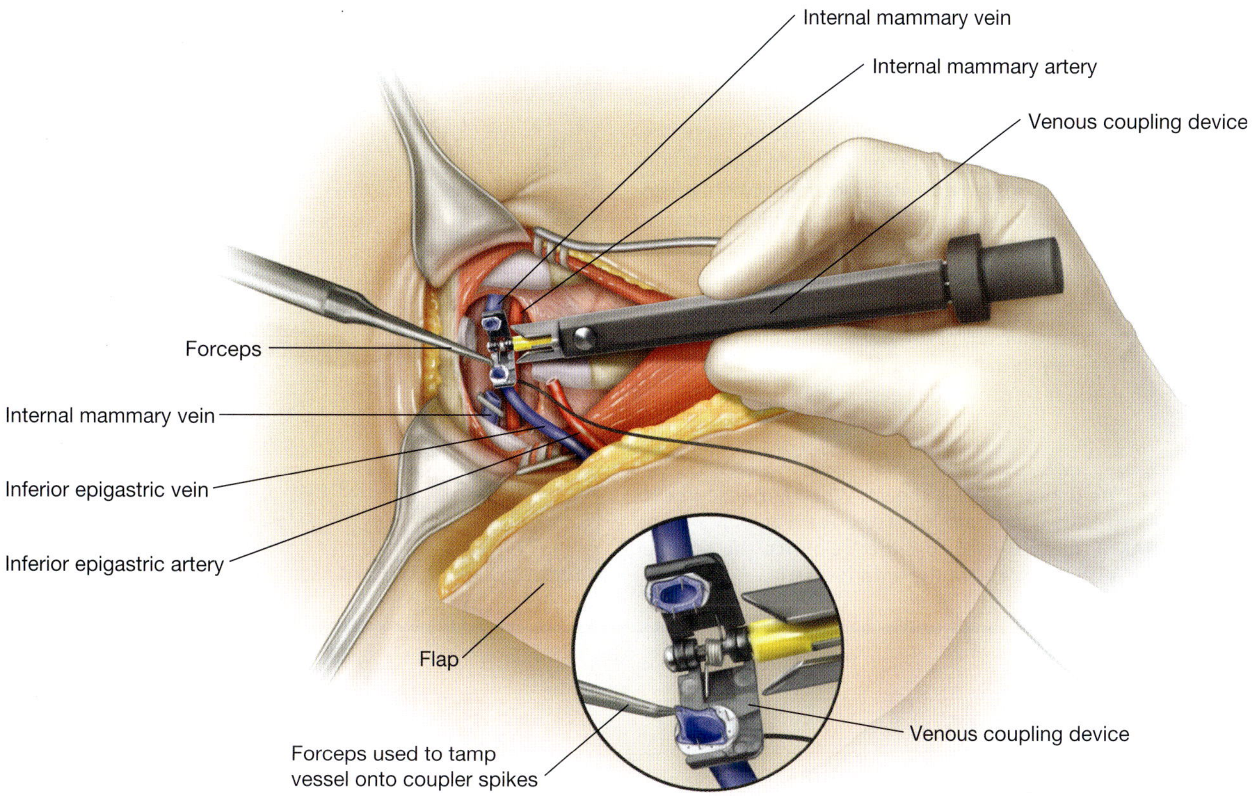

FIG 18 • When the venous coupler is chosen to perform the venous anastomosis, proper orientation of the coupler device will ensure an efficient anastomosis. Performing the donor vein first will allow for reorientation of the device prior to performing the recipient side. The tamping forceps have a small central hole that allows correct positioning of the vein on the coupler spikes.

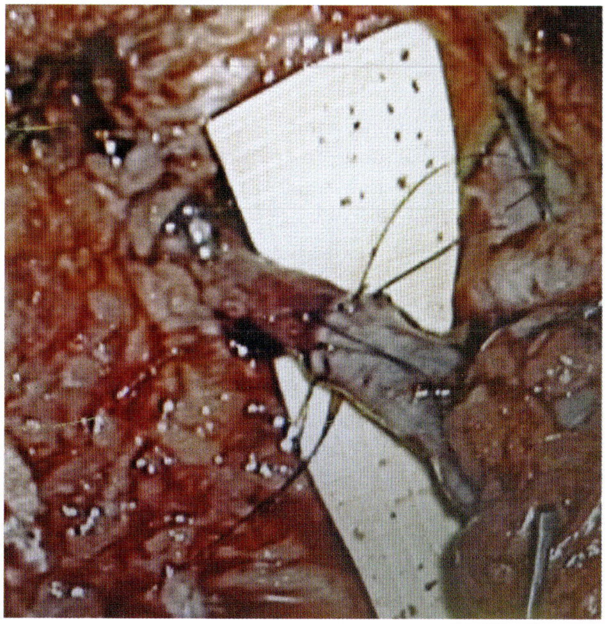

FIG 19 • The medially located vein is usually anastomosed first with interrupted microsutures.

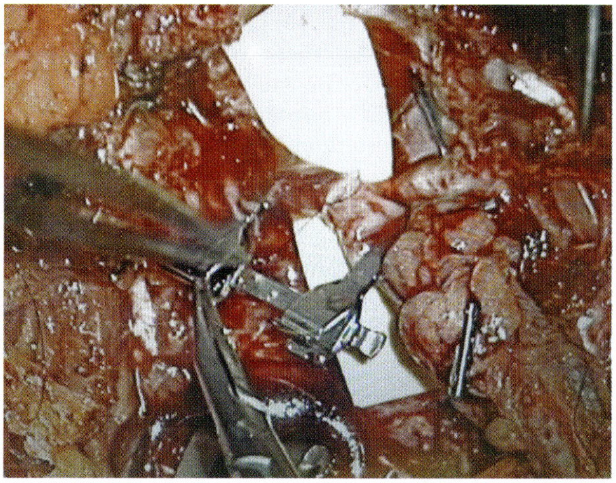

FIG 20 • Arterial anastomosis is then performed using the same microanastomosis techniques.

with free flaps, there are no points that tether the flap and mobility of the flaps is maintained for optimal shaping.

- The abdominal donor site closure is an important phase of the breast reconstruction. With the DIEP flap, there is no muscle removed and usually no fascia; therefore, the closure consisted of a primary closure using a nonabsorbable monofilament. Reinforcement with a synthetic mesh is rarely necessary. With the muscle-sparing free TRAM, muscle and fascia are removed; therefore, it is sometimes necessary to replace the fascia with a synthetic or biologic mesh. This is more common with bilateral reconstructions compared to unilateral (**FIG 21**).
- Two drains are usually placed in the donor site and one drain in the reconstructed breast.

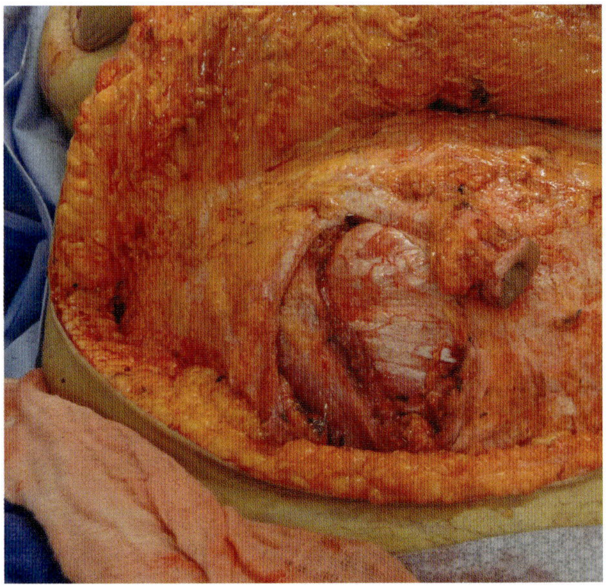

FIG 21 ● The donor defect is shown. When larger segments of anterior rectus sheath are harvested (such as in MS-0 and MS-1 TRAMs), mesh is used to either reinforce the anterior abdominal wall or to replace the anterior fascia.

PEARLS AND PITFALLS

Flap dissection	■ Finger palpation of the pedicle pulse is crucial during muscle-sparing harvest techniques. ■ A longer pedicle will allow for a larger vessel internal diameter that more closely matches the internal mammary vessel diameter.
Microanastomosis techniques	■ Secondary venous drainage may be helpful for larger flaps. ■ Radiated internal mammary vessels are less pliable and may tear more easily when using a venous coupler device.
Flap insetting	■ Excising radiated mastectomy flap skin may prevent tightness of the flap inset and later contour irregularities. ■ Suture tacks in the superior portion of the flap will maintain contour of the superior pole of the breast.

POSTOPERATIVE CARE

- Close flap monitoring occurs in the first 72 hours to ensure flap viability. A strict nursing flap check protocol includes frequent Doppler examination, color, and capillary refill assessments. Tissue oximetry is used on almost all flaps.
- Patients are maintained on postoperative antibiotic therapy for approximately 5 days and aspirin for 1 to 2 weeks to prevent anastomotic thrombosis.
- Ambulation is encouraged on postoperative day 1 or 2.
- Patients usually stay in the hospital for 3 to 4 days following surgery and are discharged home. They are encouraged to shower on postoperative day 3.

OUTCOMES

- The free TRAM reconstruction has been demonstrated to result in high levels of patient satisfaction and quality of life.[4] In long-term evaluation, autologous tissue reconstruction maintains a more natural-appearing breast as compared to implant-based reconstruction.[5]
- Abdominal donor site morbidity is relatively low.[6,7] Bulge/hernia formation may occur in approximately 3% to 5% of patients. In the event that surgical repair is necessary, this is usually achieved with fascial plication and reinforcement with a synthetic mesh.
- The free TRAM and DIEP flaps for breast reconstruction are valuable options for breast reconstruction following mastectomy.
- Free tissue transfer techniques are useful in complex situations such as prior radiation therapy, prosthetic failure, and in overweight and obese patients.
- Microsurgical expertise is necessary to obtain predictable outcomes and a low failure rate.
- Donor site morbidity rates are acceptable. Most women will achieve an "abdominoplasty" appearance of the abdomen following free TRAM and DIEP flap reconstruction.

COMPLICATIONS

- The most relevant complications following microvascular breast reconstruction include anastomotic thrombosis, hematoma, and flap failure. Postoperative flap monitoring is necessary to ensure prompt operative exploration in cases of vascular thrombosis. This is usually accomplished using tissue oximetry or Doppler analysis. Return to the operating room is necessary when there is a disruption in flow. Revision maneuvers include mechanical thrombectomy, tissue plasminogen activator (TPA), and redo anastomosis.

- Donor site morbidities are slightly more common and include contour abnormalities (hernia/bulge), incisional dehiscence, delayed healing, hematoma, and seroma. These complications can be managed conservatively but sometimes require operative intervention.

REFERENCES

1. Nahabedian MY, Tsangaris T, Momen B. Breast reconstruction with the DIEP flap or the muscle-sparing (MS-2) free TRAM flap: is there a difference? *Plast Reconstr Surg*. 2005;115:436.
2. Nahabedian MY, Momen B, Manson PN. Factors associated with anastomotic failure after microvascular reconstruction of the breast. *Plast Reconstr Surg*. 2004;114:74–82.
3. Nahabedian MY. Secondary operations of the anterior abdominal wall following microvascular breast reconstruction with the TRAM and DIEP flaps. *Plast Reconstr Surg*. 2007;120:365–372.
4. Yueh JH, Slavin SA, Adesiyun T, et al. Patient satisfaction in post-mastectomy breast reconstruction: a comparative evaluation of DIEP, TRAM, latissimus flap, and implant techniques. *Plast Reconstr Surg*. 2010;125:1585–1595.
5. Hu ES, Pusic AL, Waljee JF, et al. Patient-reported aesthetic satisfaction with breast reconstruction during the long-term survivorship period. *Plast Reconstr Surg*. 2009;124:1–8.
6. Selber JC, Nelson J, Fosnot J, et al. A prospective study comparing the functional impact of SIEA, DIEP, and muscle-sparing free TRAM flaps on the abdominal wall: part I. unilateral reconstruction. *Plast Reconstr Surg*. 2010;126:1142–1153.
7. Selber JC, Fosnot J, Nelson J, et al. A prospective study comparing the functional impact of SIEA, DIEP, and muscle-sparing free TRAM flaps on the abdominal wall: part II. Bilateral reconstruction. *Plast Reconstr Surg*. 2010;126:1438–1453.

Chapter 19

Deep Inferior Epigastric Perforator Flap Breast Reconstruction after Mastectomy

Adeyiza O. Momoh

DEFINITION

- Autologous reconstruction techniques after mastectomy are well-established options for breast reconstruction. Although over the years multiple flap options for reconstruction have been described, abdominal-based flaps continue to be the workhorse for autologous breast reconstruction. Abdominal flaps provide distinct advantages over implant-based reconstruction including a natural contour, superior symmetry and appearance of the reconstructed breast mound, and higher patient satisfaction.[1,2] A secondary benefit of these flaps is the improvement they provide to the abdominal contour. Hartrampf et al.[3] first described the pedicled transverse rectus abdominis myocutaneous (TRAM) flap in 1982, with its benefits of providing a soft, ptotic, aesthetically pleasing reconstruction that closely approximates the natural breast. Technical advancements and the continued quest to improve on flap perfusion and minimize donor site morbidity led to the introduction of the deep inferior epigastric perforator (DIEP) flap by Koshima and Soeda[4] in 1989 with later popularization by Allen and Treece[5] in 1994. The DIEP flap has gained in popularity over the years, and the potential benefits it offers include less abdominal wall weakness, bulging, and hernias.[6–8]

ANATOMY

- The DIEP flap is an adipocutaneous flap based on intramuscular perforators from the deep inferior epigastric artery (DIEA) and deep inferior epigastric vein (DIEV).
- The DIEA and DIEV originate from the external iliac vessels in the groin and course superomedially toward the lateral border of the rectus abdominis muscle.
- Deep to the rectus abdominis muscle, the DIEA and DIEV most commonly bifurcate (type II branching pattern) in the vicinity of the arcuate line and join up with the superior epigastric vessels above the umbilicus.
- Other encountered branching patterns are the type I with no branching and type III with trifurcating vessels (**FIG 1**).
- Perforators to the lower abdominal skin and adipose tissue come off the pedicle at multiple levels and are referred to as medial or lateral rows of perforators, indicating their relative position within the rectus/entry point into the flap.
- Most perforators are found within a 10-cm radius from the umbilicus.
- Zones of perfusion based on fluorescent perfusion studies[9] are illustrated in **FIG 2**—illustration with zones transposed onto rectus/pedicle.
- In general, perfusion of the hemiabdominal flap ipsilateral to the perforators (zones I and II) is stronger than it is to the contralateral abdominal flap across the midline (zones III and IV).
- Medial row perforators have a greater likelihood of perfusing tissue across the midline than do lateral row perforators.
- In contrast, lateral row perforators have a greater likelihood of perfusing the most lateral extent of the ipsilateral hemiabdominal flap than do medial row perforators.
- Medial and lateral rows of perforators communicate via a subdermal plexus.
- There is also communication between DIEA and DIEV system and the superficial inferior epigastric artery (SIEA) and superficial inferior epigastric vein (SIEV) system.
- The SIEV is the dominant outflow vessel for the lower abdomen in many patients.

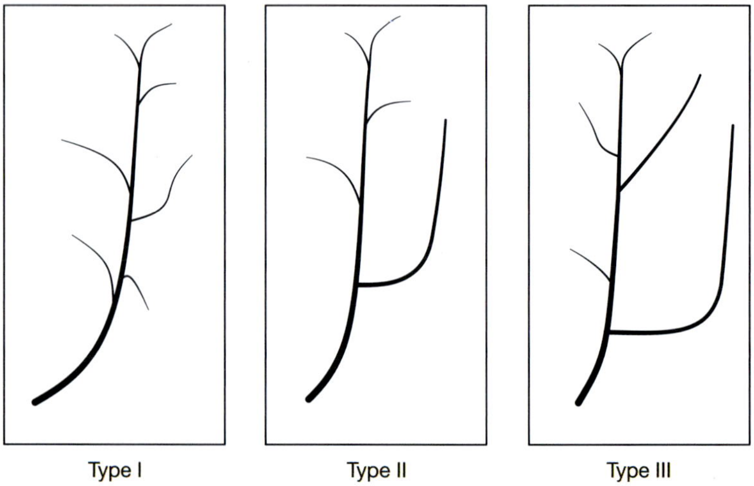

FIG 1 • Type I, type II, and type III vascular branching patterns.

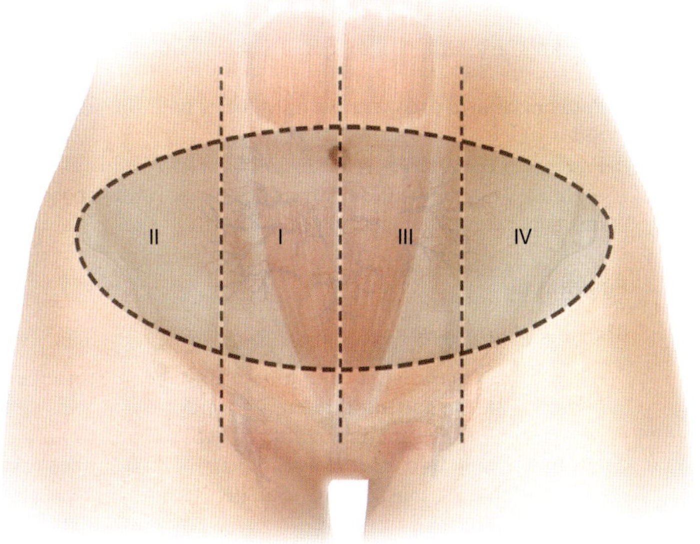

FIG 2 • Zones of perfusion of the lower abdomen based on fluorescent perfusion studies.

PATIENT HISTORY AND PHYSICAL FINDINGS

- A thorough history and physical examination are critical in preparing for reconstruction.
- Pertinent aspects of the history include previous abdominal or chest wall operations and medical conditions that would preclude patients from a lengthy operation under general anesthesia.”
- A focused abdominal examination evaluating the amount of lower abdominal adipose tissue and the location of surgical scars if present
- A team-based approach involving surgeons, anesthesiologists, primary care physicians, and other specialists such as cardiologists, as needed, ensures that patients are evaluated as a whole and all key concerns are addressed.

IMAGING AND OTHER DIAGNOSTIC STUDIES

- Preoperative computed tomography (CT) angiography of the donor site has been advocated in recent years. The preoperative scans provide a road map for flap perforators, with information on perforator location, size, and distribution (**FIG 3**).
- In patients with long low transverse abdominal incisions, the scans also allow for the assessment of continuity of the flap pedicle beyond the incision.
- Information gathered from scans has been shown to decrease operative times.[10] CT scans, however, are not an absolute requirement for preoperative planning.

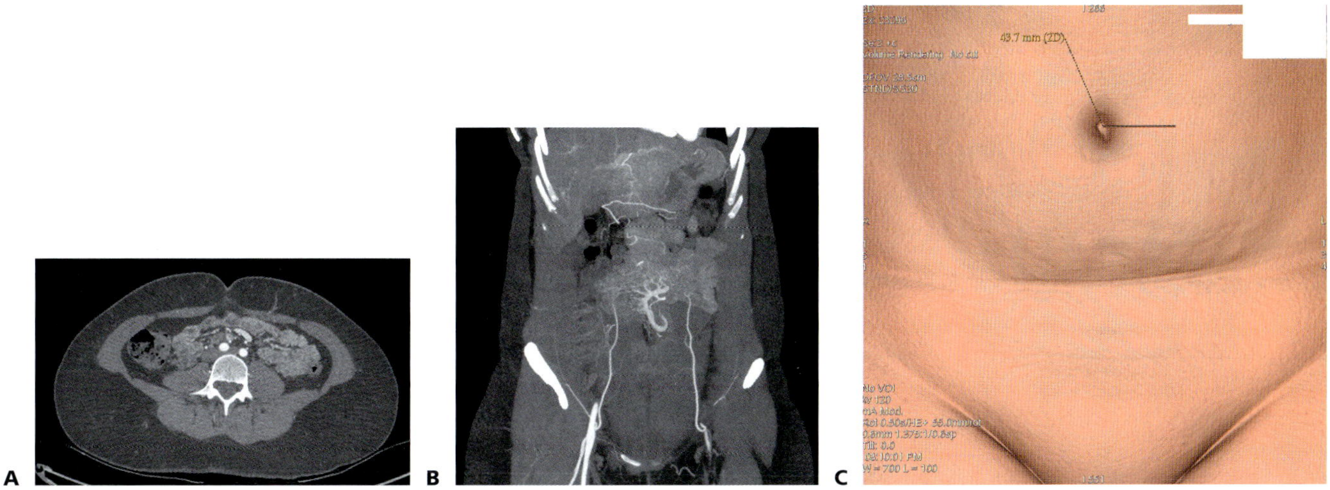

FIG 3 • **A,B.** Preoperative CT angiography of the lower abdomen. **C.** A 3-D rendering of the abdominal soft tissue. Perforator locations based on axial cuts are transposed to the skin surface to enhance preoperative planning.

SURGICAL MANAGEMENT

- In consulting with patients, decisions about the timing of reconstruction (immediately after mastectomy or delayed) and the type of reconstruction are made, taking patient factors and tumor characteristics into consideration.
  - Patient factors of significance include the following:
    - Patient preference
    - Body habitus or the availability of abdominal donor tissue
    - Body mass index
    - Smoking history
    - History of previous abdominal operations that compromise the vascular pedicle or donor site
    - Medical comorbidities that would preclude patients from undergoing a lengthy operation
  - Tumor characteristics as they relate to the following:
    - The need for postmastectomy radiation therapy or
    - The need for close postmastectomy surveillance prior to reconstruction
    - In general, patients known to require postmastectomy radiation therapy are reconstructed in a delayed fashion to avoid the detrimental effects of radiation on flaps. A history of radiation therapy also serves as a relative indication for use of an autologous form of reconstruction, as implant reconstructions in the setting of radiation are prone to higher rates of complications and failure.

Preoperative Planning

- In addition to basic labs, patients should be type and screened, particularly in cases of bilateral reconstructions.
- All anticoagulant and antiplatelet medications should be stopped a week prior to the operation. Warfarin can be bridged with enoxaparin also a week prior.
- Smokers are required to quit for a minimum of 4 weeks prior.
- Patients receive preoperative antibiotics with intraoperative redosing.
- Patients receive deep vein thrombosis (DVT) prophylaxis with use of a pneumatic compression device and subcutaneous heparin at the beginning of the case.

Positioning

Marking/positioning

- Preoperative markings of the breast and abdomen are performed with the patient in the upright position.
- Key landmarks for the breast marked are the chest midline, inframammary fold, and a periareolar marking in the case of a skin-sparing mastectomy. The breast base width is also measured (**FIG 4A**).
- The upper marking for the abdominal flap is made at or just above the umbilicus with the location of perforators on preoperative imaging, providing some guidance. The breast base width is used to mark the potential vertical height/distance from the upper marking to the lower marking. The lower marking is then made to complete the elliptical pattern (**FIG 4B**).
- Patient positioning in the operating room (OR) is supine and the table is turned 180 degrees from the anesthesiologist, providing better access for two surgical teams (**FIG 5**).

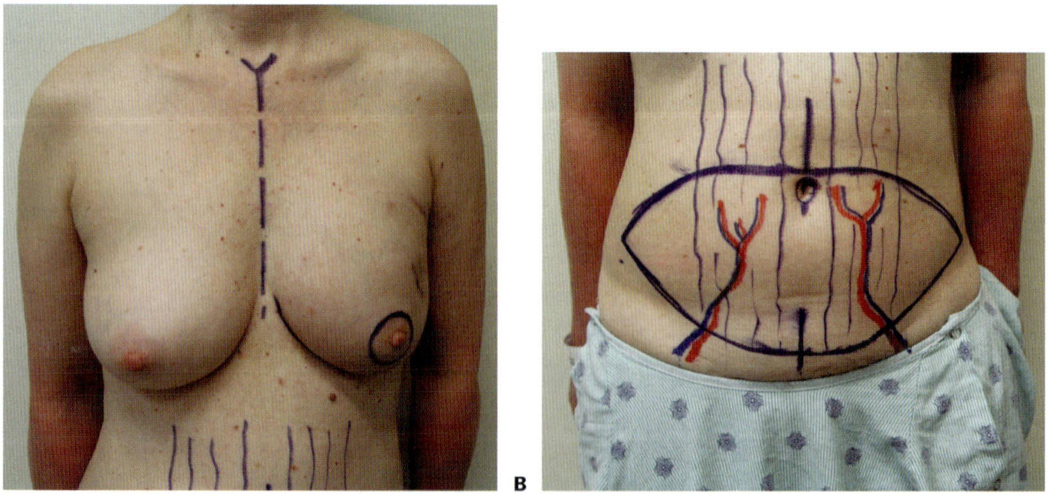

A B

FIG 4 • **A.** Breast preoperative marking. **B.** Abdominal preoperative marking.

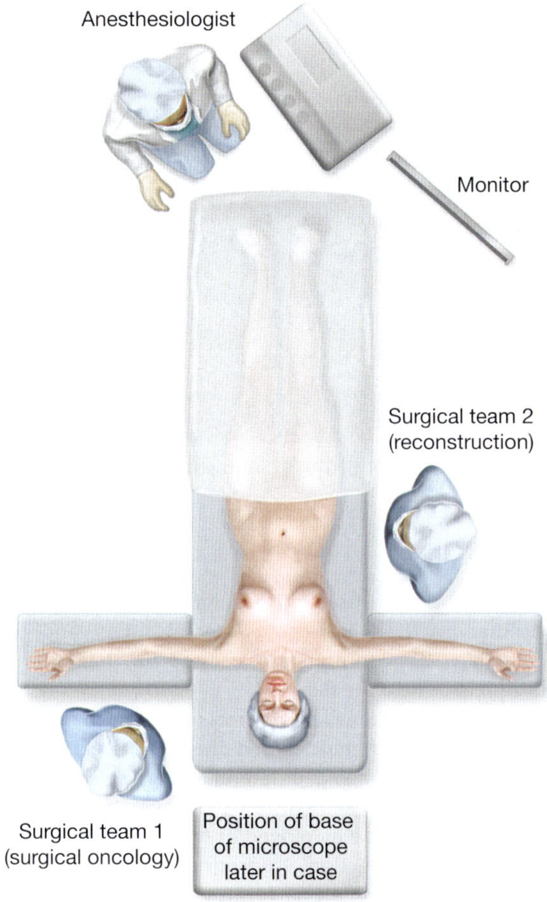

FIG 5 • Patient positioning in the OR.

FLAP HARVEST

- Skin preparation with clipping is performed as needed.
- The breasts and abdomen are prepped and draped in a sterile fashion.
- The upper abdominal incision is made with a scalpel, and dissection through the adipose tissue down to anterior abdominal wall fascia is performed with electrocautery.
- An adipocutaneous flap is elevated cephalad with the electrocautery, ending at the xiphoid centrally and at the costal margins laterally. Less elevation may be needed in patients with ample skin laxity.
- The OR table is reflexed and the raised upper abdominal flap is transposed downward to assess the ability of this skin edge to meet the lower abdominal markings for closure. The lower abdominal markings are at this time adjusted as needed and the table returned to its original position.
- The lower abdominal incision is made superficially with a scalpel and careful dissection through the adipose tissue is performed, anticipating the presence of the SIEA and SIEV, typically above Scarpa's fascia (**FIG 6**).
- Once the superficial vessels are visualized, a Weitlaner retractor is introduced to provide further exposure and

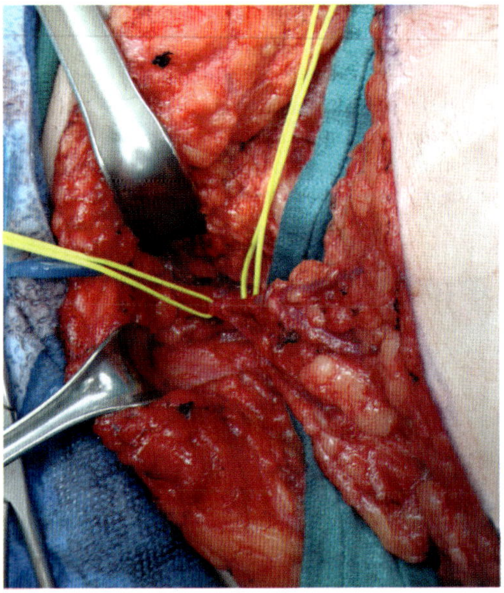

FIG 6 • Dissection of the SIEV within the lower abdominal incision.

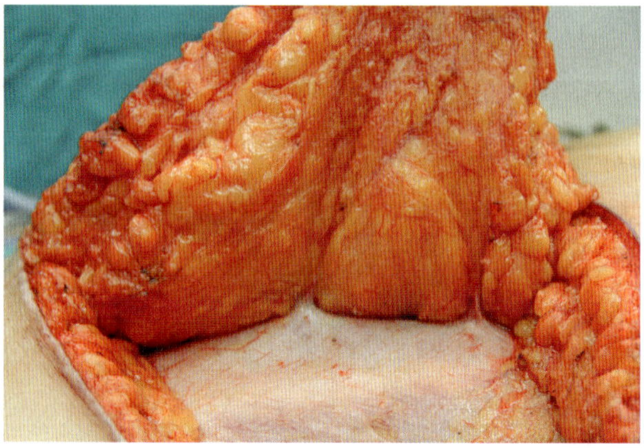

FIG 7 ● The lateral row of perforators visualized with suprafascial flap elevation.

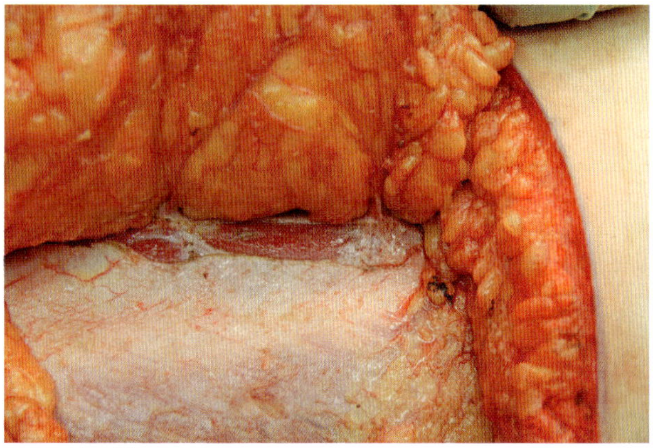

FIG 9 ● Subfascial exposure of flap perforators.

the vessels are dissected out toward the femoral vessels with use of tenotomy scissors and bipolar electrocautery. In patients who are not good candidates for the SIEA flap (SIEA) based on the absence of adequate-sized vessels, the vein is dissected to a length greater than or equal to 5 cm prior to ligating it with hemoclips and dividing it.

- Dissection down to the anterior abdominal wall fascia is then completed with electrocautery.
- Flap elevation is performed in the suprafascial plane from lateral to medial with electrocautery until the lateral row of perforators are encountered just medial to the edge of the rectus fascia (**FIG 7**).
- An incision is made around the umbilicus and along the midline of the flap in bilateral reconstruction cases or in cases with hemiabdominal flaps large enough for a unilateral reconstruction.
- The umbilical stalk is dissected out with blunt-tipped scissors and division of the flap down the midline is completed with electrocautery.
- In unilateral reconstructions that require use of portions of the flap that cross the midline, the umbilicus is dissected out without splitting the flap.
- Suprafascial elevation of the flap from its medial edge is performed with electrocautery until the medial row of perforators are encountered.

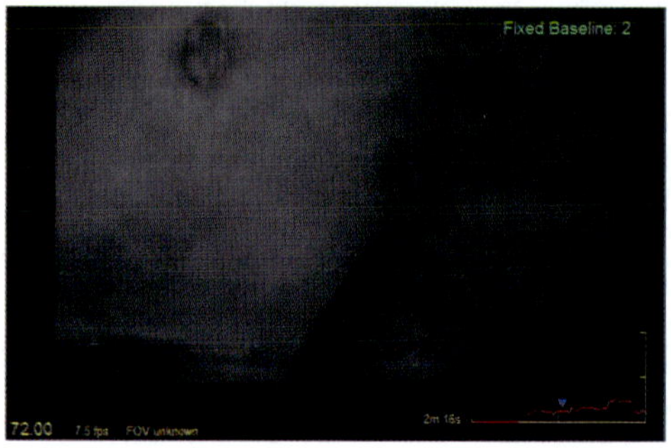

FIG 8 ● Perfusion map with laser-assisted indocyanine green fluorescent dye with dark areas indicating poor perfusion.

- Dissection around the perforators is performed with a low-energy electrocautery, and at this time, all perforators are assessed for their size and location within the flap.
- Small perforators (<1.5 mm in diameter) are ligated with hemoclips and one or more perforators within either the medial or lateral row are selected for use.
- Laser-assisted indocyanine green fluorescent dye can be employed at this point to assist with perforator selection. Appropriate-sized Acland clamps are placed on all perforators excluding the few selected and the dye is administered by the anesthesiologist intravenously. Within a few minutes of the dye administration, a real-time perfusion map of the flap is visualized (**FIG 8**).
- Alternatively, capillary refill can be assessed with the Acland clamps in place for a few minutes to determine adequacy of flap perfusion based on the few selected perforators.
- The anterior rectus fascia adjacent to the selected row of perforators is incised with electrocautery in a craniocaudal orientation (**FIG 9**).
- A millimeter cuff of fascia is cut with a tenotomy around the perforator, freeing it from the surrounding anterior rectus fascia.
- Two to 3 mL of heparinized saline is then injected into the rectus muscle adjacent to the individual perforators with an olive-tipped cannula. The heparinized saline used in this fashion hydrodissects the surrounding soft tissue away from the perforator and aids with visualization of the perforator course. This technique is repeated as needed throughout the course of the intramuscular dissection (**FIG 10**).
- The perforators are dissected through the rectus muscle with the aid of a bipolar electrocautery down to the larger deep inferior epigastric arterial and venous system that runs beneath the muscle.
- The continuation of the DIEA and DIEV system to the superior epigastric vessels is encountered above the most cephalad perforator and these vessels are ligated with

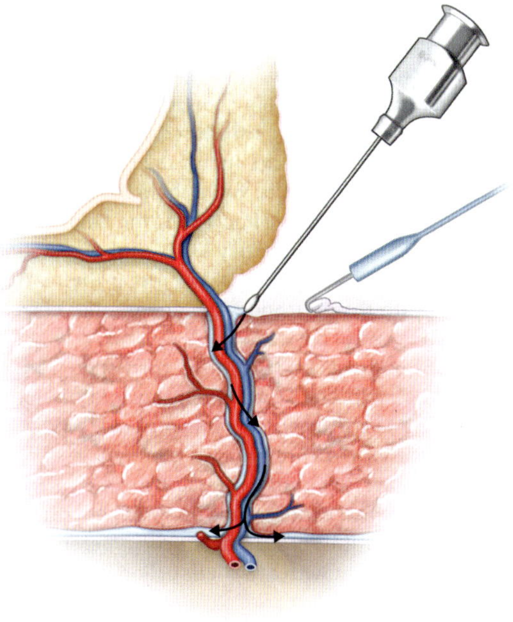

FIG 10 ● Hydrodissection technique for intramuscular perforator dissection illustrated. Heparinized saline is injected adjacent to the perforator and creates a dissection plane between the perforators and muscle. The *arrows* illustrate the course of the heparinized saline, which tracks along the perforator with each injection.

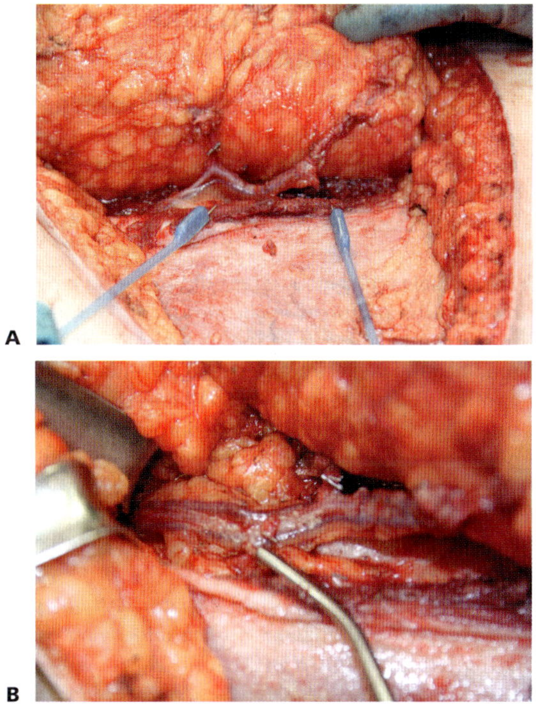

FIG 11 ● **A.** Intramuscular and submuscular dissection of perforators and vascular pedicle. **B.** DIEP flap pedicle prior to ligation.

appropriate-sized hemoclips 1 to 2 cm cephalad to the perforator.

- The submuscular dissection proceeds toward the external iliac vessels in the pelvis and is performed with the electrocautery, leaving a cuff of adipose tissue around the vessels.
- The DIEA and vein are dissected to a point where their length and size are appropriate for the recipient vessels in the chest (FIG 11).
- Once ready for transfer to the chest, the artery is first ligated distally with hemoclips followed by the vein(s).
- A tenotomy scissors is used to divide the vessels proximal to the clips.
- The harvested flap (FIG 12) is prepared on a back table by flushing the flap from its arterial end with heparinized saline until the venous outflow clears up and is less bloody.

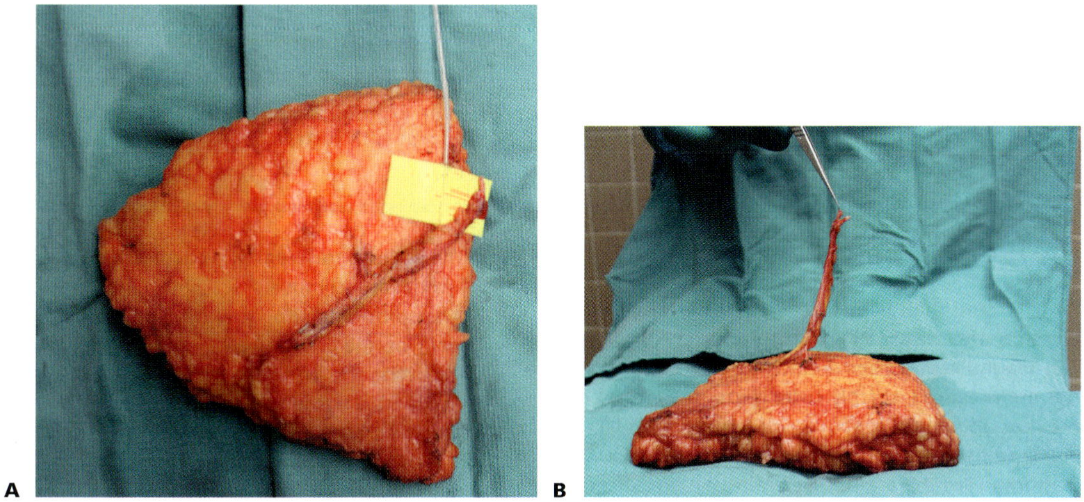

FIG 12 ● **A,B.** Flap harvested and prepped on a back table.

RECIPIENT VESSEL EXPOSURE (INTERNAL MAMMARY)

- A common choice and the author's preference for recipient vessels are the internal mammary artery and vein. Alternatively, the thoracodorsal artery and vein can be used.
- Once the mastectomy is complete, the defect is irrigated and hemostasis with electrocautery is performed as needed.
- The medial cartilaginous aspect of the 3rd rib is palpated through the pectoralis major muscle. The muscle fibers over this medial aspect of the rib are split (ideally along the fibers) with electrocautery and a Weitlaner retractor is introduced between the muscle fibers to provide exposure. The muscle split is performed from the lateral edge of the sternum to a point approximately 6 cm lateral.
- The anterior costal perichondrium is scored along its length with the electrocautery and also perpendicular to the lengthwise incision at the medial and lateral extents of the exposed cartilage.
- A freer or narrow periosteal elevator is then used to elevate the perichondrium off the underlying cartilage circumferentially (**FIG 13**).
- The cartilage is then excised with a rongeur from lateral to medial, exposing the posterior perichondrium. The internal mammary artery and vein are sometimes visible through the posterior perichondrium at this point.
- A second Weitlaner is introduced perpendicular to the first using the lateral cut end of the rib as an anchor for one end of the retractor while the opposite end retracts the medial mastectomy flap out of the field.
- An incision is made laterally through the posterior perichondrium with a scalpel and a freer is then introduced underneath the perichondrium and used to push all soft tissue and vessel downward.
- The posterior perichondrium is then split from lateral to medial, exposing the underlying internal mammary artery (IMA) and internal mammary vein (IMV).
- The posterior perichondrium is bluntly dissected off the underlying vessels with a freer and excised completely to provide optimal exposure of the recipient vessels.
- The IMA and IMV are dissected circumferentially and a background mat with attached suction is placed beneath both vessels (**FIG 14**).

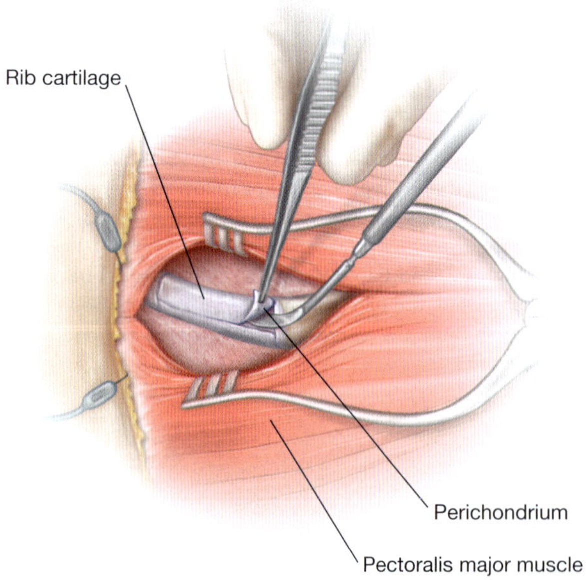

FIG 13 ● Elevation of the rib perichondrium.

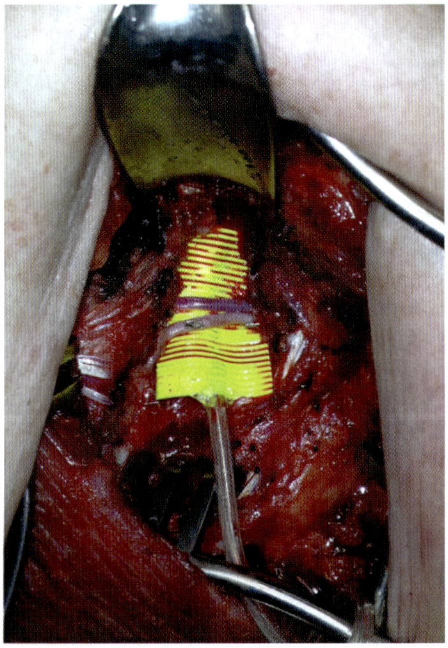

FIG 14 ● Exposed IMA and IMV with placement of a background mat with suction.

MICROVASCULAR ANASTOMOSIS

- The harvested DIEP flap is transferred to the chest and secured to the chest wall with sutures.
- With magnification from a microscope, the flap vessel ends are prepared, sharply cutting irregular vessel ends and loose adventitia.
- Similar preparation of the IMA and IMV are performed.
- Anastomosis of the arteries and veins can be performed in whichever order based on the surgeon's preference. The author preferentially couples the veins prior to the arterial anastomosis.
- An appropriate-sized single Acland clamp is placed proximally on the IMV and a hemoclip is applied distally prior to cutting the IMV with tenotomy scissors. The cut vessel end is then flushed with heparinized saline.
- A vessel sizer is used to determine the approximate vein diameter for both the flap vein and the IMV and the smaller of the two vessels determines the coupler size to be used.

- The flap vein is first placed in one end of the coupler followed by the IMV and the coupler is closed without placing tension on either vessel. The previously placed clamp is then taken off the IMV.
- One end of an appropriate-sized, double opposing Acland clamp is placed proximally on the IMA and hemoclips are applied distally prior to cutting the IMA. The flap artery is then introduced into the opposite end of the double-opposing Acland clamp.
- An end-to-end anastomosis of the arterial ends is performed with 8-0 or 9-0 nylon sutures in an interrupted or running fashion (**FIG 15**).
- Once the anastomosis is complete, the flap end of the clamp is taken off first prior to taking off the end on the IMA.
- With flow reestablished, papaverine is infiltrated into the adventitia of the arteries to prevent spasm.
- The flap and anastomosed vessels are warmed with warm saline and allowed to reperfuse for a few minutes.
- Doppler signals are identified on the flap skin and marked with sutures.
- Fat grafts obtained from either the abdominal donor site or flap edge are placed around the anastomosis to help secure the desired position of the vessels and reduce kinking.

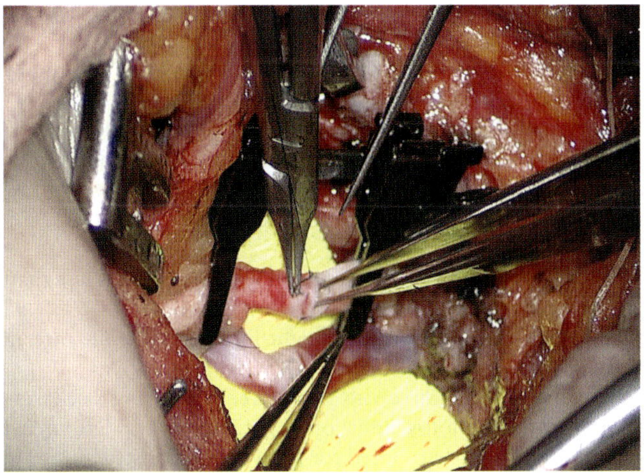

FIG 15 • Microvascular anastomosis under an operating microscope. A double opposing Acland clamp holds the arterial ends in place and an end-to-end anastomosis is being performed with interrupted 8-0 nylon sutures. The DIEV has been coupled to the IMV in the background.

FLAP INSET/DONOR SITE CLOSURE

- Peripheral zones of the flap that may be less optimally perfused are excised.
- The flap is then placed within the mastectomy defect and interrupted absorbable sutures are used to secure the flap to the medial aspect of the chest wall.
- The pattern of the skin paddle is marked and all skin (epidermis and dermis) outside of the paddle is excised with electrocautery (**FIG 16**). De-epithelialization here is also an option.
- A drain is placed along the inferior aspect of the mastectomy defect and exits the skin along the anterior axillary line.
- Skin closure for the flap inset is performed in layers with absorbable interrupted deep dermal sutures and a running subcuticular suture.
- The OR table is reflexed; two drains are placed in the abdominal donor site; and closure of the defect is performed with approximation of Scarpa's fascia, the deep dermis, and subcuticular layer.
- The umbilicus is delivered through the skin flap above the horizontal abdominal closure along the midline by creating an appropriate-sized defect with a full-thickness excision. The umbilicus is then inset with a layered closure.
- Minimal dressings in the form of a skin glue product, Steri-Strips, or an ointment are then applied to all suture lines.

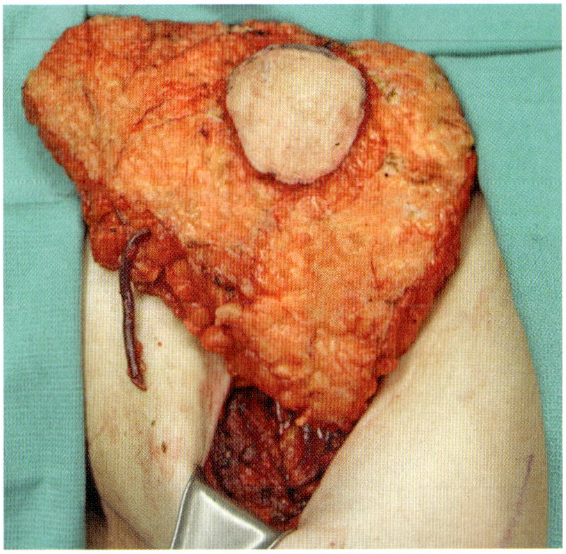

FIG 16 • Flap with all skin outside of the skin paddle excised; preserved SIEV can be seen on the medial aspect of the flap.

PEARLS AND PITFALLS

Preoperative evaluation	■ Preoperative CT angiography is a useful tool to assist with perforator selection—It provides information on perforator location and size but does not give information on flow/perfusion. ■ Flap perfusion based on a few perforators is better assessed by laser-assisted indocyanine green fluorescents dye or by physical examination with occlusion of all perforators with the exception of the few selected perforators.
Patient positioning	■ With the patient in supine position, the table can be turned 180 degrees from the anesthesiologist, providing better access for two surgical teams.
Dissection of the vessels	■ Preserve as long a length of the SIEV (≥5 cm) as possible for use as an additional outflow vessel in flaps with venous congestion after elevation or transfer to the chest. ■ The hydrodissection technique used for the intramuscular perforator dissection simplifies this portion of the operation, creating dissection planes and allowing for better visualization of the perforators and small vascular branches.

POSTOPERATIVE CARE

- Patients can be transferred from the OR to a postanesthesia care unit (PACU) or directly to a unit with nursing capabilities for flap monitoring.
- Flaps are monitored by physical examinations (color, temperature, capillary refill, and handheld Doppler signals) performed every hour for the first 24 hours and then checks can be spaced out to every 2 hours and 4 hours over subsequent hospital days.
- Additional flap monitoring with continuous near-infrared spectroscopy (NIRS) tissue oximetry is employed for 72 hours postoperatively.
- DVT prophylaxis is the only form of anticoagulation used routinely.
- The patient's bed is kept in semi-Fowler's position at all times.
- Diet is advanced from clear liquids to regular on postoperative day (POD) 1 with restrictions to caffeine intake.
- Patients are assisted out of bed to a chair on POD 1 and they ambulate beginning on POD 2.
- Foley catheters and intravenous (IV) fluids are discontinued and IV medications/patient-controlled analgesias (PCAs) are converted to orals on POD 2.
- Patients are typically ready for discharge home from POD 3 to POD 5.
- Surgical drains are discontinued once the output is less than 30 mL for two consecutive days.
- Activities are limited and weight-lifting restrictions are in place for 6 weeks postoperatively.
- The first postoperative visit is at 1 week following discharge.
- Preoperative photographs of a patient with a left breast invasive cancer who opted for DIEP flap reconstructions are presented in **FIG 17A,B**.

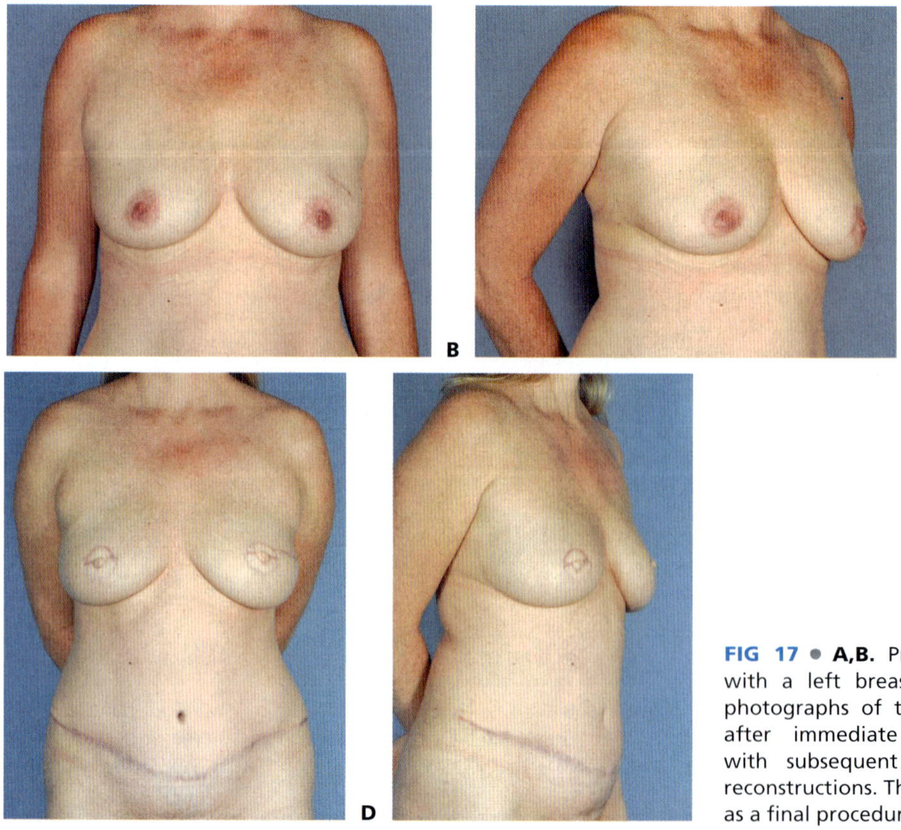

A B C D

FIG 17 ● **A,B.** Preoperative photographs of a patient with a left breast invasive cancer. **C,D.** Postoperative photographs of the breasts and abdominal donor site after immediate bilateral DIEP flap reconstruction with subsequent revisions including bilateral nipple reconstructions. The patient will undergo nipple tattooing as a final procedure.

- The same patient's postoperative results after immediate bilateral DIEP flap breast reconstruction and subsequent revisions are presented in **FIG 17C,D**.

OUTCOMES

- The goals of breast reconstruction are to create breast mounds that are aesthetically pleasing, symmetric, and similar to the natural breast in appearance and feel.
- Patient satisfaction is of great importance in assessing outcomes of reconstruction.
- Breast reconstruction patients are typically satisfied in the short term (<5 years) with their choice of reconstruction across implant-based to autologous forms of reconstruction.[11]
- Over the long term (>8 years), satisfaction with abdominal-based flap reconstruction is maintained, whereas satisfaction with implant-based techniques tends to depreciate.[11]
- Studies have also shown greater satisfaction with autologous reconstruction in patients requiring unilateral reconstructions.[12] This is likely the result of better symmetry with the natural contralateral breast.
- Patient satisfaction in bilateral reconstructions has been found to be similar across all techniques provided that the same technique is used on both sides,[12] highlighting again the importance of symmetry.

COMPLICATIONS

Flap-Related Complications

- Infections—Surgical site infections are rare as these are clean cases and the autologous tissue transferred to the chest offer greater resistance to infection than do prostheses.
- Delayed wound healing—This complication typically occurs at the interface between the mastectomy flap and DIEP flap skin paddle. It often is a result of marginal mastectomy flap necrosis from poor skin perfusion, which is more likely in smokers and in the previously radiated breast skin.
- Fat necrosis—Varying degrees of fat necrosis are encountered in 10% to 15% of reconstructions; it occurs in small segments of flap adipose tissue with poor perfusion. This complication is apparent within a few weeks of the operation and presents as a firm palpable nodule, which occasionally causes some discomfort. These areas of necrosis can be directly excised or managed with liposuction (ultrasound assisted or suction assisted) during revision procedures.
- Partial flap loss—an uncommon complication that is also related to poor perfusion. Here, a segment of the flap is lost. It can be the result of poor perforator selection or thrombosis of one or more of the selected perforators. An excision of the necrotic segment is usually required.
- Total flap loss—This is one of the most devastating complications encountered and it occurs in less than 2% of reconstructions. The ultimate cause of flap loss is a thrombosis of the vascular pedicle, which could be brought about by a variety factors ranging from technical problems to hypercoagulable conditions. Early detection of thrombosis with a return to the OR and correction of the inciting problem leads to flap salvage in most cases.

Donor Site Complications

- Hernias/bulges—the result of abdominal wall weakness; this complication is seen with much less frequency when compared to the TRAM flap, which by definition takes muscle and fascia as part of the flap harvest. The incidence of this complication has been shown to decrease with use of mesh reinforcement in TRAM flap harvests.
- Delayed wound healing—Wound healing problems are encountered often in morbidly obese patients, diabetics, and smokers. Perfusion to the infraumbilical portion of the abdominal donor site is marginal in some patients; fat necrosis occurs in this area and ultimately results in a wound dehiscence. These wounds are managed by debridement and dressing changes with healing by secondary intention.

REFERENCES

1. Kroll S, Baldwin BA. A comparison of outcomes using three different methods of breast reconstruction. *Plast Reconstr Surg.* 1992;90:455–462.
2. Alderman AK, Wilkins EG, Lowery J, et al. Determinants of patient satisfaction in post-mastectomy breast reconstruction. *Plast Reconstr Surg.* 2000;106:769–776.
3. Hartrampf CR, Scheflan M, Black PW. Breast reconstruction with a transverse abdominal island flap. *Plast Reconstr Surg.* 1982;69:216–225.
4. Koshima I, Soeda S. Inferior epigastric artery skin flaps without recuts abdominis muscle. *Br J Plast Surg.* 1989;42:645–648.
5. Allen RJ, Treece P. Deep inferior epigastric perforator flap for breast reconstruction. *Ann Plast Surg.* 1994;32:32–38.
6. Blondeel N, Vanderstraeten GG, Monstrey SJ, et al. The donor site morbidity of free DIEP flaps and free TRAM flaps for breast reconstruction. *Br J Plast Surg.* 1997;50:322–330.
7. Nahabedian MY, Dooley W, Singh N, et al. Contour abnormalities of the abdomen after breast reconstruction with abdominal flaps: the role of muscle preservation. *Plast Reconstr Surg.* 2002;109:91–101.
8. Momoh AO, Colakoglu S, Westvik TS, et al. Analysis of complications and patient satisfaction in pedicled transverse rectus abdominis myocutaneous and deep inferior epigastric perforator flap breast reconstruction. *Ann Plast Surg.* 2012;69(1):19–23.
9. Holm C, Mayr M, Hofter E, et al. Perfusion zones of the DIEP flap revisited: a clinical study. *Plast Reconstr Surg.* 2006;117:37–43.
10. Smit JM, Dimopoulou A, Liss AG, et al. Preoperative CT angiography reduces surgery time in perforator flap reconstruction. *J Plast Reconstr Aesthet Surg.* 2009;62:1112–1117.
11. Hu ES, Pusic AL, Waljee JF, et al. Patient-reported aesthetic satisfaction with breast reconstruction during the long-term survivorship period. *Plast Reconstr Surg.* 2009;124:1–8.
12. Craft RO, Colakoglu S, Curtis MS, et al. Patient satisfaction in unilateral and bilateral breast reconstruction. *Plast Reconstr Surg.* 2011;127:1417–1424.

Chapter 20 Nipple–Areolar Reconstruction

Anita R. Kulkarni Amy K. Alderman Andrea L. Pusic

DEFINITION

- Nipple–areolar reconstruction (NAR) is typically performed as the final stage of breast reconstruction after mastectomy. The nipple is reconstructed to give three-dimensional projection, and the areola is reconstructed separately to mimic a natural nipple–areolar complex (NAC).

PATIENT HISTORY AND PHYSICAL FINDINGS

- NAR is an elective stage of breast reconstruction that can be performed after any type of primary breast mound reconstruction. Published studies indicate that approximately 50% of breast reconstruction patients elect to undergo NAR.[1,2]
- NAR is performed at least 3 months after breast reconstruction is complete. This allows the final breast shape and position to be obtained prior to placement of the NAC.
- NAR can also be performed in a delayed fashion at any time a patient decides, including months or years after breast mound reconstruction.

SURGICAL MANAGEMENT

- There are many described techniques for nipple reconstruction, including nipple sharing, local flaps, cartilage grafts, dermal grafts, and prostheses.[3] Local flaps are the most popular option and are described in detail in this chapter.
- Reconstructed nipples lack the rigid ductal and smooth muscle elements of a natural nipple; therefore, the long-term maintenance of nipple projection continues to be the most challenging aspect of NAR.[4]
- Multiple autologous and prosthetic materials (auricular cartilage, rib cartilage, toe pulp, acellular dermal matrix, calcium hydroxylapatite, polytetrafluoroethylene implants, etc.) have been attempted to give permanent rigidity to the nipple; however, no single technique has demonstrated definitive superiority.[3]
- Areolar reconstruction is primarily done by skin grafting, tattoo, or both.
- The first described technique in this chapter is a skate flap for nipple reconstruction with a full-thickness skin graft for areolar reconstruction. This procedure is typically done in the operating room under sedation or general anesthesia.
- The second described technique is a C-V flap for nipple reconstruction, which can be used in combination with a tattoo for areolar reconstruction. This procedure can be done in the office under local anesthesia.

Preoperative Planning

- In unilateral NAR, the position, size, and shape of the opposite nipple are taken into consideration to design the reconstruction in addition to anatomic landmarks. In bilateral NAR, anatomic landmarks and standard measurements are used to position and design the NAC.
- Anatomically, the NAC is located at the anterior-most projecting part of the breast mound at the level of the inframammary fold, centered on the reconstructed breast mound.
- The nipple has an average projection of 5 mm and the areola has an average diameter of 35 to 45 mm.

POSITIONING

- In the operating room, patients are positioned supine with arms at 90 degrees secured to arm boards. Both breasts are prepped into the field to allow for evaluation of symmetry. Patients are secured to the operating table to allow upright evaluation intraoperatively.
- In the clinic, patients are positioned supine with arms at sides.

Skate Flap (Nipple) and Full-Thickness Skin Graft (Areola)

- The patient is placed in supine position with arms abducted at 90 degrees. Arms are secured on arm boards.
- The NAC position is selected at the anterior-most projecting part of the reconstructed breast with the patient in an upright position. In unilateral nipple reconstruction, the NAC is placed symmetrically to the opposite side (**FIG 1**).
- A donor site is chosen for the full-thickness skin graft, which will be used to reconstruct the areola. Commonly used sites include the lateral edge of the mastectomy scar, the lower abdomen, and the groin crease. Additionally, the areolar graft can be taken adjacent to any of the patient's existing scars.
- A 38- or 42-mm nipple sizer is used to mark the areolar skin graft. An ellipse is drawn tangent to the areolar graft to allow linear closure of the donor site.
- The areolar skin graft is scored with a knife prior to harvest. The ellipse is then excised as a full-thickness skin graft (**FIG 2**).
- The areolar graft is aggressively defatted with a small sharp scissor, leaving only full-thickness skin behind (**FIG 3**).
- The skate flap is designed at the previously marked site (**FIG 4**).
  - A 1- to 1.5-cm circle is drawn at the planned location of the nipple.

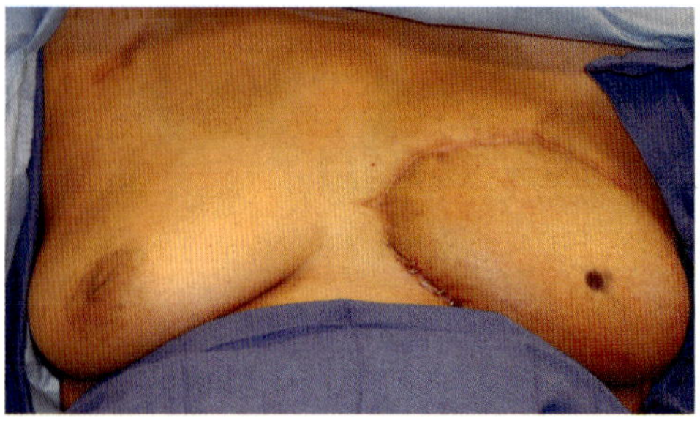

FIG 1 • Nipple position is selected symmetrically to the native nipple.

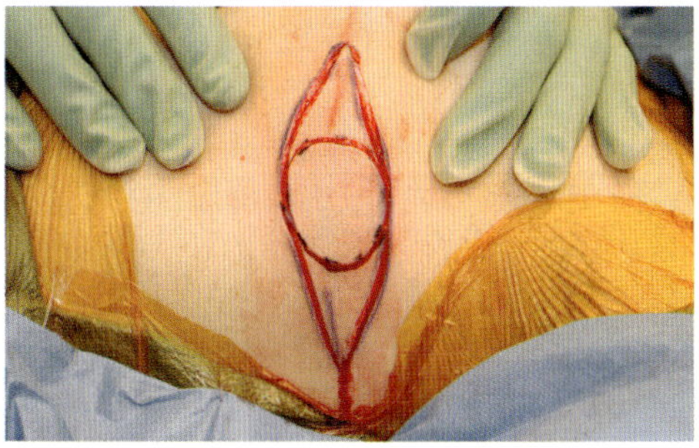

FIG 2 ● Areolar skin graft is marked with a 38-mm nipple sizer. An ellipse is drawn tangentially to facilitate linear closure.

  - A 38- or 42-mm nipple sizer is used to mark the areola centered around the nipple.
  - A horizontal line is drawn across the circle at the superior edge of the marked nipple.
  - The upper portion of the circle is crosshatched to mark the area that will be de-epithelialized.
  - The lower portion of the circle will be raised as the "skate flap" to create the new nipple.
- The epidermis is scored along all incisions.
- The crosshatched semicircle is de-epithelialized (**FIG 5**).
- The flap is then raised from the edges at the level of the mid-dermis. The deepest layer of dermis is left down in order to provide a vascularized bed for the areolar skin graft (**FIG 6**).
- The flap remains attached to the deep dermis at the marked nipple. The flap is raised in a slightly deeper plane at the center in order to include some fat with the flap to provide bulk (**FIG 7**).
- The corners of the flap are centralized and sutured to the underlying dermis using 5-0 Vicryl Rapide (**FIG 8**).
- The edges of the flap are sutured together using interrupted 5-0 Rapide (**FIG 9**).
- The cap is sutured down to close off the nipple (**FIG 10**).
- The full-thickness skin areolar skin graft is sutured to the bed using 4-0 chromic half-buried horizontal mattress sutures. The buried portion of suture is placed along the native breast skin to avoid scarring on the breast (**FIG 11**).
- A 1-cm hole is cut in the center of the areolar graft to expose the nipple (**FIG 12**).

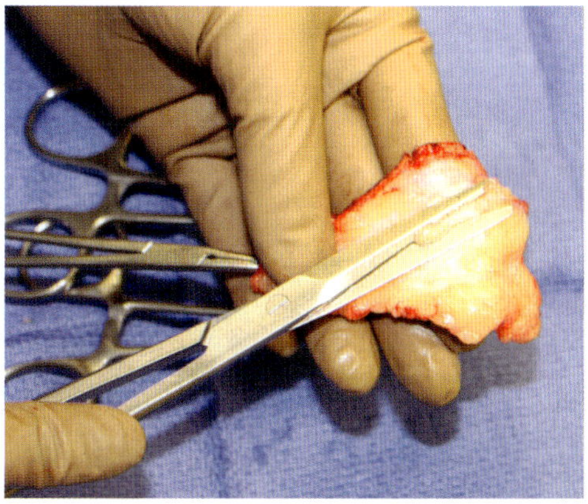

FIG 3 ● Areolar skin graft is aggressively defatted.

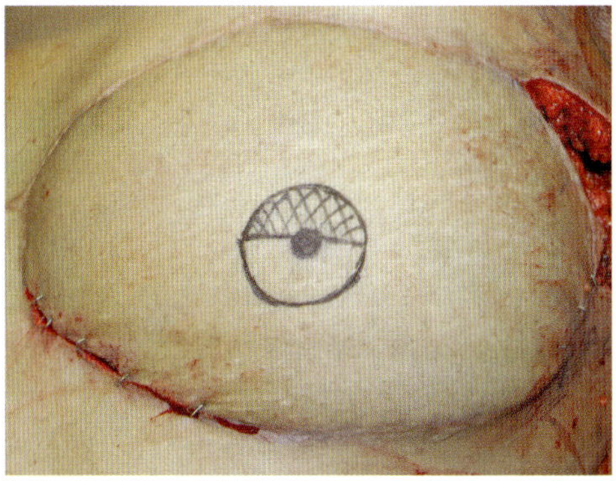

FIG 4 ● Skate flap design.

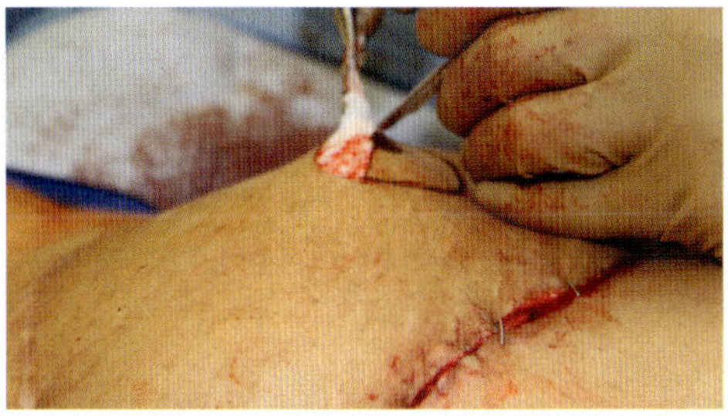

FIG 5 ● Crosshatched area is de-epithelialized.

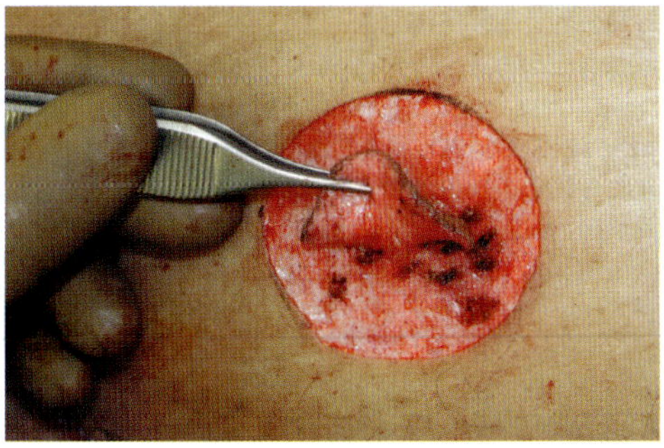

FIG 6 ● Skate flap is raised in the middermal plane, leaving central pedicle attached.

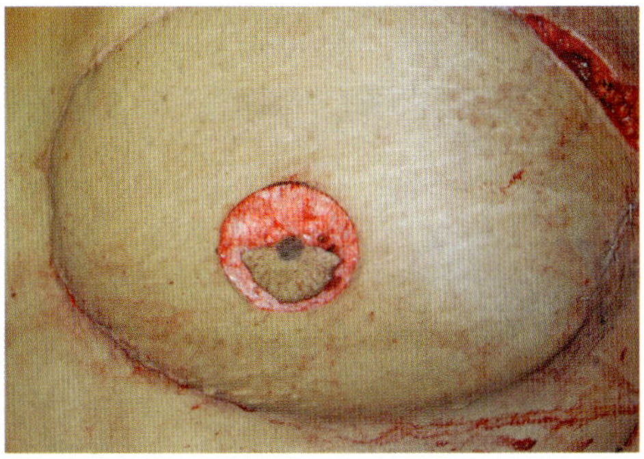

FIG 7 ● Skate flap is shown raised.

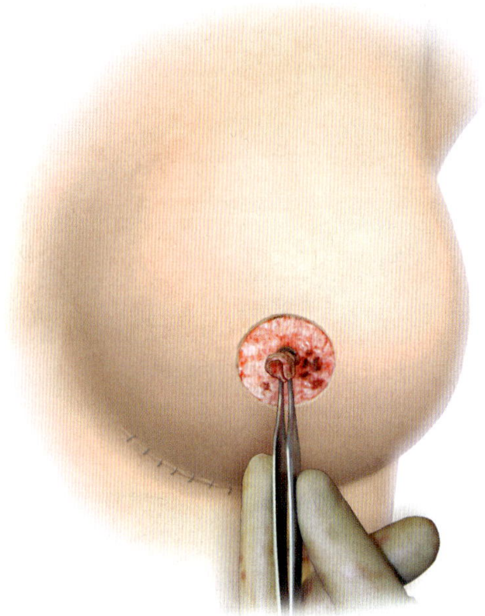

FIG 8 • Edges of skate flap are brought together centrally to recreate nipple.

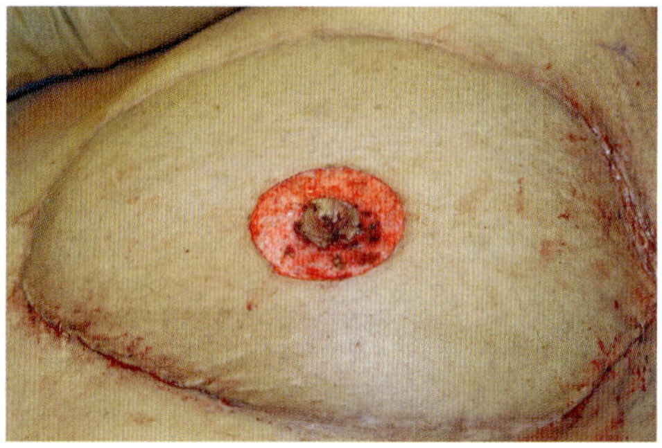

FIG 10 • Open end of nipple is sutured down as a cap.

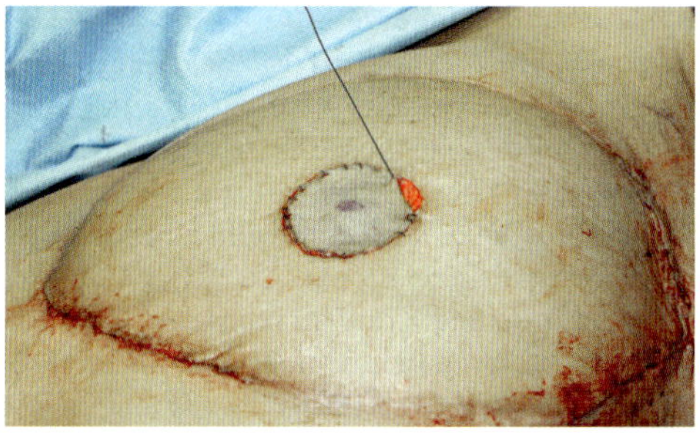

FIG 11 • Areolar skin graft is sutured to skin edges.

- The graft is secured to the nipple using interrupted 5-0 chromic sutures.
- 4-0 chromic tacking sutures and piecrust incisions are placed in the areolar graft (**FIG 13**).
- A protective dressing is applied using Mastisol on the native breast, crisscrossed Steri-Strips, 2 × 2 fluffed gauze, and foam tape (**FIG 14A–D**). The goal of the dressing is to protect the NAR without putting any pressure on the skate flap.
- The dressing is kept in place for 5 to 7 days after surgery, at which time it is removed in clinic.

C-V Flap

- This procedure can be performed under local anesthesia with the patient awake.
- With the patient in a seated upright position, the NAC position is marked at the anterior-most projecting part of the breast (**FIG 15**).

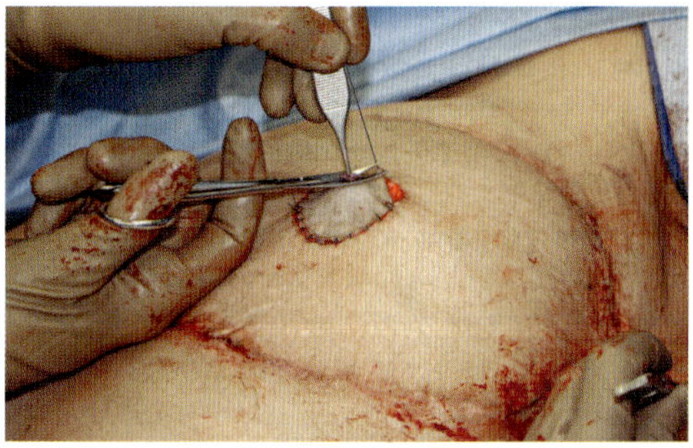

FIG 12 • Central hole is cut in areolar skin graft to allow nipple to protrude.

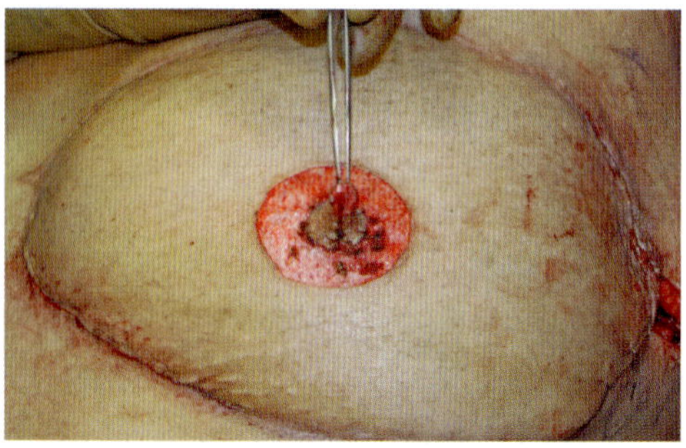

FIG 9 • Edges are sutured together in midline.

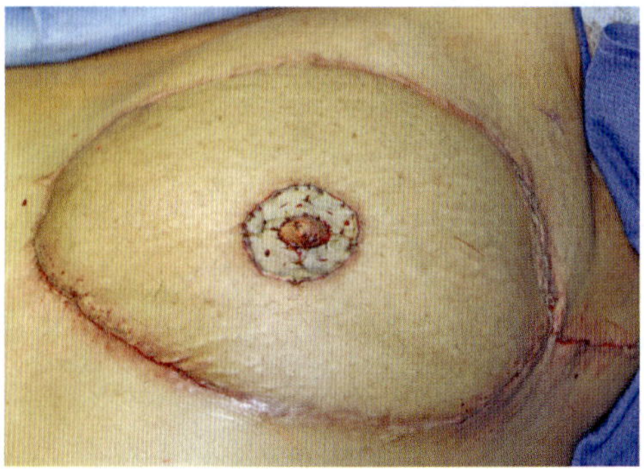

FIG 13 • Tacking sutures and piecrust incisions are placed in areolar skin graft.

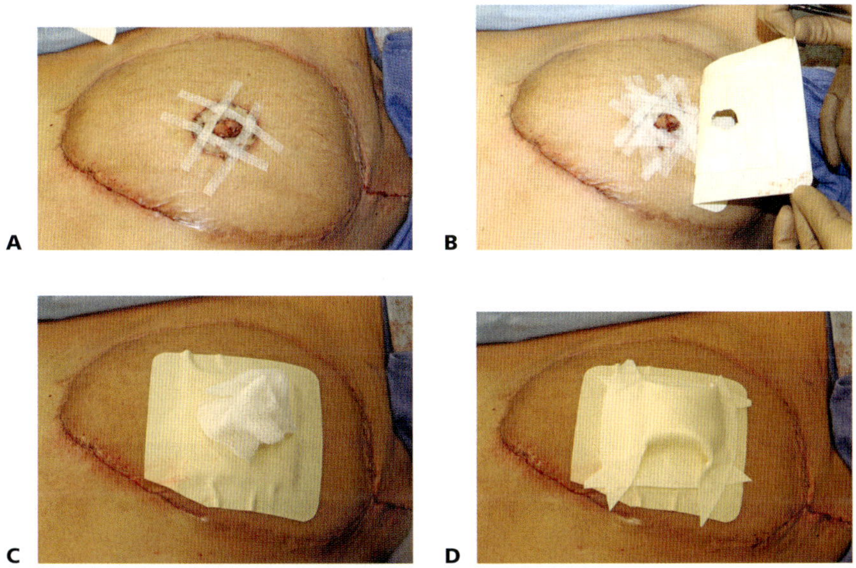

FIG 14 • Bolster dressing. **A.** Mastisol is applied to surrounding breast skin, followed by tightly adherent Steri-Strips placed in crosswise fashion to apply pressure to graft. **B.** Foam tape dressing with a central hole for nipple is placed over crosswise Steri-Strips. **C.** 2 × 2 fluffed gauze is placed over the nipple. **D.** Additional foam tape is tented over the fluffed gauze without putting any pressure on nipple reconstruction.

- C-V flap is drawn as shown. The length of the flap is approximately 5 cm (*A* to *F*), and the width is approximately 1.5 cm. The width of the flap (*BD* to *CE*) determines the projection of the nipple (**FIG 16**).
- The subcutaneous tissue is infiltrated with 1% lidocaine with 1:100,000 epinephrine (**FIG 17**).
- Incisions are made along all edges *except* points *B* to *D* at the base of the nipple. This area is left attached and serves as the blood supply to the flap (**FIG 18**).
- The flap is raised from both sides in the midsubcutaneous fat plane (**FIG 19A,B**).
- The incision is closed from point *B* to *C* and *D* to *E* (**FIG 20**).
- One flap edge (point *A*) is brought to the center and sutured in place with 5-0 Vicryl Rapide (**FIG 21**).
- The opposite flap edge (point *F*) is brought to the center and sutured to the first flap edge (**FIG 22**).
- The cap is sutured down to close the top of the nipple and the remainder of the incision is closed with 4-0 Vicryl deep and 4-0 Monocryl running subcuticular (**FIG 23**).
- Nipple projection is shown with both reconstructions complete (**FIG 24**).

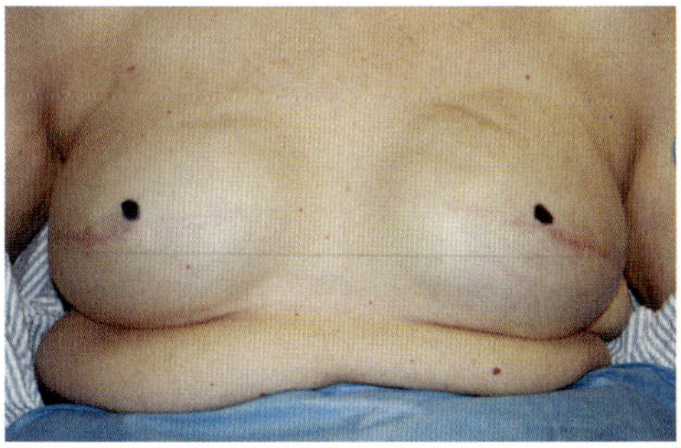

FIG 15 • Bilateral nipple position marked at the anterior-most projecting part of breast mounds adjacent to mastectomy scars.

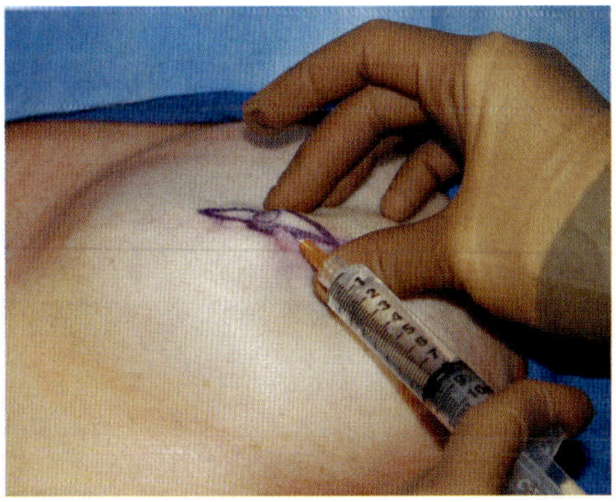

FIG 17 • 1% lidocaine with 1:100,000 epinephrine is injected subcutaneously.

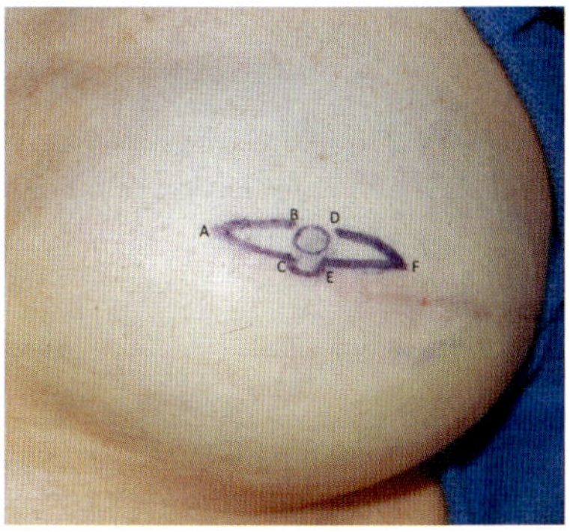

FIG 16 • Markings for C-V flap. Length from *A* to *F* is approximately 5 cm, width from *BD* to *CE* is approximately 1.5 cm.

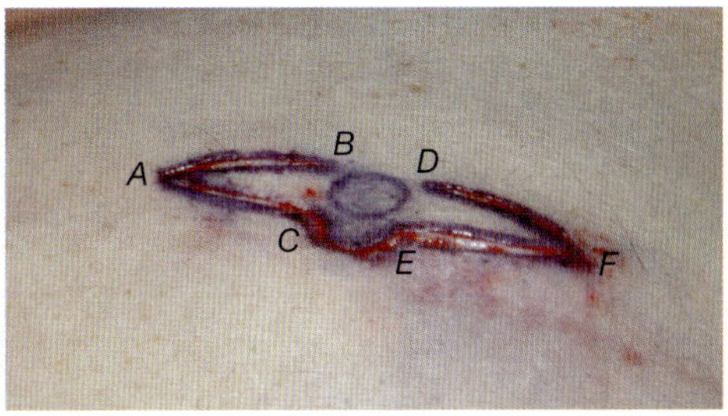

FIG 18 • C-V flap is incised through to midfat level along all incisions except *B* to *D*.

A

B

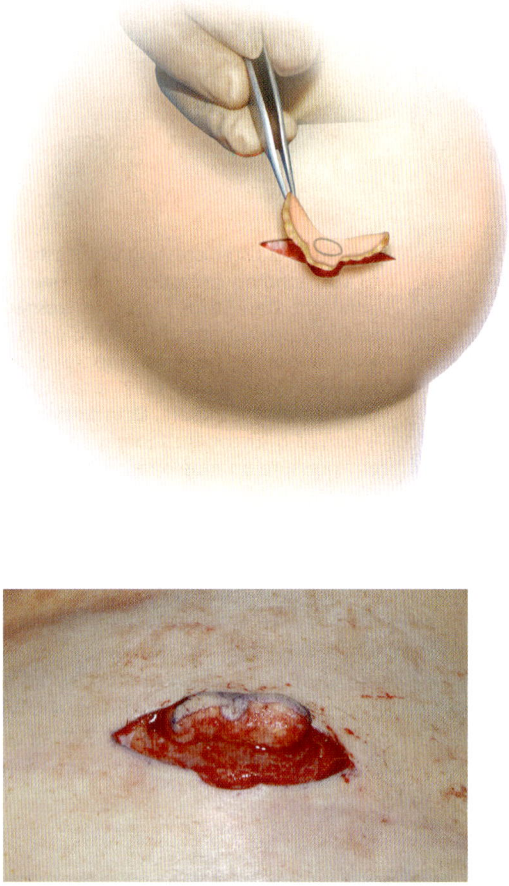

FIG 19 • **A.** C-V flap is raised in the midfat plane. **B.** C-V flap is shown raised.

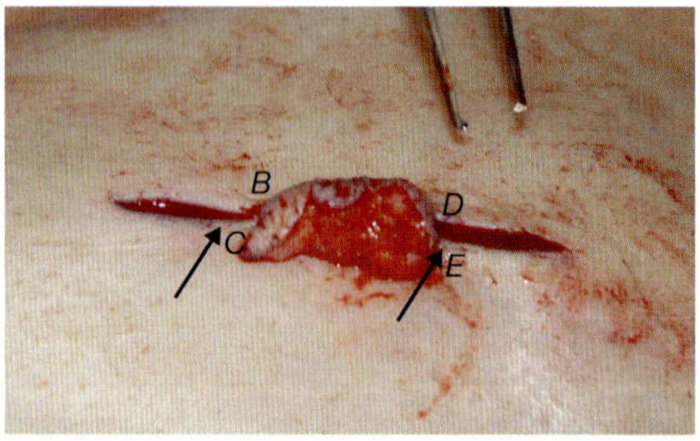

FIG 20 • Incision is closed *(point B* to *C* and *D* to *E)*.

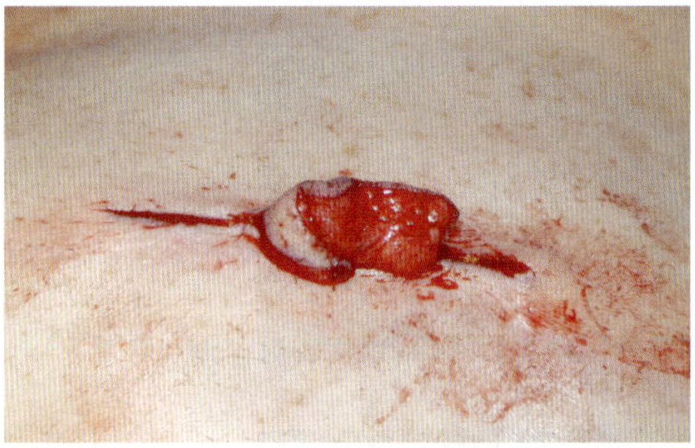

FIG 21 • One flap edge *(point A)* is centralized and sutured to the deep surface.

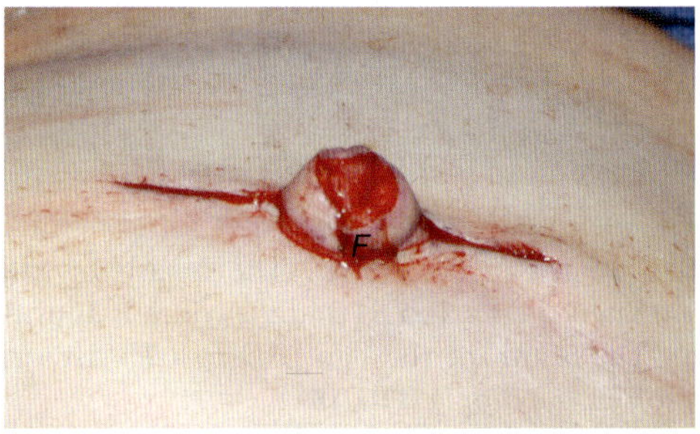

FIG 22 • Opposite flap edge *(point F)* is centralized and sutured to point *A*.

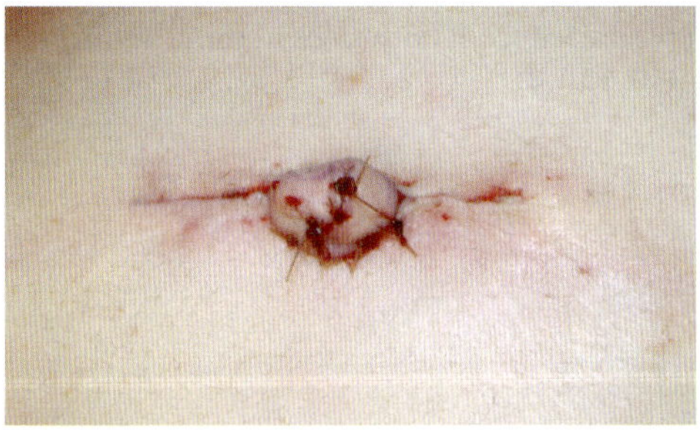

FIG 23 • Cap is sutured down to close off nipple, and all incisions are closed with interrupted sutures.

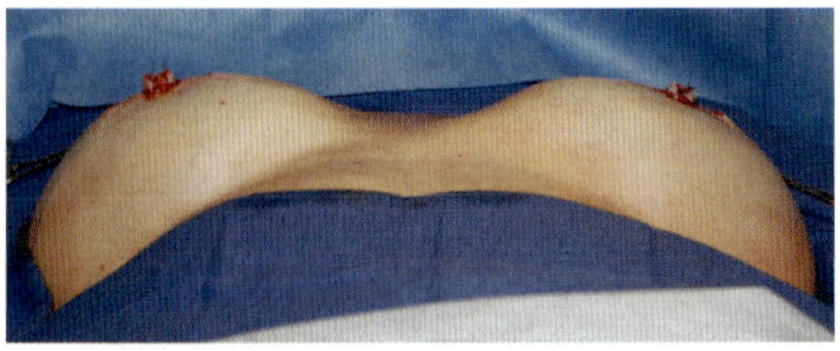

FIG 24 • Final result showing projection of bilateral C-V flaps.

PEARLS AND PITFALLS

Indications	■ Nipple–areolar reconstruction should be deferred until the final breast mound shape is obtained.
Placement of incision	■ Flaps should be based adjacent to the mastectomy scar whenever possible to avoid additional scarring.
Projection	■ Nipple projection will decrease by 50% in the first year; therefore, projection should be overestimated at the time of reconstruction. ■ Projection can be increased later with dermal fillers such as collagen or hyaluronic acid.
Areola	■ Areolar tattoo is often used as an addition to skin grafting or as a primary modality for areolar reconstruction. ■ Tattoos often need more than one application spaced over several months in order to achieve the final desired color.

POSTOPERATIVE CARE

- After nipple reconstruction, a protective dressing should be applied and maintained in place for 1 week postoperatively. Brassieres should be avoided for the first 6 weeks to prevent pressure on the nipple flap.
- If no skin graft is used, patients may shower after the dressing is removed 1 week postoperatively.
- If a skin graft is used for areolar reconstruction, the bolster is removed 1 week postoperatively in the clinic, and daily Xeroform dressing changes are performed for 1 week. After 2 weeks, patients may shower and apply moisturizer to the graft.

OUTCOMES

- All modes of nipple reconstruction result in some degree of loss of projection over time, up to 50%.[5] Most loss of projection occurs within the first 3 months, and final nipple shape and size is typically achieved by 1 year.[6] C-V flaps tend to lose more projection than skate flaps over time.
- Dermal fillers such as collagen and hyaluronic acid can be injected into the nipple to increase projection.

COMPLICATIONS

- Loss of nipple projection
- Partial or complete flap necrosis
- Partial or complete loss of areolar skin graft
- Infection

REFERENCES

1. Andrade WN, Baxter N, Semple JL. Clinical determinants of patient satisfaction with breast reconstruction. *Plast Reconstr Surg*. 2001;107(1):46–54.
2. Schover LR, Yetman RJ, Tuason LJ, et al. Partial mastectomy and breast reconstruction. A comparison of their effects on psychosocial adjustment, body image, and sexuality. *Cancer*. 1995;75(1):54–64.
3. Boccola MA, Savage J, Rozen WM, et al. Surgical correction and reconstruction of the nipple-areola complex: current review of techniques. *J Reconstr Microsurg*. 2010;26(9):589–600.
4. Farhadi J, Maksvytyte GK, Schaefer DJ, et al. Reconstruction of the nipple-areola complex: an update. *J Plast Reconstr Aesthet Surg*. 2006;59(1):40–53.
5. Shestak KC, Gabriel A, Landecker A, et al. Assessment of long-term nipple projection: a comparison of three techniques. *Plast Reconstr Surg*. 2002;110(3):780–786.
6. Few JW, Marcus JR, Casas LA, et al. Long-term predictable nipple projection following reconstruction. *Plast Reconstr Surg*. 1999;104(5):1321–1324.

Chapter 21

Reduction Mammoplasty

Sebastian Winocour Valerie Lemaine

DEFINITION

- Reduction mammoplasty is defined by the removal of expendable breast skin and parenchyma, and repositioning the nipple–areolar complex (NAC) in patients who suffer from breast hypertrophy. The goal is to achieve an overall reduction in breast volume in an aesthetic manner without sacrificing breast sensation or function. Other terms for reduction mammoplasty include breast reduction and reduction mammoplasty.

DIFFERENTIAL DIAGNOSIS

- The differential diagnoses of breast hypertrophy include breast carcinoma, phyllodes tumors, benign breast masses (including fibroadenomas, neurofibromas, lymphangiomas, and breast cysts), hematomas, ectopic tumors producing sex steroids, pregnancy, lactation, and virginal hypertrophy. It is of paramount importance to distinguish benign breast hypertrophy from breast carcinoma, which is much less common, tends to be unilateral, is usually eccentric with respect to the NAC and typically presents as a defined lesion firm to touch.

PATIENT HISTORY AND PHYSICAL FINDINGS

- A thorough history should be performed prior to treatment, identifying physical, functional, and psychological symptoms. It is also important to obtain a detailed past medical and surgical history, reproductive history, family history, social history, and current medications and allergies from the patient.[1]
- Physical and functional problems associated with macromastia include pain (neck, back, and shoulder), mastodynia, shoulder grooving, intertriginous rashes and/or infections, physical activity restriction, and difficulty fitting into clothing. Patients often suffer from psychological symptoms related to breast size, including feelings of physical unattractiveness and embarrassment in both private and social settings.[2,3]
- Past medical history should screen for any diseases that would impact the patient's ability to recover from the reduction mammoplasty, such as heart or lung disease, or impact the viability of the NAC postoperatively, such as collagen vascular diseases.[1] A history of previous benign or malignant breast masses should also be elicited. Obtaining a thorough past surgical history should identify any previous breast or chest wall incisions that may influence planning of either the skin pattern incision or the pedicle to the NAC.[1]
- Because childbearing can affect the size and shape of a woman's breasts, the reproductive history of the patient is important to understand and anticipate the effect reduction mammoplasty will have on the future breast.[1] Inquiring about plans for future pregnancies and breastfeeding is important to inform patients of the risks of the procedure. Finally, in patients who have recently given birth and who may be currently breastfeeding, it is important to discuss timing of surgery because it is ideal to delay surgery for at least 1 year after completing either.
- Obtaining a thorough family history is important to identify patients at increased risk for breast carcinoma. Younger patients with a family history of breast cancer, in addition to any patient older than the age of 40 years, should undergo a preoperative mammogram in order to identify any suspicious lesions prior to surgery.[2] Some surgeons routinely obtain a bilateral mammogram in all patients considering reduction mammoplasty.
- Smokers are at increased risk of compromise of the blood supply to the NAC and for poor wound healing.[1] Therefore, eliciting a smoking history may alter the timing of surgery. Current recommendations indicate that a period of at least 4 weeks of smoking cessation prior to surgery is ideal for best outcomes.
- Macromastia can present at different periods in a woman's life and therefore surgical timing is important. When present during adolescence, the timing of reduction mammoplasty needs to be balanced with the effects of macromastia on self-esteem and physical activity restriction with ongoing pubertal breast development and potential future childbearing.[4] In older patients who have encountered recent significant changes in overall weight, it is prudent to delay surgery for at least 1 year until their weight has stabilized, as this can translate into disproportionate changes in breast volume.
- A bilateral breast examination should be performed in every patient, including examination of the axillary and supraclavicular lymph node basins. The patient's height, weight, body mass index, and body surface area, as well as appropriate breast measurements should be taken, including breast width, sternal notch/clavicle to nipple distance, midline inframammary fold to nipple distance, and the dimensions of each areola.[2] In addition, breast characteristics should be noted including symmetry, upper pole contour and fullness, presence of breast ptosis, skin quality including presence of striae, and breast tissue density (**FIG 1**).[1]

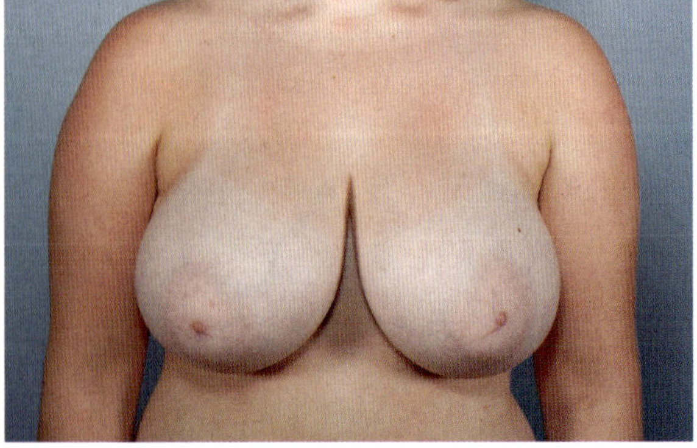

FIG 1 • A typical patient suffering from macromastia.

- A discussion of patient's desires and expectations following surgery is essential to avoid dissatisfaction and misunderstandings. In addition, the patient should be informed about possible complications associated with reduction mammoplasty, including changes in nipple sensation, asymmetry, unappealing breast size or shape, scarring, fat necrosis, NAC loss, inability to breastfeed, hematoma, and infection.

IMAGING AND OTHER DIAGNOSTIC STUDIES

- The American Cancer Society recommends screening mammograms starting at age 40 years in patients with average risk of developing breast cancer.[5] These patients, and younger patients at increased risk of breast cancer, should therefore undergo a preoperative mammogram prior to reduction mammoplasty. Many plastic surgeons routinely perform a preoperative screening mammogram in all patients undergoing this procedure.

SURGICAL MANAGEMENT

- There are multiple surgical approaches to reduction mammoplasty; however, all must deal with the following four considerations: (1) reduction in the parenchymal volume of the breast, (2) creation of the NAC pedicle, (3) reduction of expendable skin followed by redraping, and (4) repositioning of the NAC.[3] This chapter will describe the most commonly practiced Wise pattern (inverted T) technique, which reduces the medial, lateral, and superior breast parenchymal volume and maintains blood supply to the NAC by an inferior pedicle. Other techniques include the superior medial breast reduction,[3] short scar periareolar inferior pedicle reduction (SPAIR),[1] and the liposuction breast reduction,[6] among others.
- Advantages to the Wise pattern technique include its reproducibility, popularity, and applicability to a wide range of breast shapes and sizes, whereas disadvantages include longer scars and a tendency toward developing breast ptosis over the long term.

Preoperative Planning

- Preoperative markings with a permanent marker should be performed in the upright position in the preoperative holding area on the day of surgery.
- The chest midline, breast meridian, and inframammary creases are initially marked. The inframammary crease should then be transposed onto the anterior breast to mark the desired new nipple position.[7] The distance from the sternal notch/clavicle to this point is measured and transposed symmetrically to the other breast. Eight-centimeter obliquely vertical limbs are then drawn medially and laterally from this point. They should be separated by a distance of 8 to 10 cm between their inferiormost points, depending on the desired breast width reduction. The bases of the vertical limbs are subsequently connected medially and laterally with a curvilinear line that joins the inframammary crease. Minor adjustments are made to account for breast asymmetry and minimize the appearance of standing cones (**FIG 2**).

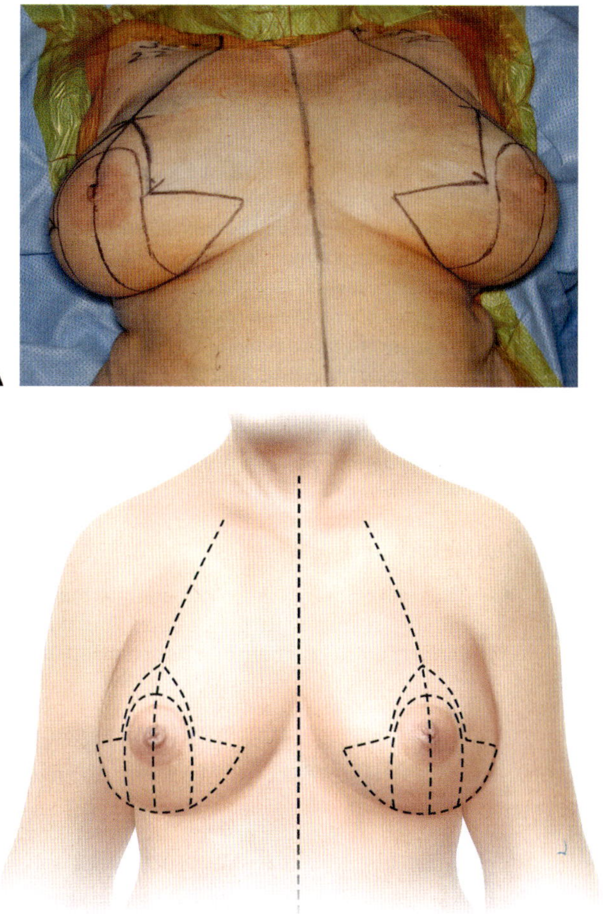

A

B

FIG 2 • **A,B.** Preoperative markings are made with the patient in the standing position prior to surgery.

- Although there is limited data to support the use of preoperative antibiotics for reduction mammoplasty, the general consensus among plastic surgeons is that prophylactic antibiotics covering skin flora should be administered at least 30 minutes prior to skin incision.[8] Data can be also be extrapolated from several general surgery mastectomy studies demonstrating that antibiotic prophylaxis reduces the incidence of postoperative wound infections.[9]

Positioning

- Reduction mammoplasty is performed under general endotracheal anesthesia.
- Because the procedure requires intraoperative assessment of breast symmetry, shape, and contour in the semi-upright position, the patient should be placed in the supine position with the bed break at the hips. The patient's arms should be securely padded on adjustable arm boards, ready for repositioning.
- Sequential compression devices are applied to the lower extremities and a Foley catheter is inserted.

PREINCISION INFILTRATION AND MARKINGS

- The breast bases and planned incisions may initially be infiltrated with 1% Xylocaine with 1:100,000 epinephrine. Then, an 8- to 10-cm–wide inferiorly based dermal pedicle is marked on the skin of each breast, extending in a circular fashion above the NAC all the way down to the chest wall. Using a cookie cutter centered on the nipple, a 40- to 44-mm circular marking is made with the breast skin under minimal to no tension to reduce the diameter of the NAC (**FIG 3**). Tourniquets may then be placed around each breast base to assist with hemostasis (**FIG 4**). After the skin incisions and de-epithelialization of the dermal pedicles are completed, the tourniquets are removed.

Initial Incisions

- The markings of the NAC and dermal pedicle are initially scored with the scalpel. The skin of the inferior pedicle is then de-epithelialized down to the inframammary line, leaving the NAC intact. The dermis between the vertical limbs is preserved to maintain the dermal and subdermal plexus blood supply to the NAC. Incisions are made around the neo-NAC and along the vertical limbs down to the subcutaneous tissue isolating the inferior pedicle from the surrounding breast parenchyma (**FIG 5**).

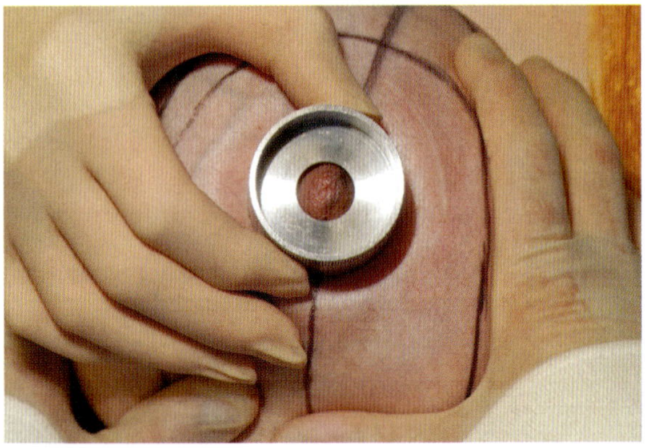

FIG 3 • A 40- to 44-mm cookie cutter is centered on the nipple with the breast skin under minimal to no tension to mark the neo-NAC.

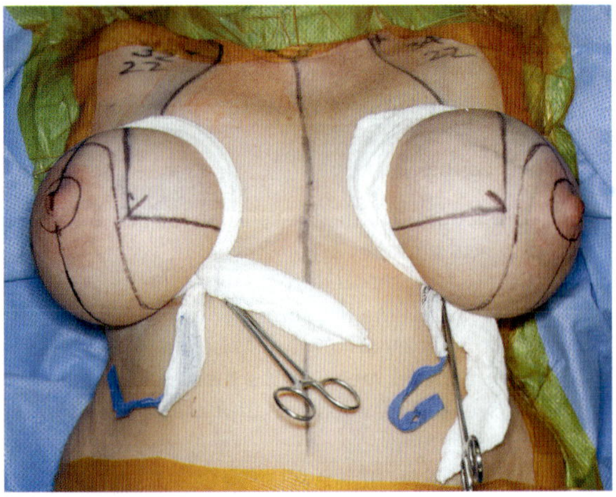

FIG 4 • Tourniquets are placed around each breast base to minimize blood loss and are removed after skin incisions and de-epithelialization of the dermal pedicles.

A

B

C

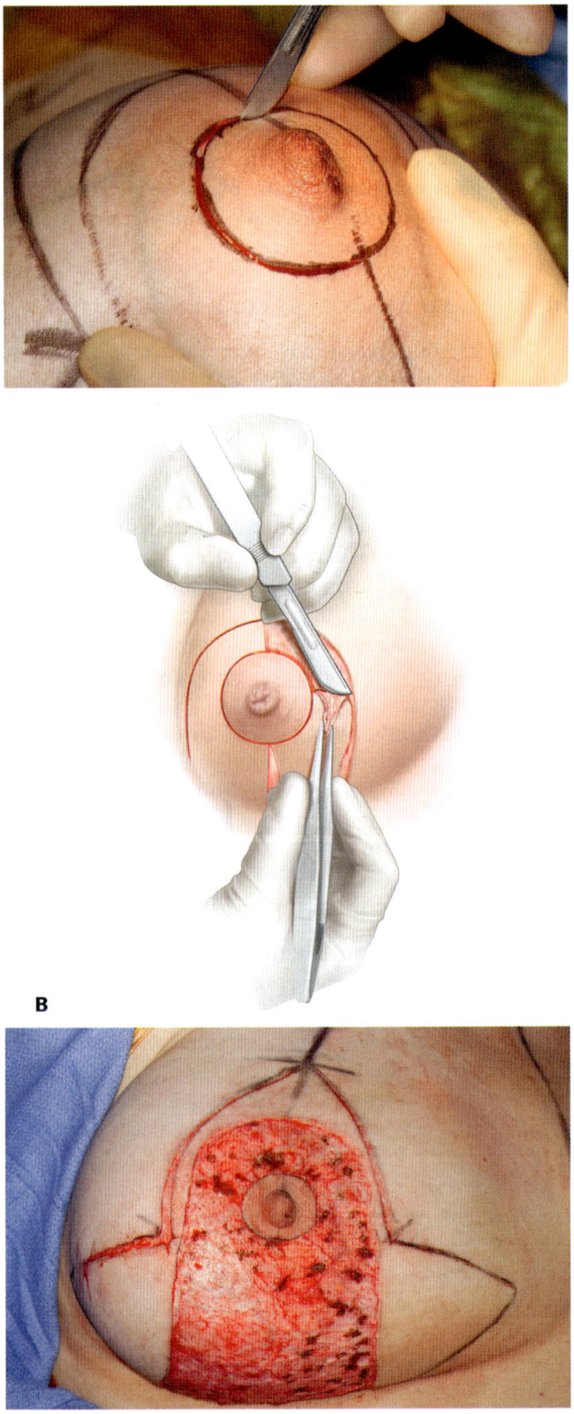

FIG 5 • **A–C.** The skin markings are scored with the scalpel after which the inferior pedicle is de-epithelialized down to the inframammary line, leaving the neo-NAC intact.

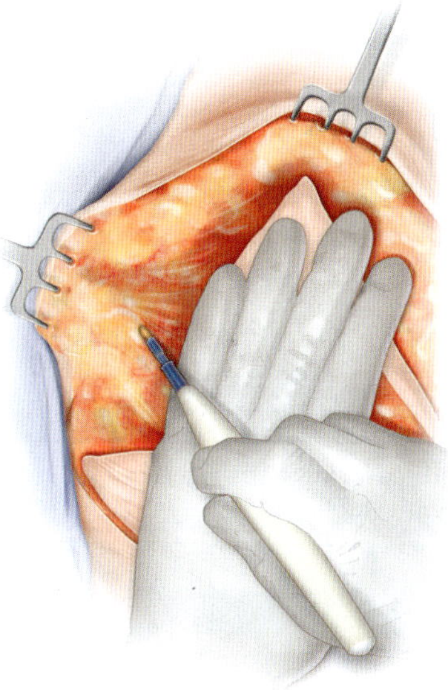

A

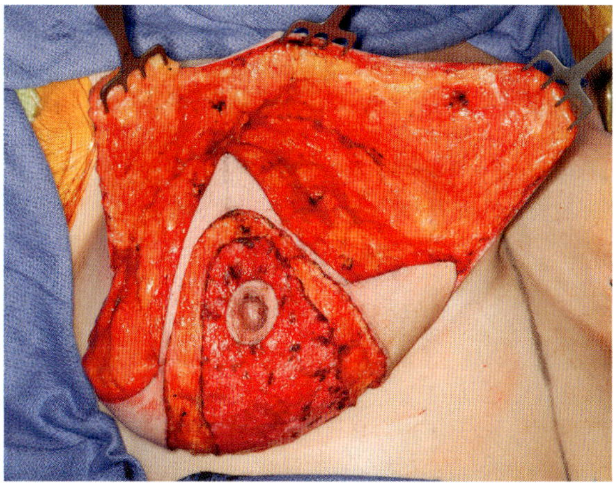

B

FIG 6 • A,B. Skin flaps are raised medially, laterally, and superiorly around the pedicle.

Creation of Skin Flaps

- Medially, laterally, and superiorly based skin flaps are then raised to separate the skin from the breast parenchyma. The flaps are designed to gradually increase in thickness as one approaches the chest wall to ensure a smooth breast contour when the skin is eventually redraped over the breast. They should measure 1 to 2 cm in thickness (FIG 6).[1]

Creation of the Nipple–Areolar Complex Pedicle and Parenchymal Excision

- The inferior pedicle is then created without undermining the blood supply to the NAC. The excess breast parenchyma is systematically excised medially, laterally, and superiorly. Superiorly, breast tissue is removed down to the chest wall extending up to the level of the clavicle, whereas medially, it is removed down to the pectoral fascia but stopping short of midline. Finally, a layer of breast tissue is left on the chest wall laterally in an attempt to preserve the innervation to the NAC (FIG 7). Wound irrigation and meticulous hemostasis is achieved prior to proceeding.
- All breast parenchyma removed from the breast is initially weighed and subsequently sent to pathology for evaluation (FIG 8).

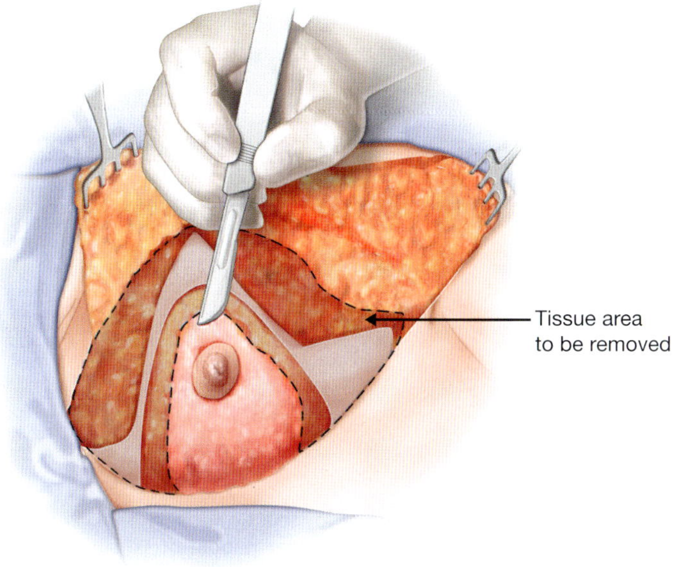

A

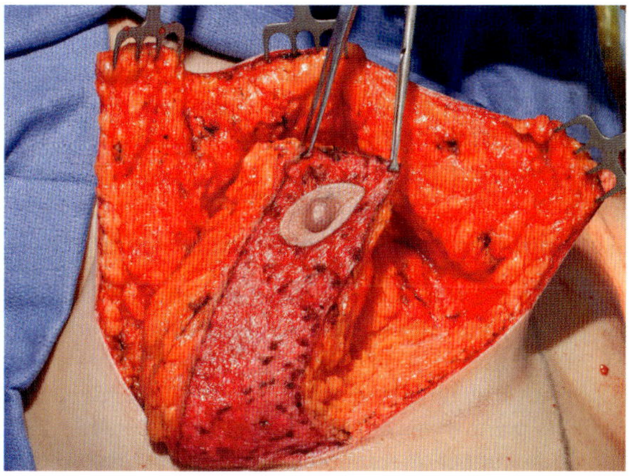

B

FIG 7 • A,B. The inferior pedicle is created without compromising the blood supply to the NAC by excising breast parenchyma in the medial, lateral, and superior quadrants.

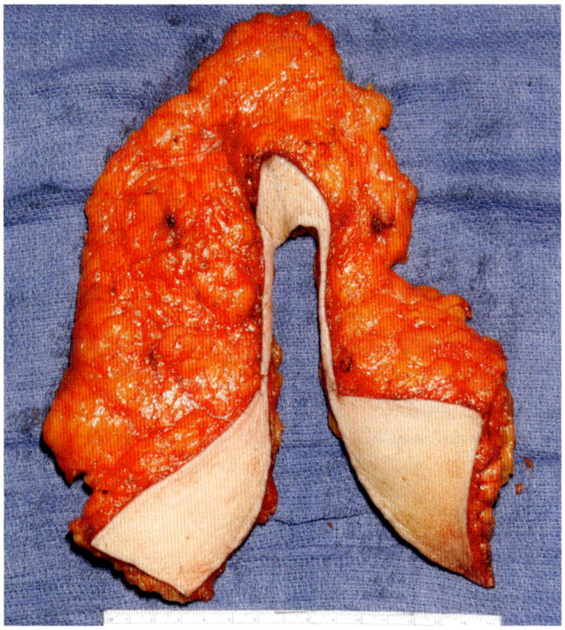

FIG 8 ● The excised specimen includes skin and parenchyma and should be weighed prior to having it sent to pathology.

- The same procedure is repeated on the opposite breast with the goal of achieving breast symmetry in shape and size.

Skin Reduction and Redraping

- The skin flaps are redraped over the breast and temporarily approximated using staples (FIG 9). The patient is then placed in the sitting position and minor adjustments can be made to skin approximation to achieve symmetry and improve aesthetics. The final markings for the medial and lateral inframammary margins can then be made; after which, the skin is excised as needed.
- Once symmetry is achieved, and with the patient still in a sitting position, the final NAC position is determined with a 38- to 42-mm cookie cutter and marked on the breast (FIG 10). The skin is then excised and the NAC is exteriorized (FIG 11).

Repositioning of the Nipple–Areolar Complex

- Once the NAC is exteriorized, the position and orientation of the inferior pedicle is verified to ensure that it is not distorted. A Gillies suture using absorbable monofilament may be placed at the inverted T junction, which is the point of maximal tension. The NAC is then secured in its correct orientation with buried dermal absorbable monofilament sutures in four quadrants. All incisions are then closed in layers with deep dermal interrupted absorbable monofilament sutures, followed by an absorbable running subcuticular monofilament suture (FIG 12). A dry dressing is applied to all wounds.
- Bulb suction drains may be left prior to closure.

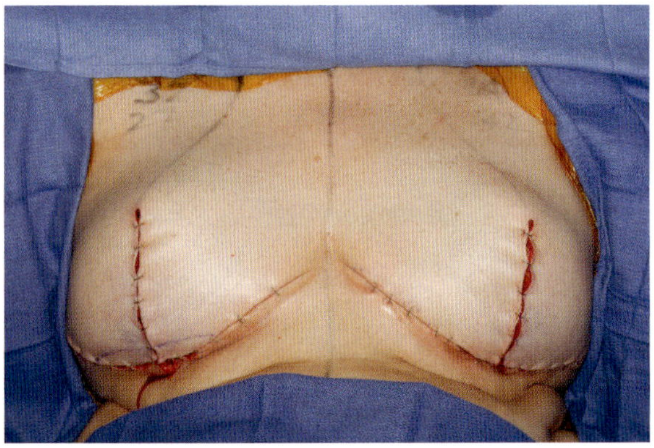

FIG 9 ● The breast skin flaps are redraped over the pedicle and secured with staples.

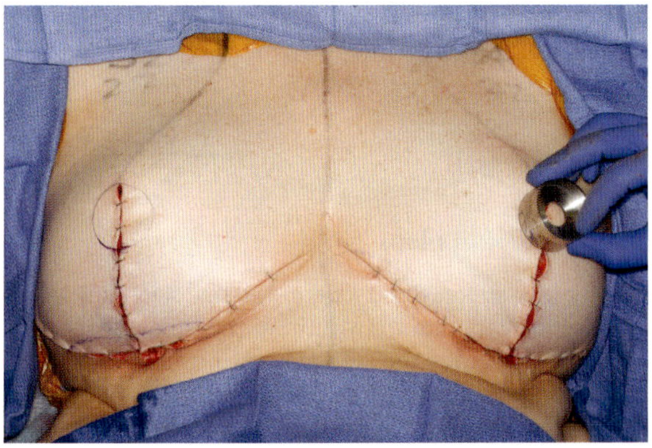

FIG 10 ● The final NAC position is chosen and marked with a 38- to 42-mm cookie cutter.

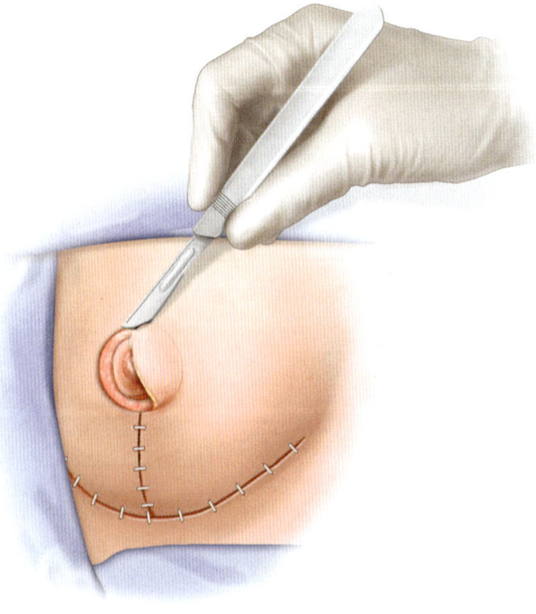

FIG 11 ● The NAC is exteriorized by incising the circular marking and removing the circular paddle of skin and soft tissue. Care is taken not to injure the underlying NAC.

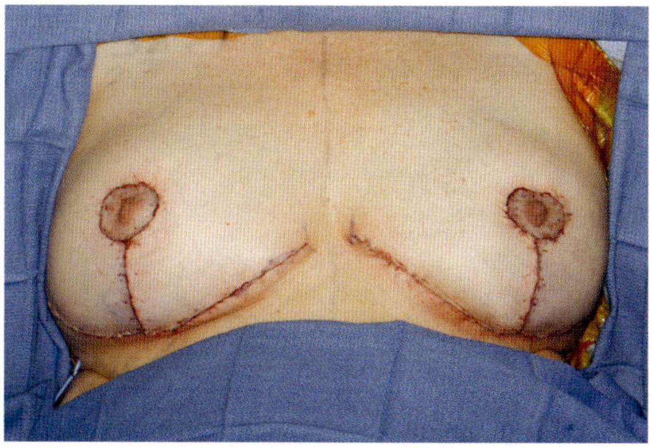

FIG 12 ● The final result after all skin incisions are closed.

PEARLS AND PITFALLS

Preincision infiltration	■ A spinal needle is helpful for thorough infiltration of the breast bases with anesthetic and epinephrine solution.
Initial incisions	■ Only the dermis of the vertical limbs should initially be incised to allow for better traction during de-epithelialization. ■ De-epithelialization can be more efficiently performed with Kaye scissors as compared to a scalpel blade.
Creation of skin flaps	■ Appropriate flap thickness is critical for good blood supply to the skin and to maintain smooth breast contour. The skin flaps should gradually increase in thickness as one approaches the chest wall.
Creation of the NAC pedicle and parenchymal excision	■ Avoid dissection below the inframammary fold medial and lateral to the NAC pedicle to prevent inferior migration of tissue and breast ptosis postoperatively.
Skin reduction and redraping	■ Staples can be an effective alternative to skin approximation clamps when redraping the skin flaps over the breast. ■ Crosshatched orientation marks can be placed after the skin is redraped to ensure skin segments are accurately approximated when staples are removed.
Repositioning of the NAC	■ Verify that the pedicle is not distorted prior to skin closure to avoid ischemia to the NAC due to unusual positioning.

POSTOPERATIVE CARE

- After reduction mammoplasty, the patient should be placed in either a breast binder/wrap or supportive brassiere that should be worn regularly for 2 to 4 weeks after surgery. This maintains pressure on the breasts, minimizing hematoma and seroma formation, and also relieves tension on the skin incisions, preventing wound dehiscence and unfavorable scarring (**FIG 13**).

OUTCOMES

- Outcomes following reduction mammoplasty are excellent with high overall patient satisfaction rates.[8] The complications most frequently reported are (1) symptomatic scarring (6%), (2) wound dehiscence (5%), and (3) infection (1.2%).[10] Patients also report high reduction or resolution of common preoperative symptoms including neck pain (91%), back pain (96%), shoulder grooving (100%), as well as a subjective improvement in perception of self-image (92%).[10]

COMPLICATIONS

- Undesirable scarring
- Wound dehiscence
- Infection (cellulitis or abscess)
- Decreased NAC sensation
- Breast asymmetry
- Unappealing size and/or shape
- Fat necrosis
- NAC loss
- Difficulty or impossibility to breastfeed
- Hematoma

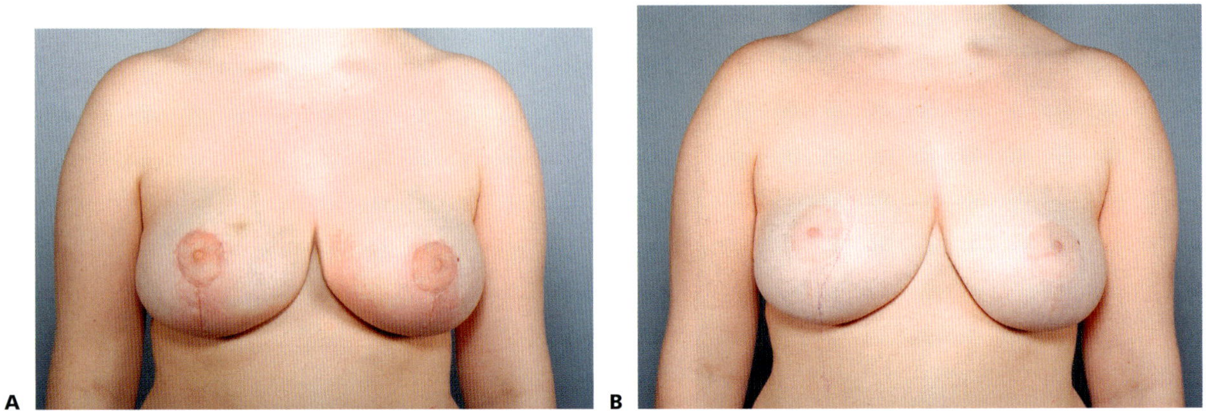

FIG 13 • Postoperative result at **(A)** 1 month and **(B)** 1 year after surgery, respectively.

REFERENCES

1. Hammond DC. *Atlas of Aesthetic Breast Surgery*. Philadelphia, PA: Saunders/Elsevier; 2009.
2. Jones G, ed. *Bostwick's Plastic and Reconstructive Surgery*. 3rd ed. St. Louis, MO: Quality Medical Publishing, Inc; 2010.
3. Hall-Findlay E, Evans GRD, eds. *Aesthetic and Reconstructive Surgery of the Breast*. Philadelphia, PA: Saunders/Elsevier; 2010.
4. Hoppe IC, Patel PP, Singer-Granick CJ, et al. Virginal mammary hypertrophy: a meta-analysis and treatment algorithm. *Plastic Reconstr Surg*. 2011;127(6):2224–2231.
5. Smith RA, Cokkinides V, Brooks D, et al. Cancer screening in the United States, 2010: a review of current American Cancer Society guidelines and issues in cancer screening. *CA Cancer J Clin*. 2010;60(2):99–119.
6. Adam WP. Reduction mammaplasty and mastopexy. *Select Read Plast Surg*. 2002;9(29):1–36.
7. Guyuron B, Eriksson E, Persing JA, et al, eds. *Plastic Surgery Indications and Practice*. Philadelphia, PA: Saunders/Elsevier; 2009.
8. Kalliainen LK. ASPS clinical practice guideline summary on reduction mammaplasty. *Plast Reconstr Surg*. 2012;130(4):785–789.
9. Bunn F, Jones DJ, Bell-Syer S. Prophylactic antibiotics to prevent surgical site infection after breast cancer surgery. *Cochrane Database Syst Rev*. 2012;(1):CD005360.
10. DeFazio MV, Fan KL, Avashia YJ, et al. Inferior pedicle breast reduction: a retrospective review of technical modifications influencing patient safety, operative efficiency, and postoperative outcomes. *Am J Surg*. 2012;204(5):e7–e14.

Chapter 22

Wide Excision of Primary Cutaneous Melanoma

Russell S. Berman   Jeffrey E. Gershenwald

DEFINITION

- Wide excision (WE) of a primary cutaneous melanoma is the term used to describe the definitive surgical management of the primary melanoma site. It is defined as the surgical removal of the primary tumor and/or the biopsy site that includes a defined radial margin of normal-appearing skin and underlying subcutaneous tissue. The appropriate margin of resection is determined by the Breslow thickness as discussed in this chapter.
- Depending on primary tumor characteristics and clinical nodal status, WE may be performed concomitantly with either intraoperative lymphatic mapping and sentinel lymph node biopsy (SNB) (for patients with clinically negative nodes and a primary tumor suggesting sufficient risk of occult regional node metastasis) or regional lymphadenectomy (for patients with clinically involved regional lymph nodes without distant metastasis)[1] (refer to Chapters 31, 32, and 34).
- The main function of the WE is to remove the primary tumor along with any nearby microscopic melanoma cells. In addition to following oncologic principles, the surgeon should also aim to simultaneously minimize dysfunction or disfigurement. This procedure is also known as a wide local excision.

DIFFERENTIAL DIAGNOSIS

- A WE should not be performed unless a definitive pathologic diagnosis of melanoma has been obtained.

PATIENT HISTORY AND PHYSICAL FINDINGS

- A patient with newly diagnosed melanoma should undergo a comprehensive history that includes assessment of age, gender, personal or family history of melanoma or other malignancy as well as history of any nevus syndromes. The patient should also be assessed for any other significant medical and surgical history or issues, medications used, and allergies.
- History of sun exposure and use of tanning beds, if any, should also be obtained. A thorough history may also provide clinical clues as to the extent of disease present at diagnosis. Symptoms such as worsening headaches or abdominal cramps may suggest distant metastatic disease and warrant additional workup.
- A physical examination is extremely important in the newly diagnosed patient with melanoma. If a biopsy has been performed, the anatomic site and orientation of the biopsy should be documented along with the presence or absence of any residual pigmented lesion.
- Skin and soft tissue between the primary site and draining regional nodal basin(s) should be examined for any signs of satellite metastases or in-transit disease. Melanoma most commonly metastasizes via regional lymphatics to regional lymph nodes. Nonetheless, because melanoma may metastasize to both regional and distant nodes, all palpable lymph nodes should be carefully examined in the new melanoma patient, including cervical, supraclavicular, axillary, epitrochlear, inguinal, and popliteal nodes. For patients with a melanoma in a region of ambiguous drainage (typically considered to be the head and neck and trunk regions), multiple nodal basin drainage is possible. Given the importance of the lymphatics in melanoma, meticulous attention to the lymphatic exam is essential. Evidence of lymphedema in the melanoma-bearing extremity may also suggest regional nodal disease.
- It is imperative to confirm the specific site(s) of any primary melanoma to be treated. Although this may seem obvious, many patients have had concomitant and/or prior skin biopsies, and further clarification with source information, including pre-biopsy photographs and/or direct consultation with the referring clinician, may be necessary. Because biopsy sites may heal prior to treatment, photographic images are often obtained to document location(s) of all biopsy sites for which treatment is/may be planned.
- The clinician should document the presence of any lymphadenopathy along with details such as firm, fixed, or matted nodes. Clinically suspicious lymph nodes should be evaluated by fine needle aspiration biopsy (often performed with ultrasound guidance) and cytologic analysis. Biopsy-proven regional metastasis renders a sentinel node biopsy (SNB) procedure unnecessary to diagnose stage III disease in the involved basin.
- Importantly, palpable "reactive" lymphadenopathy may sometimes develop following biopsy of the primary melanoma, thus highlighting the importance of pathologic confirmation of metastatic melanoma before definitive treatment of the basin—for example, lymphadenectomy—is considered.
- Newly diagnosed melanoma patients should also undergo a head-to-toe skin examination to identify the presence of other suspicious skin lesions. Although it is beyond the scope of this section to review biopsy techniques in detail, an appropriate biopsy should include the epidermis, dermis, and at least a cuff of subdermal fat. This allows the dermatopathologist to accurately report the essential components of primary melanoma tumor histopathologic microstaging, including, at a minimum, Breslow thickness (in millimeters), presence or absence of ulceration, mitotic rate, Clark level, status of peripheral and deep margins, and presence or absence of satellite lesions.
- When signs and/or symptoms are suggestive of additional disease, a well-performed physical examination may raise suspicion for distant metastasis. Particular attention should be paid to the neurologic examination, assessing for any localizing symptoms or mental status changes. The finding of hepatomegaly, abdominal mass, or a rectal exam significant for mass or occult blood should prompt further workup. Finally, distant dermal or subcutaneous nodules or distant adenopathy also warrant investigation.

IMAGING AND OTHER DIAGNOSTIC STUDIES

- Treatment planning for patients with primary melanoma is based largely on primary tumor histologic microstaging.
- In the absence of symptoms, the use of imaging studies as part of a staging workup has not been shown to significantly impact survival or the treatment algorithm of the newly diagnosed, clinically node-negative melanoma patient. For asymptomatic preoperative stages I and II melanoma patients, preoperative cross-sectional imaging has a very low yield.[2] In one study, only 1 of 344 (0.3%) studies correlated with confirmed melanoma metastasis; no significant impact on proposed surgical management or staging was noted.[3]
- Even among asymptomatic microscopic stage III patients (i.e., sentinel-node positive), cross-sectional imaging studies infrequently identify distant metastatic melanoma.[4] Although positron emission tomography (PET)/computed tomography (CT) generally includes images of the extremities, regions not typically imaged during standard CT or magnetic resonance imaging (MRI), a benefit for routine use of PET/CT has yet to be demonstrated in this patient population.
- In the otherwise asymptomatic patient with clinically palpable adenopathy, the detection rate of asymptomatic distant metastasis is higher and baseline imaging for staging (CT, PET/CT, MRI) is recommended.[5]
- There is no specific tumor marker or biochemical parameter that has been validated and employed for melanoma screening or recurrence. Elevated serum lactate dehydrogenase (LDH) level is an adverse prognostic factor in patients with distant metastatic melanoma and is included in the American Joint Committee on Cancer (AJCC) staging system for stage IV disease. Patients with elevated serum LDH levels LDH levels are classified as M1c regardless of distant anatomic site(s) involved.[6]

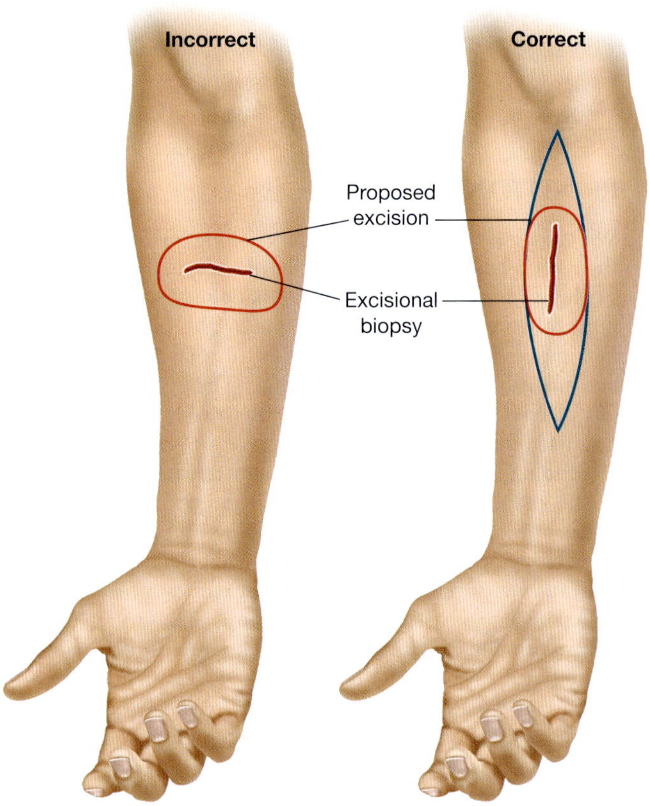

FIG 1 • Importance of orientation of excisional biopsy. An excisional biopsy of the extremity is typically oriented parallel to the long axis of the extremity (right panel). In this example, incorrect orientation (left panel), would likely result in the need for skin graft closure, while primary closure could be likely be achieved if the biopsy had been correctly orientated (right panel). Note the in the right panel example, the overall excision has been extended to accommodate primary closure. It is always important to consider next steps when performing a biopsy.

SURGICAL MANAGEMENT

Preoperative Planning

Biopsy

- Most cutaneous lesions suspicious for melanoma have been biopsied by a dermatologist or other health care provider prior to treatment referral.
- If the biopsy of a lesion suspicious for melanoma has not yet been performed, the surgeon should plan and perform a biopsy: to establish a definitive histologic diagnosis, to obtain appropriate microstaging of the lesion (if melanoma is confirmed), and to maximize the potential for primary closure of the subsequent WE.
- An excisional biopsy should include a narrow margin of normal-appearing skin around the suspicious lesion along with a cuff of underlying subcutaneous fat to provide the dermatopathologist with sufficient material to fully diagnose and, if melanoma, to histologically microstage the primary tumor.
- An excisional biopsy of the extremities is typically oriented parallel to the long axis of the extremity (**FIG 1**). On the trunk and head and neck, the orientation of the biopsy should ideally follow the lymphatic drainage of the involved skin while also being mindful of the lines of tension for optimal closure.
- Incisional biopsies are sometimes necessary for large lesions, especially in cosmetically sensitive areas. Such a biopsy approach does not always reflect the full primary tumor microstaging of the lesion, including margin assessment, and such limitations need to be considered during definitive treatment.
- Shave biopsies are not generally recommended when a cutaneous lesion is suspicious for melanoma, because the full extent of the lesion (especially Breslow thickness) may not be included in the biopsy and the approach may limit accurate microstaging of the primary tumor.
- Confirmation of the melanoma biopsy site(s) must be performed prior to any planned definitive treatment.

Histopathologic microstaging of primary melanoma

- In order to determine the appropriate extent of surgery for a patient with a primary melanoma—including WE margin and whether to offer/perform intraoperative lymphatic mapping and SNB—assessment of several of the primary tumor's histopathologic features is essential.

- Breslow thickness (in millimeters), mitotic rate (expressed in mitoses/mm^2), presence or absence of primary tumor ulceration, and the biopsy margin status (peripheral and deep margins) are all essential to define T stage and to guide appropriate surgical therapy; they should be assessed by a dermatopathologist. Additional primary tumor information that may be useful to the operative surgeon includes the presence or absence of lymphovascular invasion, neurovascular invasion, regression, extent of tumor-infiltrating lymphocytes, histologic subtype, and Clark level.

Margins of excision

- WE includes a radial margin of skin and underlying subcutaneous tissue, with margins appropriate for tumor thickness.
- The radial margin chosen for the WE is based on the primary tumor (Breslow) thickness. At least five prospective randomized trials conducted over the past three decades informed an evidence-based approach. Although detailed discussion is beyond the scope of this section, the recommendations from the National Comprehensive Cancer Network (NCCN) for the radial margin are as follows:[5]
  - Melanoma in situ: 0.5-cm margin (Note: For large diameter melanoma in situ, for example, lentigo maligna type, margins >0.5 cm may sometimes be considered to adequately treat occult early invasive disease).
  - Less than or equal to 1.0 mm: 1.0 cm
  - 1.01 to 2.0 mm: 1.0 to 2.0 cm
  - 2.01 to 4.0 mm: 2.0 cm
  - Greater than 4.0: 2.0 cm

Positioning

General positioning strategies

- Depending on primary tumor characteristics and other considerations, lymphatic mapping and SNB are most often performed in the same operative setting as a WE. For this reason, proper patient positioning should account for both the location of the primary melanoma and the location(s) of draining regional nodal basins. This may become challenging when the primary melanoma drains to multiple nodal basins and/or to interval, ectopic, and/or in-transit sites. Skin graft donor sites or other reconstructive issues must also be considered when positioning the patient.

Proximal extremity

- For proximal upper extremity lesions, a supine position is generally appropriate for WE and SNB. For more posterior lesions near the shoulder, a modified supine position using a shoulder roll or a lateral decubitus position provides easy access for WE and closure. The arm, prepped circumferentially, should be supported to prevent injury to the brachial plexus and/or shoulder.
- For proximal lower extremity lesions, the supine position provides excellent exposure of anterior or lateral sites, allowing both WE and SNB. When the melanoma is on the posterior proximal leg or the buttock, the WE may be performed with the patient in the lateral or prone position. Pressure points need to be padded and axillary and chest rolls need to be appropriately positioned. Some surgeons are comfortable performing both WE and inguinal SNB in the lateral position; a potential advantage is that repositioning is not required. Alternately, SNB can be performed in the supine position, and the patient repositioned for the WE.

Distal extremity

- In general, a supine position is appropriate for most distal extremity lesions. If SNB is also to be performed, access to the axillary, epitrochlear, and inguinal nodal basins is readily achieved. If a patient's melanoma drains to the popliteal nodal basin, then an alternative position other than the supine approach should be used. The prone position is sometimes used so as to allow the sentinel node to be removed through an incision that could be incorporated into a full popliteal node dissection incision if evidence of metastasis were to be identified.
- Heel melanomas not only have the potential to drain to the popliteal basin but may also require specialized reconstructive approaches (e.g., wound vac device, rotational flaps, and/or vascularized free flaps). In this situation, use of a beanbag on the operating room table allows for repositioning as indicated.

Truncal sites

- When an SNB is performed with WE of a truncal melanoma, the possibility of multiple nodal basin drainage patterns must be considered when devising an operating room positioning strategy. A preoperative lymphoscintigraphy will demonstrate afferent lymphatic drainage patterns to major and unusually situated (e.g., ectopic, interval) nodal basins.
- For most anterior truncal melanomas (e.g., chest and abdomen), the supine position allows for access to the primary and draining regional nodal basins. For lateral truncal melanomas, ideal positioning for the WE may include placing the patient in a partial or formal lateral position (with appropriate padding and brachial plexus protection).
- When performing a WE only (e.g., for a thin melanoma without adverse risk features), back melanomas may be performed in the prone (e.g., for medial lesions) or lateral (e.g., for most back lesions) position at the discretion of the surgeon. Appropriate padding and brachial nerve protection must be employed and airway protection is essential. If SNB is being performed in the same operative setting, patient positioning must foster access to draining nodal basins including multiple and/or unusually situated nodal basins. It may be necessary to reposition the patient after the SNB and before the WE (**FIGS 2** and **3**).

Head and neck sites

- Head and neck melanoma patients must also be carefully positioned with consideration of the WE, reconstructive requirements, and in continuity access to draining regional nodal basins if SNB is to be performed. Whether in a supine, prone, or lateral position, the head and neck must be appropriately supported and padded. Additionally, the airway, eyes, and ears must be protected.

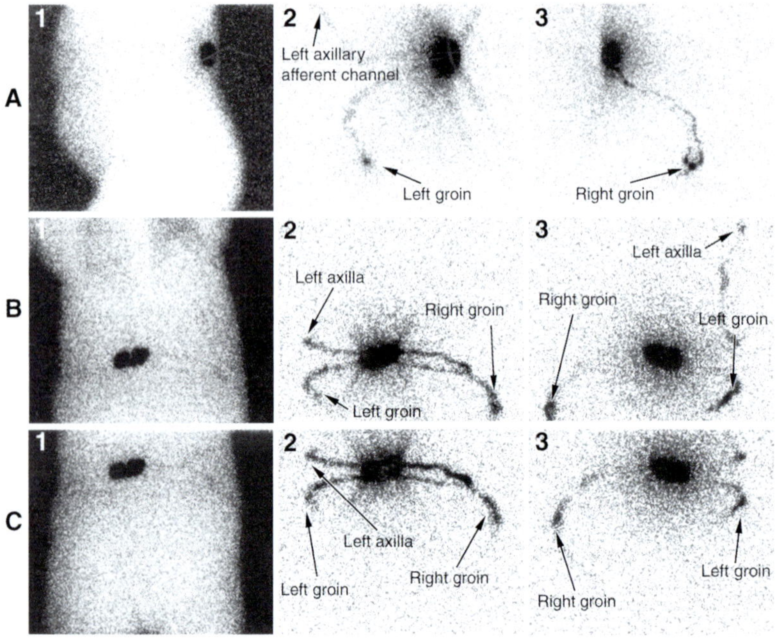

FIG 2 • Lymphoscintigraphic images of a patient with a primary cutaneous melanoma of the midline mid back demonstrates radiotracer uptake activity in the bilateral groins and the left axilla.

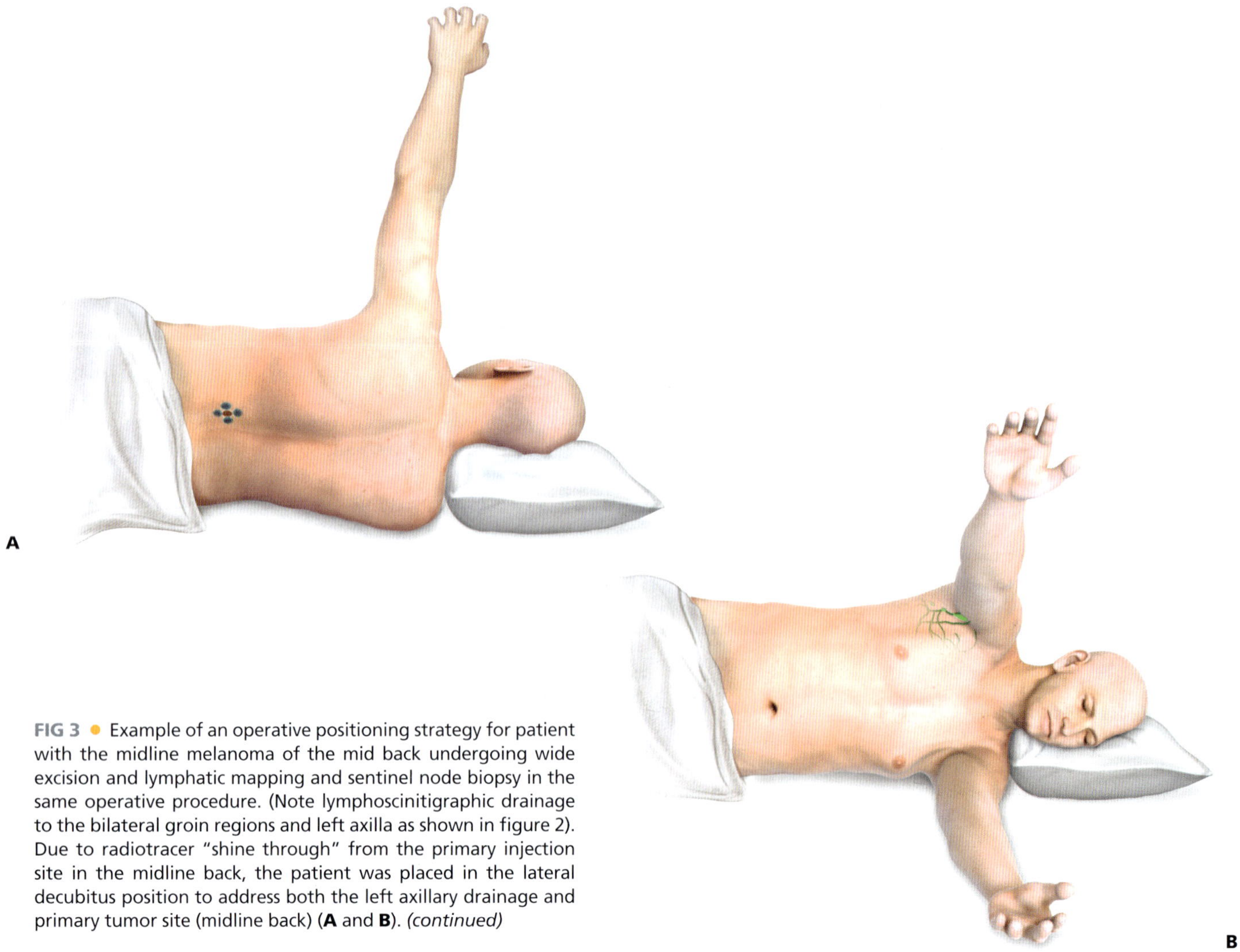

FIG 3 • Example of an operative positioning strategy for patient with the midline melanoma of the mid back undergoing wide excision and lymphatic mapping and sentinel node biopsy in the same operative procedure. (Note lymphoscinitigraphic drainage to the bilateral groin regions and left axilla as shown in figure 2). Due to radiotracer "shine through" from the primary injection site in the midline back, the patient was placed in the lateral decubitus position to address both the left axillary drainage and primary tumor site (midline back) (**A** and **B**). *(continued)*

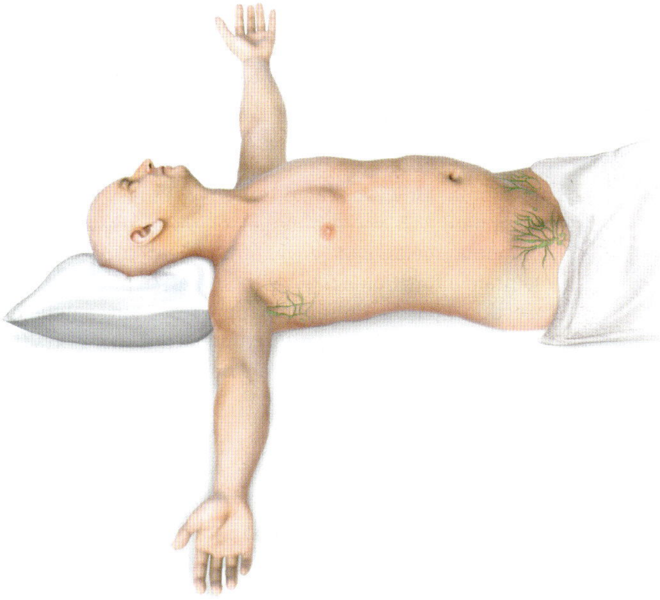

C

FIG 3 ● *(continued)* The patient was then repositioned to supine to perform bilateral inguinal sentinel node biopsies **(C)**. Note that if radiotracer shine through was not a problem, then the patient could have been initially positioned in the supine position (after injection of both isosulfan blue dye and radiocolloid) to address the bilateral inguinal nodal basins as well as left axillary nodal basin and then repositioned into the lateral decubitus position to perform the wide excision of the back melanoma. Regardless of approach, it is important to scan intervening regions with the gamma probe.

WIDE EXCISION MARGIN

- The planned margin of excision of the primary melanoma is based on the Breslow tumor thickness as described above and refers to the radial margin of normal-appearing skin to be resected. If the primary melanoma is entirely or partially intact, the margin should be measured from the periphery of the visible lesion. When the entire pigmented lesion has been excised by the previous biopsy, the margin should be measured from the periphery of the biopsy scar.

PLACEMENT AND ORIENTATION OF INCISION

- Proper planning of the incision is critical. The surgeon must consider the required radial margin (i.e., margin of excision), the specific anatomic primary site involved, as well as the quality and quantity of local soft tissue.
- Because the resulting final incision may be significantly longer than what the patient might have otherwise anticipated, based on the usually "small" biopsy site, we strongly recommend that this theme be integrated into the surgical consultation and preoperative visits: a "scale" drawing presented to the patient at the time of initial and/or preoperative visit is often very instructive.
- The recommended margin of excision is based on primary tumor thickness (described above) and is measured from either the edge of the intact melanoma or biopsy scar, generally resulting in the proposed circular or oval defect marked on the skin (**FIG 4A,B**). When a primary closure is planned, the circle or oval can be modified into

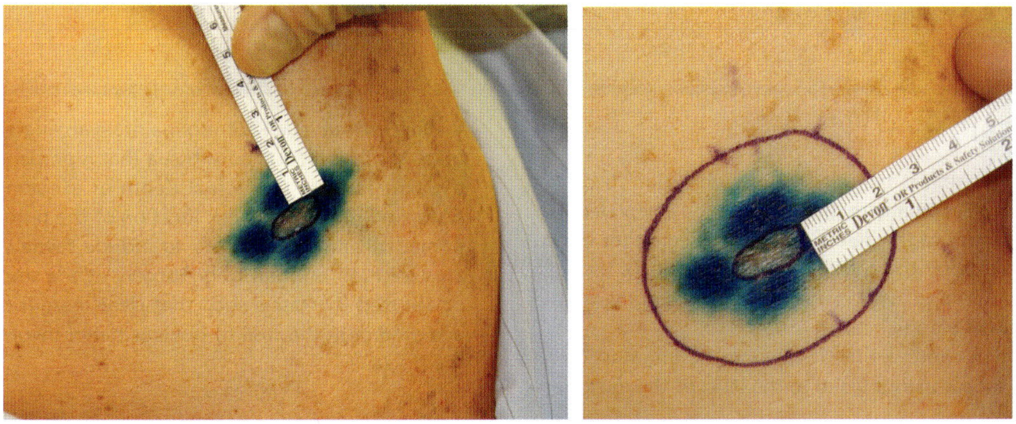

A B

FIG 4 ● **A,B.** In this example, the patient has already been injected with both Tc-99 sulfur colloid and isosulfan blue intradermally around the biopsy site for a lymphatic mapping and sentinel biopsy procedure at the time of wide excision in the same operative setting. The recommended margin of excision is based on primary tumor thickness and is measured from either the edge of the intact melanoma or biopsy scar, generally resulting in the proposed circular or oval defect marked on the skin.

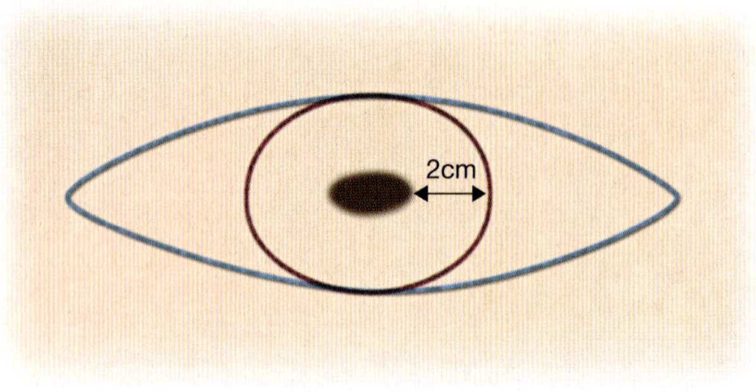

FIG 5 ● When a primary closure as planned, the circle or oval is generally fashioned into an ellipse prior to wide excision to improve cosmetic outcome and facilitate primary closure.

an ellipse prior to WE to improve cosmetic outcome and facilitate primary closure (FIG 5). Excision of an ellipse of tissue results in a more gradual transition in wound contour and minimizes "dog ears" at the poles of the incision.

- Creation of an ellipse three to four times as long as it is wide has often been recommended in textbooks; cosmetically acceptable closure can sometimes be achieved with a smaller ratio and should be individualized.
- Alternatively, tissue that may contribute to dog ears can be resected after the oncologic portion of the WE. Depending on the lines of tension of the skin, a modified ellipse such as lazy S or "hurricane"-type (FIG 6) incision may facilitate closure, generally as triangular-shaped segments of skin and underlying subcutaneous tissue.
- When feasible, the incision should be oriented to facilitate primary closure. On the extremities, for example, the WE incision is usually oriented parallel to the long axis of the limb. This facilitates primary closure, results in greater excision of lymphatics that are at risk for melanoma tumor cell emboli, and may decrease subsequent lymphedema.
- Breast—Primary cutaneous melanoma of the skin of the breast should be managed with similar principles as cutaneous melanoma elsewhere. A mastectomy is not required to achieve oncologic control.
- Hand, foot, and digits—General margin guidelines for cutaneous melanoma should be followed and consideration for preservation of function should be maximized. As a general principle, it is not usually necessary to remove bone to obtain oncologic control of the primary melanoma. However, amputation is usually necessary if standard WE for subungual or distal digit invasive cutaneous melanoma leaves insufficient soft tissue to maintain a functional digit without partial phalanx bony resection. Phalanx-preserving approaches can sometimes be employed for distal digit/subungual melanoma in situ.
- Perianal skin melanomas should be treated as cutaneous melanomas.

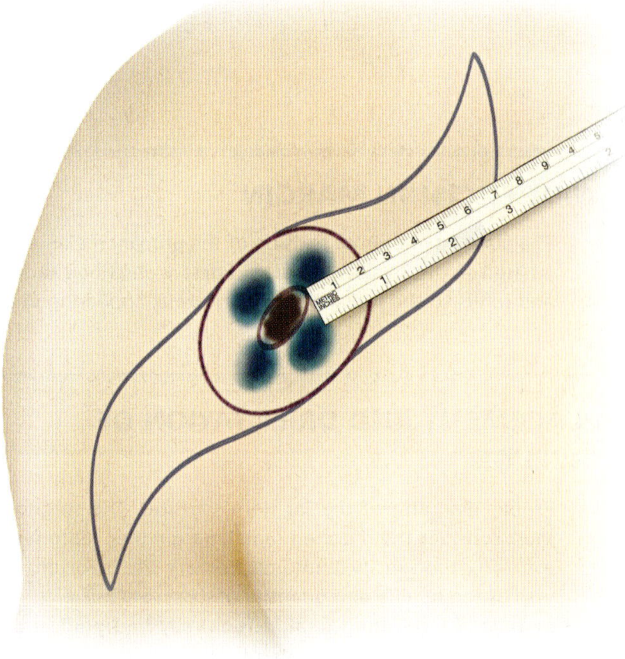

FIG 6 ● Depending on the lines of tension of the skin, a modified ellipse such as lazy S or hurricane-type incision may facilitate closure.

SKIN INCISION

- The skin incision is typically made with a no. 10 or 15 blade scalpel, initially to the level of the deep dermis. The remainder of the dermis can be divided either using the electrocautery on cutting mode or by using a scalpel. Care is required to avoid cautery to the skin edges, as this may result in wound healing issues.
- The excision continues by deepening the initial incision into the subcutaneous tissue to the level of the muscular fascia; care must be taken to maintain an angle of attack through the subcutaneous tissue that is perpendicular to the skin surface. The actual depth of excision will vary according to the anatomic location of the primary melanoma. It is rarely necessary to include fascia with WE[5]; an exception is when prior surgery at the site included or abutted the fascia such that clear margin cannot be achieved or in the case of obvious tumor involvement at the fascia.

EXCISION OF SPECIMEN

- Once the depth of the resection has reached the underlying muscular fascia, the WE is completed by dissecting skin and soft tissue from the underlying fascia using the electrocautery (**FIG 7**).
- WE specimens are almost always submitted for permanent section analysis; intraoperative frozen section analysis is the exception. When reconstruction may be significantly impacted by an involved margin, "rush" permanent pathology (turnaround about 24 to 48 hours) may be coordinated with the pathology team (see also "Delayed Wound Closure" later in this chapter).
- It is important to properly orient the specimen in the event that final margins are involved and an additional resection (usually as a separate operative procedure) is required (**FIG 8**).

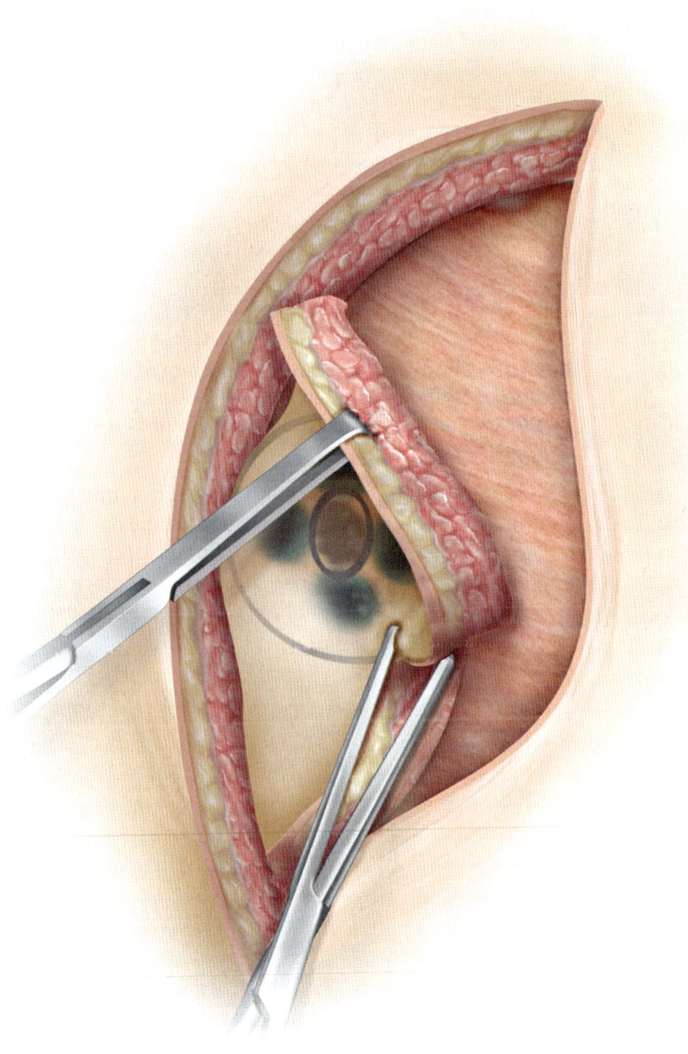

FIG 7 • The depth of wide excision down to the muscular fascia is demonstrated. Once this depth is reached, the skin and soft tissue is dissected off the underlying fascia, completing the wide excision.

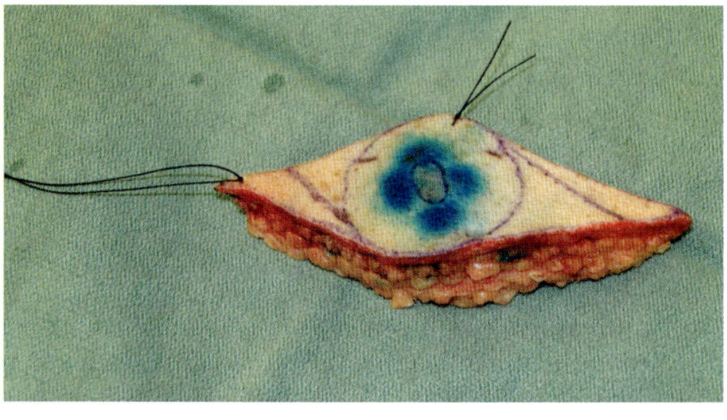

FIG 8 • The resected specimen is carefully oriented to ensure accurate margin assessment by the pathologist. It is also important to orient in such a fashion that re-excision of involved margins can be accurately mapped back to the patient.

CLOSURE

- The majority of 1-cm margin defects and many 2-cm margin defects can be closed primarily. Recruitment of adjacent tissue by fashioning local flaps often facilitates primary closure and is dependent on the primary tumor location, margin, and the laxity of adjacent skin. Surgical defects may often be closed by mobilizing tissue flaps that have been created by undermining in a suprafascial plane and include full-thickness skin and underlying subcutaneous fat (**FIG 9A,B**).
- Complex closure of a WE defect involves placement of one or two layers of deep absorbable sutures (**FIG 10**), followed by placement of an intradermal layer of a buried absorbable suture. Skin closure can be carried out using a number of techniques, depending on the tissue tension, anatomic location, mobility, and surgeon preference. A subcuticular skin closure may be performed using an absorbable monofilament suture or a nonabsorbable pull-through suture that requires removal. Interrupted or running nonabsorbable sutures and skin staples may also be used as per surgeon preference (**FIG 11**). Dermal adhesives or adhesive bands may be used to directly cover the skin.

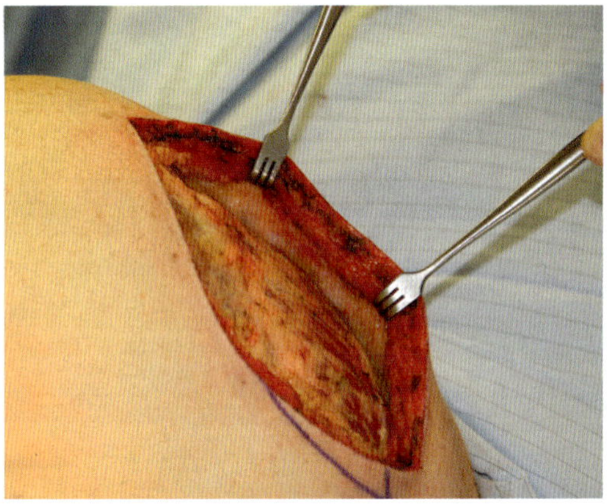

A

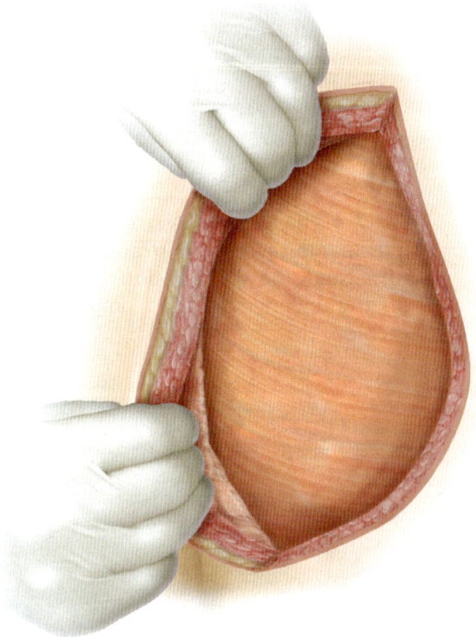

B

FIG 9 • Photo **(A)** and illustration **(B)** demonstrating the mobilization of tissue flaps by undermining the full thickness of skin and subcutaneous fat at a level just superficial to the muscular fascia.

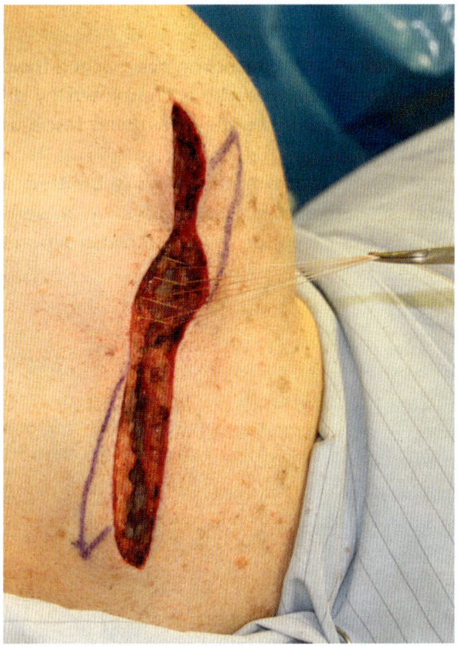

FIG 10 • Photo demonstrating placement of deep absorbable sutures to facilitate complex primary closure of a WE. Typically one or two layers of deep absorbable sutures are used.

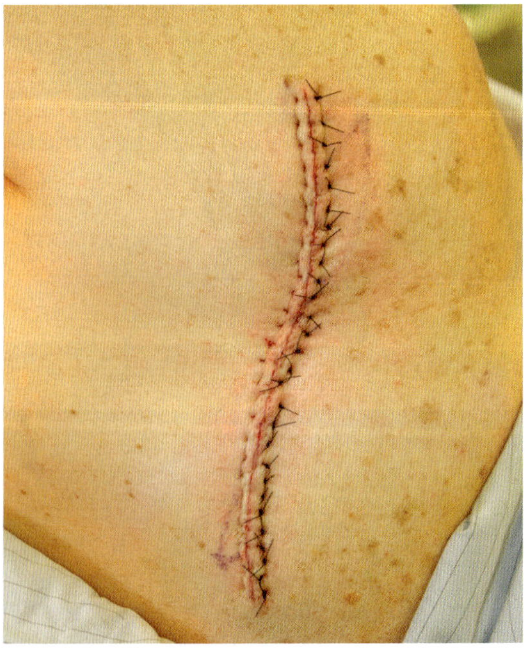

FIG 11 • After reapproximation of deep layer(s), the skin may be closed using a number of different techniques and sutures depending on location, tension, and surgeon preference. In this photograph, interrupted vertical mattress sutures were used.

- At the discretion of the surgeon, closed suction drainage may be used when extensive undermining or large flaps are necessary or when considerable dead space persists after layered closure. If a drain is used, the exit site should be placed in line with the incision so that any potential recurrence can be reexcised without jeopardizing subsequent wound closure. Alternatively, suture plication of the more superficial tissue to the underlying fascia may sometimes be used and obviate the need for drainage, even when larger flaps are used.

RECONSTRUCTION

- When primary closure is not feasible, consideration should be given to skin grafts or local tissue flaps. The advantage of a skin graft is that it is a relatively straightforward procedure that minimizes adjacent tissue manipulation, allows for easy long-term monitoring of the primary melanoma site, and does not disrupt lymphatic drainage pathways. Skin grafts, however, are insensate, provide little protection to underlying tissue, and may result in a more pronounced contour defect. Furthermore, compared to local tissue flaps, skin grafts may result in more disfigurement and prolonged healing. Skin grafts are discussed in detail in Chapter 24.
- Typically, split-thickness skin grafts are harvested from the posterior or proximal lateral thigh. Of note, when a lower extremity melanoma requires a skin graft closure, the graft should be harvested from the contralateral extremity.
- Full-thickness skin grafts can be harvested from multiple locations, allowing for better skin color and texture matching to skin adjacent to the melanoma excision. Full-thickness skin grafts may be harvested from the inguinal groin crease, the lower neck region overlying the clavicle, or behind the ear. After an appropriately sized ellipse of skin is excised down into the subcutaneous fat, the donor site is primarily closed, resulting in less morbidity than the typical split-thickness skin graft donor site. The full-thickness harvested skin is de-fatted and prepared as a skin graft.
- The decision to proceed with a local tissue or rotational flap should be made after careful consideration of the features of the local tumor, including risk of satellite or in-transit metastases, the potential benefit to the patient from the functional and cosmetic perspective, the comorbidities of the patient, and the local tissue options available. The advantages of local flaps include durable, sensate, similar thickness, and textured skin. Disadvantages include rearrangement of regional soft tissue at risk for in-transit/satellite metastatic disease. Advancement and rotational flaps are discussed in detail in Chapter 23.

DELAYED WOUND CLOSURE

- The majority of WE defects are closed or reconstructed during the same operation as the WE. There are circumstances, however, when delayed reconstruction is the most appropriate course of action. These situations may include delaying reconstruction in the setting of large diameter or poorly defined melanomas where margins are clinically equivocal at time of WE. Unlike its common use for assessment of margins for nonmelanoma skin cancer, intraoperative frozen section margin assessment is infrequently employed for intraoperative margin assessment of melanoma WE.
- Delayed reconstruction may also be beneficial when time is needed for a granulation bed to form in order to facilitate grafting, such as after excision of a heel melanoma where skin grafting onto a granulating bed is often performed in such a fashion (**FIG 12**).
- When wound closure is delayed, options for wound coverage include temporary wound dressings with routine dressing changes or a vacuum-assisted sponge dressing device (e.g., vacuum-assisted closure [VAC] device). VAC devices are sometimes not available until negative margins are confirmed.
- In some situations, a request for rush permanent pathology of the WE specimen may be coordinated in advance with the pathology team, thus facilitating advance surgical planning (often at 48 hours postoperative) both in terms of operating room space and collaboration with the reconstructive team. In such cases, a temporary occlusive dressing is often used to protect the WE site until final margins are available.

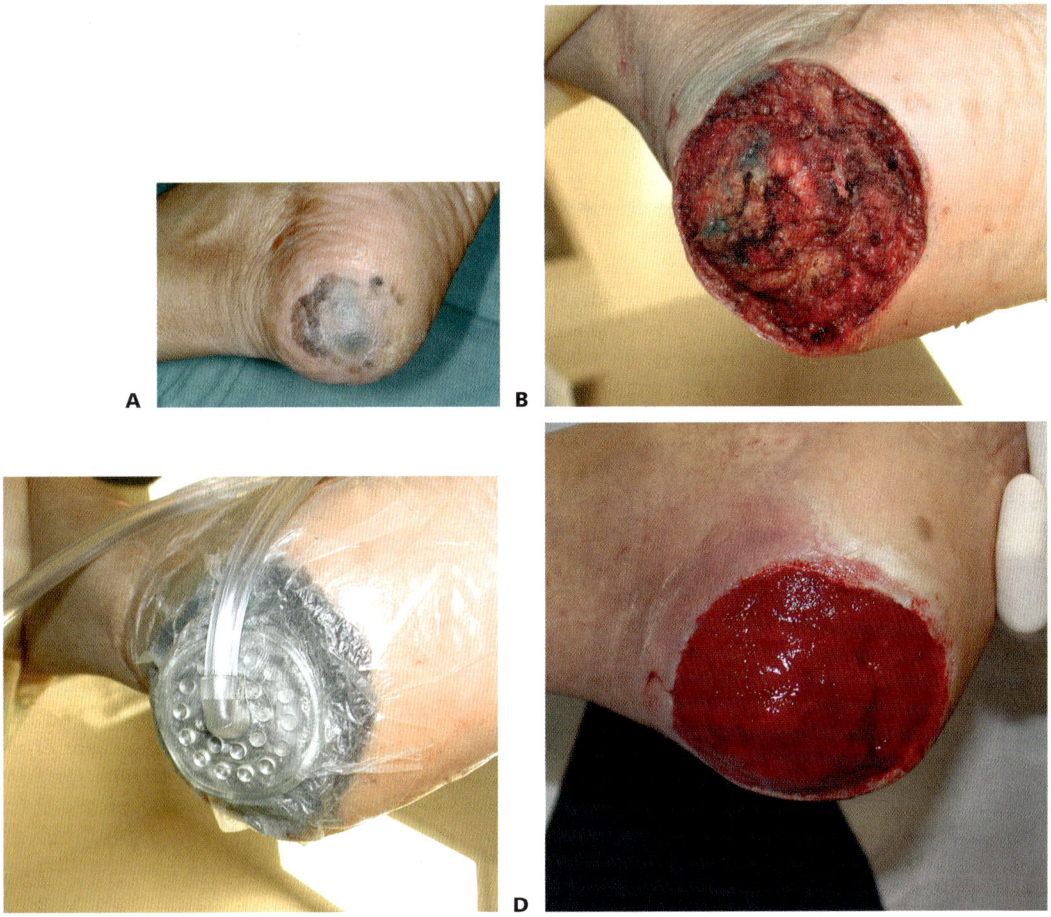

FIG 12 ● Photographs demonstrating use of delayed reconstruction for a large heel melanoma **(A)**. Upon completion of the WE **(B)**, a vacuum-assisted sponge dressing device is placed intraoperatively **(C)**. The recipient granulation bed, shown here after use of a vacuum-assisted device for approximately 3 weeks, is now optimized for skin grafting **(D)**.

PEARLS AND PITFALLS

Preoperative strategies	■ Orientation of biopsy is important whenever performed. ■ Healing of biopsy—Photo document biopsy site for later site confirmation whenever it may be possible that site will be healed prior to definitive WE. ■ Complete history and physical essential to identify additional suspicious primary lesions as well as potential sites of in-transit metastasis, satellites, and clinical nodal disease.
Operative positioning	■ Pad all pressure points. ■ Include potential interval and/or in-transit drainage sites within operative field if SNB is to be performed. ■ Do not harvest skin grafts from in-transit region (i.e., between primary tumor and draining nodal basin); as a practical approach, it is generally not prudent to harvest skin grafts from ipsilateral extremity.
Placement of incision	■ Extremities—Incision is generally oriented parallel to the long axis of extremity. ■ Always consider reconstructive options when placing and planning incision for WE. ■ Use radial margins appropriate for tumor thickness. ■ Be aware of superficial (subcutaneous) motor nerves (e.g., superficial peroneal and portion of spinal accessory)
Intraoperative considerations	■ Excision should be performed to, but not include, level of the underlying muscular fascia, unless the fascia itself is involved with tumor or the prior biopsy procedure. ■ Maintain perpendicular orientation through subcutaneous tissue. ■ Frozen section margin analysis is rarely employed. ■ Proper orientation of WE specimen is essential to facilitate reexcision of involved margins when necessary.
Closure	■ Consider overall risks of locoregional and other metastases with any extensive reconstruction option employed. ■ Consider closing dead space where appropriate to reduce likelihood of seroma formation.

POSTOPERATIVE CARE

- Specific postoperative care is dependent on the type of closure, the use of absorbable or permanent suture material, the extent of tension on the wound, and the presence or absence of a drain.
- In general, the patient can shower in 24 to 48 hours unless skin grafts are used.
- Drains (if used) usually stay in place until collected volumes remain 30 mL or less for 2 consecutive days.
- Specific restrictions may apply depending on anatomic location (e.g., restrictions on weight bearing for melanomas on the plantar surface of foot) and type of closure (e.g., skin graft).
- Progressive increase in activity, weight bearing, or lifting over a 4- to 6-week period

OUTCOMES

- After an appropriate WE based on tumor thickness, true local melanoma recurrences are uncommon and likely represent lymphatic tumor emboli. Some "local recurrences" are a result of an incompletely or inadequately excised primary melanoma.
- Functional outcome is critical and early use of physical therapy is encouraged when appropriate.

COMPLICATIONS

- Infection (cellulitis or abscess)
- Seroma
- Hematoma/ bleeding
- Wound dehiscence or separation
- Failure of take of skin graft or flap
- Poor functional or cosmetic outcome
- Numbness and/or hyperesthesia and/or pain
- Edema/lymphedema

REFERENCES

1. Gershenwald JE, Ross MI. Sentinel-lymph-node biopsy for cutaneous melanoma. *N Engl J Med.* 2011;364:1738–1745.
2. Sabel MS, Wong SL. Review of evidence-based support for pretreatment imaging in melanoma. *J Natl Compr Canc Netw.* 2009;7(3):281–289.
3. Buzaid AC, Sandler AB, Mani S, et al. Role of computed tomography in the staging of primary melanoma. *J Clin Oncol.* 1993;11:638–643.
4. Aloia TA, Gershenwald JE, Andtbacka RH, et al. Utility of computed tomography and magnetic resonance imaging staging before completion lymphadenectomy in patients with sentinel lymph node-positive melanoma. *J Clin Oncol.* 2006;24:2858–2865.
5. NCCN clinical practice guidelines: melanoma. http://www.nccn.org/professionals/physician_gls/pdf/melanoma/pdf Accessioned 08/08/2014
6. Balch CM, Gershenwald JE, Soong SJ, et al. Final version of 2009 AJCC melanoma staging and classification. *J Clin Oncol.* 2009;27(36):6199–6206.

Chapter 23 Advancement and Rotational Flaps

Jeffrey H. Kozlow

DEFINITION

- Advancement and rotational flaps are tissue transfer techniques used in reconstructive surgery for the closure of acquired defects.
- A flap is an area of tissue designed for movement to another area while remaining vascularized. This is in contrast to a graft, which is transferred in a nonvascularized fashion and becomes revascularized only with local incorporation and vascular neogenesis.
- Advancement and rotation flaps are both considered local flaps because they borrow from the tissue adjacent to the defect. Distant flaps use tissue from areas away from the defect, and free flaps involve the transfer of tissue from a distant site by means of a microsurgical anastomosis.
- Local flaps can be defined by their vascularity. Random flaps are based on blood flow through the subdermal plexus to provide vascularity to the distal end of the flap (**FIG 1**). Axial flaps are based on a longitudinal blood vessel incorporated into the flap design that can extend the effective length of a flap (**FIG 2**). Perforator flaps are based on underlying septocutaneous or musculocutaneous perforators into the central area of the flap (**FIG 3**).
- Local flaps can also be defined by the geometry of the incisions used with example of common designs shown in the following text.
- Flap design includes evaluation of tissue laxity, optimization of scar position, and management of standing cutaneous deformities.

PATIENT HISTORY AND PHYSICAL FINDINGS

- The choice and design of local flaps is dependent on multiple factors including the region on the body for reconstruction, local and regional soft tissue laxity, relationships with underlying critical anatomy, relaxed lines of skin tension for scarring, and underlying flap vascularity.
- Poor quality of tissue adjacent to the defect may preclude the use of local flaps.
- Local radiation damage will often limit the pliability of tissues for transfer and inhibit the healing potential of tissue.
- Each patient is different and flap choice must be tailored to the individual, the size of the defect, and the location of the defect.
- There are often multiple different flaps that will adequately reconstruct a defect; there is no "one right answer" for any given case.
- Flap design should also consider potential oncologic implications including the need for recurrence monitoring, secondary reconstruction techniques, and margin management when reconstruction is done immediately after resection and margin status cannot be confirmed.
- For patients with lower extremity defects, an evaluation of arterial status and venous insufficiency should be considered.

IMAGING AND OTHER DIAGNOSTIC STUDIES

- In general, local flaps do not require preoperative imaging or diagnostic studies.
- Doppler can be used to identify either axial or perforating blood vessels if clinically indicated.

SURGICAL MANAGEMENT

Preoperative Planning

- A reconstructive plan can only be made after the resection is designed. In cases that may require a plastic and reconstructive surgeon for advanced reconstructive techniques, it is always best to plan accordingly ahead of time and not consult intraoperatively.

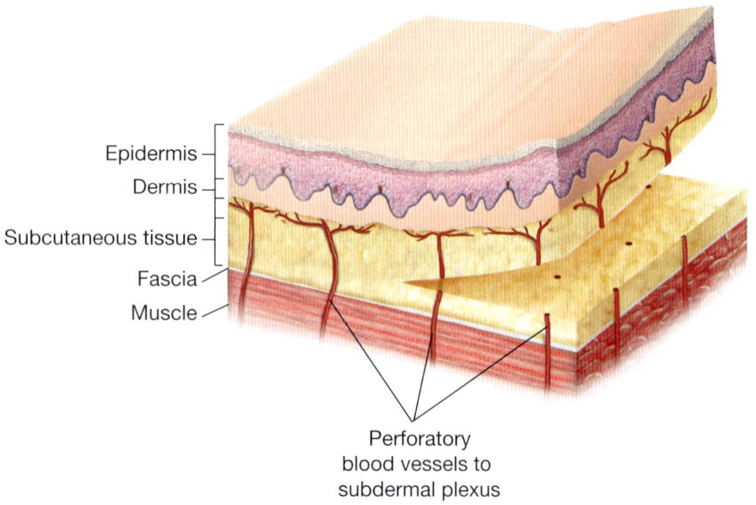

FIG 1 • Demonstration of a "random" pattern flap based on the subdermal plexus—The distal aspect of the flap remains vascularized through the small vessels running underneath the dermis only. As the length of the flap increases, the blood flow through the subdermal plexus decreases.

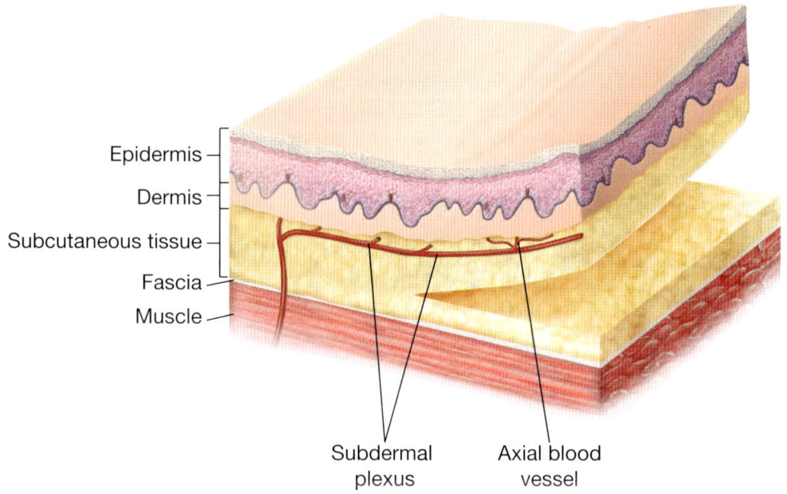

FIG 2 • Demonstration of an axial pattern flap—The flap design incorporates a named arterial supply along the length of the flap, which increases perfusion to the distal aspect of the flap compared to a random pattern flap.

- Preoperative markings may include important regional anatomic landmarks (such as facial rhytids) that may be obscured with the injection of local anesthetic intraoperatively.

Positioning

- Patients should be positioned to optimize not only surgical access for tumor resection but also for access to any local areas potentially usable for the subsequent reconstruction.
- All areas should be prepped widely to allow for access to all local and regional flap option. All extremities should be prepped and draped circumferentially. For areas where symmetry is important (such as the face or breasts), it is important to have the contralateral side in the operative field as well.

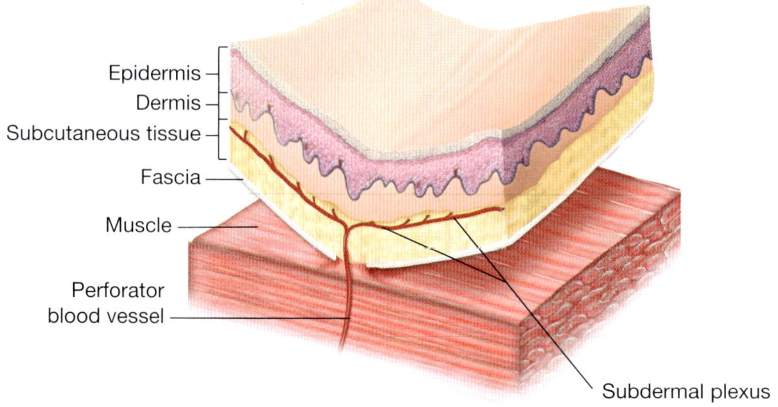

FIG 3 • Demonstration of a perforator-based flap—The flap is centered around a single blood vessel, which perforates through the fascial layer from the underlying muscle or muscular septa to then supply the subdermal plexus.

- There are multiple local flaps that are available for use in reconstruction. Not all of them can be highlighted in this text; however, the most common flaps for general reconstruction are described in the following text. In some cases, multiple local flaps are required and techniques can be combined to achieve closure of the defect.
- In most flaps, the area is often infiltrated with local anesthesia including 1:100,000 to 1:200,000 parts epinephrine to help with hemostasis and minimize electrocautery injury to dermal edges. However, overinjection of local anesthesia can result in tissue edema that decreases flap mobility.
- Skin hooks are used on the margins of a flap for handling; the use of forceps is discouraged due to injury to the flap edges from overzealous pressure.
- Drains are typically not used unless flaps are large.
- Flaps designed around joints should be inset under the greatest tension of the joint to avoid postoperative dehiscence.

SIMPLE ADVANCEMENT FLAPS

Flap Design

- Based on either the subdermal plexus as a vascular supply from the base of the flap to the distal end or can include an axial vessel for additional length and degrees of freedom
- Incisions are designed in a parallel fashion equal to the dimensions of the defect (**FIGS 4A** and **5A**); choice of direction is based on local tissue laxity.
- Classic teaching is that a maximum 3:1 ratio of length to width can be used when the flap is based on the subdermal plexus.

Flap Elevation

- Incisions are made extending from the defect in a parallel fashion toward base of flap.
- Dissection is carried down to the depth of defect or deeper in order to match volumetric dimensions of reconstruction.
- The central portion of the flap is undermined either in the deep subcutaneous level or below the fascia, depending on flap design and reliance on subdermal only versus axial-based blood supply (**FIGS 4B** and **5B**).

Defect Closure

- Careful hemostasis is assured after flap elevation; hematomas under the flap can compromise vascularity and overall outcome.
- Once flap has adequate advancement to fill defect, closure often occurs from the base of the flap to help "push" the flap into the defect, which can help alleviate tension over the distal closure (**FIG 4C**).
- Standing cutaneous deformities can occur as the base is advanced. These areas can be resected with a scar perpendicular to the direction of the flap.
- Dermal closure is performed using an absorbable suture followed by either a subcuticular or simple external suture (**FIG 5C**).

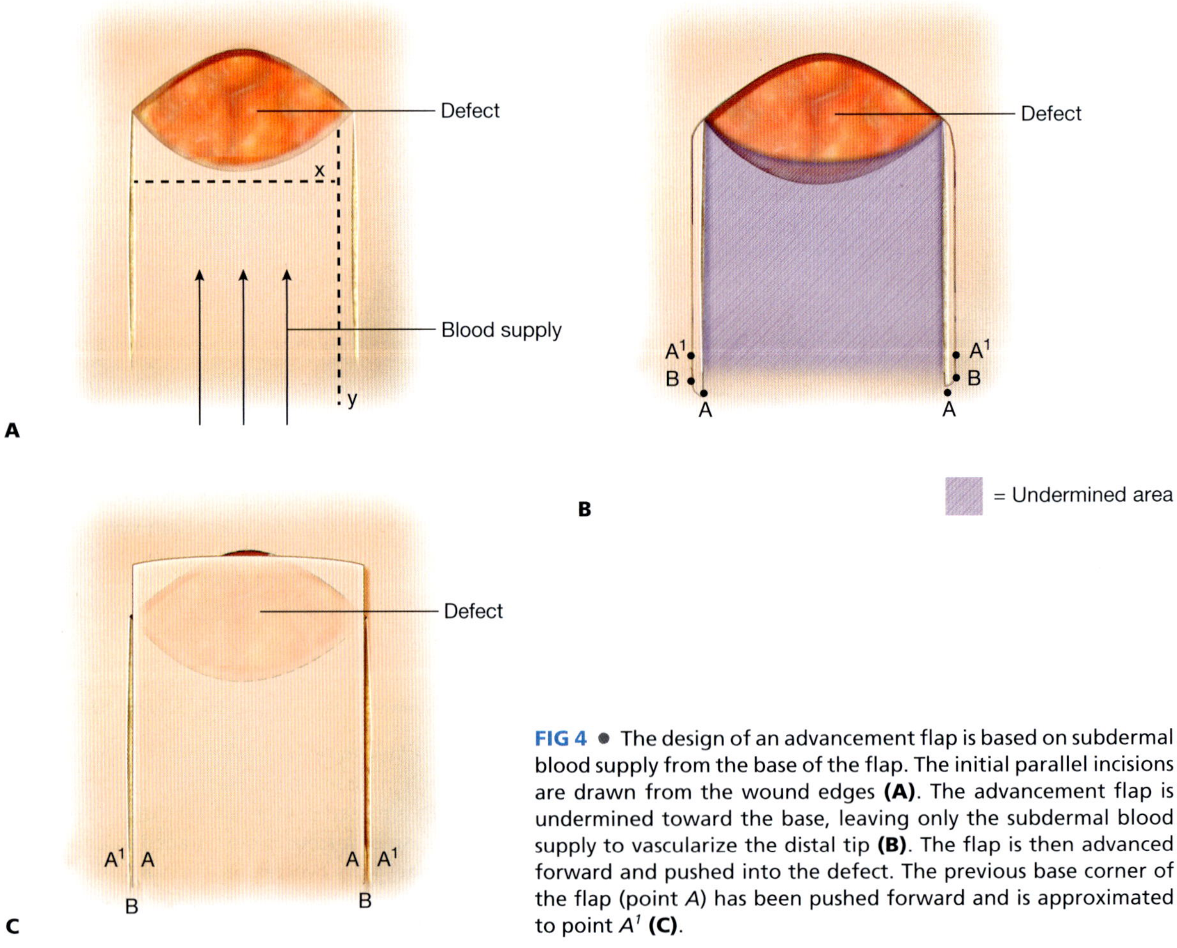

FIG 4 ● The design of an advancement flap is based on subdermal blood supply from the base of the flap. The initial parallel incisions are drawn from the wound edges **(A)**. The advancement flap is undermined toward the base, leaving only the subdermal blood supply to vascularize the distal tip **(B)**. The flap is then advanced forward and pushed into the defect. The previous base corner of the flap (point *A*) has been pushed forward and is approximated to point *A*[1] **(C)**.

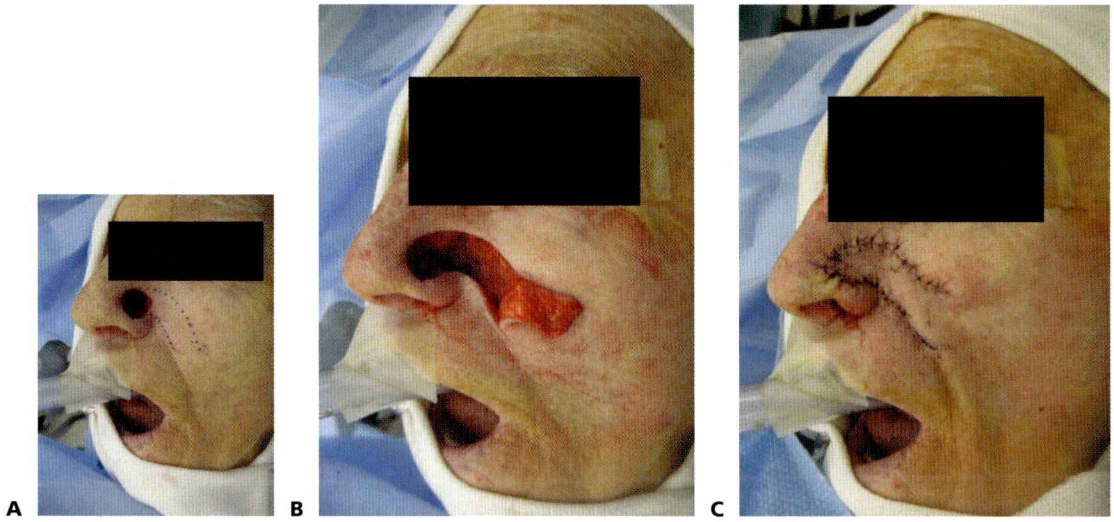

FIG 5 ● **A.** In this case, an axial-based advancement flap for nasal reconstruction is designed to incorporate the angular artery for additional length. This undermining is seen in **B** as the flap is fold back toward its base prior to advancement. The final advancement and closure of the advancement flap is demonstrated in **C**.

ROTATIONAL/TRANSPOSITION FLAPS

Flap Design

- Designed as a semicircle extending from one corner of the defect (FIGS 6A and 7A)
- Direction and orientation of flap is based on local areas of laxity.
- Based on a pivot point at "base" of flap that determines amount of rotation available

Flap Elevation

- Incision is made through skin and subcutaneous tissues to depth of defect or greater.
- Flap is undermined in same or deeper plan up to the base (FIG 6B).
- Careful hemostasis is assured in undermined area to avoid a hematoma that may compromise flap.

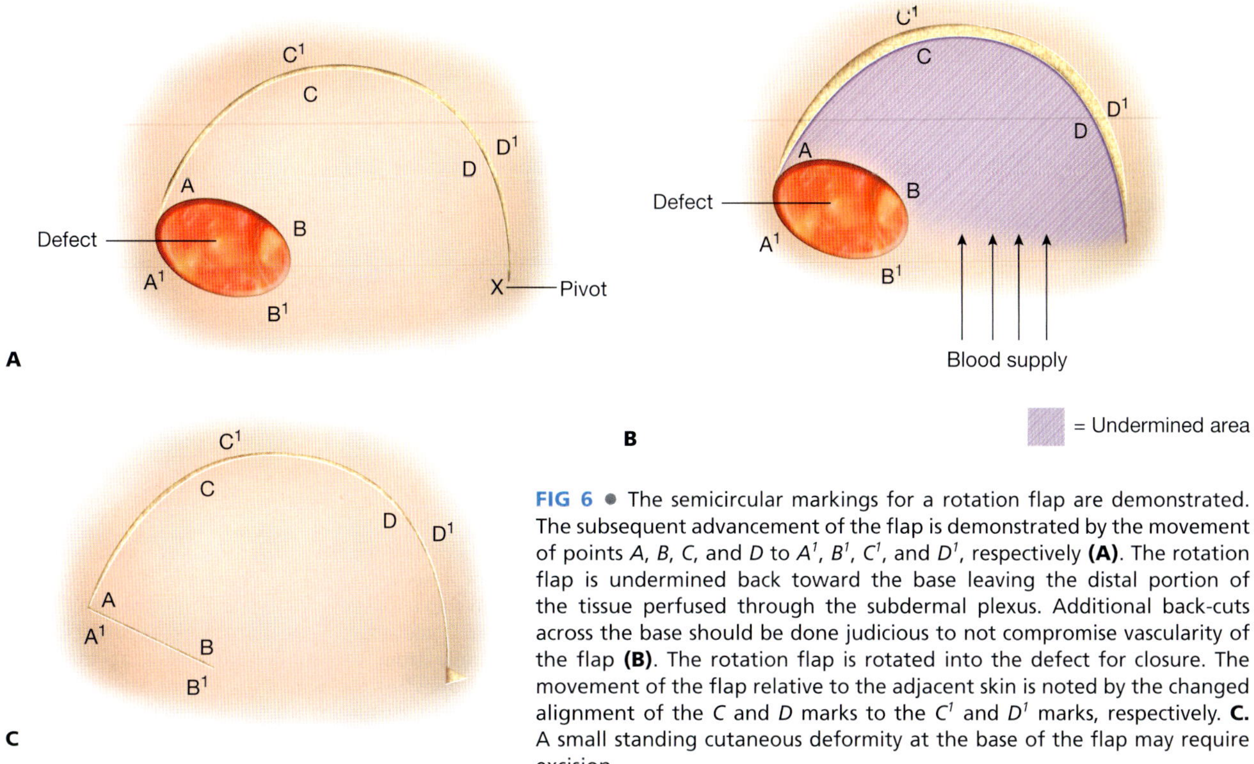

FIG 6 ● The semicircular markings for a rotation flap are demonstrated. The subsequent advancement of the flap is demonstrated by the movement of points *A*, *B*, *C*, and *D* to A^1, B^1, C^1, and D^1, respectively **(A)**. The rotation flap is undermined back toward the base leaving the distal portion of the tissue perfused through the subdermal plexus. Additional back-cuts across the base should be done judicious to not compromise vascularity of the flap **(B)**. The rotation flap is rotated into the defect for closure. The movement of the flap relative to the adjacent skin is noted by the changed alignment of the *C* and *D* marks to the C^1 and D^1 marks, respectively. **C.** A small standing cutaneous deformity at the base of the flap may require excision.

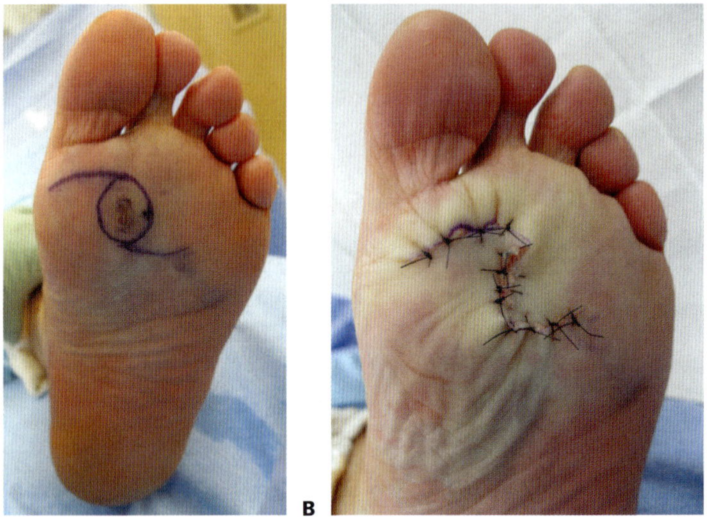

A B

FIG 7 • **A.** In this clinical case, opposing advancement flaps have been designed for reconstruction of a plantar foot wound. **B.** In this case, the opposing flaps have both been advanced to reconstruct the defect.

Defect Closure

- Flap is advanced and rotated into defect with closure often starting at base of defect to help push and rotate flap into defect (**FIG 6C**).
- Dermal closure is performed using an absorbable suture followed by either a subcuticular or simple external suture (**FIG 7B**).
- Excision of standing cutaneous deformities should be away from the base of the flap to avoid decreasing flap vascularity.

Additional Designs

- Multiple variations in flap design are commonly used but based on the same principle as earlier. For example
  - A bilobed flap uses two adjacent rotation/transposition flaps. The flap directly adjacent to the defect is used to close the primary defect and the other flap is then used to close the donor site for the first flap (**FIG 8A–C**).
  - A rhomboid flap is designed along the longer edge of a defect and transposes skin from an area of laxity to the defect, allowing for primary closure of the donor site (**FIG 9A–C**).

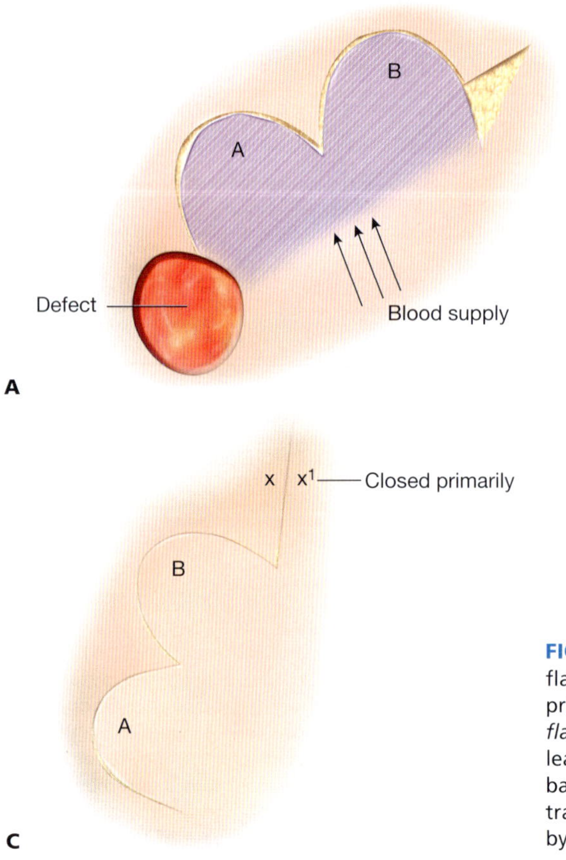

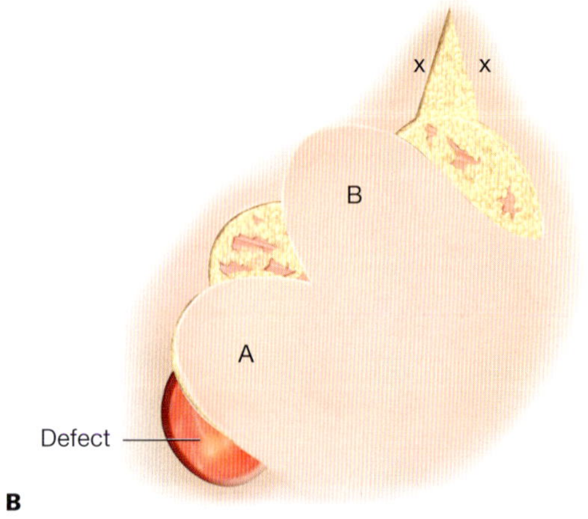

FIG 8 • The bilobed flap uses two rotation-transposition flaps for closure of a defect. **A.** *Flap A* is used to close the primary defect and *flap B* is used to close the donor site from *flap A*. **B.** The flap is elevated in the subcutaneous tissues leaving blood supply from the subdermal plexus at the base of the both "lobes" of the flap. **C.** The flaps are then transposed with primary closure of the donor site for *flap B* by reapproximation of *x* to *x*^{1}.

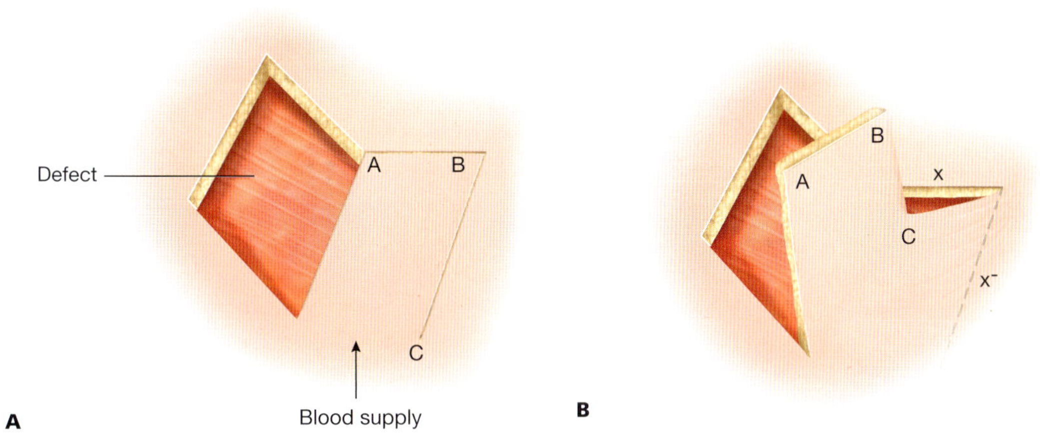

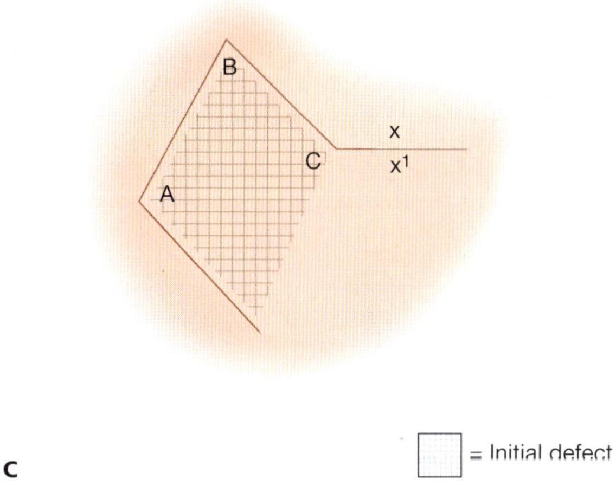

FIG 9 ● The rhomboid flap is another variation on the rotation-transposition flap and works well with elliptical- or rhomboid-shaped defects. The flap is designed off the "oblique" angle of the defect directly perpendicular to the defect. An additional incision designed parallel to the side of the defect is used to create a mirror image of the defect through the shared border of the flap and the defect **(A)**. The flap is then elevated in the subcutaneous tissues leaving blood supply from the subdermal plexus **(B)**. The flap is then rotated and transposed to fill the defect with the flap donor site closed primarily with approximation of *x* to x^{1} **(C)**.

V-Y ADVANCEMENT FLAP

Flap Design

- The vascularity of the V-Y advancement flap is based on the central perforating vessels.
- Orientation is designed on areas of local laxity and mobility.
- Incisions are designed from wide part of defect and then gently tapered into a triangle perpendicular to wound edge (**FIG 10A** and **FIG 11A**).
- Care is taken to design large enough flap to allow for some undermining at base of flap for additional advancement while still leaving enough central contact with deeper tissues for vascularity.

Flap Elevation

- Incisions are made through skin and subcutaneous tissues. Dissection through the subcutaneous tissues should be beveled away from the flap in order to increase the area for capture of underlying perforators into the central flap.
- The fascia can also be divided to allow for additional flap mobility.
- Can undermine the distal and proximal one-fourth of flap to allow for additional advancement but must *not* undermine centrally because this area is key to vascularity (**FIG 10B**). This is often done by spreading with a scissors vertically to preserve any potential blood vessels entering the flap.

Defect Closure

- Careful hemostasis is assured after flap elevation; hematomas under the flap can compromise vascularity and overall outcome.
- Closure starts at the "point" of the triangle where the donor site is closed primarily to form the vertical limb of the "Y." This also helps push the flap forward into the defect (**FIG 10C**).
- The flap is then pushed forward into the defect by closure of the sides of the triangle (**FIG 11B**).

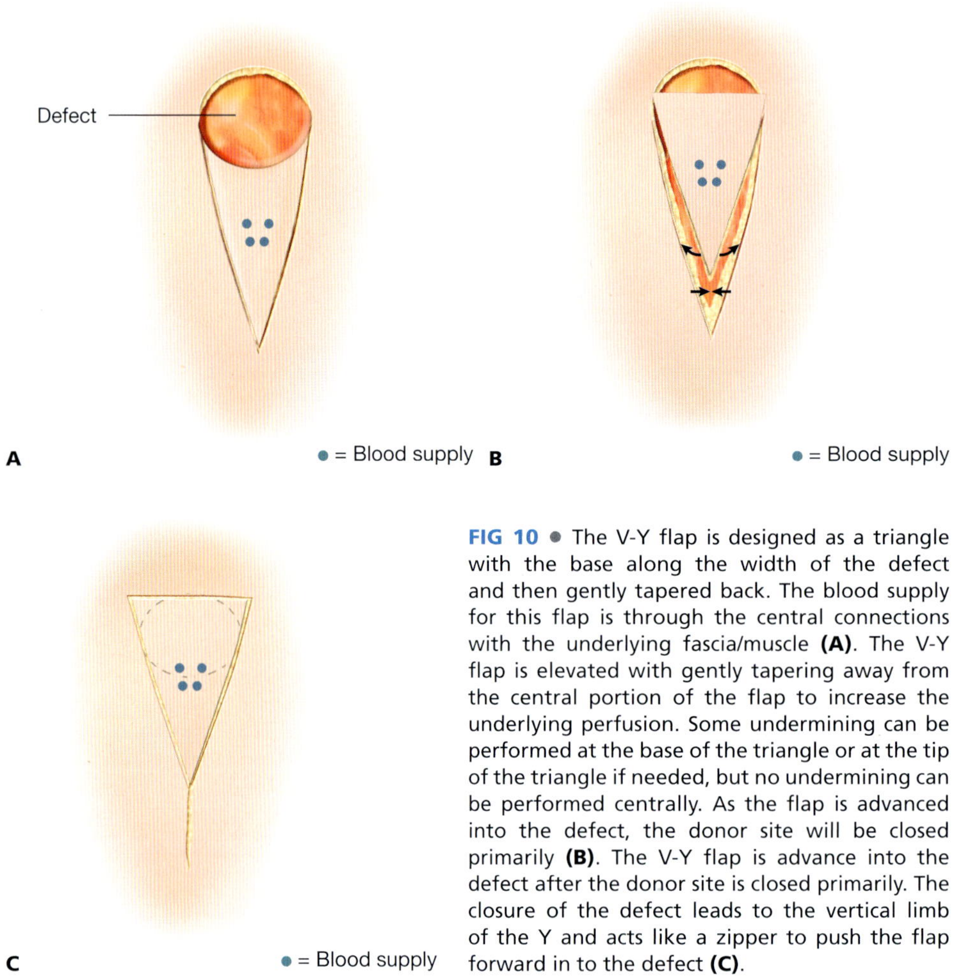

FIG 10 ● The V-Y flap is designed as a triangle with the base along the width of the defect and then gently tapered back. The blood supply for this flap is through the central connections with the underlying fascia/muscle **(A)**. The V-Y flap is elevated with gently tapering away from the central portion of the flap to increase the underlying perfusion. Some undermining can be performed at the base of the triangle or at the tip of the triangle if needed, but no undermining can be performed centrally. As the flap is advanced into the defect, the donor site will be closed primarily **(B)**. The V-Y flap is advance into the defect after the donor site is closed primarily. The closure of the defect leads to the vertical limb of the Y and acts like a zipper to push the flap forward in to the defect **(C)**.

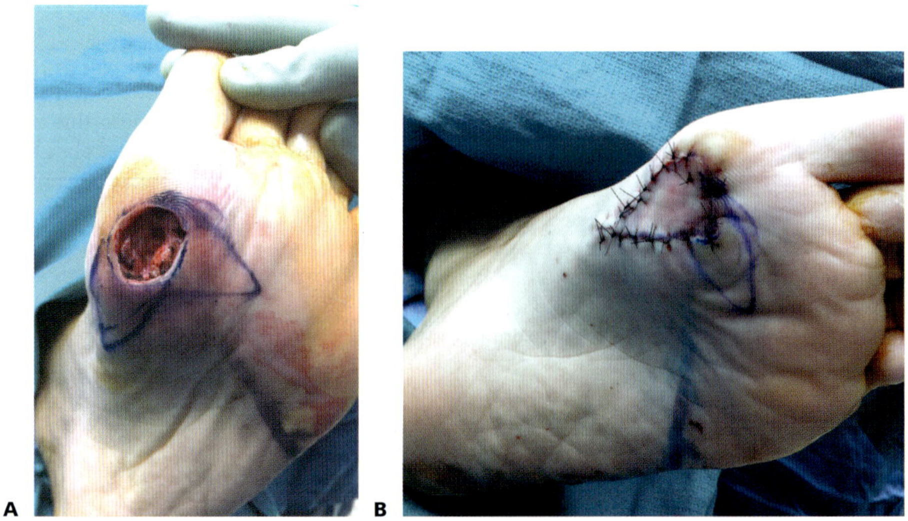

FIG 11 ● **A.** In this clinical case, two potential options for a V-Y flap have been designed with the decision to use the flap designed back toward the heel selected due to the relative laxity of that donor site compared to the flap running transversely across the plantar foot. **B.** In this case, the flap has been nicely advanced into the defect with the resultant Y closure demonstrated.

KEYSTONE FLAP

Flap Design

- Flap design is based on central perforators and use of "V-Y" closures to gain local tissue for advancement into the defect.
- A handheld Doppler can be used to identify specific large central perforators for preservation if additional mobilization is expected.
- The flap is most often designed from the longer border of a defect by first marking out the lateral borders of the flap at a 90-degree angle to the defect (**FIG 12A**).
- The flap width is then determined to be at least the width of the defect if not large. The flap is designed to remain this width along the entire length to each of the lateral borders (**FIGS 12B** and **13A**).

Flap Elevation

- Incisions are made through skin and subcutaneous tissues. This dissection is carried perpendicular to the skin with minimal beveling.
- The underlying fascia may also be divided for additional mobility and can be especially helpful in larger flaps.
- A small amount of subcutaneous or subfascial undermining can be performed, but this must be done judiciously unless large perforators have been knowingly included in the flap design.

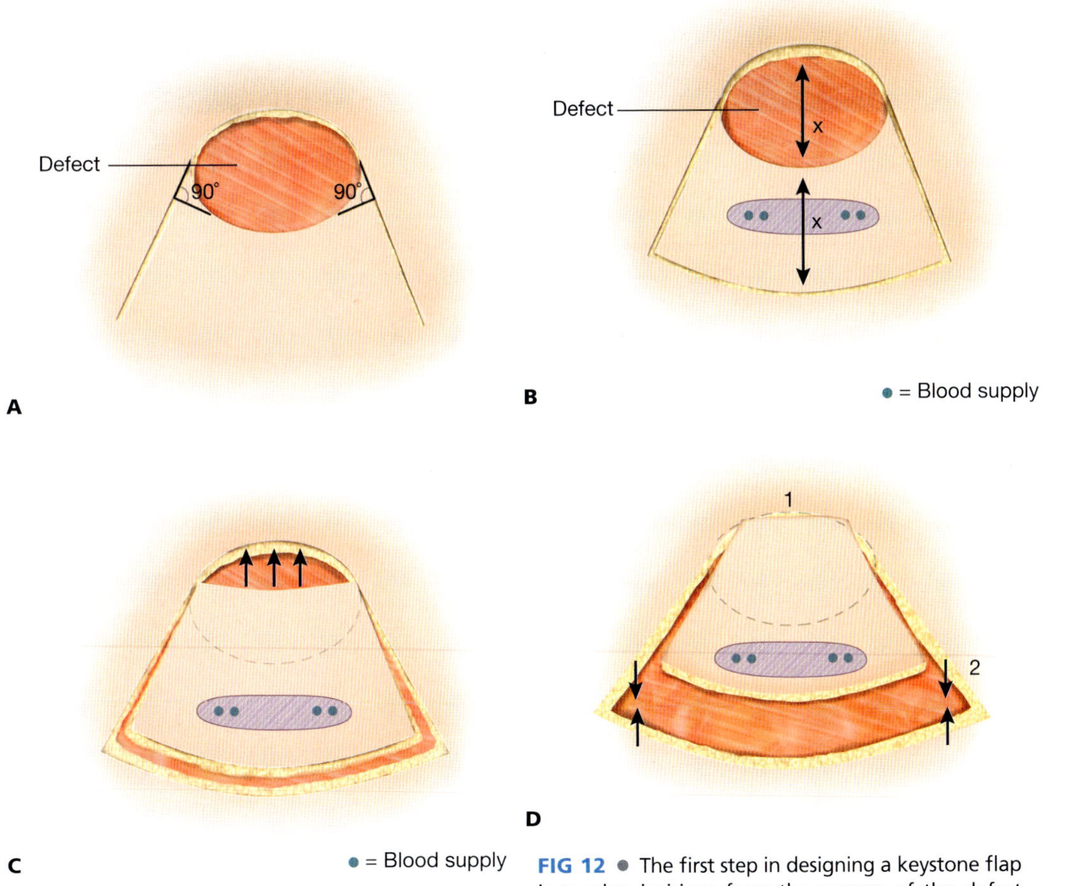

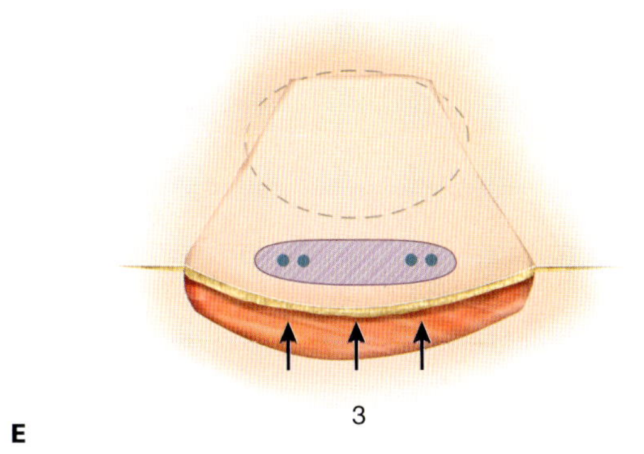

FIG 12 • The first step in designing a keystone flap is to plan incisions from the corners of the defect perpendicular to the defect **(A)**. Next, the flap is designed to be at least the width of the defect with the central blood supply from the underlying tissue providing the vascularity to the flap **(B)**. The flap is elevated by incising through the skin, subcutaneous tissues, and fascia. The flap is then advanced into the defect and closure occurs first in this area of maximal tension **(C)**. After the flap has been advanced into the defect, the corners of the donor site are closed in a V-Y fashion, which also help push the flap into the defect and transitions the flap into a rounder shape **(D)**. The incision along the flap border opposite the initial defect is then closed by advancing the adjacent skin flap, which is often undermined **(E)**.

Defect Closure

- The leading edge of flap is advanced into the defect with deep dermal sutures. In situations where this may be initially under significant tension, one can start away from this area and work from peripheral to central, helping push the flap toward the defect (**FIG 12C**).
- The defect tissue margin opposite the flap can also be undermined to provide some advancement. Alternatively, an opposing keystone flap may also be designed along this border to provide additional tissue laxity.
- The lateral ends of flap donor site are then closed in a V-Y fashion to help recruit additional tissue centrally as the flap transitions from a hemi-arc shape to an ellipse (**FIG 12D**).
- Finally, the trailing edge of the flap opposite the defect is sutured back the edge of the donor site. This may require undermining of adjacent skin flaps to ease the overall tension on the closure (**FIGS 12E** and **13B**)

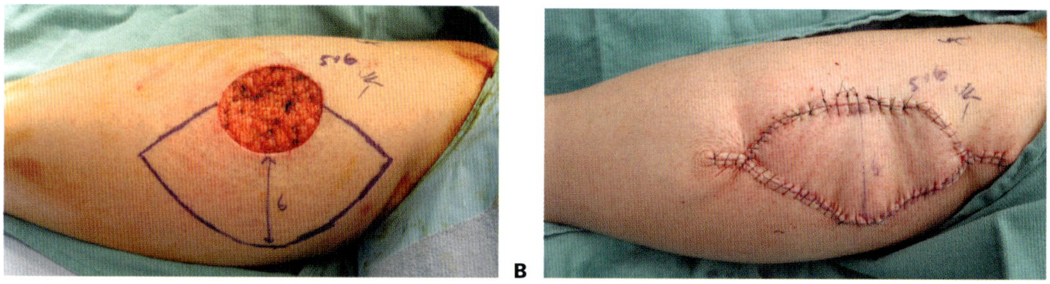

A B

FIG 13 ● In this case, a 6-cm wide flap has been designed to match the 6-cm width of the defect **(A)**. In this case, the flap has been advanced and reconstructed the defect. The corners of the flap donor site have been closed in a V-Y fashion and the flap shape has changed from a "keystone" or semi-arc shape to a more round shape **(B)**.

PEARLS AND PITFALLS

Flap selection	■ Flaps that are not undermined (e.g., keystone flaps) should be considered when margin status is unknown.
Flap design	■ Flaps should be large enough for readvancement if necessary.
Flap elevation	■ Care must be taken with perforator-based flaps to avoid central undermining because the subdermal plexus is transected circumferentially around the flap.
Defect closure	■ Care must be taken to avoid hematomas or infections, which can compromise a flap. ■ Postoperative immobilization should be considered for flaps around movable areas. ■ Excision of residual standing cutaneous deformities should be done judiciously to avoid compromise of flap vascularity and can be done at a later operative date if necessary.

POSTOPERATIVE CARE

- Flaps near joints should be immobilized with splinting to prevent mechanical dehiscence.
- Elevation for flaps on the extremities is critical for postoperative edema control.

COMPLICATIONS

- Marginal flap ischemia
- Delayed wound healing
- Infection (cellulitis or abscess)
- Hematoma
- Poor cosmetic outcome
- Flap failure/loss

OUTCOMES

- Outcome data for cutaneous reconstruction are quite heterogeneous due to the multiple body areas, flap techniques, and individual surgeon preferences.
- In general, the average incidence of a major complication is low but increases with the size of the defect and reconstruction. Minor complications include delayed wound healing, nonoperative infections, and need for secondary revision surgery.[1–3]
- The incidence of total flap failure is low when appropriate reconstructive principles are followed.

REFERENCES

1. Griffin GR, Weber S, Baker SR. Outcomes following V-Y advancement flap reconstruction of large upper lip defects. *Arch Facial Plast Surg*. 2012;14(3):193–197.
2. Coombs CJ, Ng S, Stewart DA. The use of V-Y advancement flaps for closure of pretibial skin defects after excision of cutaneous lesions. *Ann Plast Surg*. 2013;71(4):402–405.
3. Khouri JS, Egeland BM, Daily SD, et al. The keystone island flap: use in large defects of the trunk and extremities in soft-tissue reconstruction. *Plast Reconstr Surg*. 2011;127(3):1212–1221.

Chapter 24 Skin Grafts

David L. Brown

DEFINITION

- A graft, unlike a flap, does not bring an independent blood supply with its tissue to the recipient site. Skin grafts can be defined based on their origin: autograft (same individual), allograft/homograft (another individual of the same species), or xenograft (from another species).
- Skin grafts represent a rung on the proverbial reconstructive ladder above those of primary closure and healing by secondary intention and below local flaps (**FIG 1**).

PATIENT HISTORY AND PHYSICAL FINDINGS

- Skin grafting should only be considered once a viable recipient bed is obtained. This includes debridement of nonviable tissues, elimination of active infection, assurance of good vascularization to the wound bed, lack of significant fluid efflux from the wound (i.e., edema or bleeding), and coverage of vital structures (exposed bone, vessels, tendons, nerves, etc.).
- Indications include inability to perform primary closure or insufficient tissues for local skin flap coverage, uncertainty of tumor clearance, and comorbid conditions.
- Contraindications include active infection (i.e., bacterial counts $>10^5$ CFU/g via quantitative culture), poor vascularity of recipient bed (i.e., history of radiation to the area), and anticipation of further underlying reconstruction (i.e., nerve or tendon grafting).

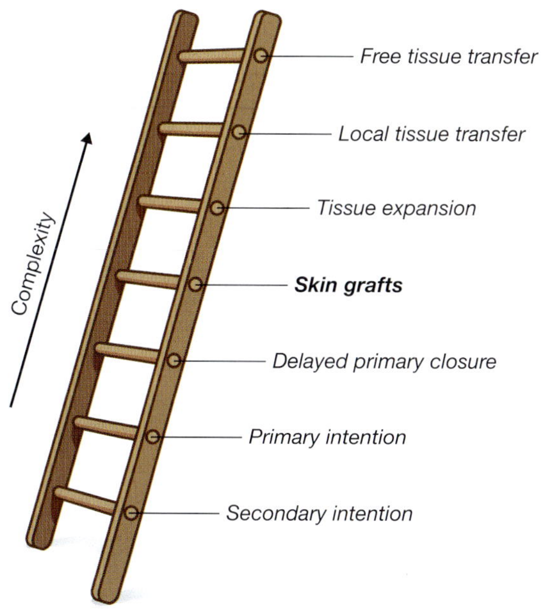

FIG 1 • The reconstructive ladder. Skin grafts occupy an intermediate position in the heirarchy of complexity of closure technique.

- Relative contraindications: comorbidities that can affect the healing of skin grafts such as diabetes, smoking, and venous insufficiency.

SURGICAL MANAGEMENT

Preoperative Planning

- Patients should be counseled regarding postoperative expectations, wound management, and restrictions so that they can make preparations prior to the operation.
  - Care of the donor site
    - Split-thickness grafts—Xeroform versus OpSite versus other coverings. May shower; more pain with Xeroform; watch for leaks and infection with OpSite
    - Full-thickness grafts—Steri-Strips. May shower; some bruising; minimal pain
  - Care of the graft site—bolster dressing. May shower if bolster is exposed, but do not let water run through the bolster continuous as this will wash out mineral oil (if used on cotton inside) and allow bolster to dry out over graft. Bolsters are usually taken down in 4 to 6 days, unless infection is suspected, then earlier.
- Choice of graft thickness
  - Split-thickness skin grafts (STSGs)
    - 12/1,000 inch is standard, with 6–16/1,000 inch being used for special situations.
    - Thinner grafts: more assured healing at the recipient site; the more dermis is left behind for subsequent harvest as necessary and the less primary contraction and greater secondary contraction.
    - Thicker grafts: more durable, as they carry more dermis with them.
    - "Sheet" (unmeshed) grafts have the advantage of better cosmesis but are encumbered by seroma or hematoma formation underneath, which can lead to local failure of the graft. These grafts should be inspected early at approximately 24 to 48 hours and any underlying fluid removed via aspiration. "Pie crusting" is unaesthetic and is not associated with higher graft survival.
    - Meshing of grafts can be performed with two advantages. One is coverage of greater recipient surface area with less donor graft. The ratios 1:2 or 1:1.5 are more commonly used, whereas 1:4 is typically reserved for extreme cases only. The larger the graft expansion, the more tenuous the coverage, and the more secondary contraction will occur. The second advantage is wound bed drainage and prevention of seroma or hematoma formation resulting in graft failure. A common method is meshing 1:1.5 but applying the graft to the recipient site in an unmeshed fashion.
  - Full-thickness skin grafts (FTSGs)
    - Primary contraction is greater (about 40%), but secondary contraction is less (about 15%), making them a good choice for joints, neck, eyelids, and so forth.

- Donor sites from FTSGs (usually straight-line layered closures) have the benefits of little postoperative pain and minimal scarring compared to STSGs.
- Choice of meshing versus sheet grafts
  - Meshing: allows for egress of wound fluids and lessens the risk of seroma and hematoma. As interstices must heal via secondary contraction and re-epithelialization, meshed grafts will contract more over time and be less durable. More wound area is able to be covered with less donor site.
  - Sheet grafts: prone to hematoma and seroma but are aesthetically more pleasing and exhibit less secondary contraction. Useful on hands and feet, across joints, and on the face and neck.

SPLIT-THICKNESS SKIN GRAFTS

Patient Positioning and Setup

- The patient is positioned either prone or supine, so that the lateral or anterolateral thigh is accessible for graft harvesting.
- The approximate donor site is marked out from several inches below the trochanter to several inches above the knee (smaller if less is needed).
- The donor site is injected with local anesthetic in the subdermal space, using a 22-gauge spinal needle. A mixture of 0.5% lidocaine with 1:200,000 concentration of epinephrine and 0.25% bupivacaine works nicely for providing both hemostasis and postoperative pain relief.
- Mineral oil is spread over the area to allow for smooth gliding of the dermatome over the skin (**FIG 2**).

Preparing the Dermatome

- The dermatome is assembled, and the appropriate width guard is attached (**FIG 3A**). A 3-in guard is appropriate for most applications and fits the contour of the thigh well in most adult patients.
- Proper seating of the blade in the machine and underneath the guard is assured; uneven seating can cause an excessively thin graft at one edge and overly thick at the other.
- The desired thickness of skin harvest is selected via the dial on the side (12/1,000 inch is shown here) (**FIG 3B**).

Harvesting the graft

- Either the surgeon (using his nondominant hand) or an assistant hold manual countertension on the skin (**FIG 4A**).
- The dermatome is pressed against the skin at a 45-degree angle and, with moderate down force, is slowly advanced the length of graft harvest (**FIG 4B,C**).

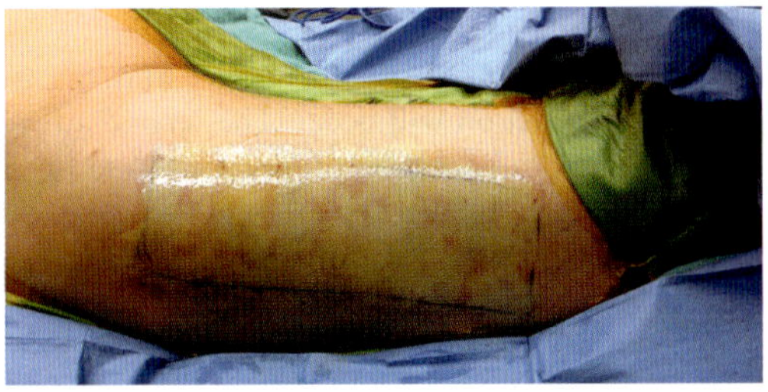

FIG 2 • Prone patient, with the lateral thigh showing from buttock crease (left) to knee (right). Note blanching of skin from epinephrine injection and glossiness of mineral oil application.

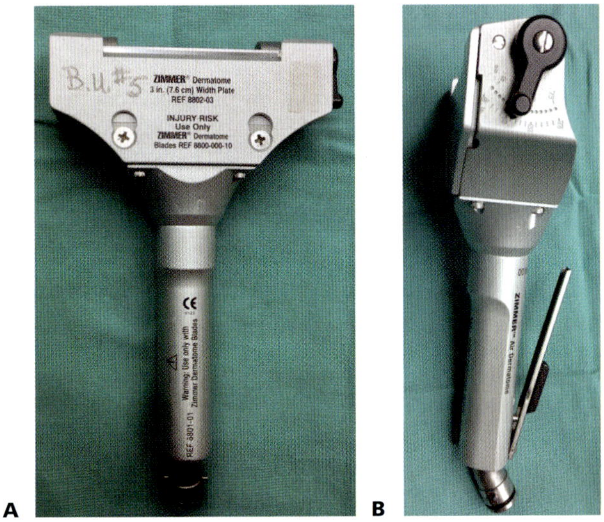

FIG 3 • **A.** Underside of dermatome, with blade and 3-in guard attached. Blade and guard are flush against machine, as assembled. **B.** Dermatome set to 12/1,000 inch thickness.

- To complete the harvest and separate the end of the graft from the patient, the surgeon lowers the handle of the dermatome toward the patient (decreasing the angle of attack) and slowly lifts off the skin surface (**FIG 4D**).

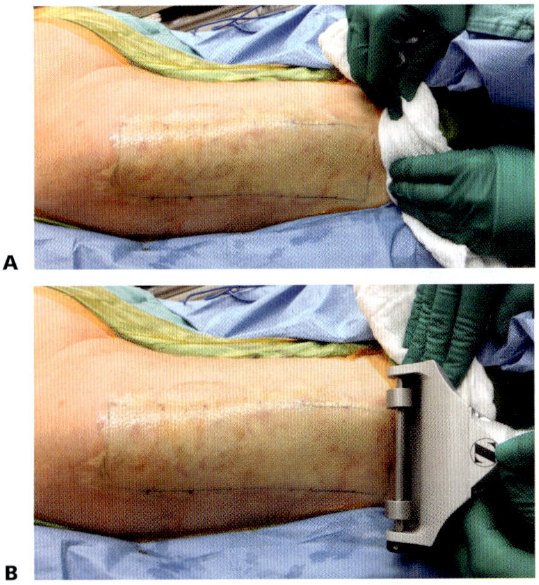

FIG 4 • **A.** Assistant holding countertraction on skin with the use of laparotomy sponge. **B.** Dermatome is placed on skin, running at a 45-degree angle. *(continued)*

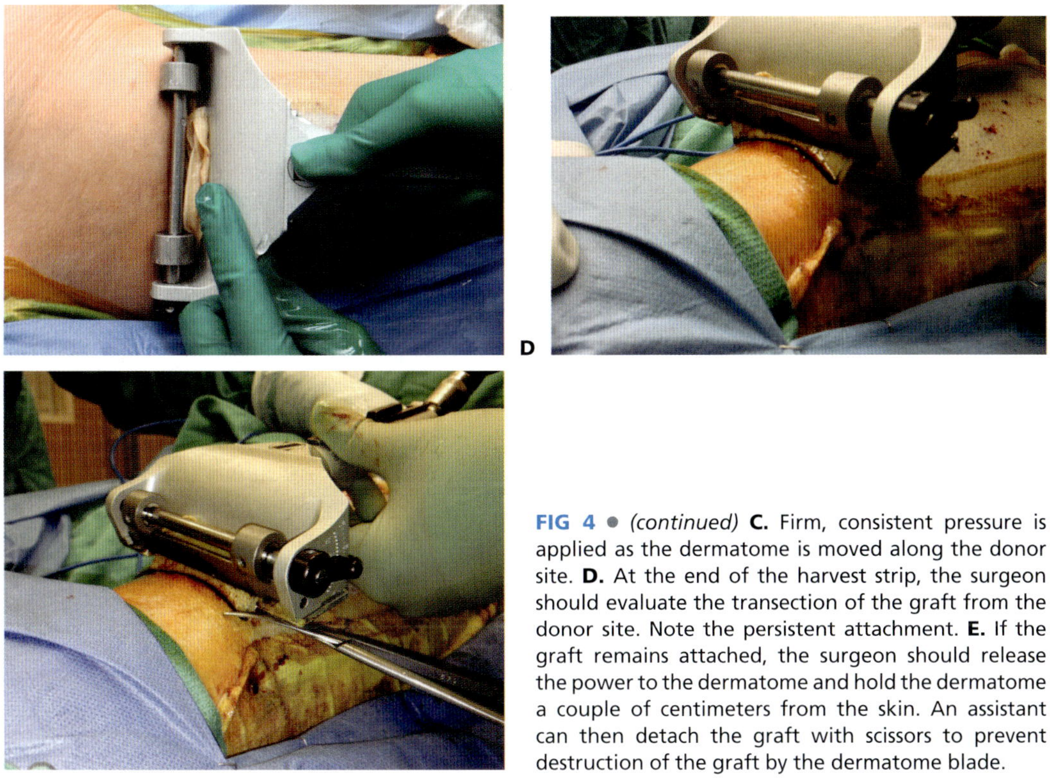

C D E

FIG 4 • *(continued)* **C.** Firm, consistent pressure is applied as the dermatome is moved along the donor site. **D.** At the end of the harvest strip, the surgeon should evaluate the transection of the graft from the donor site. Note the persistent attachment. **E.** If the graft remains attached, the surgeon should release the power to the dermatome and hold the dermatome a couple of centimeters from the skin. An assistant can then detach the graft with scissors to prevent destruction of the graft by the dermatome blade.

- Power is released on the dermatome when it rises 1 cm above the skin, in case the graft remains attached.
- If the graft is not immediately separated from the donor site at the end of the run with the dermatome, the surgeon should release power to the dermatome and hold it a couple of centimeters over the skin until an assistant can cut it free with a Metzenbaum scissor. Otherwise, the graft is pulled back out through the blade entrance and can result in mangling of the graft (FIG 4E).

Meshing the Skin Graft

- For meshed grafts, the mesher is assembled, and an appropriate cutting wheel is chosen. 1:1.5 (shown here, FIG 5A) is a standard ratio but can be varied up to 1:4 depending on the amount of donor sites available compared to the area needing coverage as well as the specific application.
- The graft is placed superficial side down on the carrier and run through the mesher (FIG 5B,C).

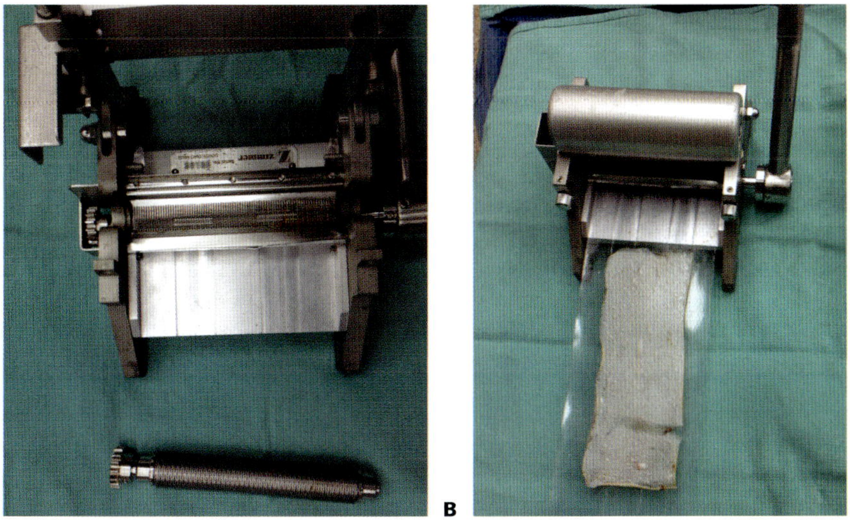

A B

FIG 5 • **A.** View of an opened mesher with space to place the chosen cutting wheel (in this case 1:1.5 ratio). **B.** Graft placed dermal side up on the carrier, which is positioned within the mesher entrance. *(continued)*

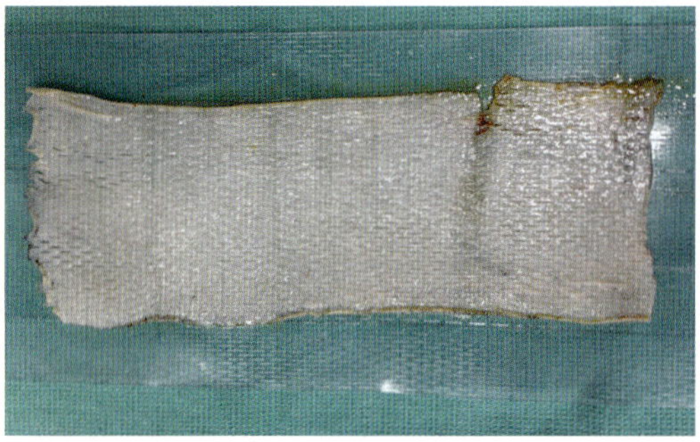

C

FIG 5 • *(continued)* **C.** Graft, postmeshing.

Insertion of the Graft into the Wound Site

- The graft is placed in the wound bed, trimmed appropriately, and secured to the wound edges with surgical clips or sutures (4-0 chromic work well) (**FIG 6A,B**).
- A nonstick dressing is applied. A bolster consisting of mineral oil– and saline-soaked cotton balls or batting will provide pressure on and moisture to the graft (**FIG 6C**). Trunk wounds can be covered with Allevyn (Smith and Nephew) foam, whereas tie-over's with interrupted silk are suitable for the face and hand, or wrapping with gauze and an elastic bandage for the extremities (**FIG 6D**).

Other Considerations

- Excess ("left over") skin graft can be preserved in tissue culture media at 4°C for application to the wound should original graft loss occur. Graft survival diminishes with storage time and is generally considered to be poor after 10 to 14 days.
- Some clinical situations call for delayed graft placement (24 to 48 hours postoperatively) due to wound fluid seepage. In cases such as coverage of muscle and omental flaps, or recently debrided wounds over edematous tissues, graft application can be performed at the bedside. This saves a return trip to the operating room (OR) for the patient.

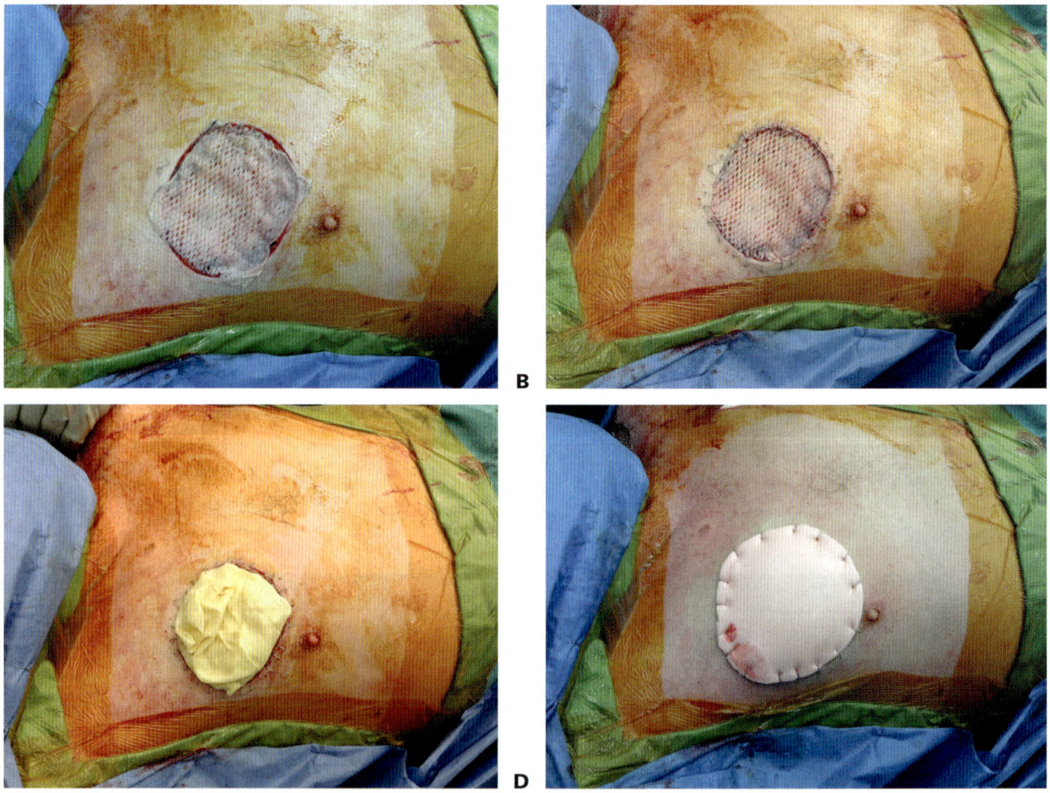

A B C D

FIG 6 • **A.** Patient with right superior chest wound. Meshed graft placed within wound, dermal side down, and minimally expanded. **B.** The graft is trimmed appropriately and secured with stainless steel clips. **C.** Mineral oil– and saline-soaked cotton batting, wrapped in Xeroform, is shaped to the size of the wound. **D.** A foam bolster is used to secure the dressing over the graft.

PEARLS AND PITFALLS

Harvesting the graft	▪ Proper seating of the blade in the machine underneath the guard should be assured; uneven seating can cause an excessively thin graft at one edge and an overly thick one at the other. ▪ If the graft is not immediately separated from the donor site at the end of the run with the dermatome, the surgeon should release power to the dermatome and hold it over the skin for an assistant to cut it free with a Metzenbaum scissor. Otherwise, the graft can be pulled back out through the blade entrance, mangling the graft. ▪ Rinsing the graft washes away vital procoagulant factors and should be avoided, if possible.
Placing the graft in the wound bed	▪ To assure consistent application of the graft to the wound bed dermis-side down and to transfer it without bunching, it should be placed on the carrier dermis side up. ▪ If the graft is not immediately needed for wound coverage, it can be stored on the back table (appropriately marked to avoid disposal), wrapped in moistened gauze, or left on the carrier and covered with the same. ▪ Care should be taken to avoid "tenting" a graft over an uneven wound bed. Extra graft should be placed to allow for complete contour touchdown. ▪ Placement of a meshed graft does not need to involve full expansion of the graft; leaving it relatively unexpanded will allow for egress of wound fluids while speeding healing. ▪ "Pie-crusting" of sheet (unmeshed) grafts is thought to be superfluous, as it will likely not prevent a hematoma or seroma from forming between slits and is aesthetically unappealing.
Donor site	▪ Some surgeons apply epinephrine-soaked sponges to the fresh donor site to limit bleeding. This is obviated with the use of local anesthetic.

POSTOPERATIVE CARE

Patient Expectations

- Patients should be told that the donor site is likely to cause more pain than the wound site postoperatively.
- Healing stages of the graft and donor site are discussed to educate the patient.
- Over large areas of grafting and/or uneven surfaces, some graft loss is to be expected.

Wound Management

- Dressings
  - Bolsters should be left in place, barring complications such as fever and so forth, for 5 to 8 days.
  - Patients may shower and get the bolsters wet with incidental water contact. Soaking or significant water rinsing of the bolster is discouraged, as this washes out the mineral oil and allows the bolster to dry out.
  - Following bolster removal, the graft is protected with once-daily dressing changes with petrolatum gauze until it is more fully healed (usually another 7 to 10 days). After this point, the patient should moisturize the graft (and donor site) twice daily for a few months to prevent desiccation, as oil and sweat glands are not transferred with the graft.
- Donor site care
  - Typically, split-thickness donor sites are covered with petrolatum gauze, which is loosely attached to the skin with surgical clips around the perimeter. An ABD pad and a gauze wrap are applied in the OR.
    - On postoperative day 1, the wrap and ABD are removed, and the attached gauze is left open to the air. It can get wet in the shower, but afterward, and several times per day, is dried with the use of a hair dryer set on cool air only.
    - Rewrapping with gauze is performed for the patient to get dressed. The attached petrolatum gauze will form an artificial "scab" on the wound, and re-epithelialization will cause the gauze to become nonadherent at its edges over the next 10 days or so. Trimming of the gauze so that it does not catch and get pulled off is recommended.
  - Other dressings are used for donor site care, each for a specific quality. Silver-impregnated dressings help to prevent infection. Occlusive dressings are significantly less painful but are plagued by infection.

Restrictions

- Judgment is exercised to determine the degree of immobilization prescribed, depending on graft location. It is not necessary to splint the foot for grafts on the lower leg, but patients should keep the extremity elevated to prevent swelling and edema and thus graft loss.

COMPLICATIONS

- Seroma and hematoma are the most common complications. If left untreated, they will lead to graft loss due to lack of contact with the wound surface.
- Infection can destroy a graft, particularly in the early postoperative period, prior to revascularization. In the case of unexplained postoperative fevers, the dressings should be removed early and the wound inspected for infection, which can be potentially treated, with graft salvage.
- Secondary contraction of skin grafts is increased with thinner grafts and with greater expansion of meshed grafts. This can affect underlying joint mobility and aesthetics.
- Incompletely debrided or poorly vascularized wound beds can lead to nonadherence and ultimate loss of the graft.

Chapter 25 Digit Amputations

Steven C. Haase

DEFINITION

- Digital amputation refers to the removal of a finger or thumb, most commonly at the level of the phalanges or interphalangeal joints (**FIG 1**). More proximal amputations that include a significant portion of the metacarpal are referred to as ray amputations. The techniques found in this chapter have been described chiefly for the hand, although similar procedures can be used on the foot in many cases.
- Digital or ray amputation may be indicated for subungual melanoma, or for other large, invasive melanomas of the finger or thumb.

PATIENT HISTORY AND PHYSICAL FINDINGS

- It is important to assess how long the lesion has been present; how fast it has grown; and whether there has been any history of ulceration, bleeding, or pain. Lesions exhibiting rapid growth in addition to these other findings may require more aggressive treatment.
- A patient's age, handedness, occupation, and hobbies should be considered carefully in planning an operation that might significantly affect their function. In some cases, preoperative consultation with a physiatrist and/or occupational therapist may help a patient mentally prepare for what is a sometimes emotionally difficult operation.
- Physical examination should include both the epitrochlear and axillary lymph nodes. For lesions on the toes, examination should include the popliteal and inguinal basins. Clinically node-negative patients with melanoma greater than or equal to 1 mm in thickness, or thin lesions with other worrisome histologic features, may be candidates for sentinel lymph node biopsy at the time of amputation (see Chapter 27). Patients with clinically involved nodes should undergo fine needle aspiration (FNA) biopsy and staging for distant metastases. These patients may require lymph node dissection at the time of amputation.

IMAGING AND OTHER DIAGNOSTIC STUDIES

- Suspicious lesions require biopsy to establish diagnosis. This should include a full-thickness sampling of the skin and/or nail matrix for accurate assessment of depth of the lesion. Increased depth of invasion is consistently associated with worse prognosis.[1]
- For large or fixed lesions, radiographs of the digit should be obtained to assess for the presence of bone involvement. If radiographs demonstrate significant bone destruction, additional imaging with magnetic resonance imaging (MRI) may be required to assess the full extent of tumor spread in the hand.

SURGICAL MANAGEMENT

Positioning

- For hand operations, patients are positioned supine, with the affected extremity extended on a hand table attached to the operating room table.

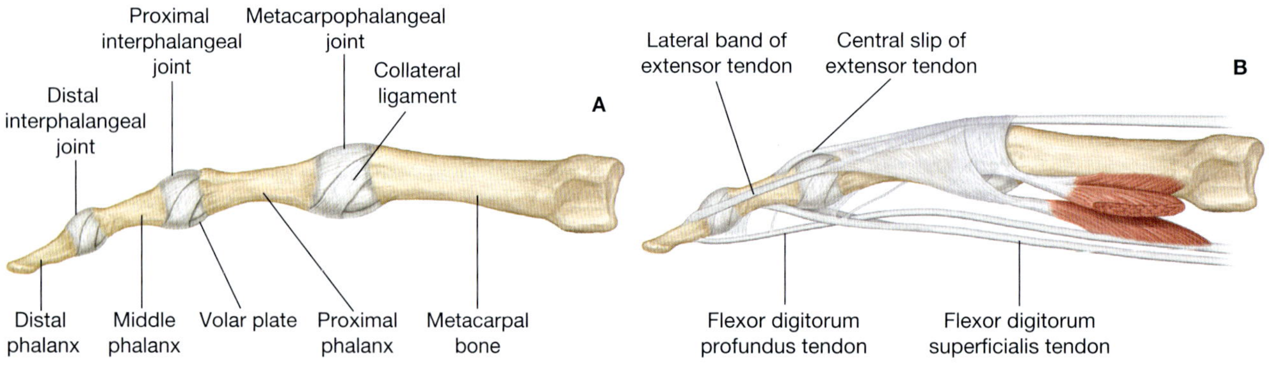

FIG 1 • **A,B.** Anatomy of the digit.

TECHNIQUES

DIGITAL AMPUTATION

Skin Incision

- The skin incision should be designed as a "fish mouth," such that dorsal and volar flaps are created that close in a more or less transverse line of closure that gives a smooth, rounded contour to the amputation stump.
- The skin flaps should be designed with enough laxity to close over the underlying skeleton to be preserved. Typically, the level of disarticulation or osteotomy should be a few millimeters proximal to the level of the skin incision.
- Ideally, the volar flap can be designed a bit longer than the dorsal flap (**FIG 2A**) to allow resurfacing of the entire

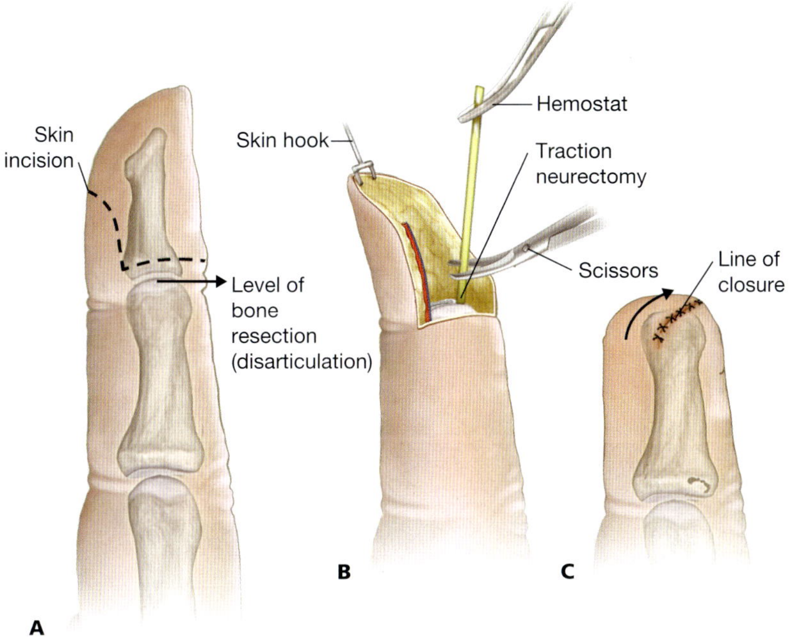

FIG 2 • Digital amputation technique. **A.** The skin incision is designed just distal to the level of planned bone resection or disarticulation. The volar flap is designed longer than the dorsal flap to allow for coverage of the fingertip with more durable, well-innervated volar skin. **B.** After removal of the skeletal elements and nail complex, the neurovascular bundle is identified on the volar flap, and the nerve is gently dissected proximally, ultimately dividing the nerve while on traction, and allowing the stump to retract proximally. **C.** The volar skin is advanced to cover the wound, and a smooth, rounded closure is performed.

opposition surface (contact surface) of the fingertip with the thicker, more densely innervated palmar skin.

Soft Tissue Dissection

- The soft tissue should be divided in a way that minimizes devascularization of the tissues or skin flaps. Sharp scalpel dissection directly to the bone can be performed both dorsally and volarly, dividing the neurovascular bundles, tendons, and periosteum.

Bone Dissection and Osteotomy

- The periosteum should then be sharply elevated proximally using an elevator or scalpel, circumferentially around the digit. This will allow the bone cut to be positioned slightly proximal to the soft tissue dissection.
- Bone division is most efficiently accomplished with a small oscillating power saw. Instruments such as bone cutters or rongeurs tend to crush and fracture the proximal bone stock and are not recommended.
- If disarticulation is planned, the collateral ligaments should be detached from the proximal aspect of the joint, so this bulky, poorly vascularized tissue is discarded with the amputated part.

Traction Neurectomy

- The neurovascular bundle should be identified with delicate dissection. The artery may be cauterized; the nerve should be dissected away from the artery and followed proximally several millimeters. The nerve should be placed on traction, divided proximally, and allowed to retract (FIG 2B). This will ensure that the neuromas that inevitably form at the end of each digital nerve will be located proximally to the contact surface of the fingertip.

Closure

- Closure is usually performed with a single layer of nonabsorbable sutures (FIG 2C), which are removed about 2 weeks later. Do *not* suture the extensor tendon to the flexor tendon over the end of the exposed bone; this will functionally shorten the flexor tendon to that digit, resulting in weakened grip strength due to the quadrigia effect.

RAY AMPUTATION

Skin Incision

- Incisions are designed to avoid a scar in the webspace. Conceptually, the goal is to preserve one webspace and resect the other, rather than having a webspace at the operative site with a contracted scar in its midline (FIG 3A–E).
- Usually the dissection is performed mostly through a dorsal incision, which extends longitudinally from the base of the finger. Palmar incisions are limited to avoid the possibility of sensitive scarring in that location.

Dorsal Dissection

- Major sensory nerves in the subcutaneous tissue are preserved when possible. The extensor tendon is divided proximally and the metacarpal exposed.
- The periosteum of the metacarpal is incised longitudinally and subperiosteal dissection carried out circumferentially along the shaft of the bone. The attachments of

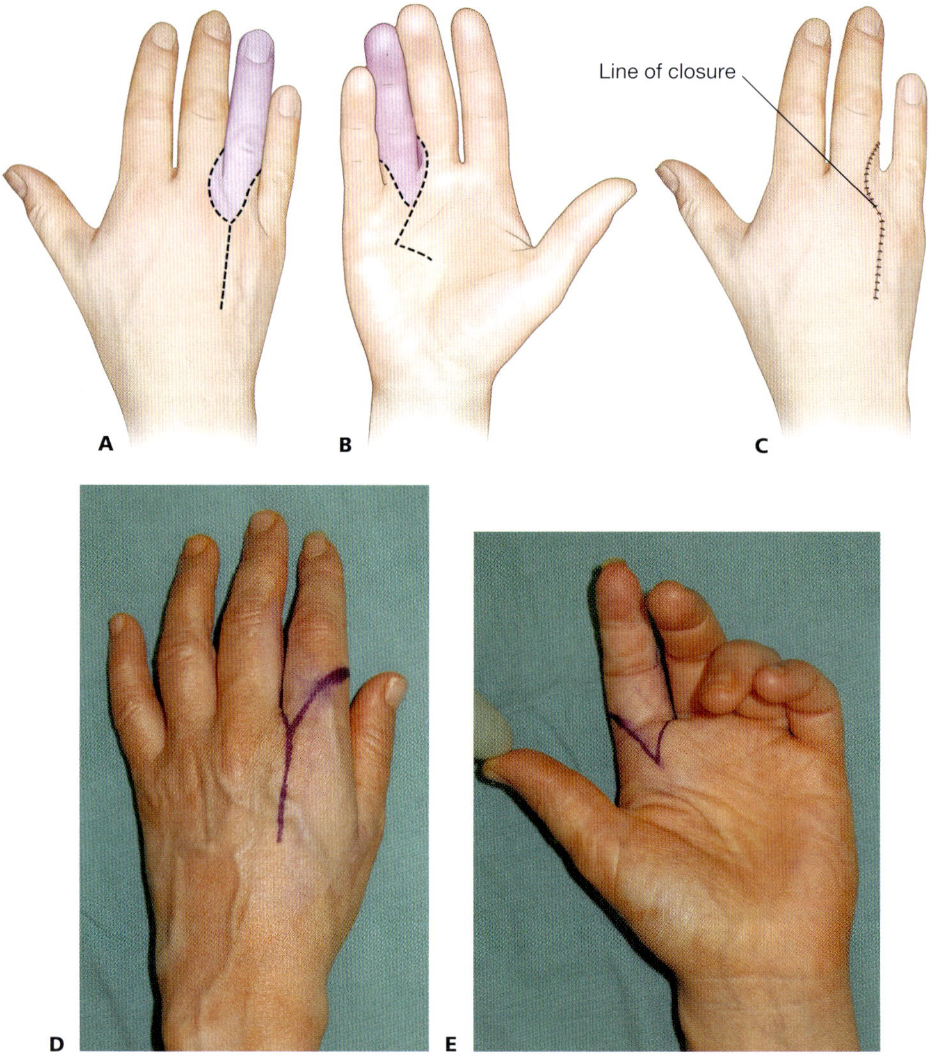

FIG 3 • Skin incision for ray amputation. **A.** Dorsal incision can be designed proximally as a straight line, or as a zigzag, extending distally to encircle the base of the finger to be removed. Note the preservation of an intact webspace for closure, rather than dividing the web with the incision. **B.** Volar incision must be a zigzag or chevron-style incision to avoid longitudinal scars crossing the flexion creases of the palm. **C.** Closure is shown, with preservation of the delicate webspace skin. **D.** Dorsal and **(E)** volar skin markings for index finger ray amputation.

the intrinsic muscles are disrupted with this dissection; most of these do not require transfer or repair, with the exception of the origin of adductor pollicis (FIG 4). When removed from the middle metacarpal during ray amputation, this muscle origin should be reattached to the index metacarpal with bone anchors or transosseous sutures.

Bone Dissection

- For index, middle, and small finger ray amputations, the osteotomy should be performed distal to the insertion of the wrist extensors: extensor carpi radialis longus, extensor carpi radialis brevis, and extensor carpi ulnaris, respectively (refer to FIG 5).
- For the ring finger metacarpal, which has no extrinsic tendon attachments, the entire metacarpal can be disarticulated at the base and removed (if no transposition is planned).
- For middle or ring finger ray amputations, some effort should be made in eliminating the troublesome gap between digits that can result.[2,3] This can be accomplished by two principle methods:
  - Meticulous soft tissue repair, including permanent sutures in the intermetacarpal ligaments and careful postoperative splinting (FIG 6)

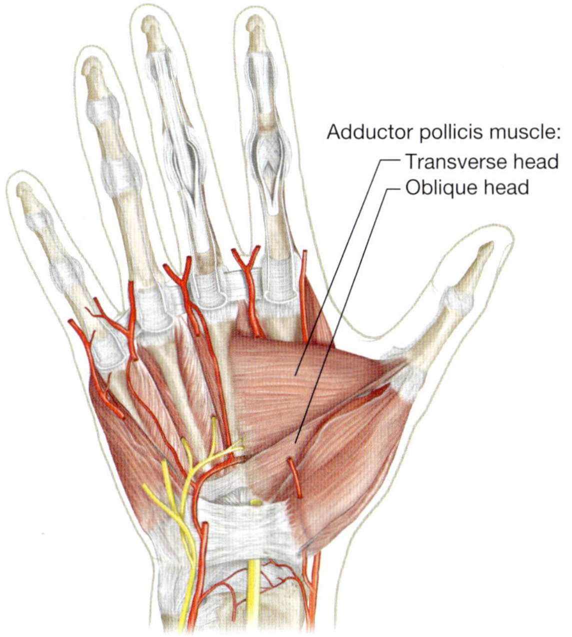

FIG 4 ● Anatomy of the adductor pollicis.

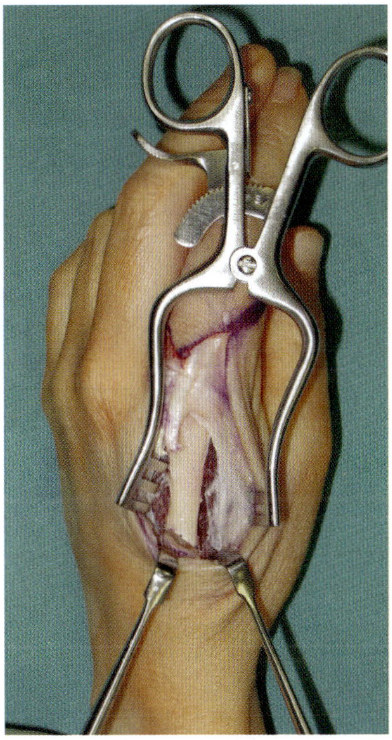

FIG 5 ● Dorsal dissection completed, with division of the metacarpal at the proximal shaft, preserving the base with its tendon attachments.

- Transposition of the adjacent border digit, requiring bony fixation of the metacarpal, and often longer postoperative immobilization (FIG 7)
- Once the bone has been transected, dissection proceeds around the side(s) of the metacarpal head to divide the intermetacarpal ligaments.

Volar Dissection

- The volar dissection is usually done last. The digital neurovascular bundles are identified and transected distally, keeping them rather long, in contrast to the shortening that is done for phalangeal-level amputations (FIG 8A,B).
- Once the ray amputation is complete, the digital nerves are folded dorsally into the periosteal sleeve left behind after metacarpal removal (FIG 9). The nerves are secured in this deep, padded area, surrounded by healthy interosseous muscle, where they are protected from trauma during routine hand function.

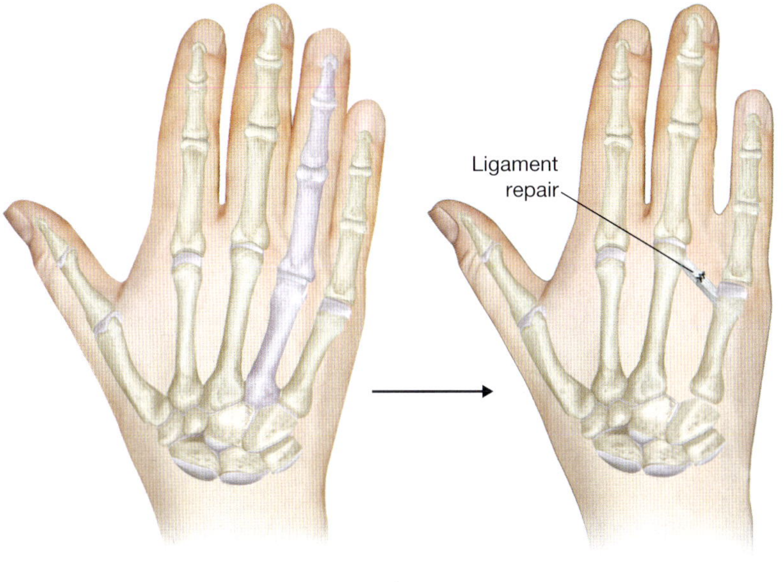

FIG 6 ● Ray resection without transposition. Using permanent sutures to reapproximate the intermetacarpal ligament, as well as meticulous skin closure, the finger "gap" can be closed with soft tissue repair alone.

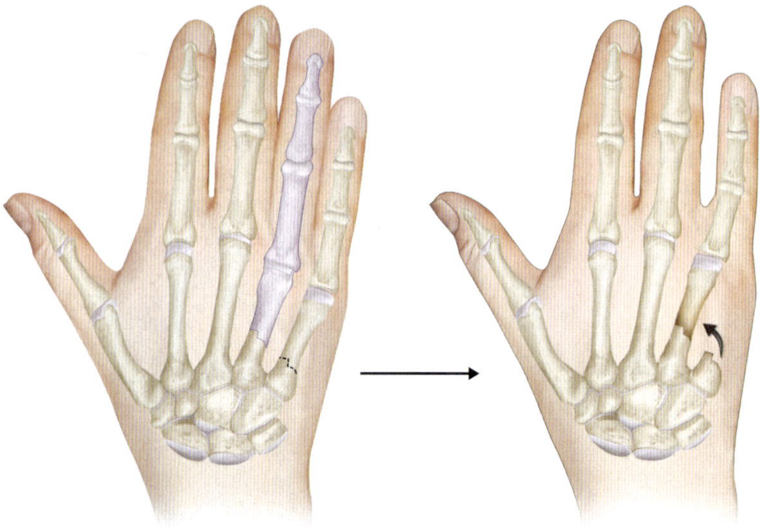

FIG 7 • Ray resection with transposition. Transposition requires osteosynthesis of the involved metacarpals with wires, pins, or plate and screws. One advantage is the potential to minimize length discrepancy of the small finger by preserving added length at the base of the ring metacarpal, as illustrated here.

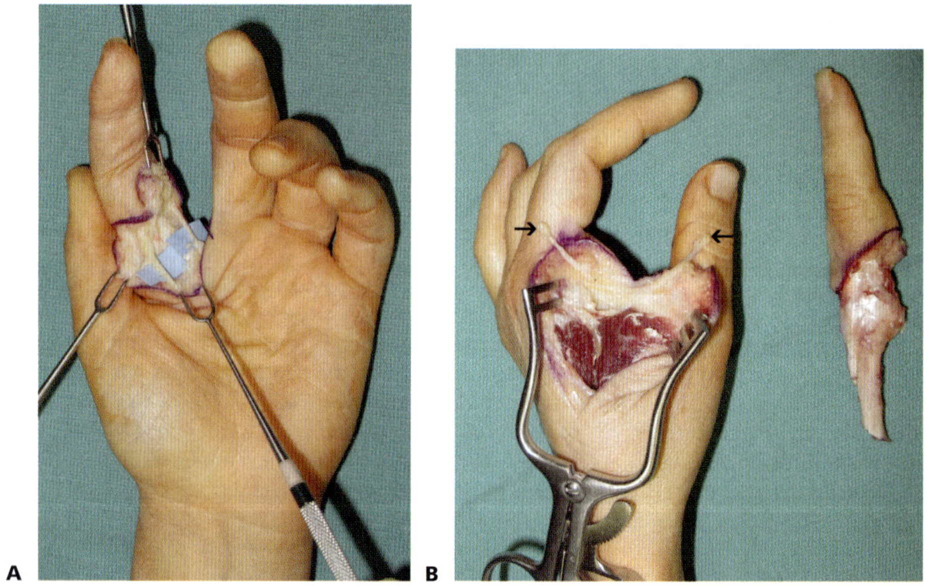

FIG 8 • **A.** Volar dissection with identification of the digital nerves, which are preserved with some length, so they can be relocated in the deeper dorsal tissues at the time of closure. **B.** Ray resection completed, with digital nerves transected *(black arrows)*.

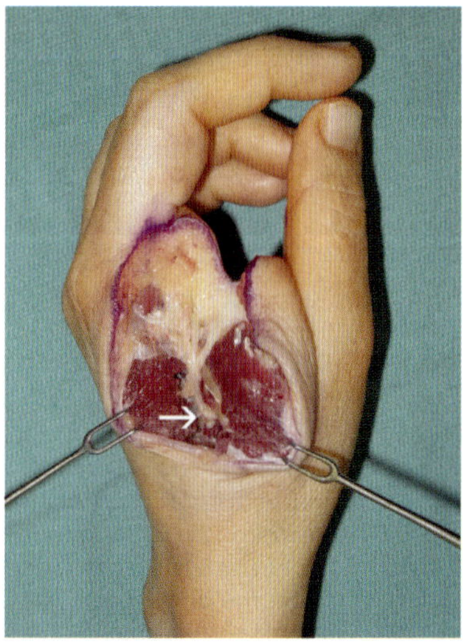

FIG 9 • Digital nerves *(white arrow)* transposed deep into the periosteal sleeve between the interosseous muscles.

Closure

- Skin closure should be meticulous, addressing excess laxity and/or standing cutaneous deformities ("dog ears") if encountered (**FIG 10A,B**). The relative tightness or looseness of the dorsal skin closure, in particular, can help maintain proper orientation of the adjacent digits and help avoid malalignment or "scissoring."

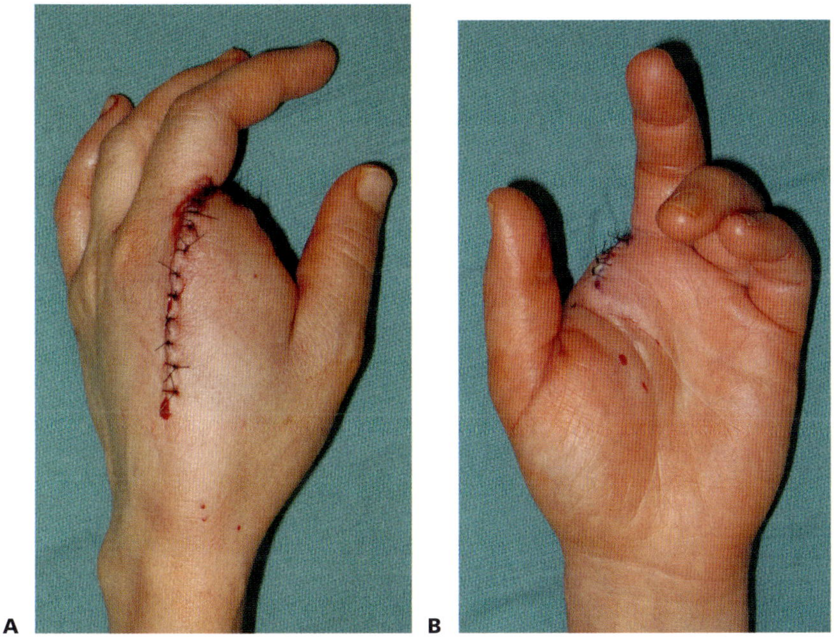

FIG 10 ● **A,B.** Final wound closure, which avoids extensive incisions on the sensitive palmar skin.

PEARLS AND PITFALLS

Digital amputations	■ When required, retract the skin edges with skin hooks only. This avoids tissue damage that can occur from repeated grasping of the tissues with forceps.
Quadrigia effect	■ Because the flexor digitorum profundus tendons share a common muscular origin, effectively shortening any one of the tendons can lead to an overall decrease in grip strength. During force generation, the foreshortened tendon becomes tight early, preventing transmission of force to the adjacent digits.
Neuroma detection	■ It can be difficult to differentiate symptomatic neuroma from ordinary hypersensitivity after finger amputation. A diagnostic injection of local anesthetic into the specific area of the neuroma, to anesthetize the nerve in isolation, can confirm the diagnosis of neuroma.

POSTOPERATIVE CARE

- For digital amputations, the postoperative dressing should be amply padded to allow for postoperative swelling. A hand-based splint for a short time (1 or 2 weeks) can be used if desired. Prolonged immobilization should be avoided so that the remaining finger joints (including the adjacent digits) do not become stiff.
- For ray amputations, the hand should be splinted for the first 2 weeks, taking care to maintain proper alignment of the digits in the splint, to avoid divergence or convergence of the fingers on either side of the amputation site. Sometimes, temporary pinning of the fingers is warranted to maintain good alignment in this early postoperative period, as the soft tissues are healing. Splinting beyond 2 weeks may still be required for comfort and protection, but the orthosis use should not interfere with early mobilization of the interphalangeal and metacarpophalangeal joints, which may become permanently stiff if immobilized for too long.
- In all cases, consultation with a certified hand therapist may be of benefit to the patient, for help with orthosis fabrication, edema control, joint mobilization, scar massage, desensitization, and molding of the finger stump for prosthesis wear, if desired.

OUTCOMES

- Compared to the contralateral hand, patients with single-ray amputations have on average 13% less key pinch strength, 26% less oppositional strength, and 28% less grip strength at long-term follow-up.[4,5]

COMPLICATIONS

- Acute complications such as bleeding, infection, and delayed healing should be uncommon.
- Chronic complications include phantom pain and painful neuromas.
  - Persistent sensation in an amputated part is common (over 80% in one prospective study) but is not always painful.[6]
  - Neuromas will form at the stump of divided nerves but are not usually symptomatic if the nerve endings are properly padded and located away from contact surfaces.

REFERENCES

1. Warso M, Gray T, Gonzalez M. Melanoma of the hand. *J Hand Surg Am*. 1997;22(2):354–360.
2. Colen L, Bunkis J, Gordon L, et al. Functional assessment of ray transfer for central digital loss. *J Hand Surg Am*. 1985;10(2):232–237.
3. Steichen JB, Idler RS. Results of central ray resection without bony transposition. *J Hand Surg Am*. 1986;11(4):466–474.
4. Peimer CA, Wheeler DR, Barrett A, et al. Hand function following single ray amputation. *J Hand Surg Am*. 1999;24(6):1245–1248.
5. Melikyan EY, Beg MS, Woodbridge S, et al. The functional results of ray amputation. *Hand Surg*. 2003;8(1):47–51.
6. Jensen TS, Krebs B, Nielsen J, et al. Phantom limb, phantom pain and stump pain in amputees during the first 6 months following limb amputation. *Pain*. 1983;17(3):243–256.

Chapter **26**

Resection of Head and Neck Melanoma

Scott A. McLean

DEFINITION

- Resection of head and neck cutaneous melanoma is performed with wide surgical margins intended to achieve histologically negative margins. Current guidelines for wide excision of the primary lesion, with an adequate margin of surrounding normal skin and deep soft tissue necessary to achieve clear surgical margins, are based on depth of invasion of the primary lesion (Table 1).[1] However, given the complex anatomic and functional nature of the head and neck, resection margins are sometimes modified to preserve normal function. Reconstruction of complex head and neck defects is often delayed until final histopathologic evaluation of margins is deemed negative. Reconstruction can be accomplished with primary closure, split- or full-thickness skin grafts, local or regional adjacent tissue transfer, or free tissue transfer.
- Patients with invasive melanoma and no clinical evidence or regional metastatic disease may warrant assessment of regional lymph nodes via sentinel lymph node (SLN) biopsy. SLN biopsy has been shown to be both accurate and prognostic in head and neck melanoma.[2,3] Current recommendations on use of SLN biopsy are based on depth of invasion of the primary lesion as well as the presence of adverse histologic features such as ulceration and mitotic rate. Patients with melanoma measuring 1 mm or greater should be offered SLN biopsy. SLN biopsy should also be considered in patients with a thickness of between 0.76 and 0.99 mm if they have any of the following adverse features: greater than or equal to 1 mitotic figure per square millimeter, lymphovascular invasion, satellitosis, or young patient age. SLN biopsy may also be considered with thin melanoma when the deep margin was broadly transected.[1–5]
- Patients who present with clinical evidence of regional metastatic disease and patients who are found to have micrometastatic disease on sentinel lymph node biopsy (SLNB) are offered completion lymph node dissection (CLND). Based on the site of the primary lesion, the nodal basins included in the CLND may include the postauricular and suboccipital lymph nodes, the parotid gland and its associated lymph nodes, and the cervical lymph nodes levels I to V (Table 2) (see Chapter 31).[6]

Table 1: Surgical Margin Recommendations for Cutaneous Melanoma

Primary Tumor Thickness	Clinically Measured Surgical Margin
In situ	0.5–1.0 cm
≤1 mm	1 cm
1.01–2.0 mm	1–2 cm
2.01–4 mm	2 cm
>4 mm	2 cm

From National Comprehensive Cancer Network. Guidelines version 4.2014. http://www.nccn.org. Accessed August 2014.

Table 2: Nodal Basins Included in Therapeutic Lymph Node Dissection

Primary Cutaneous Lesion Location	Nodal Basins Included in Therapeutic Lymph Node Dissection
Anterolateral scalp, temple, lateral forehead, lateral cheek, and ear: all arising anterior to coronal plane through the external auditory canal	Parotid and cervical lymphatic levels I–V
Chin and neck	Cervical lymphatic levels I–V
Scalp and occiput posterior to coronal plane through the external auditory canal	Postauricular, suboccipital, and cervical lymphatic levels II–V

DIFFERENTIAL DIAGNOSIS

- Cutaneous melanoma of the head and neck usually presents as a pigmented lesion of varying size, shape, and color. Other benign and malignant cutaneous lesions can present in a similar fashion and include the following:
  - Seborrheic keratosis
  - Junctional nevi
  - Compound nevi
  - Dermal nevi
  - Hemangioma
  - Blue nevus
  - Pyogenic granuloma
  - Spitz nevus
  - Pigmented actinic keratosis
  - Pigmented or nonpigmented basal cell carcinoma
  - Squamous cell carcinoma

PATIENT HISTORY AND PHYSICAL FINDINGS

- A thorough history of the lesion of concern should include the duration of clinical symptoms; the presence of pruritus; bleeding; and any changes in the size, shape, or color of the lesion.
- Most cutaneous melanomas will present as either a new pigmented lesion or changes in an existing lesion that exhibit the ABCDs of melanoma: A–Asymmetry, B–Border, C–Color, D–Difference (a change in the lesion).
- A thorough past medical history should be performed and include information regarding any previous malignancies, past surgical procedures, current medications and allergies, family history of cancer, problems with anesthesia, and social history—including smoking history, occupation, sun exposure, and history of blistering sunburns.

- A focused review of systems should also be completed and include review of any constitutional, musculoskeletal, neurologic, respiratory, gastrointestinal, hepatic, skin, and lymphatic signs or symptoms.
- All newly diagnosed melanoma patients should undergo full body skin evaluation.
- A complete head and neck exam should be performed on every patient and include a thorough skin exam and palpation of the suboccipital, postauricular, parotid, and cervical nodal basins to rule out the presence of clinically palpable regional metastatic disease.
- A detailed cranial nerve exam should be performed to document preoperative cranial nerve function.

IMAGING AND OTHER DIAGNOSTIC STUDIES

- Newly diagnosed patients with localized cutaneous melanoma are not recommended to undergo distant metastatic workup. In the absence of clinical signs or symptoms of distant metastatic disease, no imaging modality has been shown to be useful in detecting occult metastatic disease and in fact more often lead to false-positive findings, requiring further unnecessary invasive procedures.[1]
- Chest x-ray and serum lactate dehydrogenase are also both insensitive for the detection of occult metastatic disease.
- Many patients will require preoperative chest x-ray, complete blood count (CBC), and electrocardiogram (EKG), depending on age, health status, and need for general anesthesia.

SURGICAL MANAGEMENT

Preoperative Planning

- Prior to proceeding to the operating room, the primary cutaneous lesion should be reexamined and confirmed with the patient. The surrounding skin should also be reexamined to make sure no new lesions have developed. In addition, the plan regarding surgical margins and primary closure versus delayed reconstruction should be confirmed with the patient. All cranial nerve functions in the operative field should also be retested prior to surgery.
- Patients who are scheduled for SLN biopsy in conjunction with excision of their primary cutaneous lesion will undergo lymphoscintigraphy prior to their definitive excision. This procedure is done in the nuclear medicine department and is enhanced by the use of single-photon emission computed tomography–computed tomography (SPECT-CT) imaging.[7] Prior to proceeding to the operating room, the SPECT-CT/lymphoscintigraphy should be reviewed to determine the likely location of the SLN(s) (**FIGS 1** and **2**). These locations should then be discussed with the patient and marked appropriately. If the location of a likely SLN is in close proximity to a cranial nerve, this should be discussed with the patient and the cranial nerve function should be well documented.
- Appropriate use of antibiotics and deep vein thrombosis (DVT) prophylaxis should also be discussed prior to proceeding to the operating room.
- In addition, it is crucial to have a thorough discussion with the anesthesia team regarding the use of long-acting paralytics. If cranial nerves are likely to be in the operative field, as is almost always the case in the resection of head and neck melanoma, the anesthesia team must be aware to avoid the use of long-acting paralytics.

Positioning

- Patients who are scheduled for wide local excision alone (melanoma in situ or T1a lesions) often can tolerate surgery under sedation with monitored anesthesia. In these cases, the head of the bed is often rotated 90 degrees away from the anesthesia cart to allow for easy access to the surgical field. Oxygen delivery methods can be designed to avoid

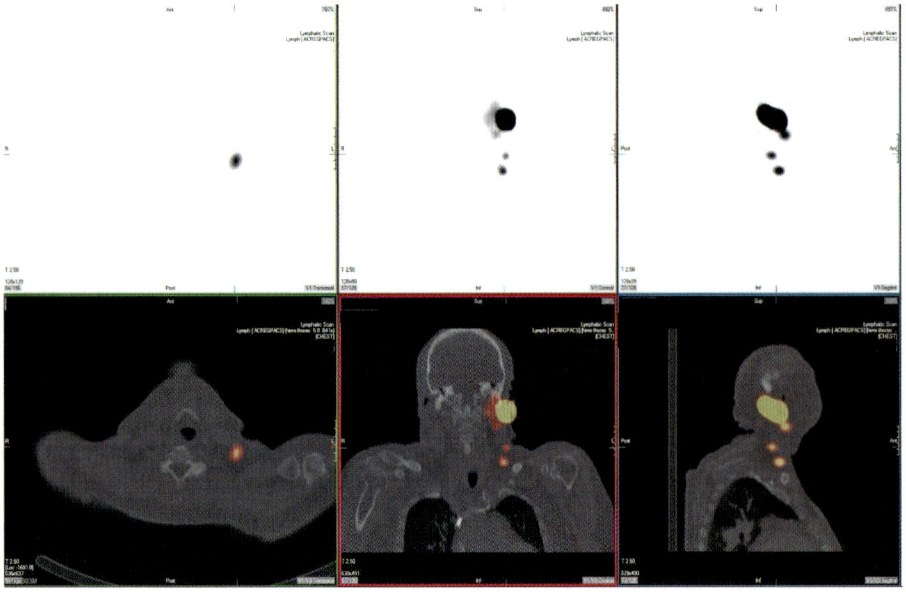

FIG 1 • Lymphoscintigraphy with SPECT-CT imaging after injection of left postauricular primary melanoma site. Imaging reveals a left level II lymph node as well as secondary drainage to left levels Va and Vb.

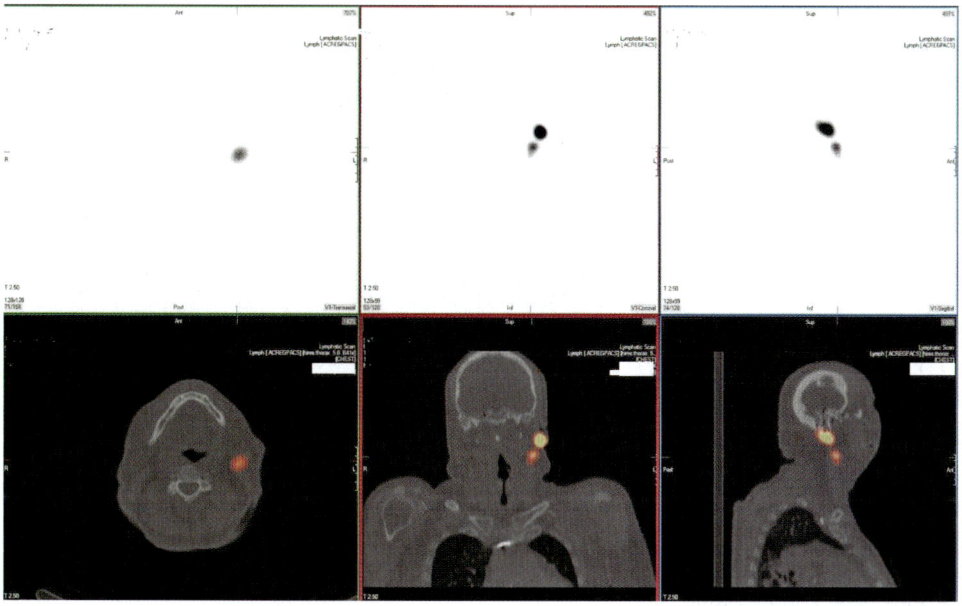

FIG 2 • Lymphoscintigraphy with SPECT-CT imaging after injection of left postauricular primary melanoma site. Careful observation reveals the level II lymph node to be located just inferior to the tail of the parotid and just anterior to the sternocleidomastoid muscle. Likely, this represents an external jugular lymph node.

crossing the surgical field and may include either nasal cannula or mask. In these cases with free-flowing oxygen, it is very important to discuss the risk of fire with the entire operating room team. The entire face and neck can be prepped into the operative field. Wide draping can then be used with attention to avoid any tenting of drapes, which could lead to pooling of oxygen in the operative field (**FIG 3**).

- Patients who are scheduled to undergo SLN biopsy in conjunction with the primary excision are almost always placed under general anesthesia. Again, the use of long-acting paralytics must be avoided. The head of the bed can be rotated 180 degrees away from the anesthesia cart to allow for easy surgical access to the operative field. Most primary lesions can be excised with the patient in the supine position. Rarely, the patient may need to be turned prone to allow access to the posterior scalp or suboccipital nodal basin. With the patient intubated, either half of the face and neck or the entire face and neck can be prepped and draped, depending on the need for surgical access.

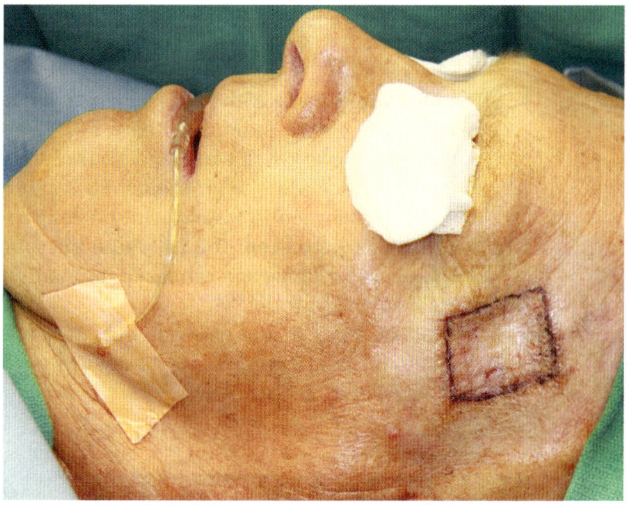

FIG 3 • Patient is under sedation with the entire face prepped to allow for wide draping and to avoid pooling of oxygen within the surgical field.

TECHNIQUES

PLACEMENT OF PLANNED INCISIONS

Primary Lesion Excision Site

- The primary lesion is carefully inspected and cleaned with a moist sponge. The lesion should be marked out with careful attention to include any evidence of dermal extension. This may include any pale, erythematous, or lightly pigmented extension from the primary lesion (**FIG 4**).
- With the primary lesion now marked, the appropriate margin is then marked circumferentially around the visible lesion. The excision margin is most often 1 to 2 cm, depending on the depth of invasion of the primary lesion.
- In certain functional situations, the excision margin may be left a little short of standard margins. For example, if a lower eyelid lesion requires 2-cm margins, but at 1 cm the excision would cross the lid margin, it may be acceptable to use 1 cm (**FIG 5**). In this case, the surgeon must be willing to reexcise this margin should it return positive on final histopathologic review.

Injection of Methylene Blue Dye

- To assist with SLN identification, the dermis surrounding the primary lesion is injected with methylene blue dye. Usually only 1 or 2 mL of dye is injected (**FIG 6**).

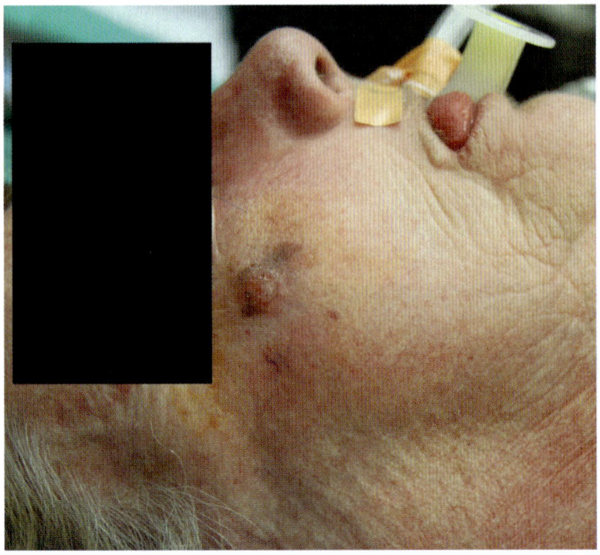

FIG 4 • The main lesion is pink and raised. Notice the pigmented extension into the surrounding skin. The entire pigmented area must be marked out prior to marking out circumferential margins.

- The injection is made with a 30-gauge needle with the bevel of the needle facing up. There should be slight pressure as the dye is injected and visually the dermis should begin to turn blue. If the dermis is not turning blue or the injection is passing with no resistance, the needle is likely too deep. This will cause the subcutaneous tissue to turn blue and can make recognition of tissue planes more difficult.
- Several injections should be made into the dermis surrounding the primary lesion until the lesion is surrounded by blue dye (**FIG 7**).

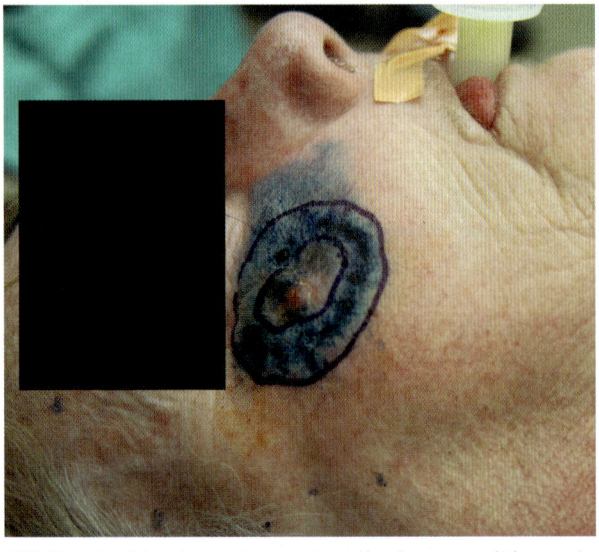

FIG 5 • In this planned resection, the lower eyelid margin is left a little narrow in the hopes of avoiding postoperative ectropion. The margins must be carefully examined by pathology and reexcised should they return positive.

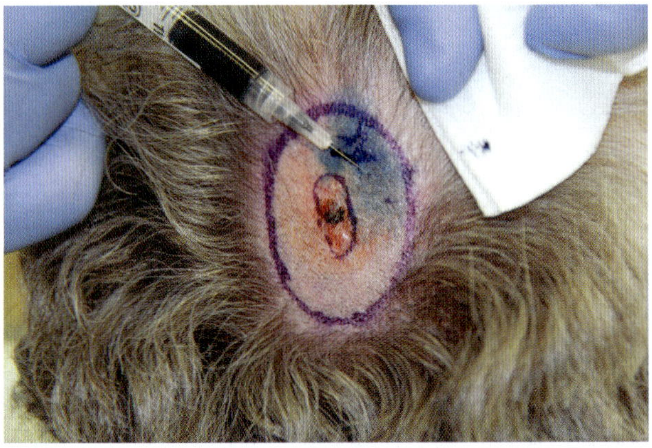

FIG 6 • Methylene blue dye injected circumferentially into the dermis surrounding the lesion. A 30-gauge needle is used and effort is made to inject directly into the dermis only.

Placement of Incisions for Sentinel Lymph Node Biopsy

- The preoperative lymphoscintigraphy/SPECT-CT is again reviewed to help determine the approximate location of the SLNs in relation to visible or palpable anatomic structures. The intraoperative gamma probe can then be used to confirm the site of the sentinel nodes. Once the location is confirmed, incisions are marked to allow access to remove the sentinel nodes (**FIG 8**).
- Marking the planned incisions should take into account placement along relaxed skin tension lines. In addition, consideration should be given to any future potential procedures such as rotation flap reconstruction sites or the need for parotidectomy and cervical lymphadenectomy (**FIG 9**).
- At this point, all planned incisions are usually injected with local anesthesia. Typically 1% lidocaine with 1:100,000 epinephrine solution is used. A small volume should be used to help avoid inadvertent paralysis of cranial nerves close to the operative sites.

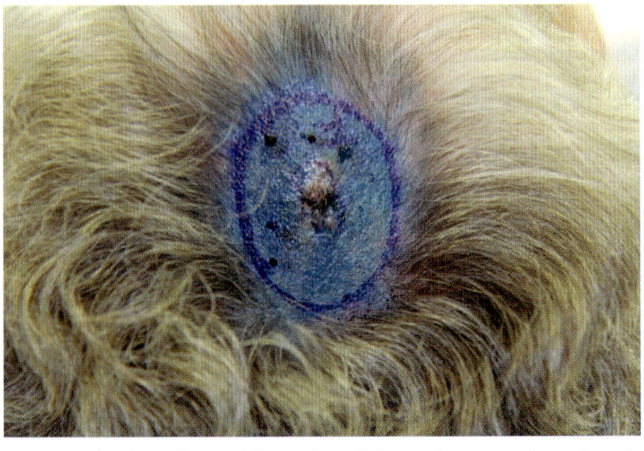

FIG 7 • Methylene blue dye injected into the dermis circumferentially around the lesion.

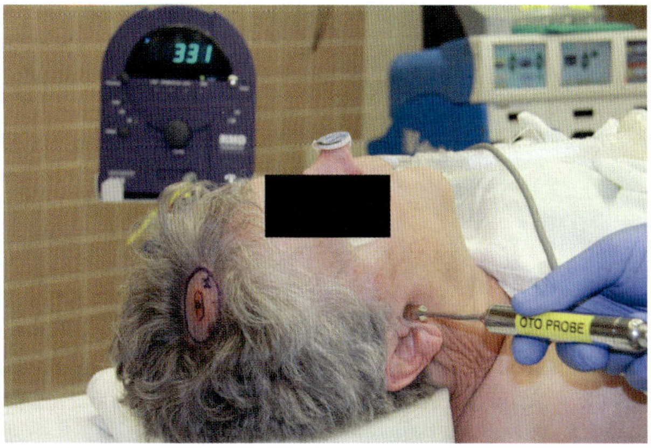

FIG 8 ● The intraoperative gamma probe is used to confirm the sites of the potential SLNs.

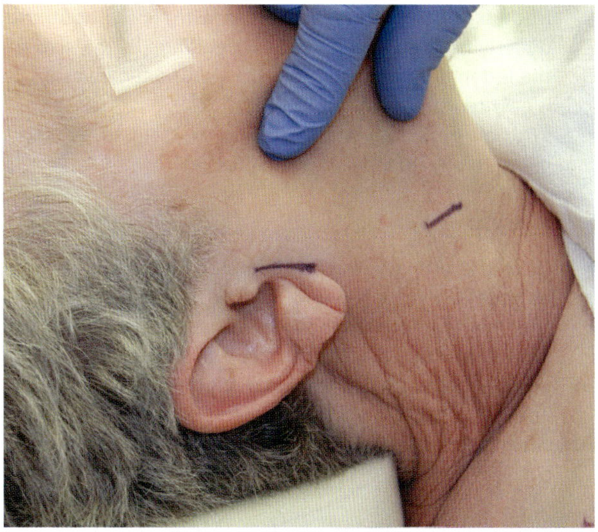

FIG 9 ● Small incisions are planned along relaxed skin tension lines.

EXCISION OF THE PRIMARY LESION

Skin Incision

- The skin surrounding the primary lesion is now sharply incised, being careful to follow the exact marking. The incision is carried thru the subcutaneous tissue, now being careful to avoid beveling the cut toward the primary lesion.

Determining the Depth of the Excision

- Once the peripheral incisions are made around the primary lesion, the depth of the excision must be determined. In general, the depth of the excision is carried to the fascial plane deep to the subcutaneous tissue. The depth of the excision is highly dependent on the location of the primary lesion, the size and depth of the lesion, and the amount of subcutaneous tissue deep to the lesion.
- For facial lesions, the excision is most often carried to a plane just above the facial musculature (**FIG 10**).
- Preauricular lesions are excised to a depth of the parotid fascia (**FIG 11**).
- Nasal lesions are excised above the level of the nasal cartilages.
- Auricular lesions are removed either with or without the underlying cartilage, depending on the size of the primary lesion. In many cases, the underlying cartilage should be removed to ensure adequate negative margins.
- Scalp lesions are usually excised in a subgaleal plane with the underlying pericranium left intact. In large bulky lesions, the underlying pericranium can also be removed to allow for wider clear margins (**FIG 12**).

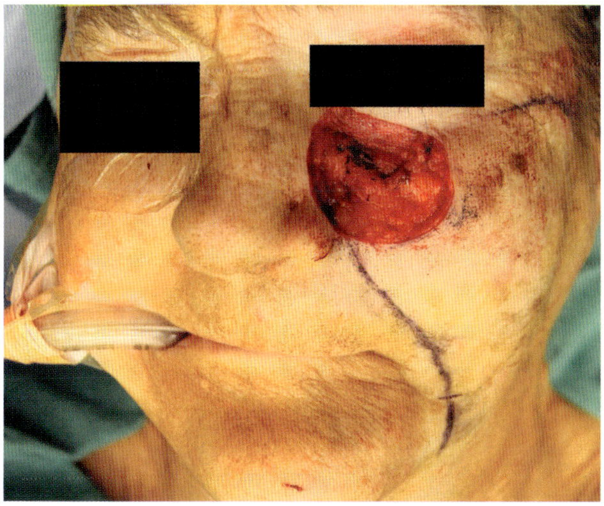

FIG 10 ● The facial lesion has been excised to a depth just above the facial musculature.

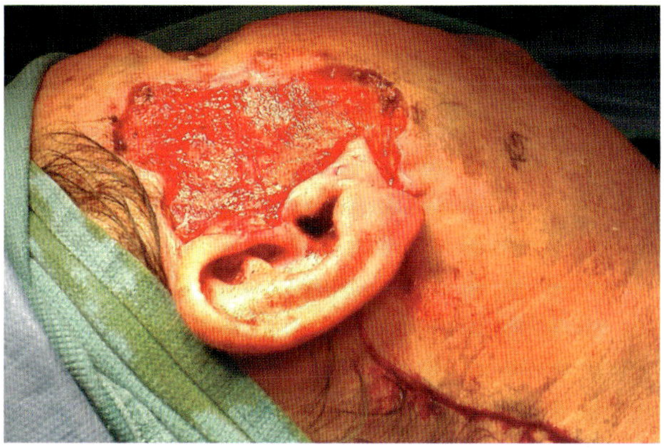

FIG 11 ● Preauricular lesions are excised to a depth just above the parotid fascia.

- Neck skin can be excised either with or without the underlying platysma muscle, depending on the size of the lesion. If there is any concern about deep invasion, it is easy to remove platysma.
- With all excisions, attention must be paid to avoiding injury to any underlying cranial nerves.

Orientation

- Once the primary lesion is completely excised, it must be carefully oriented and marked for permanent pathology. Marking stitches should be easily understood and allow for easy communication between surgeon and pathologist. Any areas of special concern should also be noted on the pathology request, such as when margins are less than ideal due to functional considerations.

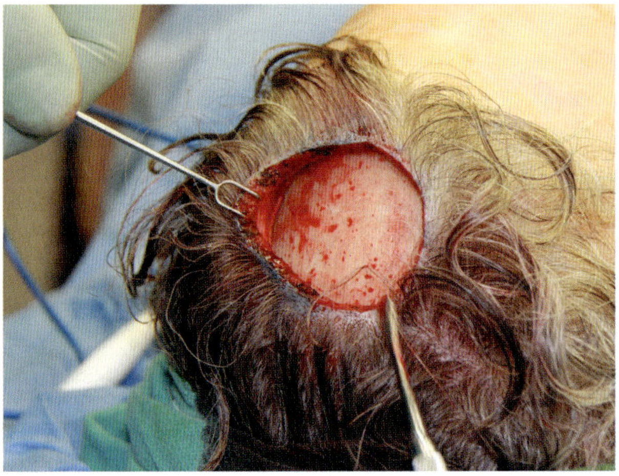

FIG 12 ● Scalp lesions are usually excised in a subgaleal plane with the underlying pericranium left intact.

SENTINEL LYMPH NODE BIOPSY

Intraoperative Gamma Probe

- The intraoperative gamma probe is now used to confirm the site of the SLN. In some cases, the primary excision site should be surveyed to look for potential SLNs, which may be deep to the primary excision site. These nodes may not appear on the SPECT-CT due to the shadowing caused by the high intensity of the primary lesion injection site. Sometimes, a blue lymphatic channel can be seen at the edge of the excision site and can be followed to an SLN (**FIG 13**).

Incision and Node Dissection

- Before proceeding with lymph node dissection, it is important to confirm that the patient has not been given any paralytic agents.
- After confirming the previously marked SLN sites with the gamma probe, the incision is made and carried to the deep soft tissue. Usually a 2- to 3-cm incision is long enough to allow for easy dissection and visualization.
- With the incision made, skin hooks are used to retract the skin edges. Blunt dissection is then used to enter the deeper soft tissue. In the neck, dissection will go deep to the platysma muscle. In the preauricular region, the dissection will often proceed deep to the parotid fascia into the parotid parenchyma.
- The intraoperative gamma probe is used frequently to help determine the direction of further dissection. As the tip of the probe gets closer to the sentinel node, the gamma counts will increase.
- Oftentimes, a blue lymphatic channel can be identified and can then be followed to the SLN (**FIGS 14** and **15**).
- Once the node is identified, it is carefully removed with blunt dissection and judicious use of bipolar electrocautery.
- The node is then examined away from the patient to document the gamma count and the presence of blue dye. The node is labeled with the anatomic

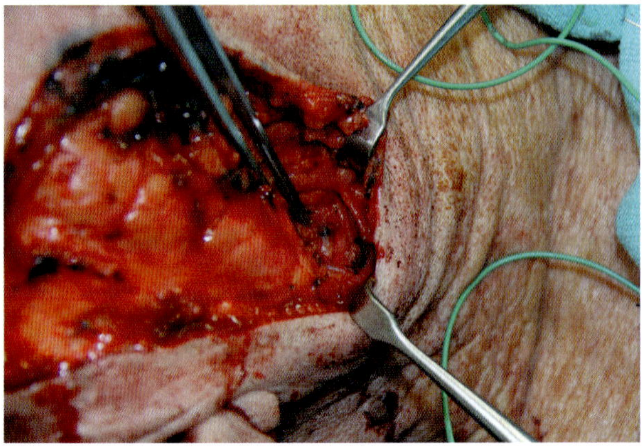

FIG 13 ● The SLN is identified deep to the primary excision site.

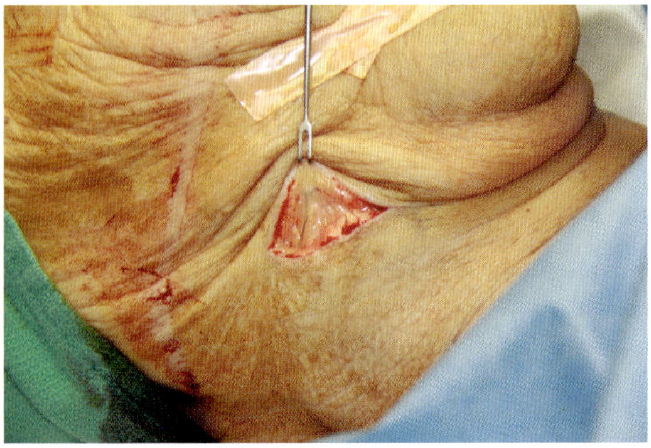

FIG 14 ● Oftentimes, a blue lymphatic channel can be identified.

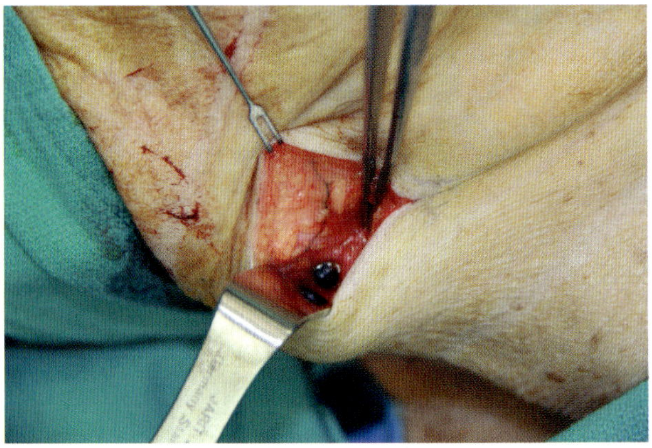

FIG 15 ● Lymphatic channels can then be followed to the SLN.

location, gamma count, and presence of blue dye and sent for histopathology.

Confirmation and Closure

- After removing the SLN, the gamma probe is then used to reexamine the surgical bed. The area where the node was removed should now have a very low count compared to the count prior to node removal. As a general rule, the count should drop to less than 10% of the count prior to node removal. If the count remains elevated, further dissection is warranted to remove any other SLNs identified.
- Once all potential SLNs are removed, the surgical bed is irrigated with saline. A Valsalva maneuver should be performed to confirm there is no ongoing bleeding. The incision can be closed in standard fashion and a small pressure dressing applied.

PRIMARY CLOSURE VERSUS DELAYED RECONSTRUCTION OF THE PRIMARY SITE

Primary Closure

- After the primary lesion has been resected and the SLN biopsy completed, it is time to determine the best method of closing the primary site. If the primary site can be closed without distorting the surgical margins and without the use of rotation flaps or grafts, this can be done immediately. Should a margin return positive on permanent pathology, it would still be easy to return for wider excision.
- This is usually the case for small lesions or for lesions on the neck where excess skin can easily be advanced.
- In these cases, bilateral Burrow's triangle excisions can be performed along the direction of relaxed skin tension lines. The skin is then undermined, advanced, and closed with deep absorbable suture and superficial suture at the skin edge.
- The wound is then dressed with a small pressure dressing, which can be removed after 24 hours.

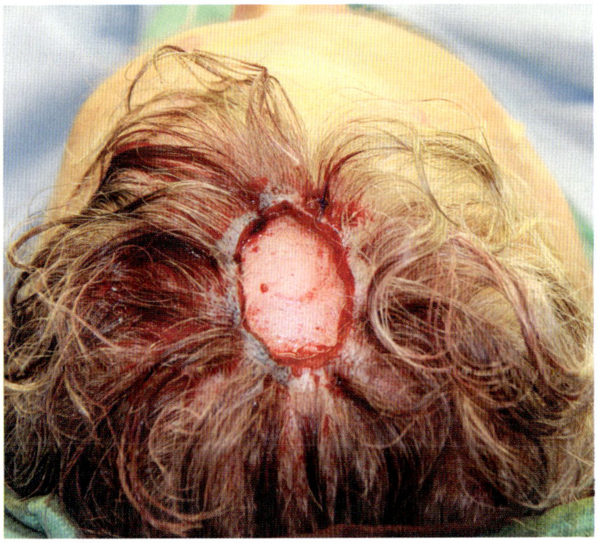

FIG 16 ● Circumferential purse-string suture is used to decrease the size of the wound.

Delayed Reconstruction

- In many cases, reconstruction of the primary resection site will require significant tissue rearrangement, skin grafting, or even free tissue transfer. In these situations, it is preferable to wait for final histopathologic confirmation of negative surgical margins prior to proceeding with definitive reconstruction.
- In these cases, the size of the wound can often be decreased with use of a circumferential purse-string suture (FIG 16).
- The wound can then be dressed with a moist bolster dressing using Vaseline or Xeroform gauze, bacitracin, cotton balls (FIG 17), or a foam-type dressing (FIG 18). The bolster dressing can be secured with either silk suture or surgical staples.
- Wound infections are very rare in the head and neck and therefore postoperative antibiotics are not routinely used even in the setting of an open wound with a bolster

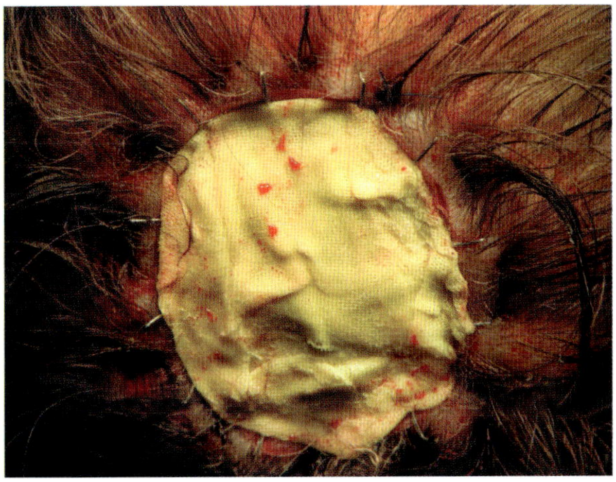

FIG 17 ● A Xeroform gauze dressing is placed over the resection site.

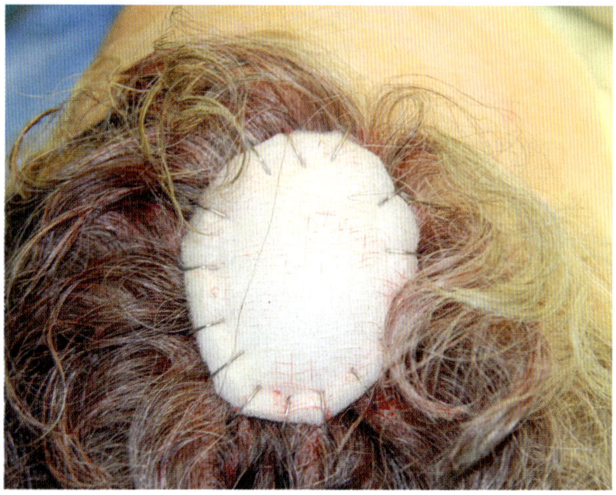

FIG 18 • A Reston foam bolster is secured to the scalp to apply pressure after either resection or skin graft reconstruction.

applied. In some cases, such as immune suppression or previous infection, antibiotics may be indicated.

Skin Graft and Rotation Flap Reconstruction

- Once the final surgical margins have returned clear, definitive reconstruction can be completed. The method of reconstruction is dependent on the site of the defect and the goals of the patient. Complex facial defects should be addressed by colleagues with experience in facial plastic and reconstructive surgery.
- Facial skin and preauricular skin defects are most often closed with the use of cervicofacial rotation flaps and transposition flaps. Incisions are planned along relaxed skin tension lines when possible and are carried to postauricular and posterior cervical skin. These flaps create standing cutaneous deformities along the arc of rotation, which will need to be excised. Very large defects can be closed and achieve excellent cosmetic outcomes (**FIGS 19–21**).
- Eyelid defects can be very difficult to repair without causing significant ectropion. Lid-tightening procedures can be done in conjunction with skin grafts, transposition flaps, and rotation flaps. Oculoplastic surgeons should be involved if there is concern about postoperative eyelid function (**FIGS 22–24**).
- Nasal defects can be closed with skin grafts, composite grafts, transposition flaps, advancement flaps, and the interpolated paramedian forehead flap. Each technique can yield excellent results when used in the proper clinical setting (**FIGS 25–27**).
- Auricular defects are most easily closed with wedge excision and advancement flap closure. Transposition flaps can be used to reconstruct large defects and achieve acceptable cosmetic results (**FIGS 28** and **29**).

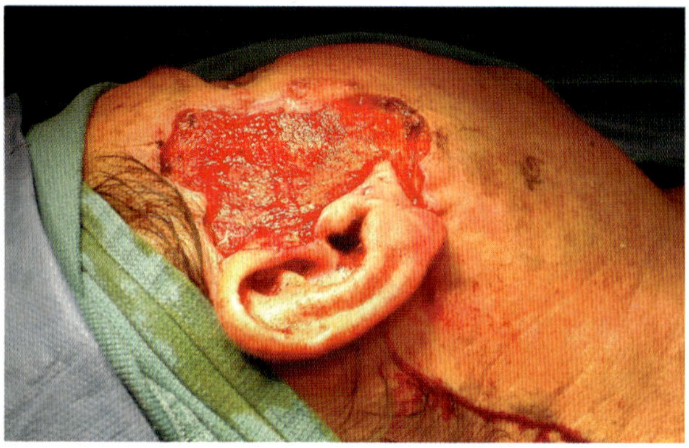

FIG 19 • Large facial defect with posterior cervical incision made to allow for cervicofacial rotation flap reconstruction.

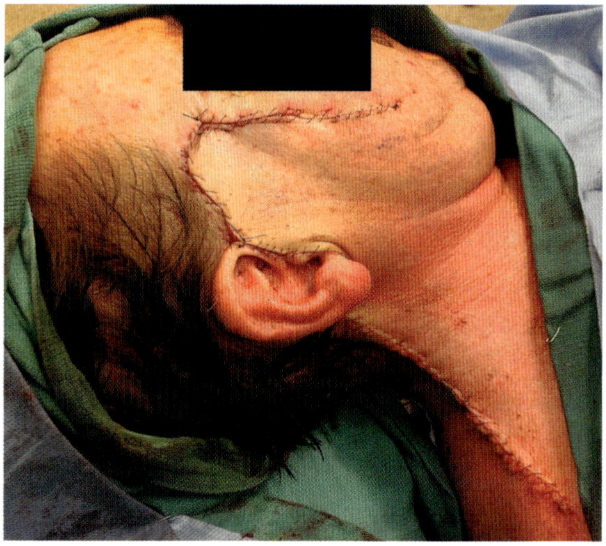

FIG 20 • Cervicofacial rotation flap brought into position.

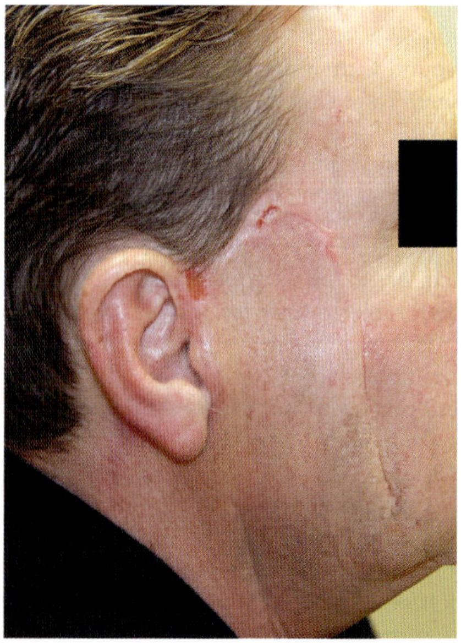

FIG 21 • Excellent cosmetic result several weeks after cervicofacial reconstruction of large facial defect.

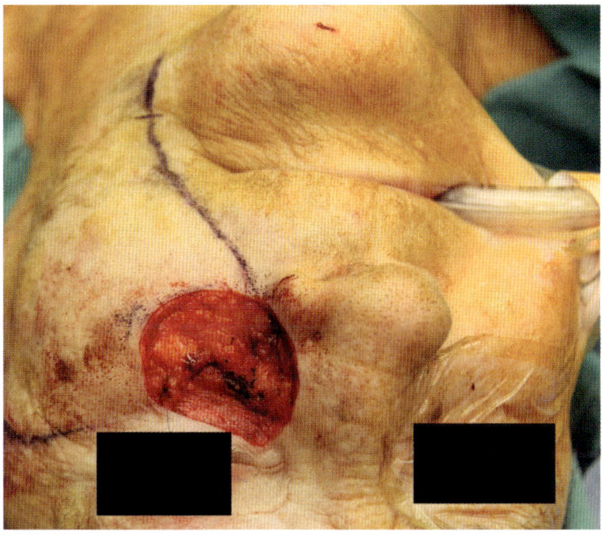

FIG 22 • Large rotation flap designed for reconstruction of lower eyelid defect.

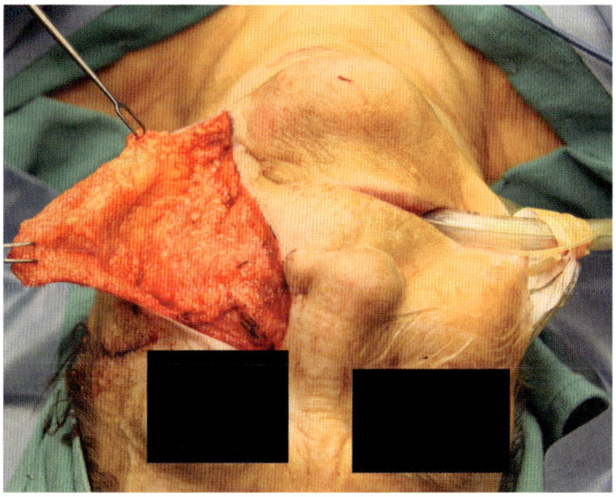

FIG 23 • The flap is raised far enough to allow for tension-free closure.

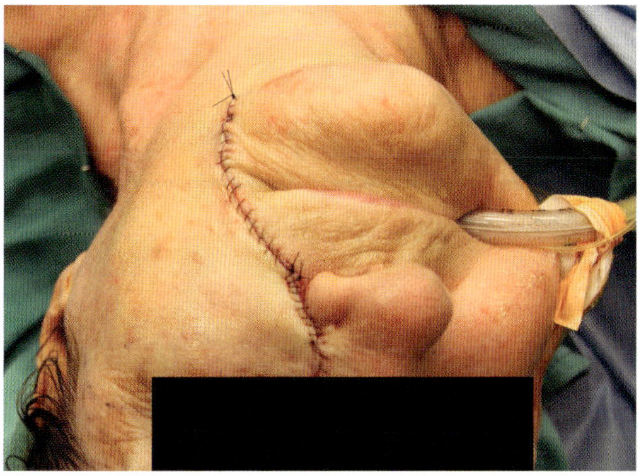

FIG 24 • The rotation flap is sewn into place with no tension inferiorly, thus avoiding postoperative ectropion.

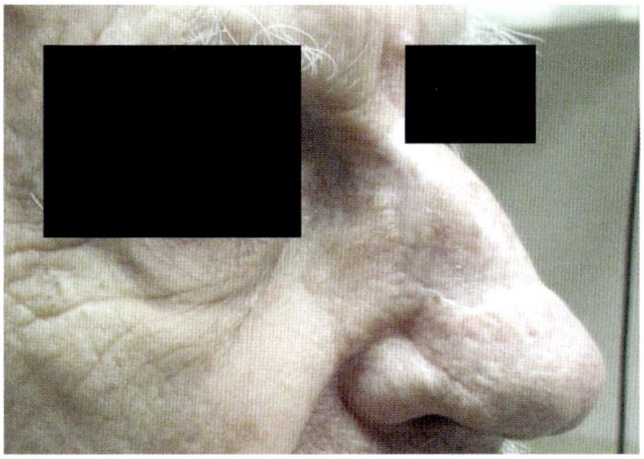

FIG 25 • Postoperative result after full-thickness skin graft reconstruction of the nasal dorsum.

- Scalp defects are most easily closed with the use of full-thickness or split-thickness skin grafts. In older patients, large amounts of supraclavicular skin can be harvested and used to graft large scalp defects. The skin is thinned to the dermal layer, making sure to remove all subcutaneous tissue. The skin graft can be placed over intact periosteum or can be grafted directly to exposed bone. In this case, a burr can be used to burr down the bone until punctate vessels are seen. The graft is then secured with a bolster dressing and left intact for 7 to 10 days.
- Neck skin defects can almost always be closed with adjacent tissue transfer reconstruction as described earlier.

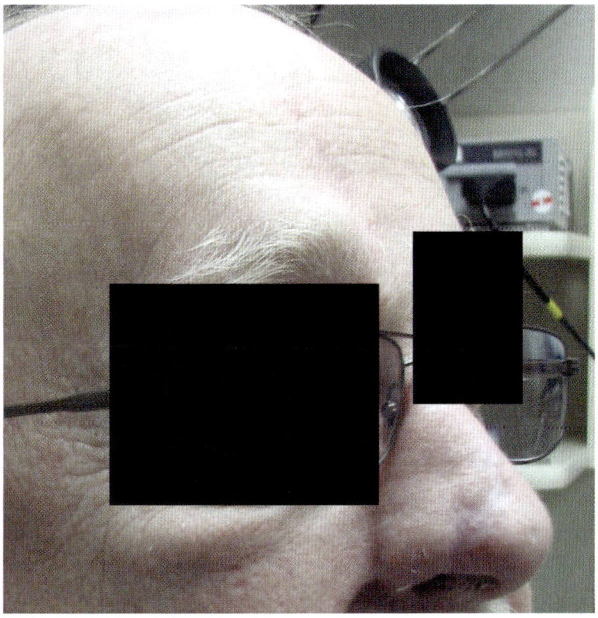

FIG 26 • Postoperative result after paramedian forehead flap reconstruction of right lateral nasal wall and alar rim with use of ear cartilage grafting to alar rim (lateral view).

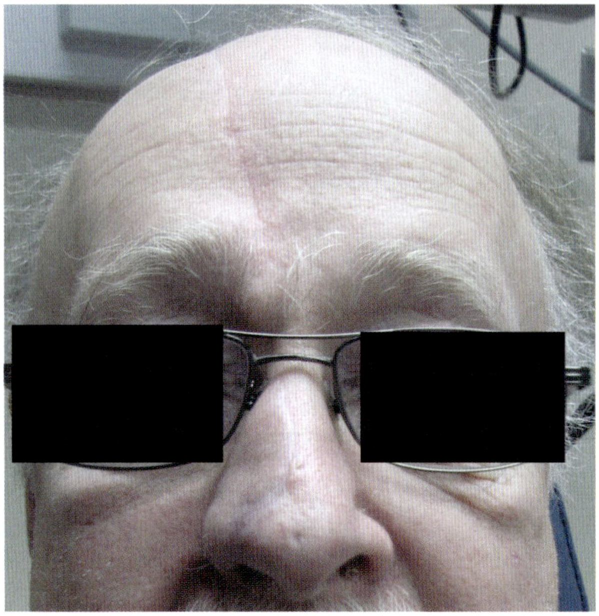

FIG 27 ● Postoperative result after paramedian forehead flap reconstruction of right lateral nasal wall and alar rim with use of ear cartilage grafting to alar rim (frontal view).

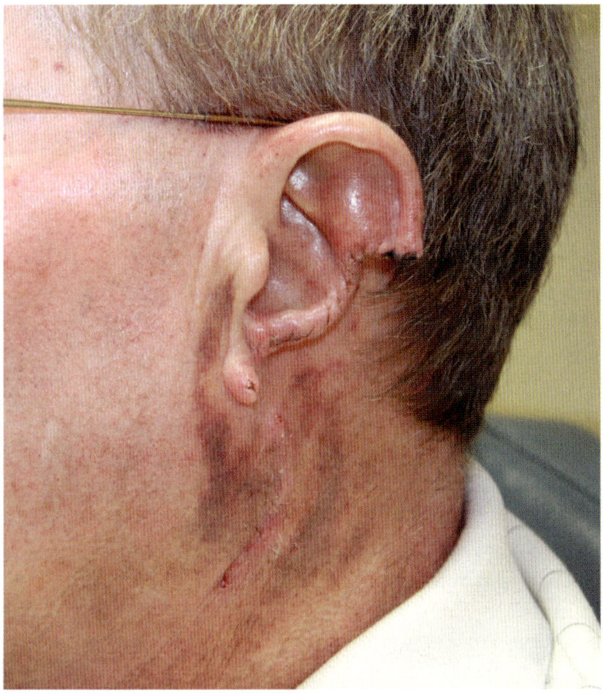

FIG 28 ● Resection of left lower ear and helical rim.

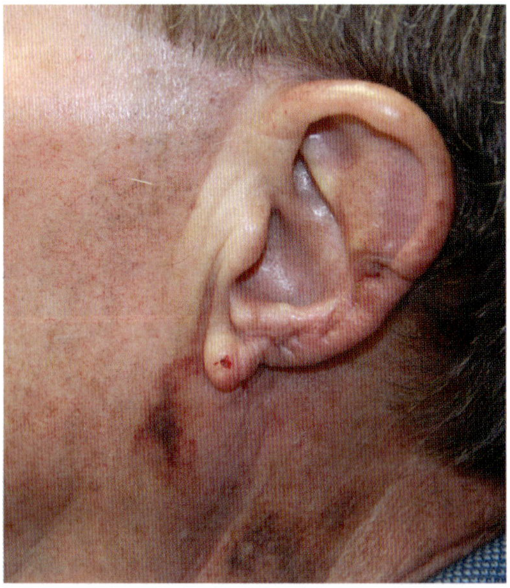

FIG 29 ● Reconstruction of left ear with postauricular transposition flaps.

PEARLS AND PITFALLS

Indications and preoperative workup	■ A complete history and physical exam should be performed including full body skin check. ■ If SLN biopsy is indicated, lymphoscintigraphy with SPECT-CT imaging should be reviewed prior to surgery. ■ A detailed cranial nerve exam should be completed prior to proceeding with surgery.
Excision of primary lesion	■ The primary lesion should be marked to include any pale, erythematous, or pigmented adjacent skin. One to 2-cm circumferential margins are marked depending of depth of invasion of the primary lesion. ■ The depth of excision needs to include enough normal tissue to ensure complete surgical excision. ■ Mark the specimen with clear orientation sutures to allow for definitive margin analysis.

SLNB	▪ Review preoperative lymphoscintigraphy/SPECT-CT to identify likely sites of SLNs. ▪ Carefully, inject methylene blue dye circumferentially into the dermis surrounding the primary lesion. ▪ Ensure anesthesia has not paralyzed the patient prior to lymph node surgery. ▪ Make incisions along relaxed skin tension lines and keep in mind the possible need for rotation advancement flap reconstruction or future parotid/neck dissection incisions. ▪ Use the intraoperative gamma probe to localize SLNs and make sure that all potential SLNs are removed.
Closure vs. delayed reconstruction	▪ If wound can be closed by simple advancement flap without reorienting margins, then wound can be closed primarily. ▪ If rotation/transposition flap or skin graft is needed, it may be wise to delay reconstruction until final surgical margins are clear. ▪ Facial plastic and oculoplastic colleagues should be consulted for closure of complex wounds.

POSTOPERATIVE CARE

- Small pressure dressings are usually applied to small advancement flap reconstruction sites as well as SLN biopsy sites and are left intact for 24 hours. Larger cervicofacial advancement flap reconstruction sites are dressed with Jobst pressure dressings and are left intact for 2 to 3 days. When the dressings are removed, the incisions should be kept clean with half-strength peroxide and moist with Vaseline. Topical antibiotic ointment may be used for 2 to 3 days but can cause skin irritation with longer use. When skin grafts are used, the bolster dressing is left intact for 7 to 10 days. After the bolster is removed, the graft is kept moist with Vaseline for 1 to 2 weeks or until the wound has completely healed.

OUTCOMES

- In the hands of experienced head and neck surgeons, an SLN can be identified in nearly all patients. In patients with cutaneous melanoma of the head and neck with Breslow depth of 1 mm or greater or with Breslow depth between 0.75 mm and 0.99 mm with other adverse features, approximately 20% are found to have a positive SLN. Upon completion lymphadenectomy, 25% of patients with a positive SLN will have at least one more positive non-SLN. Approximately 4% of patients with negative SLNs will fail regionally within the sentinel node basin.[2]
- Positive SLN status is the factor most strongly associated with decreased recurrence-free survival (hazard ratio [HR] 4.23) and decreased overall survival (HR 3.33).[2] The estimated 4-year overall survival approaches 84% in patients with negative SLN biopsy and decreases to an estimated 58% in patients with a positive SLN.[2]

COMPLICATIONS

- Seroma or hematoma at the SLN biopsy site
- Infection at either the SLNB or primary resection site
- Wound dehiscence or epidermolysis of rotation flap reconstruction site
- Decrease in sensation at either surgical site
- Theoretical risk of cranial nerve injury
- Poor cosmetic outcome

REFERENCES

1. Bichakjian CK, Halpern AC, Johnson TM, et al. Guidelines of care for the management of primary cutaneous melanoma. *J Am Acad Dermatol.* 2011;65:1032–1047.
2. Erman AM, Collar RM, Griffith KA, et al. Sentinel lymph node biopsy is accurate and prognostic in head and neck melanoma. *Cancer.* 2012; 118:1040–1047.
3. Gershenwald JE, Thompson W, Mansfield PF, et al. Multi-institutional melanoma lymphatic mapping experience: the prognostic value of sentinel lymph node status in 612 stage I or II melanoma patients. *J Clin Oncol.* 1999;17(3):976–983.
4. Kupferman ME, Kubik MW, Bradford CR, et al. The role of sentinel lymph node biopsy for thin cutaneous melanomas of the head and neck. *Am J Otolaryngol.* 2014;35:226–232.
5. Morton DL, Thompson JF, Cochran AJ, et al. Sentinel-node biopsy or nodal observation in melanoma. *N Engl J Med.* 2006;355(13): 1307–1317.
6. Schmalbach CE, Johnson TM, Bradford CR. The management of head and neck melanoma. *Curr Probl Surg.* 2006;43:781–835.
7. Zender C, Guo T, Weng C, et al. Utility of SPECT/CT for periparotid sentinel lymph node mapping in the surgical management of head and neck melanoma. *Am J Otolaryngol.* 2014;35:12–18.

Chapter **27** # Sentinel Lymph Node Biopsy for Melanoma

Merrick I. Ross Michael Kim

DEFINITIONS

- The sentinel lymph node(s) are defined as the first nodes to receive direct lymphatic drainage from the cutaneous site of a primary melanoma and therefore the most likely lymph node(s) to harbor microscopic metastases. The technique of lymphatic mapping and sentinel lymph node (SLN) biopsy is used to determine the histologic status of the regional lymph node basin(s) in patients with early-stage (American Joint Committee on Cancer [AJCC] clinical stages I and II) melanoma without performing a formal lymph node dissection. The SLN concept as well as the minimally invasive technique, which initially used intradermal injections of vital blue dye[1] (**FIG 1**) and was later modified with the addition of radiolabeled colloid injections[2,3] at the site of the primary melanoma, was first studied and reported in detail by Morton and colleagues, demonstrating proof of concept in a large group of patients with primary melanoma and clinically negative regional lymph nodes.[1] This and several subsequent studies have confirmed that the lymphatic drainage patterns from specific regions of the skin can be accurately determined, the SLN is the most likely first site of regional lymph node metastasis, and if the SLN is histologically negative, the remaining lymph nodes in the mapped basin are unlikely to contain disease.

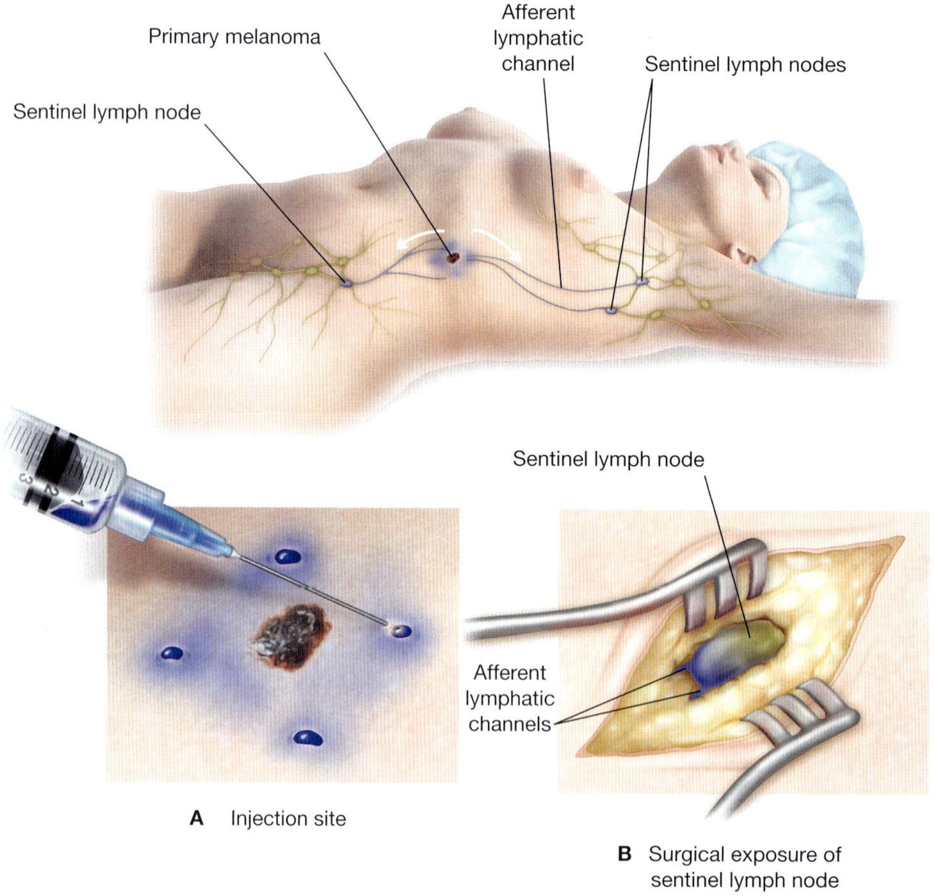

FIG 1 • Sentinel node localization using blue dye injections. An artistic rendition of the sentinel node concept and afferent lymphatic drainage patterns is depicted. After the intradermal injection of blue dye around a primary cutaneous melanoma (left abdominal wall, **Panel A**), afferent lymphatic drainage to a left inguinal sentinel lymph node and two left axillary sentinel lymph nodes is shown. **Panel B** shows surgical exposure, using a self-retaining retractor, of the first of two sentinel nodes in the left axilla. Note the two afferent lymphatic vessels entering the sentinel node. Both nodes in the axilla would be defined as "sentinel" because they each receive first (primary) echelon drainage from a specific afferent lymphatic vessel. Both nodes need to be removed from the axilla as well as the SLN in the groin to complete the surgical procedure of SLN biopsy.

The reported accuracy (sensitivity) of SLN biopsy is 95%.[1,3–5] The term "biopsy" is perhaps a misnomer (particularly to patients) because the biopsy procedure is excisional in nature in that the entire SLN is removed and subjected to rigorous histologic analysis. Alternatively, the term "sentinel lymphadenectomy" can be used to define the surgical procedure.

CLINICAL IMPORTANCE

- Improving outcomes: The sobering reality is that once patients with melanoma develop clinically apparent (palpable) nodal disease (advanced AJCC stage III), the risk of subsequent distant stage IV disease and recurrent lymph node basin disease, despite a complete therapeutic lymphadenectomy, is at least 50%[6] and 15% to 50%,[7] respectively. Therefore, the original motivation to study SLN biopsy was to establish an effective method of identifying and then treating lymph node disease early when microscopic, an approach termed "selective lymphadenectomy," not to be confused with the aforementioned "sentinel lymphadenectomy," which refers specifically to the SLN biopsy procedure. Such an approach would prevent the development of clinically palpable nodal disease and in turn improve the outcomes for the node-positive patients in terms of both regional disease control and survival. The collective experience with SLN biopsy demonstrates that these two goals have been accomplished.[8,9]
- Staging and reducing morbidity: The stages I and II melanoma patient population represent at least 85% of the newly diagnosed patients. The prognosis of this group is very heterogeneous and dependent on a variety of primary tumor factors, specifically tumor thickness, ulceration, and mitotic rate, and probably most importantly, the presence of occult lymph node involvement.[10] The role of SLN biopsy as a staging tool has been well established, as several published multivariable analyses demonstrate that the histologic status of the SLN is the strongest independent predictor of survival for stages I and II melanoma and therefore offers another motivation for SLN biopsy.[10,11] The procedure is also intended to identify patients with pathologically node-negative disease for whom additional surgery is not indicated and adjuvant systemic therapy may not be of benefit, sparing these patients the morbidity of unnecessary surgery and treatment-related toxicities.
- SLN biopsy is now accepted as a standard of care[12,13] in the surgical management of appropriately selected melanoma patients. Central to the success of this minimally invasive approach, and in turn achieving the earlier described staging and treatment goals, is the consistent and accurate identification and complete removal of the SLN(s).
- Although in simplest terms SLN biopsy is a straightforward surgical procedure, in reality, the overall approach integrates several necessary components: identification of the appropriate candidates, careful physical examination of the potential nodal basins at risk, preoperative assessment of the lymphatic drainage patterns, intraoperative localization and removal of all the SLN(s), and careful histologic assessment of the SLN(s).

IDENTIFYING THE APPROPRIATE CANDIDATES

- Primary invasive cutaneous melanoma: The selection criteria for identifying the appropriate candidates for SLN biopsy is based on the predicted risk for the presence of microscopic lymph node involvement for those patients with newly diagnosed primary melanoma and clinically negative nodes. This is best determined by the various primary tumor factors inclusive of tumor thickness, ulceration,[14] and mitotic rate, which define the five AJCC stages I and II substages of primary melanoma.[10] The consensus recommendations are to offer SLN biopsy to any patient with a thickness of 1 mm or greater as long as they are safe operative candidates. SLN biopsy should also be strongly considered in any patient with a thickness of 0.7 to 0.99 mm, particularly if they have at least one of the following adverse prognostic features: Clark level IV or V, one mitotic figure or more per square millimeter, and lymphovascular invasion or microsatellites.[12,15–17] For patients with a thickness of less than 0.76 mm, SLN can be considered if, based on other adverse risk factors, a risk of 8% to 10% of SLN involvement is anticipated. This, however, would be a minority of patients in this subset.[14] Although these patients represent the vast majority who will be offered an SLN biopsy, a variety of other clinical scenarios are encountered with some frequency where SLN may also be considered. These scenarios are described in the 6 bulleted points that follow directly.
- Primary melanoma in an ambiguous (unpredictable) lymphatic drainage site (i.e., head and neck or trunk location) and proven synchronous nodal involvement in at least one, but not all, of the potential regional lymph node basins at risk: These patients may be candidates for SLN biopsy to stage the other regional nodal basins proven to receive direct lymphatic drainage from the primary site but without clinical nodal involvement. Generally speaking, these patients will undergo treatment of the primary melanoma and the involved nodal basin with a wide excision and formal therapeutic lymphadenectomy in the same operative setting. In the event that preoperative lymphoscintigraphy (**FIG 2**) demonstrates lymphatic drainage to an additional but clinically negative regional nodal basin, SLN biopsy

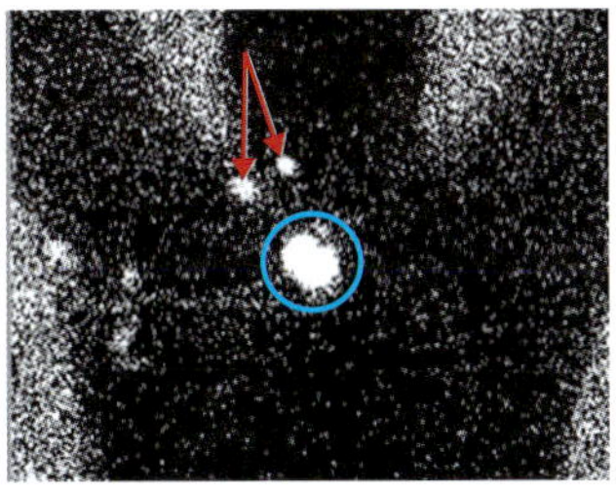

FIG 2 • Lymphoscintigraphy showing lymphatic drainage to more than one nodal basin. An anterior–posterior view of a lymphoscintigraphy is shown, demonstrating lymphatic drainage from a primary melanoma site *(blue circle)* in an ambiguous (unpredictable) drainage location. Afferent drainage is seen to the right axilla and right neck *(red arrows)*. This patient presented with a newly diagnosed melanoma in the right midback. Palpable nodes were appreciated on physical exam in the right axilla; an ultrasound-guided fine needle aspiration confirmed metastatic disease. The neck was clinically uninvolved by palpation and ultrasound. The patient underwent surgery with curative intent, which included a right axillary dissection, wide excision of the primary site, and an SLN biopsy in the right neck. Final pathology showed micrometastatic disease in both SLNs removed.

can also be performed at the same time in an attempt to be inclusive in the treatment of all nodal disease, both macro- and microscopic.

- Mucosal melanoma: Patients with primary mucosal melanomas that are in locations with easy access for direct injection with the SLN localizing agents, conjunctival and anorectal in particular, can be candidates for SLN biopsy as part of their initial surgical management strategy. Although specific primary tumor criteria for these lesions are not well established for predicting the presence of occult regional node involvement, these tumors are most often diagnosed late and likely to have a high enough inherent risk to consider SLN biopsy.
- True locally recurrent melanoma: Some patients develop recurrent melanoma at the edge of a previous wide excision site and may have one of the following three histologic features: in situ disease alone, in situ disease plus an invasive component, or invasive (dermal) component only. All three of these events are likely the result of an inadequate wide excision and an undetected positive margin and therefore represent a "true" local recurrence and have a good chance for long-term survival with surgical treatment. Most of these patients have clinically negative nodes, and in the context of a recurrent invasive component with the appropriate tumor characteristics (see earlier discussion), it is rational to offer these patients an SLN biopsy as a part of the definitive surgical therapy.
- Limited satellite/in-transit metastases: In contrast to the patients with "true" locally recurrent disease, these patients represent manifestations of the biologic disease continuum of regional cutaneous metastases (stage III). Not infrequently, these patients will present with clinically negative regional lymph nodes, stage IIIb. If the extent of the regionally metastatic disease is limited (one or two lesions), a surgical approach to the recurrence is rational. The presence of synchronous microscopic nodal disease not only impacts disease stage, advancing to IIIc and therefore the prognosis, but also the treatment strategies. Therefore, SLN biopsy could also be used in this clinical scenario in conjunction with the resection of the recurrence(s).
- After a wide excision: It is typical and preferable that the SLN biopsy be performed together in a single operative setting in conjunction with the definitive wide excision of the primary melanoma following a diagnostic incisional or excisional biopsy. Occasionally, a patient will have undergone a formal wide excision of the primary melanoma site and then be referred for consideration of an SLN biopsy. A theoretical concern is that the lymphatic drainage pattern of the skin brought together to close the surgical defect or surrounding a skin graft reconstruction has either been altered by the surgery or is far enough away from the original primary lesion that it may not accurately reflect that of the removed skin that was directly adjacent to the primary melanoma, resulting in the identification and removal of the wrong SLN(s). A few publications have put most of these concerns to rest. The data shows that although more afferent lymphatic vessels are likely to be accessed because of the broadened area injected, leading to more SLNs being removed and even the possibility of additional nodal basins explored in sites of ambiguous drainage (trunk and head and neck), the correct SLNs will likely be among the specimens removed, providing accurate nodal staging information.[18] As long as complex rotational flaps were not used for the reconstruction, SLN can be recommended to patients when this clinical setting is encountered.
- Prior surgery in a nodal basin: Occasionally, a primary melanoma will be diagnosed in a location with predicted or possible lymphatic drainage to a regional nodal basin in which surgical intervention has previously been performed, such as an SLN biopsy or lymph node dissection, as treatment for a previous melanoma or other malignancies. An SLN biopsy may still be possible, but a preoperative lymphoscintigraphy is mandated to determine how the lymphatic drainage has been affected or altered by the previous nodal surgery. Lymphatic drainage patterns may be demonstrated in one or more of the remaining nodes (if any exist) in the previously treated basin or diverted to another basin. This information is critical for appropriate surgical planning and operative positioning.

PATIENT HISTORY AND PHYSICAL FINDINGS

- Pertinent information such as a prior personal history of melanoma or other malignancies and current or recent symptoms referable to the presence of metastatic disease should be elicited from the patient during the history.
- Questions about allergic reactions to antibiotics, sulfa in particular, and intravenous (IV) contrast agents should be documented as this information may suggest an increased risk of an allergic reaction to the isosulfan blue dye and therefore may influence the decision to use a different blue dye such as methylene blue or not use any blue dye at all for the SLN procedure (see more details in the following text).
- A thorough head-to-toe skin examination should be performed with the intent of identifying additional suspicious lesions that could represent another primary melanoma or other skin cancers. Diagnostic full-thickness punch or excisional biopsies should be performed on selected lesions.
- Special attention should be paid to the region of the index melanoma. Visual inspection as well as palpation of the biopsy site and surrounding skin and soft tissues should be performed to determine the presence of any residual primary disease and/or satellite and in-transit metastases.
- Skin and soft tissues between the primary lesion and draining lymph node basins should be palpated and closely examined for in-transit disease. All suspicious cutaneous and subcutaneous lesions may undergo fine needle aspiration for pathologic diagnosis.
- All potential regional lymph node basins should be palpated for the presence of clinically apparent disease. This examination should include the epitrochlear and popliteal minor nodal basins when the primary melanoma is located distal to the elbow and knee, respectively.
- Palpable lymph nodes suspicious for metastatic disease should be assessed by either direct fine needle aspiration or further examined with ultrasound and biopsied with ultrasound guidance if confirmed to be radiographically suspicious. Such data may obviate the need for SLN biopsy in that basin and instead invoke a formal radiographic staging evaluation prior to carrying out a therapeutic lymph node dissection of the affected lymph node basin(s).

HISTOLOGIC EVALUATION OF THE PRIMARY MELANOMA

- An experienced dermatopathologist should review all pathology slides related to the melanocytic lesion in question to both confirm the diagnosis of melanoma as well as to provide the microstaging (tumor thickness, ulceration status, and mitotic rate) information and other relevant adverse histologic features (see earlier discussion).
- The decision to proceed with an SLN biopsy should be based on the earlier described established criteria. In some situations, however, the primary lesion is essentially intact and the diagnostic biopsy represents only a small sampling of the entire lesion or very superficial in depth. This type of biopsy may accurately render a definitive diagnosis of melanoma but may lack the histologic features needed to recommend an SLN biopsy. In this situation, the entire lesion should be narrowly removed as an excisional biopsy for complete histologic evaluation.

PREOPERATIVE RADIOGRAPHIC STUDIES

- Although *symptom-directed* preoperative radiographic imaging is a good practice in patients with newly diagnosed melanomas, generally speaking, most newly diagnosed early stage patients are asymptomatic; therefore, no special radiographic imaging is required or recommended prior to performing an SLN biopsy for most primary melanoma patients.[19] In the asymptomatic patient, extensive radiographic staging is more likely to result in false-positive rather than true positive findings. One possible exception would be the patients with both very thick (>4 mm) and ulcerated primary lesions. Many surgeons would obtain complete radiographic staging inclusive of computed tomography (CT) of chest/abdomen/pelvis or positron emission tomography (PET) scan and magnetic resonance imaging (MRI) of the brain routinely for this high-risk group.[19]
- In contrast, in patients with a locally metastatic lesion or a limited number of in-transit metastases for whom an SLN biopsy is being considered as part of the definitive surgical management, a thorough preoperative radiographic staging evaluation should be performed.[19]
- As mentioned earlier, ultrasound examination should be performed in patients with suspicious palpable nodes. Furthermore, ultrasound evaluation of the regional nodal basins should also be used as an adjunct to physical examination particularly of the axilla, in obese patients, with thick and ulcerated melanomas to evaluate for the presence of macroscopically involved nodes. In these situations, the sensitivity of physical examination is low and the risk of harboring synchronous macroscopically involved nodes is relatively high. Ultrasound examination suspicious for nodal involvement can be confirmed with an ultrasound-guided fine needle aspiration (**FIG 3**).
- The success of any SLN program is dependent on the preoperative determination of the lymphatic drainage patterns from the primary melanoma site. Although the nodal basins at risk in extremity melanomas are relatively predictable, such is not the case for head and neck and trunk melanomas where lymphatic drainage patterns are considered ambiguous or unpredictable. Preoperative identification of lymphatic drainage patterns is accomplished with *lymphoscintigraphy*.[20,21]

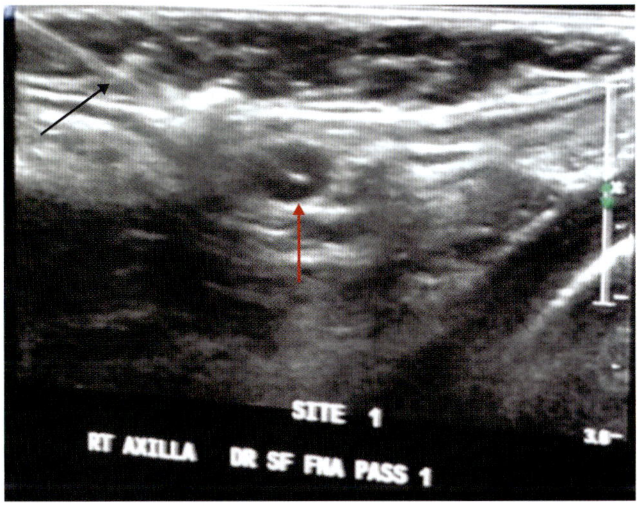

FIG 3 • Ultrasound-guided fine needle aspiration of a suspicious nonpalpable lymph node. A static ultrasound image of biopsy needle *(black arrow)* within the node *(red arrow)* is shown.

PREOPERATIVE LYMPHOSCINTIGRAPHY

- Once the decision is made to perform an SLN biopsy, the most important preoperative decision is whether or not to perform a lymphoscintigraphy.
- The technique of cutaneous lymphoscintigraphy provides an objective description of the lymphatic drainage pattern from a primary cutaneous lesion to the nodal basin(s) that receive direct afferent lymphatic drainage. Through the use of external gamma camera images, the migration of the radioactive tracer that is injected intradermally (where the invasive melanoma cells are located) at the site of the primary tumor can be visualized to determine the following: (1) the major lymph node basin(s) receiving direct lymphatic drainage, (2) number and relative location of sentinel nodes within the basin, and (3) the existence and location of SLN(s) located outside of a formal lymph node basin, referred to as either "interval" or "in-transit" SLNs that are located in the subcutaneous tissues between the primary tumor and the formal nodal basin or *ectopic* in completely unpredicted anatomic locations.[22] The lymphatic drainage patterns mimic how melanoma cells metastasize within the lymphatic compartment. Approximately 5% to 10% of the time, an interval or in-transit SLN pattern will be identified during lymphoscintigraphy on the trunk; these nodes are just as likely to be involved with metastatic disease as the SLNs in the formal nodal basins.[22] **FIG 4** provides a simplified schematic of potential lymphatic drainage patterns.
- Two radiopharmaceutical agents are now available in the United States to be used for lymphoscintigraphy and for intraoperative SLN localization, both using a dose of 0.5 to 1.0 mCi of the radiotracer technetium-99m. Radiolabelled sulfur colloid has been the historical standard and is still used commonly, to date, but not specifically approved for

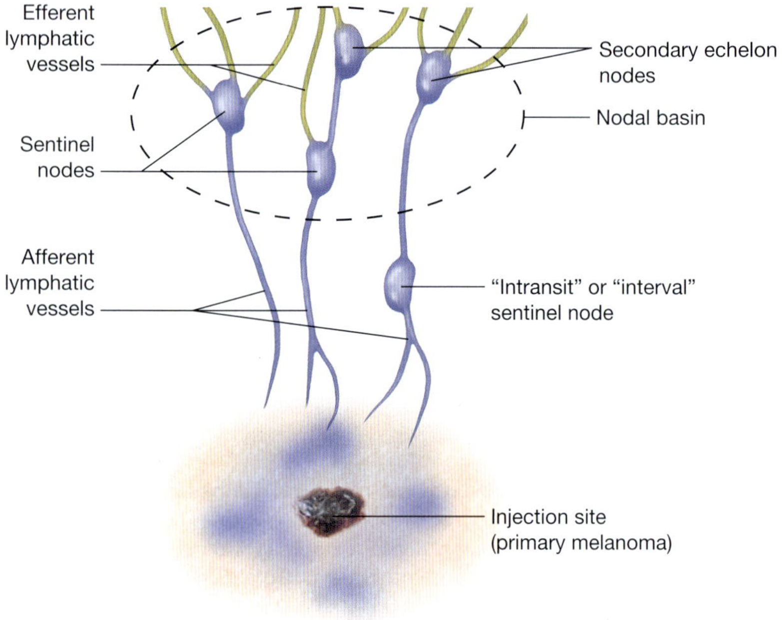

FIG 4 • Lymphatic drainage patterns. A schematic of potential lymphatic drainage patterns from the primary site to the regional nodal basin is shown. The first (primary echelon) node of drainage from a specific afferent lymphatic vessel is defined as an SLN. Up- or downstream drainage from the SLN to another node via efferent lymphatic vessels are considered secondary echelon nodes. Occasionally, primary lymphatic drainage is to a lymph node proximal to the formal basin in the subcutaneous tissue and termed as either an "interval" or "in-transit" SLN.

this use. Recently, the U.S. Food and Drug Administration (FDA) has approved the use of Tilmanocept,[23] which is a formulation of a dextran framework with several attached mannose residues and a technetium-99m binding site.

- In theory, the sulfur colloid particles migrate from the injection site through the afferent lymphatic vessels and are actively taken up by the macrophages in the first draining nodes (the sentinel nodes). Similarly, Tilmanocept migrates to the sentinel nodes from the injection site but is then covalently bound to the macrophages in the sentinel node as a result of the mannose residues, limiting significant pass through to secondary echelon nodes.
- Two types of images can be created. The routine examination is termed "planar" and provides images in two perpendicular planes: posterior–anterior (P-A) and/or anterior–posterior (A-P), or both, and lateral views[20] (**FIG 5**). These images visualize the injection site, the afferent lymphatic channels, and the accumulation of the radiotracer in the SLNs. The A-P and P-A views give the clinician medial and lateral as well as superior–inferior orientations, whereas the lateral views provide anterior and posterior localizations and also superior–inferior localizations. A transmission scan adds the contour of the body to the image and provides additional anatomic localizing information. When radioactive tracer injection sites (primary melanoma site) overlies or is in close proximity to a draining lymph node basin in at least one visual plane, the radioactivity in the sentinel node will not be visualized in that plane. Perpendicular images are necessary in order to visualize the sentinel activity separate from the injection site activity.

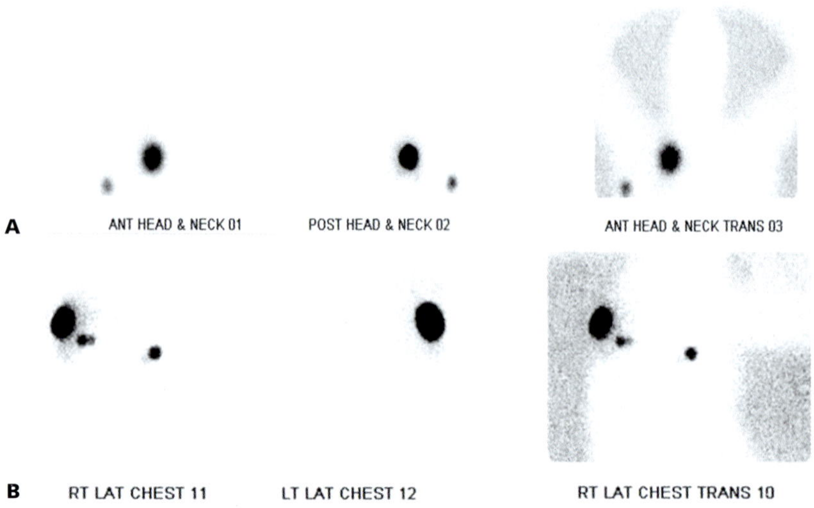

FIG 5 • Planar lymphoscintigraphy. Typical example of a cutaneous lymphatic drainage scan, obtained by injecting the technetium-99m–labelled tracer in the intradermal location at the primary melanoma site, is shown. The injection site, the afferent lymphatic vessels, and the SLNs in the regional basin nodal are visualized. A-P and P-A **(A)** as well as right and left lateral images **(B)** are taken to visualize the drainage pattern in perpendicular visual planes. The last image in both rows is the transmission scan that outlines the contour of the body to facilitate anatomic localization.

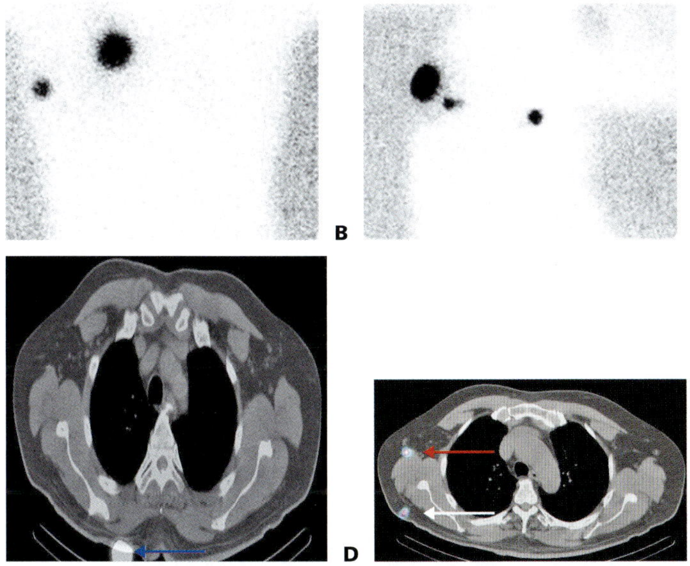

FIG 6 • SPECT-CT lymphoscintigraphy. Planar lymphoscintigraphy of primary melanoma is shown in the top row, with anterior view in **(A)** and lateral view in **(B)**. Selected SPECT-CT images of the same patient are seen in the bottom row. Only the axillary SLN is seen in **(A)** and an additional SLN is seen in **(B)**, which was obscured by the overlying activity transmitted to the axilla from the injection site. The additional SLN in **(B)** is likely an in-transit node, the exact anatomic location of which is better visualized in the transaxial view of the SPECT-CT image in **(D)**. In **(C)**, the *blue arrow* indicates the injection site and in **(D)**, a few cross-sectional images inferior the *white arrow* identifies the in-transit SLN and the *red arrow* the axillary SLN, both of which are located in the same A-P visual plane.

- More recently, single-photon emission computed tomography–computed tomography (SPECT-CT) lymphoscintigraphy[21] has been developed, providing more exact anatomic localizations. With this method, serial cross-sectional, axial, coronal, and sagittal images are obtained and fused with the nuclear images. Relatively precise locations of the SLN and injection sites can be accomplished and is therefore particularly helpful in primary tumor locations such in the head and neck regions where multiple SLNs may be present or in locations where the potential nodal basins, and therefore the SLNs, may be in close proximity to the injection's site and lie within one of the same visual planes as the injection's site. In this latter situation, the SLN radioactivity will be obscured by activity within the injection site in one or more planes and therefore possibly go undetected on a "planar" study. Although obtaining a perpendicular image may visualize the SLN activity in a different line of sight, as described earlier, the SPECT-CT provides consistent three-dimensional imaging. The SPECT-CT images are also better at determining the presence of and delineating the location of interval or in-transit SLNs (**FIGS 6** and **7**).
- In the management of primary tumors located in cutaneous regions predicted to have ambiguous lymphatic drainage, such as in the head and neck and trunk, a preoperative lymphoscintigraphy is mandated. The extent of ambiguous cutaneous lymphatic drainage includes a very large area of the trunk and head and neck regions and is underestimated by the original classic descriptions of lymphatic drainage patterns. **FIG 8** illustrates the actual regions of ambiguous drainage. **FIG 9** demonstrates an example of ambiguous drainage.
- For extremity lesions, a formal lymphoscintigraphy is not essential as the basins at risk are predictable and intraoperative scanning can be performed with the handheld gamma probe. Some clinicians, however, will obtain a preoperative study for extremity lesions as well, particularly if the primary tumor is located distal to the knee or elbow to have a preoperative assessment for the presence of popliteal (**FIG 10**) or epitrochlear drainage patterns. Even in the proximal extremity locations, a preoperative lymphoscintigraphy can provide useful information in determining whether any upstream drainage from the thigh to the pelvis or the upper arm to the neck is primary (sentinel) or secondary echelon.
- Whereas some clinicians will schedule the lymphoscintigraphy on a day prior to the surgical procedure, others will obtain the study on the day of the surgery. In the latter scenario, the injection of the technetium-99m–labeled radiotracer that is used for the scan can be used for the gamma probe–directed intraoperative localization of the SLN. Because the half-life of technetium-99m is only 6 hours, when the lymphoscintigraphy is performed on a day remote from the surgery, another injection is required on the day of surgery unless a larger (three times) dose of the radiotracer is given the evening before the surgery.
- The lymphoscintigraphic images should be viewed by the surgeon and displayed in the operating room (OR) at the time of the SLN biopsy surgery to facilitate operative positioning, the intraoperative identification of the SLNs, and subsequent removal of all of the SLNs.

SURGICAL MANAGEMENT

Preoperative Planning

- Except in situations when the patient has already undergone a wide excision of the primary melanoma and then is referred for SLN biopsy, the SLN biopsy is carried out in the same operative setting as the definitive wide excision of the primary site.
- The surgery is performed as a day surgery, most conveniently in an ambulatory OR setting, under general anesthesia or with local anesthesia supported with intravenous sedation. Therefore, the patient should be nil per os (NPO) after midnight.
- Because frequently the entire index clinical lesion has been removed with either the shave or excisional diagnostic biopsy, identifying the correct site at the time of

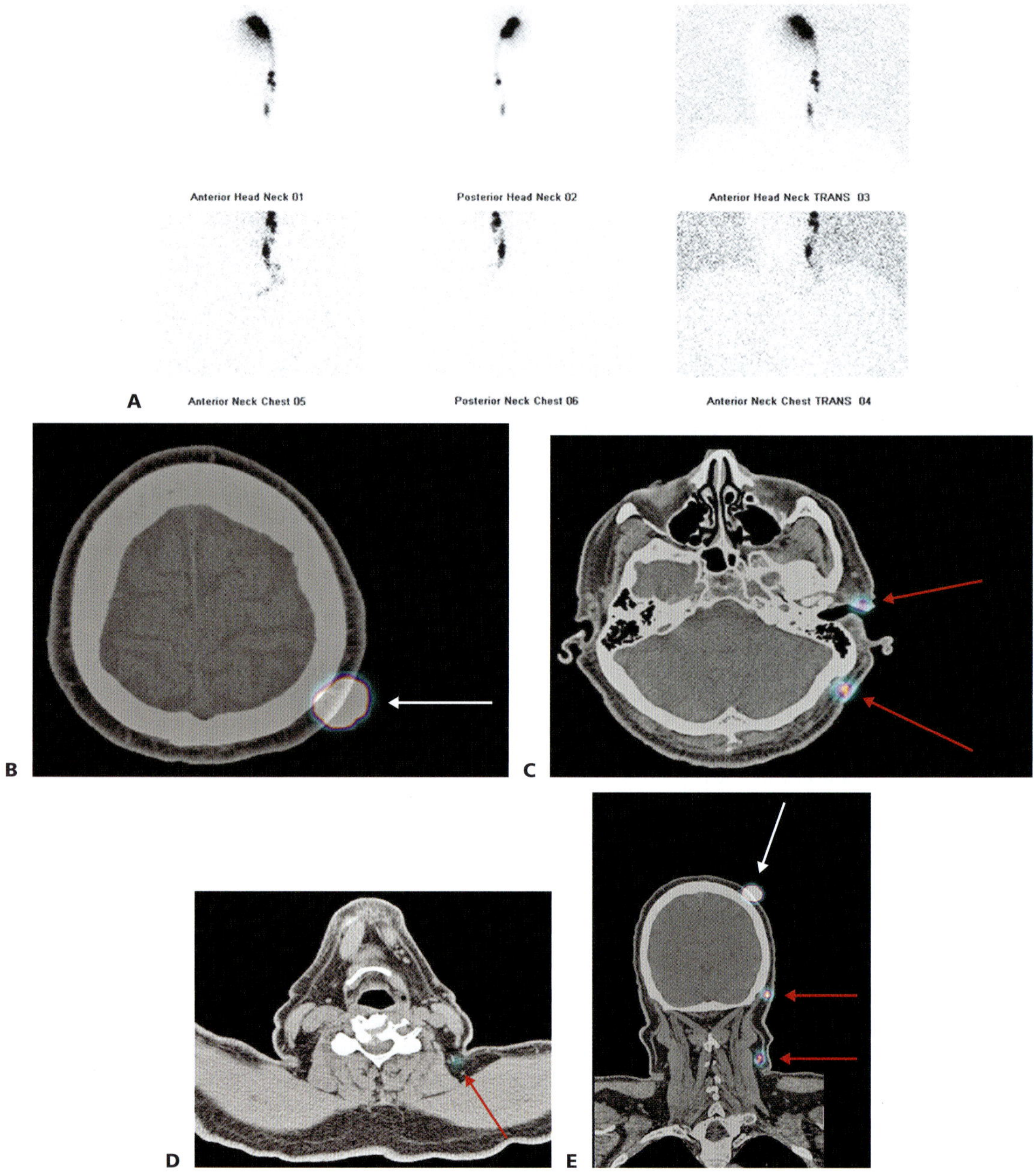

FIG 7 • SPECT-CT lymphoscintigraphy. Planar lymphoscintigraphy of a primary melanoma on the left scalp is shown in **(A)**, demonstrating multiple SLNs, the anatomic locations of which are difficult to define. In **(B–D)**, the SPECT-CT images are shown, with the *white arrows* indicating the injection site and the *red arrows* the SLNs, providing more exact localization with the use of cross-sectional (**B** and **C**) and coronal views in **(E)**.

lymphoscintigraphy or surgical procedure may be difficult. This is further complicated by the fact that these patients frequently have undergone other biopsies of skin lesions either prior to or at the time of the melanoma diagnosis. Because the accuracy of the SLN biopsy is dependent on injecting the correct site, careful documentation of the primary melanoma biopsy location to be injected should be carried out during the first clinic visit when the decision to perform the SLN biopsy is made. Digital images of this site can be obtained and downloaded in the patient's electronic medical record.

- Once the index lesion has been identified and clearly marked in the preoperative holding area and confirmed by the patient and/or family member, the patient can go to nuclear medicine for the radiotracer injection followed by the lymphoscintigraphy if not already completed on a day remote from the actual surgical procedure. The radiotracer is injected intradermally in the normal skin, just adjacent and as close as possible to the intact residual lesion (if present) or the biopsy site by the radiologist or technician. A four-point injection technique surrounding the lesion is employed with a 30-gauge needle attached to a 1-cc syringe (**FIG 11**).

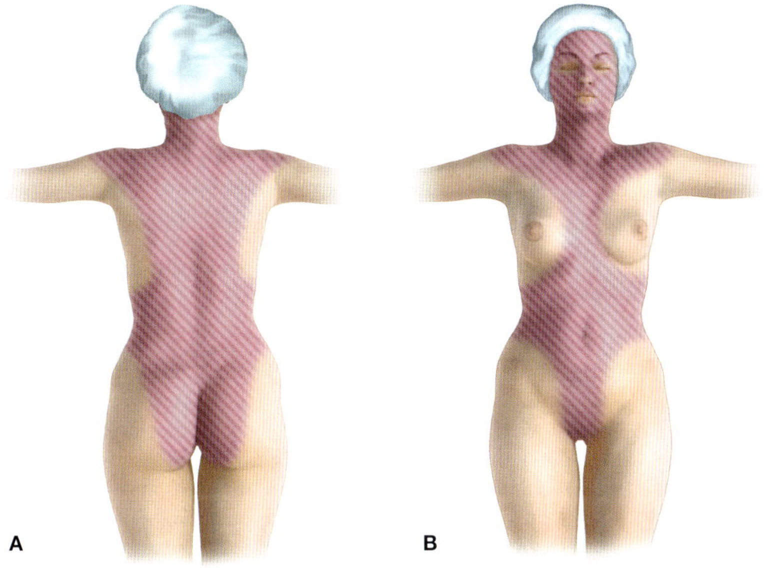

FIG 8 • Areas of ambiguous lymphatic drainage. The regions of ambiguous (unpredictable) cutaneous lymphatic drainage include broad areas of the posterior **(A)** and anterior **(B)** trunk and the entire surface area of the head and neck.

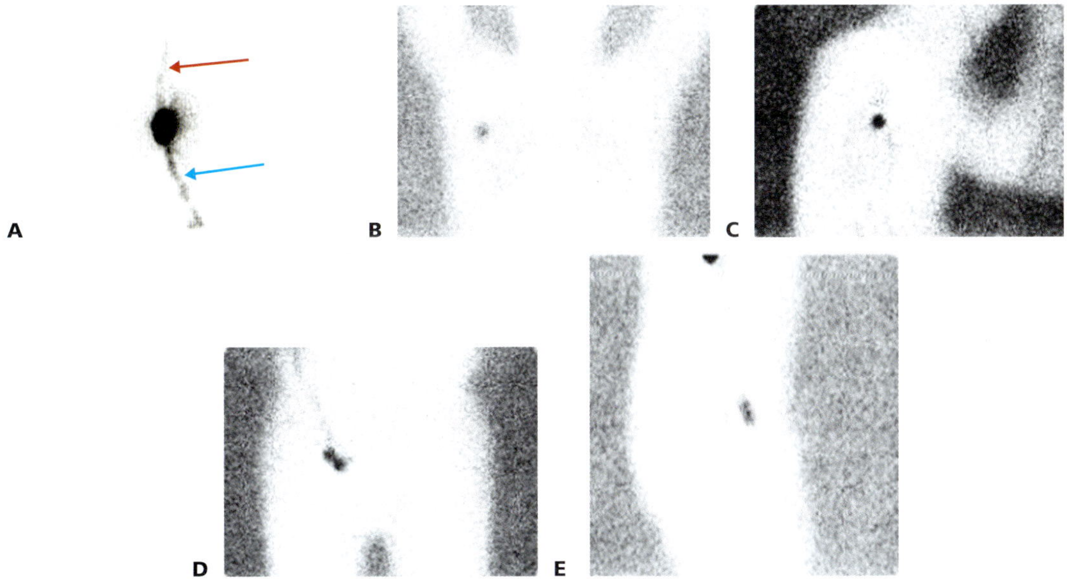

FIG 9 • Ambiguous lymphatic drainage. Lymphoscintigraphy of melanoma on the right flank is displayed. The primary injection site is shown in **(A)**, demonstrating afferent lymphatic vessels draining in a bidirectional fashion to the ipsilateral axilla *(red arrow)* and groin *(blue arrow)*. In **(B)** and **(C)**, the axillary SLN is visualized in two perpendicular planes. In **(D)** and **(E)**, the inguinal SLN is visualized in two perpendicular planes.

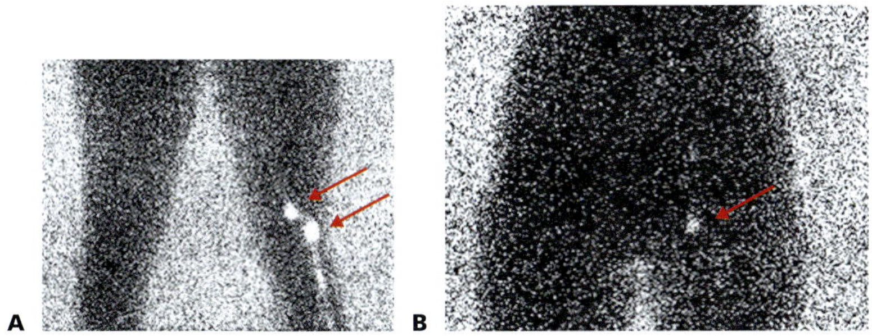

FIG 10 • Visualization of popliteal SLN. Lymphoscintigraphy of melanoma on the plantar surface of the calcaneus demonstrating both popliteal **(A)** and inguinal **(B)** SLNs *(arrows)* is shown.

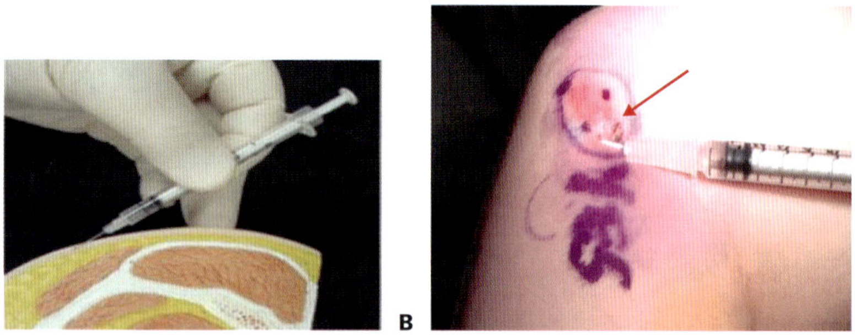

A B

FIG 11 • Radiotracer injection technique. The correct technique and needle location for an intradermal injection is shown using a soft tissue model in **(A)**. An actual intradermal injection of the radiotracer at the primary melanoma site using a 1-cc syringe and a 30-gauge needle is shown in **(B)**. Note the wheal formation *(arrow)* confirming the intradermal location.

The usual dose of the radiotracer is 0.5 to 1 mCi of technetium-99m. For extremity lesions, the surgeon may choose not to obtain a lymphoscintigraphy (see earlier discussion) and have the patient return to the preoperative holding area directly after the injection. Also for extremity primaries, if permissible by the nuclear medicine department and if a lymphoscintigraphy is not going to be obtained, the surgeon can perform the injection of the radiotracer in the OR just prior to injecting the blue dye.

- Generally speaking, scheduling the injection that will be performed by the nuclear medicine staff approximately 1 hour prior to the surgery start time is adequate, but 2 or 3 hours may be required if a SPECT-CT lymphoscintigraphy is planned.
- Open communication with anesthesia personnel should take place prior to arrival in the OR to make sure the IV is placed thoughtfully at a site removed from the planned sites of the surgical procedures.
- The patient should be administered appropriate broad-spectrum antibiotic prophylaxis to reduce the risk of surgical site infection.
- The handheld gamma probe should already be in the OR.
- If the plan is to use the vital blue dye as another SLN localizing agent, this should be drawn up in 1-cc aliquots in the OR prior to the arrival of the patient.

Operative Positioning

- Thoughtful operative positioning is more of an art than a science but is an important step that will reduce operative times, limit the number of position changes, facilitate intraoperative scanning with the handheld gamma probe, and more importantly, optimize the complete identification and removal of all SLNs.
- The lymphoscintigraphic images should be displayed in the OR.
- Once in the OR, the gamma probe is used to transcutaneously scan all the planned nodal basins and SLN locations to be explored to make sure that the radiotracer has migrated. Alternatively, the patient can be scanned with the handheld gamma probe in the holding area prior to entering the OR to make sure the radiotracer has migrated in the event that a lymphoscintigraphy was not performed on the day of the surgery or not needed (i.e., for extremity primary).
- The gamma probe should also be used to scan potential additional sites that may not have been specifically identified on the lymphoscintigraphy, such as in the epitrochlear and popliteal regions for primary lesions distal to the elbow and knee respectively, all of the major regional nodal basins in the neck for head and neck and upper trunk primaries close to the midline, contralateral axilla for mid and upper back and chest lesions close to the midline, contralateral inguinal basin for lower abdomen and lower back primaries close to the midline, and ipsilateral axilla and inguinal regions for lateralized flank primaries. Additional SLN sites may be identified and these findings may influence operative positioning and the regions to be prepped and draped. The arm(s) and leg(s) when performing SLN biopsies in the axillae and groins, respectively, should be circumferentially prepped and draped so position changes can be performed sterilely to facilitate adequate exposure of the lymph node basins intended for biopsy. Moreover, primary lesion(s) intended to undergo wide local excision should also be clearly visible and accessible.
- Whenever possible, patients should be positioned in a way to expose both the SLN and wide excision sites in one supine or lateral position. This will allow one session of prepping and draping and avoid the time it takes to change positions. This can usually be accomplished when the primary lesion is on one of the extremities, anywhere on the trunk or head and neck locations when all of the SLN sites are on the ipsilateral side of the primary, and anywhere on the anterior trunk and anterior head and neck regions even when the draining nodal are bilateral. In contrast, the most problematic locations are posterior neck and trunk lesions close to the midline when bilateral nodal basin (i.e., both axillae, both cervical, or both inguinal) drainage is identified or two or more different basins on opposite sides of the body (i.e., left axilla and right neck) contain SLNs. In these latter scenarios, at least one position change will be required.
- When foot/lower leg cutaneous lesions localize SLN(s) to the popliteal fossae, prone positioning is best suited for such patients for adequate visualization and access to the SLN(s). The patient may then be subsequently repositioned in the supine or lateral decubitus position for excision of corresponding primary lesions if that site is not accessible in the prone position. Another option for this scenario would be to place the patient in the lateral decubitus position, avoiding a position change.
- The patient should also be positioned to facilitate the surgeon in scanning the nodal basin and the intervening tissues with the handheld gamma probe positioned perpendicular to or in a direction pointed away from the injection site to limit the "shine-through" radioactivity emanating from the injection site that may obscure the radioactivity in the SLN and in turn hamper ones ability to discriminate SLN radioactivity from the injection site activity.
- After the patient is positioned, multiple steps are carried out to accomplish a complete and accurate sentinel lymphadenectomy.[24]

INJECTION OF BLUE DYE

- Once the patient is positioned, the vital blue dye is injected at the primary site using a similar four-point intradermal injection technique that was used for injecting the radiotracer. Approximately 2 to 3 cc of blue dye is injected using 1-cc tuberculin syringes and a 25-gauge needle (**FIG 12**).
- Although it is not mandatory that the blue dye be used, most surgeons feel that the two localizing agents complement each other in successfully identifying and removing the SLNs.
- The blue dyes most commonly used are isosulfan blue and methylene blue in the United States and patent Blue V in Europe and Australia. The isosulfan seems to concentrate in the SLNs in a more uniform manner compared to methylene blue, making it easier to visualize. Some surgeons prefer to use methylene blue because of the potential, albeit very low risk, of an allergic reaction to isosulfan blue.[25] However, at least one report documents increased postoperative complications with the use of methylene blue.[26]
- After the blue dye is injected, the patient is then appropriately prepped and draped. The time that transpires during the prepping and draping is long enough for the blue dye to travel through the lymphatic vessels to the SLNs.

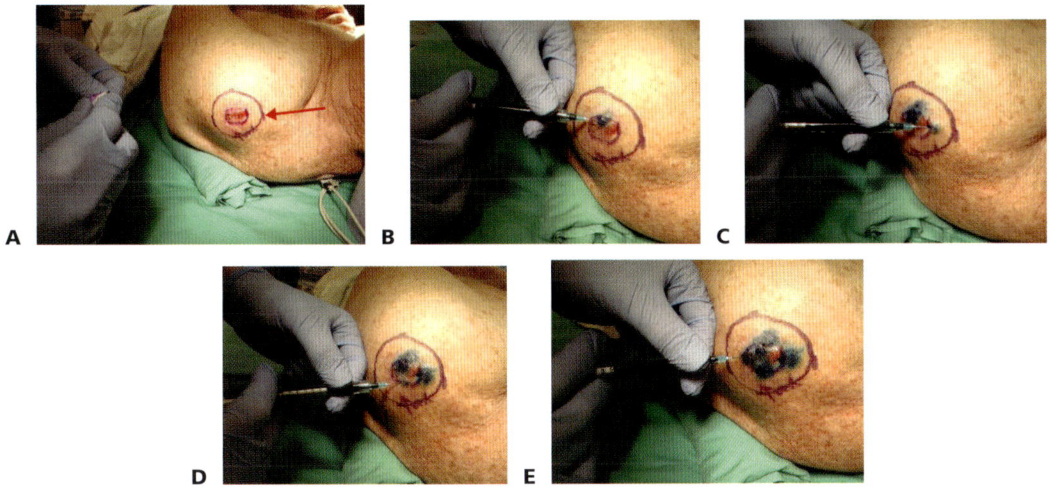

FIG 12 • Blue dye injection technique. The primary melanoma is shown **(A)** with planned margins measured and drawn *(arrow)*. The four-point intradermal injection of the blue dye is shown in images **(B–E)**.

INTRAOPERATIVE LOCALIZATION AND SURGICAL EXCISION OF THE SENTINEL NODES

- Most commonly, both the SLN biopsy and the wide excision of the primary site will be performed in the same operative setting. Generally, if the blue dye is used, the nodal basin exploration and removal of the SLN is approached first in order to take advantage of the visualization of the SLN afforded by the blue dye. If the wide excision is performed first, the blue dye will be removed as well, limiting the continued flow of dye to the SLN and in turn the visualization of the SLN.
- The use of the handheld gamma probe is central to this procedure. The probe is placed within a sterile ultrasound cover after the patient is prepped and draped.
- If the planned wide excision site (injection site) is in close proximity to the nodal basin, the shine-through activity may be greater than the sentinel activity. The following maneuvers are used to discriminate SLN activity from the shine-through activity: As the gamma probe is transcutaneously passed from the injection site to the nodal basin, the counts will diminish in proportion to the distance from the injection site. A sentinel node area is identified when the radioactive counts increase as the probe is moved further away from the injection site compared to a location that is closer to the injection site (**FIG 13**). The radioactive counts should again decrease as the gamma probe is passed further beyond the sentinel node. The use of a removable collimator can be helpful in reducing shine-through activity. Make sure that when passing the probe from the injection site to the nodal basin, the probe is positioned perpendicular to or directed away from the injection site. If none of these maneuvers are successful, the wide excision can then be performed first, which very effectively removes the background shine-through counts. This maneuver will also remove the blue dye and stop the continued flow of dye to the nodal basin and in turn significantly reduce the ability to use the blue dye as an aid in identifying the SLN.
- If the patient is positioned correctly, the surgeon will be able to transcutaneously localize the epicenter of the SLN activity with the handheld gamma (which represents a small percentage of the radioactivity at the injection site)

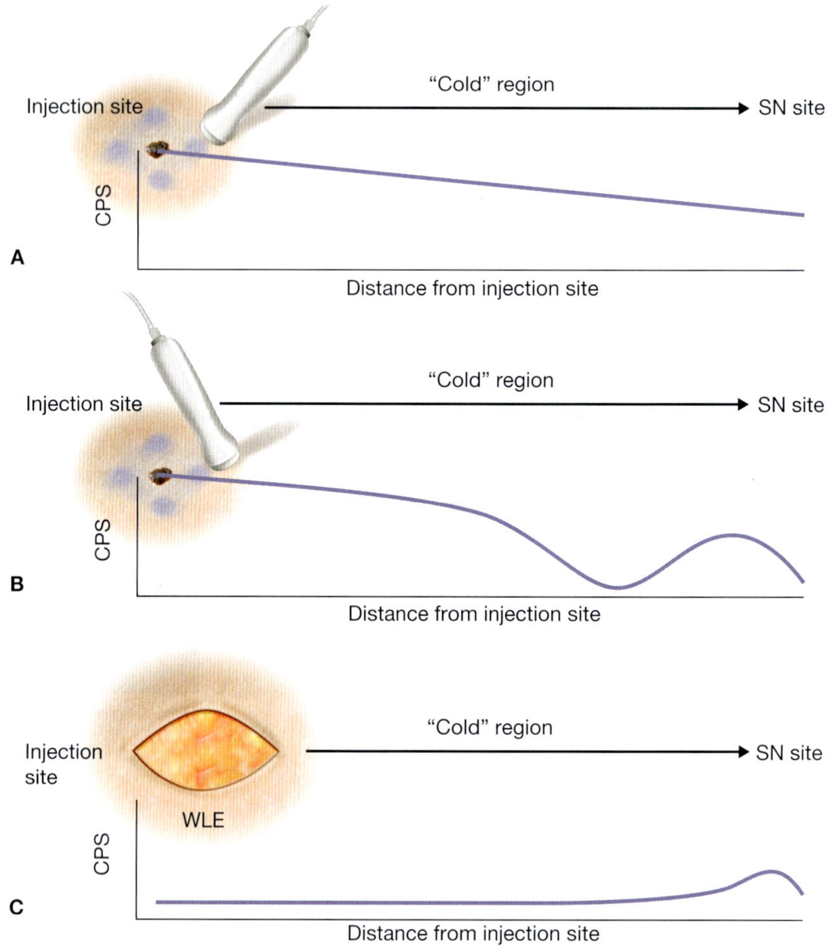

FIG 13 ● Conceptualization of intraoperative SLN scanning. Three conceptual graphs are shown, with the x-axis representing radioactive count per second (CPS) and the y-axis distance of the SLN from the injection site. The amount of radioactivity that travels to the SLN is a small percentage of the radioactivity injected. Shine-through radioactivity from the injection site may obscure the ability to detect to the radioactivity in the SLN, particularly if the injection is close to the nodal basin and/or SLNs. Although placing a collimator on the end of the probe may block out much of the shine-through activity and allow the detection of the SLN, it also narrows the exposed area of radioactivity detection crystal on the probe and in turn reduces the counts detected from the node. In **(A)**, scanning for the SLN is performed with the probe pointed at the injection site. Even though the probe is moving away from the site, shine-through counts detected may be greater than the counts in the SLN, limiting the ability to discriminate SLN activity versus shine-through injection activity. In **(B)**, the same maneuver is performed, now with the probe pointed away from the injection site, allowing the detection of a step-up in activity as one reaches the SLN. In **(C)**, the wide excision has been performed, essentially removing any shine-through activity and in turn facilitating the detection of the SLN activity. This latter maneuver is often used when trying to find the remaining SLNs with less radioactivity after the first, most radioactive SLN has been identified and removed.

within the nodal basin without too much difficulty especially if the injection site is at some distance from the nodal basin (**FIG 14**).

- The epicenter of SLN activity is marked with a sterile marking pen and used for surgical incision planning.
- The nodal basin is approached with a small biopsy incision directed by the handheld gamma probe over the epicenter of radioactivity. We make sure that this biopsy incision can be easily incorporated and excised en bloc as part of a formal lymphadenectomy incision if that is required at a later date should the sentinel node reveal metastases (**FIG 15**).
- The dermis and subcutaneous tissue is divided with cautery, advancing deeper for approximately 1 to 2 cm at a time between pauses during which time the trajectory of the line of dissection toward the radioactive signal may be confirmed with the gamma probe. Using this technique, the surgeon is able to localize and directly advance to the targeted SLN(s) with minimal tissue disruption (**FIG 16**).
- In most situations, the SLNs are deep to the subcutaneous investing fascial layer (i.e., Scarpa's in the groin and platysma in the neck), which needs to be incised in order to enter the nodal basin proper (**FIG 16C**).

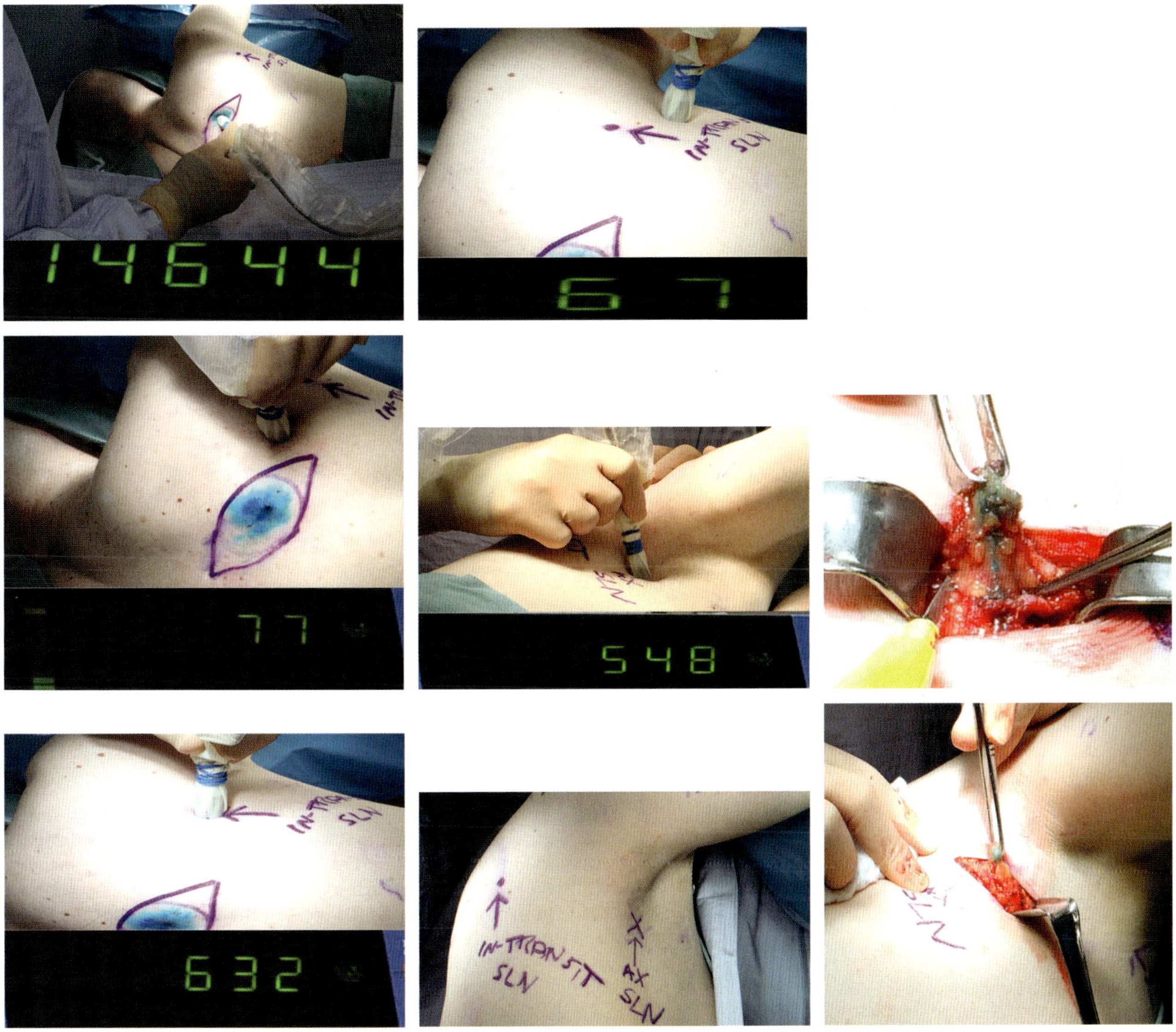

FIG 14 • Thoughtful positioning in the OR. The left lateral position is correctly chosen in this patient with a primary melanoma on the right midback with a lymphoscintigraphy showing drainage to the right axilla and a probable in-transit node over the scapula. This position facilitates not only performing the SLN biopsies and the wide excision without a position change but also scanning for the SLN nodes perpendicular to and directed away from the injection site. Under each frame, the numbers represent the counts per second of radioactivity where the gamma probe is placed. Note that the highest count is over the injection site, then counts decrease moving away from the injection until they increase to identify the in-transit node, then decrease again as the in-transit node is passed, then increase again in the axilla. The last frame in the second column shows the SLN sites marked and in the last column on the right the two frames show the in-transit SLN and the axillary SLN.

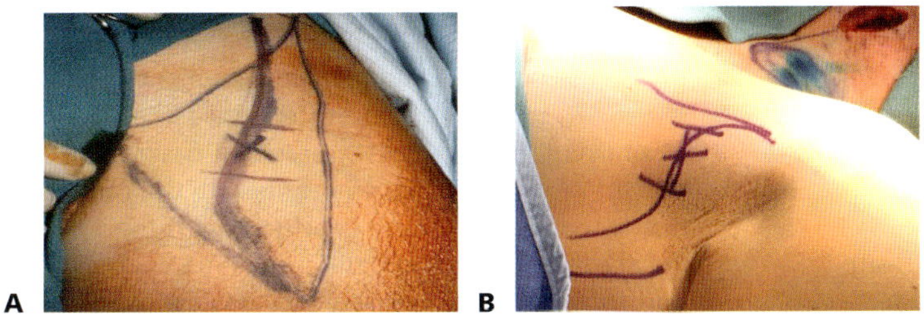

FIG 15 • Skin marking and planned SLN biopsy incision. Examples of transcutaneous SLN localization with the gamma probe in two nodal basins: **(A)** inguinal and **(B)** axillary. In each frame, the SLN biopsy incision is drawn to incorporate the location of the SLN, marked with an "X" as well as a future formal lymphadenectomy should that be required.

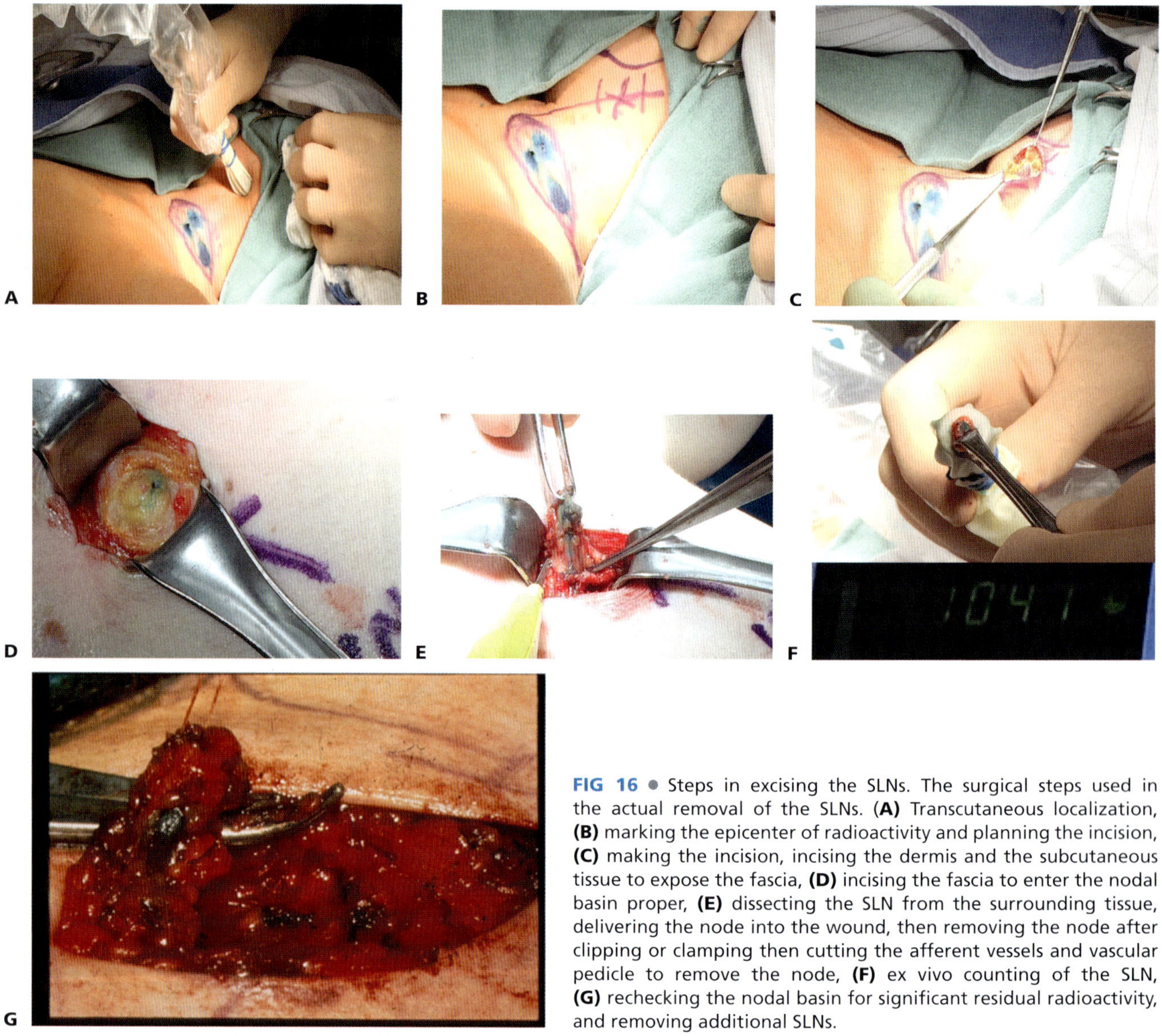

FIG 16 ● Steps in excising the SLNs. The surgical steps used in the actual removal of the SLNs. **(A)** Transcutaneous localization, **(B)** marking the epicenter of radioactivity and planning the incision, **(C)** making the incision, incising the dermis and the subcutaneous tissue to expose the fascia, **(D)** incising the fascia to enter the nodal basin proper, **(E)** dissecting the SLN from the surrounding tissue, delivering the node into the wound, then removing the node after clipping or clamping then cutting the afferent vessels and vascular pedicle to remove the node, **(F)** ex vivo counting of the SLN, **(G)** rechecking the nodal basin for significant residual radioactivity, and removing additional SLNs.

- Skin hooks, handheld Richardson-type retractors, or blunt self-retaining retractors can be used for exposure (**FIG 16D**).
- Once the nodal basin is entered, the localization of the SLN may be further facilitated by either following a blue-stained lymphatic channel toward the blue node or by direct visualization of the blue-stained lymph node (**FIG 16E**).
- The visualization of the blue dye is helpful in rapidly identifying which lymph node has accumulated the radiotracer, discriminating the SLN from the other nonstained surrounding nodes that are usually in close proximity.
- The SLN is then dissected free from the surrounding tissues. This is facilitated by gently grasping the node with a pickup and then delivering the node to a more superficial location in the basin. We prefer to use a pickup with broad and blunt jaws such as Hayes-Martin, rather than a DeBakey or Adson, to avoid tearing the node. Some surgeons place a figure-of-eight stitch in the node for this maneuver, but this can also carry the risk of tearing the node. Once mobilized and delivered, the intervening lymphatic channels can be identified because of the blue dye and are clipped or tied to limit the development of a postoperative seroma. The vascular pedicle is then clamped, cut, and then tied.
- Ex vivo counts of the node are then documented with the handheld gamma probe and recorded (**FIG 16F**). After removing the initial SLN, the nodal basin is then scanned for residual radioactive counts with the gamma probe pointed away from the injection site. If the background activity in the nodal basin is still high because of close proximity to the injection site, the wide local excision of the primary site may be performed. This removes any significant background activity (shine through) and

allows for a more complete evaluation of residual SLN counts within the nodal basin.

- Additional nodes identified by the presence of high residual radioactivity and/or blue dye staining are then removed and labeled as sentinel nodes, with numbers assigned sequentially in the order of identification. Nodes are defined as sentinel if they are blue and/or contain radioactivity significantly above background. Nodes are removed and labeled as "sentinel" until no focal basin radioactivity is greater than 10% of the "hottest" sentinel node removed.
- The skin and soft tissue between the injection site and nodal basin(s) should also be scanned to identify and subsequently remove any "in-transit" or "interval" SLNs. Similarly, if the background counts are too high because of proximity to the injection site, the wide excision can be performed to decrease the shine through and facilitate the exploration for the in-transit SLNs.

CLOSURE

- Hemostasis should be ensured and divided fascial layers closed with interrupted 3-0 absorbable sutures. Drains are usually not needed.
- Skin may then be approximated using interrupted, buried absorbable sutures in the dermis followed by a running subcuticular stitch with a 4-0 absorbable monofilament suture. Steri-Strips or a skin adhesive may then be applied.

PATHOLOGIC EVALUATION OF THE SENTINEL NODES

- A dedicated dermatopathologist should process the node and read the pathology slides.
- The SLN are serially sectioned using either along the long axis of the node or a bread-loafing technique across the short axis of the node (**FIG 17**). The width of the serially sliced sections is partly dependent on the size of the node but usually are made in 2-mm intervals.
- Frozen section evaluation of the SLNs are not recommended out of concern of leaving behind nodal tissue with small-volume diseases in the cryostat and therefore will go undetected. Such events could reduce the accuracy of the pathologic evaluation of the SLN.[27]
- The tissue slices are embedded in paraffin blocks for permanent section evaluation. All the blocks are stained with hematoxylin and eosin. If these are negative, additional sections are taken for immunostaining.

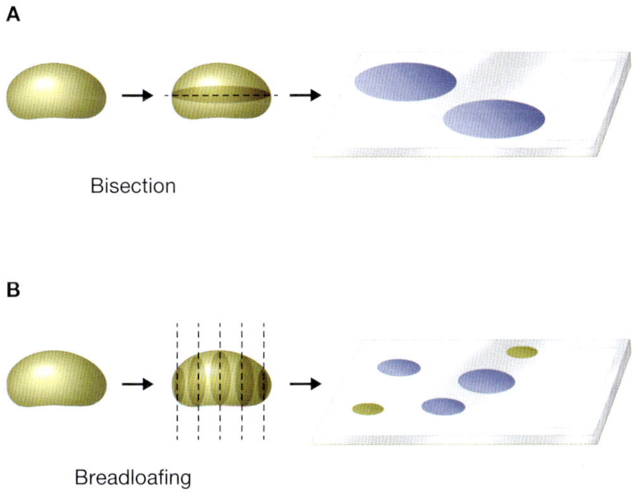

FIG 17 • Histologic examination of the SLN. Schematic representation of sectioning of lymph nodes, with routine bisection in **(A)** creating two samples to be stained and serial sectioning in **(B)**, resulting in multiple sections for staining.

COMPLICATIONS

- No identifiable drainage to SLN(s)
- Removing the "wrong" node and leaving behind the true SLN
- Hematoma
- Seroma
- Infection (cellulitis or infected seroma)
- Paresthesias
- Lymphedema

POSTOPERATIVE CARE

- Always examine the patient before discharge to make sure a hematoma has not developed.
- Instruct the patient what to look for in terms of seroma and surgical site infection.
- Remind them about the blue dye in the urine.
- Keep the SLN site dry for 48 hours.

OUTCOMES

- Using the dual localizing technique of radiotracer and blue dye injections, the SLN identification rate approaches 100%.[3]
- The frequency of a false-negative event defined as the development of clinical nodal disease in the same nodal basin subsequent to the removal of a negative SLN is 3% to 5%.[28] A false-negative event is most commonly a result of very small volume disease undetected by the original pathologic evaluation of the SLN removed, and therefore, a formal lymphadenectomy was not performed. For such an event to occur, another lymph node with subclinical disease was likely present in the same nodal basin at the time of the SLN procedure as the source of the subsequent clinical nodal recurrence. Another reason for a false-negative event leading to a nodal recurrence is the inaccurate identification of the SLN and removing a node that was not sentinel and leaving behind the true SLN that harbored microscopic disease.[28]
- Lymphedema, although rare, can occur and is most common following an SLN biopsy in the groin in conjunction with a wide excision on the thigh or lower leg.

PEARLS AND PITFALLS

Head and neck primaries	■ The lymphatic drainage from these primary lesions is the most ambiguous and least predictable. Therefore, a SPECT-CT lymphoscintigraphy is strongly encouraged. ■ Due to the close proximity to important structures when treating melanomas of the face, the excision margins for the primary lesion may have to be selectively narrowed to avoid injury to these structures and any associated functional or cosmetic impairments (see Chapter 26). It is important to note that injected blue dye at the primary site left behind in the remaining skin after the wide excision can tattoo the skin for long periods of time. Therefore, excision margins are clearly delineated with a marking pen prior to the injection of the blue dye. In this way, the volume of dye injected can be adjusted to ensure that the blue staining is limited to the skin to be excised. ■ The SLNs in the neck are surprisingly small; the use of blue dye is particularly helpful. ■ The lymphatic drainage in the head and neck region is very rapid and the flow of blue dye can be diluted out if too much time transpires between the injection and the exploration of the nodal basin for the SLN. Therefore, in contrast to other primary sites, the blue dye is injected under sterile conditions after the patient is prepped and draped. ■ The SLNs in the neck region are often adjacent to important nerves, such as the spinal accessory, great auricular, and branches of the facial nerve.
Injection of blue dye	■ An injection performed in the intradermal location creates some resistance and can result in the needle becoming separated from the syringe, splattering blue dye on oneself, the patient and OR staff. Therefore, the use of 1-cc Luer lock–type syringes is recommended. ■ Remember to tell patient that his or her urine will be blue/green colored for 24 hours. ■ Any blue dye staining of the skin not removed by the wide excision may take several months to completely fade away. ■ If the patient has already had a wide excision, a preoperative discussion should take place about whether or not to use the blue dye for the planned SLN biopsy. Another excision should not be performed just to remove the blue dye to avoid a tattooing effect. The only time that another excision should take place is when it is necessary to remove the injection site radioactivity that is obscuring your ability to adequately scan the nodal basin for the SLN.

Complications	▪ **No drainage observed from the injection site** to an SLN is almost always a result of an error in injection technique. The appropriate technique involves an intradermal injection that raises a wheel and causes some discomfort to the patient. The most common error is injecting the radiotracer too deep into the subcutaneous tissues where the concentration of lymphatic vessels is low or directly into the excisional biopsy site. Hallmarks of a subcutaneous injection include lack of pain during the injection, radiotracer activity seen in the liver on the lymphoscintigraphic images, and no drainage to a nodal basin. ▪ **Recurrent seromas** at the SLN biopsy site are conveniently handled by using a "seroma cath" system, composed of a percutaneously placed angiocatheter, a clear tubing, and a small suction bulb. This technique can also be used to treat infected seromas along with antibiotics rather than opening up the wound. ▪ **Incorrect identification of the SLN** can lead to leaving behind microscopic nodal disease, which will be the source of subsequent clinical lymph node recurrence. One important maneuver to minimize the frequency of such events is to always view the lymphoscintigraphic images prior to the surgery and display the images in the OR rather than depending on the reading by the radiologist.

REFERENCES

1. Morton DL, Wen DR, Wong JH, et al. Technical details of intraoperative lymphatic mapping for early stage melanoma. *Arch Surg*. 1992; 127:392–399.
2. Alex J, Krag D. Gamma-probe-guided localization of lymph nodes. *Surg Oncol*. 1993;2:137–144.
3. Gershenwald JE, Tseng CH, Thompson W, et al. Improved sentinel lymph node localization in patients with primary melanoma with the use of radiolabeled colloid. *Surgery*. 1998;124:203–210.
4. Thompson JF, McCarthy WH, Bosch CM, et al. Sentinel lymph node status as an indicator of the presence of metastatic melanoma in regional lymph nodes. *Melanoma Res*. 1995;5:255–260.
5. Cascinelli N, Belli F, Santinami M, et al. Sentinel lymph node biopsy in cutaneous melanoma: the WHO Melanoma Program experience. *Ann Surg Oncol*. 2000;7:469–474.
6. Balch CM, Gershenwald JE, Soong SJ, et al. Multivariate analysis of prognostic factors among 2,313 patients with stage III melanoma: comparison of nodal micrometastases versus macrometastases. *J Clin Oncol*. 2010;28:2452–2459.
7. Lee RJ, Gibbs JF, Proulx GM, et al. Nodal basin recurrence following lymph node dissection for melanoma: implications for adjuvant radiotherapy. *Int J Radiat Oncol Biol Phys*. 2000;46:464–474.
8. Gershenwald JE, Ross MI. Sentinel-lymph-node biopsy for cutaneous melanoma. *N Engl J Med*. 2011;364:1738–1745.
9. Morton DL, Thompson JF, Cochran AJ, et al. Final trial report of sentinel-node biopsy versus nodal observation in melanoma. *N Engl J Med*. 2014;370:599–609.
10. Balch CM, Gershenwald JE, Soong SJ, et al. Final version of 2009 AJCC melanoma staging and classification. *J Clin Oncol*. 2009;27: 6199–6206.
11. Gershenwald JE, Thompson W, Mansfield PF, et al. Multi-institutional melanoma lymphatic mapping experience: the prognostic value of sentinel lymph node status in 612 stage I or II melanoma patients. *J Clin Oncol*. 1999;17:976–983.
12. Wong SL, Balch CM, Hurley P, et al. Sentinel lymph node biopsy for melanoma: American Society of Clinical Oncology and Society of Surgical Oncology joint clinical practice guideline. *J Clin Oncol*. 2012;30:2912–2918.
13. Balch CM, Morton DL, Gershenwald JE, et al. Sentinel node and standard of care for melanoma. *J Am Acad Dermatol*. 2009;60(5):872–875.
14. Rousseau DL Jr, Ross MI, Johnson MM, et al. Revised American Joint Committee on Cancer staging criteria accurately predict sentinel lymph node positivity in clinically node-negative melanoma patients. *Ann Surg Oncol*. 2003;10:569–574.
15. NCCN clinical practice guidelines: melanoma. National Comprehensive Cancer Network. http://www.nccn.org/professionals/physician_gls/pdf/melanoma.pdf. Accessed August 14, 2014.
16. Paek SC, Griffith KA, Johnson TM, et al. The impact of factors beyond Breslow depth on predicting sentinel lymph node positivity in melanoma. *Cancer*. 2007;109:100–108.
17. Doeden K, Ma Z, Narasimhan B, et al. Lymphatic invasion in cutaneous melanoma is associated with sentinel lymph node metastasis. *J Cutan Pathol*. 2009;36:772–780.
18. Gannon CJ, Rousseau DL Jr, Ross MI, et al. Accuracy of lymphatic mapping and sentinel lymph node biopsy after previous wide local excision in patients with primary melanoma. *Cancer*. 2006;107:2647–2652.
19. Choi EA, Gershenwald JE. Imaging studies in patients with melanoma. *Surg Oncol Clin N Am*. 2007;16:403–430.
20. Uren RF, Howman-Giles R, Thompson JF. Patterns of lymphatic drainage from the skin in patients with melanoma. *J Nucl Med*. 2003;44:570–582.
21. Uren RF. SPECT/CT lymphoscintigraphy to locate the sentinel lymph node in patients with melanoma. *Ann Surg Oncol*. 2009;16:1459–1460.
22. Sumner W, Mansfield P, Ross MI, et al. Implications of lymphatic drainage to unusual sentinel lymph node sites in patients with primary cutaneous melanoma. *Cancer*. 2002;95:354–360.
23. Sondak VK, King DW, Zager JS, et al. Combined analysis of phase III trials evaluating [^{99m}Tc] Tilmanocept and vital blue dye for identification of sentinel lymph nodes in clinically node-negative cutaneous melanoma. *Ann Surg Oncol*. 2013;20:680–688.
24. Ross MI. Lymphatic mapping and sentinel node biopsy for early stage melanoma: how we do it at the MD Anderson Cancer Center. *J Surg Oncol*. 1997;66:273–276.
25. Leong SP, Donegan E, Heffernon W, et al. Adverse reactions to isosulfan blue during selective sentinel lymph node dissection in melanoma. *Ann Surg Oncol*. 2000;7:361–366.
26. Neves RI, Reynolds BQ, Hazard SW, et al. Increased post-operative complications with methylene blue versus lymphazurin in sentinel lymph node biopsies for skin cancers. *J Surg Oncol*. 2011;103:421–425.
27. Scolyer RA, Thompson JF, McCarthy SW, et al. Intraoperative frozen-section evaluation can reduce accuracy of pathologic assessment of sentinel nodes in melanoma patients. *J Am Coll Surg*. 2005;201:821–823.
28. Gershenwald JE, Colome MI, Lee JE, et al. Patterns of recurrence following a negative sentinel lymph node biopsy in 243 patients with stage I or II melanoma. *J Clin Oncol*. 1998;16:2253–2260.

Chapter 28 Axillary Lymph Node Dissection for Melanoma

Michael S. Sabel

DEFINITION

- Axillary lymph node dissection (ALND) involves the surgical excision of the lymph node–bearing tissue from the axilla. For melanoma patients, a complete ALND is considered the standard of care for patients with both micrometastatic disease, as demonstrated on sentinel lymph node (SLN) biopsy and clinically evident disease.
- The axilla is divided into anatomic levels based on the relationship of the nodes to the pectoralis minor muscle (**FIG 1**). Level I nodes are located lateral to the pectoralis minor, level II nodes are seated deep to the pectoralis minor, and the level III nodes are medial to the pectoralis minor. For patients with clinical evident axillary disease, a level I-III dissection is recommended. For patients with a positive axillary SLN biopsy, a level I-III dissection is often performed, but a level I-II dissection may be adequate.[1,2] This chapter will describe an ALND encompassing levels I, II, and III.

PATIENT HISTORY AND PHYSICAL FINDINGS

- The history should focus on the patient's melanoma history, including the histology of the primary tumor, disease-free interval between the primary diagnosis and the diagnosis of regional metastases, and the extent of both locoregional and distant disease. The history should also focus on comorbidities, past medical history, and medications that might impact the patient's surgical candidacy.
- The history should also include a thorough review of systems, specifically looking for symptoms suggestive of distant disease. Patients with symptoms worrisome for stage IV disease should have body imaging before proceeding with surgery.
- A complete physical examination should pay particular attention to signs of local, regional, and distant disease. The site of the primary tumor and the skin between it and the regional basin should be examined for signs of in-transit recurrences. A complete lymph node exam should be performed. This should not just be limited to the axilla of concern but bilateral cervical, supraclavicular, epitrochlear, axillary, and inguinal basins. Suspicious nodes outside of the draining basins may represent stage IV disease.
- For the involved axilla, the exam should focus on the extent of disease, including the size of the involved nodes and fixation. The ipsilateral arm should be examined for lymphedema, weakness, or sensory deficit, as these may be indicative of involvement of the axillary vein or brachial plexus. You should also document any conditions affecting the shoulder or upper extremity, which limits range of motion.
- For patients who had an SLN biopsy or excisional biopsy, it is important to document any sensory or motor deficits that may have occurred at the first surgery as well as any seroma, hematoma, or infection. It may also be helpful to note the orientation of the incision, as this may impact the orientation of the ALND incision.
- It is important to review with patients the expected postoperative course including drain management and arm exercises, as well as short-term and long-term morbidity, including the risk, prevention, and management of lymphedema.

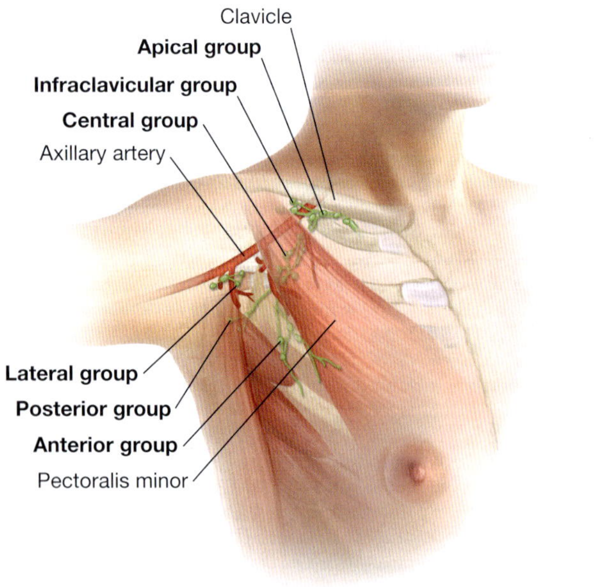

FIG 1 • Levels of axillary lymph nodes. The level I nodes are located lateral to the pectoralis minor muscle, the level II nodes are located deep to the pectoralis minor, whereas the level III nodes are located medial to the pectoralis minor.

IMAGING AND OTHER DIAGNOSTIC STUDIES

- For asymptomatic patients with micrometastatic disease identified on SLN biopsy, there are no imaging studies necessary before proceeding with ALND.[3] For patients with thick, ulcerated tumors (American Joint Commission Center [AJCC] stage T4b) and a positive SLN, the risk of distant disease may justify preoperative body imaging, with either a computed tomography (CT) scan or positron emission tomography (PET)/CT.[4] However, for patients with micrometastatic disease, preoperative staging studies have a high false-positive rate, may lead to unnecessary follow-up studies or biopsies, and rarely alter surgical decision making.
- Patients with symptoms concerning for metastatic disease should undergo staging with either a CT of the chest, abdomen, and pelvis or a PET/CT and a magnetic resonance imaging (MRI) of the brain. Patients with clinically evident regional disease should also undergo distant staging, as there

is a higher chance of detecting metastatic disease that might alter surgical decision making.[3]

- For patients with fixed, matted lymph nodes; skin involvement; or neurovascular symptoms of the involved arm (paresthesias, motor and sensory deficits, lymphedema, limited range of motion), MRI of the chest wall can be helpful in determining resectability. Unresectable or borderline resectable patients could be considered for neoadjuvant therapy with newer biologic and targeted therapies.

SURGICAL MANAGEMENT

Preoperative Planning

- In the preoperative area, the side of the ALND should be clearly marked and confirmed with the patient before proceeding to the operating room (OR).
- Intravenous (IV) antibiotics are indicated for ALND.[5] Sequential compression devices (SCDs) should be used for deep venous thrombosis (DVT) prophylaxis. Patients with a history of DVT or genetic predisposition toward clotting should receive subcutaneous heparin.
- Many surgeons prefer the use of short-acting neuromuscular blocking agents during induction, so that the patients are not paralyzed during the procedure. This allows identification of the thoracodorsal, long thoracic, and medial and lateral pectoral nerves by mechanical stimulation. However, this is not essential and some surgeons prefer paralysis with a long-acting neuromuscular blocking agent to prevent muscular contraction and allow for retraction of the pectoralis major and minor muscles. Either way, this should be discussed with the anesthesiologist prior to the case.

Positioning

- The patient should be positioned supine on the OR table, toward the edge of the side of the ALND so that the posterior axillary line is in-line with the edge of the table. The ipsilateral arm is abducted at 90 degrees on a padded arm board. It is important not to extend the arm past 90 degrees to avoid brachial plexus injury.
- The endotracheal tube should be located away from the involved arm and adequate space should be preserved above the arm for the surgical assistant.
- The chest wall, lower neck, and entire arm should be prepped and draped into the surgical field using a sterile stockinette and Kerlix wrap. This allows the arm to be rotated over the chest, relaxing the pectoralis major and minor (**FIG 2**).

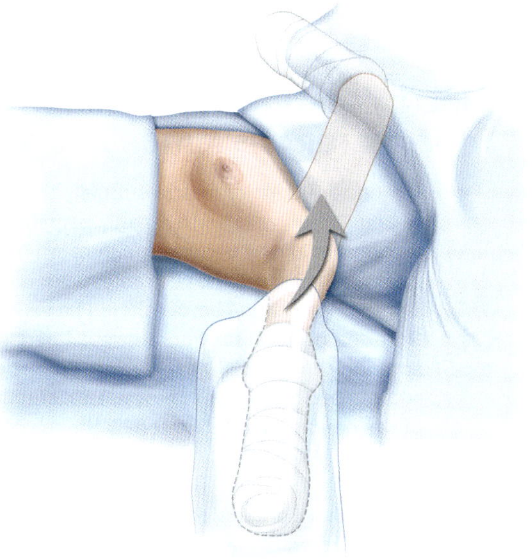

FIG 2 • Preoperative positioning and draping for an ALND. The arm should be prepped into the field with a stockinette and Kerlix wrap so it can be rotated over the chest during the procedure.

INCISION

- Typically, a "lazy S" incision is used along the pectoralis major muscle, extending posteriorly at the level of the axillary hair line, and then inferiorly along the latissimus dorsi muscle (**FIG 3**). For patients with a prior excisional or SLN biopsy incision, this should be encompassed into the ALND incision, and thus might impact the choice of incision. For patients with bulky adenopathy, particularly those with nodes close to the skin, the skin overlying the nodes should be included with the specimen. Be sure there is adequate skin to allow for a tension-free closure.
- After incising the skin with a scalpel, electrocautery is used to divide the subcutaneous tissue and elevate skin

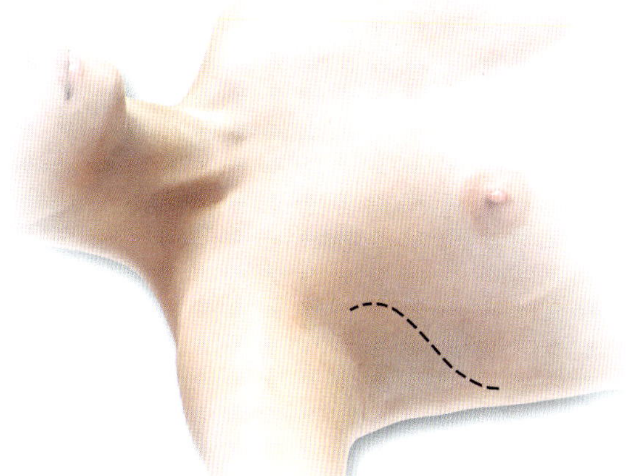

FIG 3 • The "lazy S" incision for an ALND. One can begin with the transverse incision and extend the pectoralis and latissimus arms as needed.

TECHNIQUES

flaps. Unless mandated by the presence of bulky disease, the skin flaps should not be too thin and get progressively thicker as they are raised. Thin skin flaps will increase the risk of wound complications and give the axilla a sunken-in appearance.

- The skin is elevated using skin hooks or sharp rakes. It is important that the surgical assistant holds the flaps straight up and not retract them back (which residents will sometimes do in order to get a better view). The surgeon retracts the tissue with the opposite hand in order to apply strong countertraction and identify the appropriate tissue plane.
- Surgeons are often hesitant to go too far or too deep while elevating the inferior skin flap at this initial point of the operation for fear of injuring the long thoracic nerve. However, raising an adequate inferior flap allows for greater mobility of the specimen and easier dissection. The inferior flap should be raised to approximately the level of the 5th rib.
- Once the flaps are elevated, the next step will be to identify some of the borders of the axilla: the pectoralis major and minor muscles, the latissimus dorsi muscle, and the axillary vein. Although individual surgeons have their preferences, there is no correct order, and the presence of large lymph nodes might mandate changing your approach. In this chapter, we will describe a medial-to-lateral approach.

IDENTIFICATION AND RETRACTION OF THE PECTORALIS MAJOR AND MINOR

- The pectoralis major muscle is usually the easiest margin to begin with, as it is often easily palpable upon raising the flaps (and may become apparent while elevating the superior flap). Once the pectoralis major is identified, the length of the lateral border should be exposed (**FIG 4**).
- Once the pectoralis major muscle is freed, it is retracted anteriorly and medially to expose the interpectoral nodes and the pectoralis minor muscle. This, and the remainder of the operation, is facilitated by the use of a Thompson retractor (**FIG 5**).
- The tissue between the pectoralis major and minor muscle that contains the interpectoral (Rotter's) nodes is included with the specimen, dissecting it off the pectoralis minor muscle. As the dissection proceeds onto the pectoralis minor, the medial pectoral bundle can be observed coming either through or lateral to the pectoralis minor (**FIG 6**). This should be preserved. There is often an accompanying vein with a branch going into the specimen. This will need to be clipped, taking care not to clip the medial pectoral nerve.

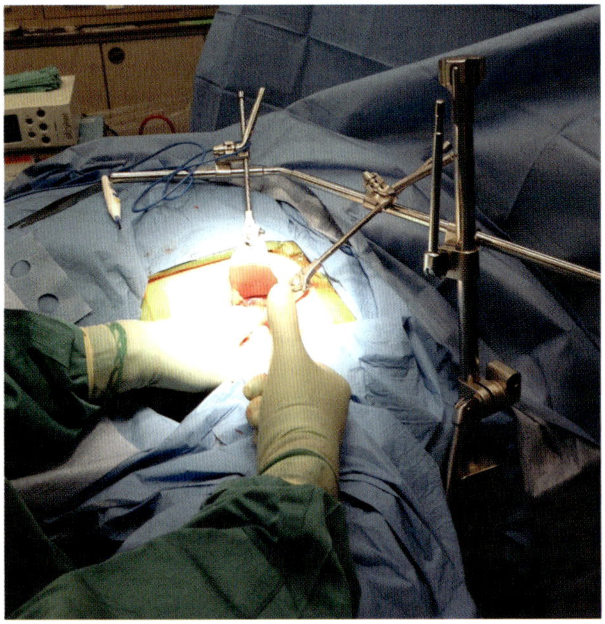

FIG 5 ● The Thompson retractor provides excellent exposure for an ALND.

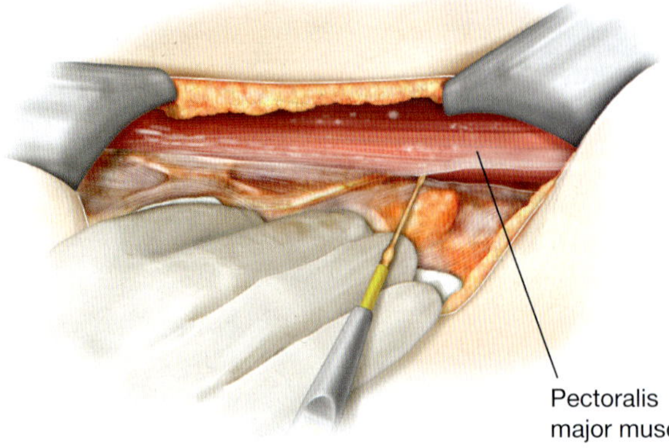

FIG 4 ● The pectoralis major muscle is identified and cleaned off along the lateral edge.

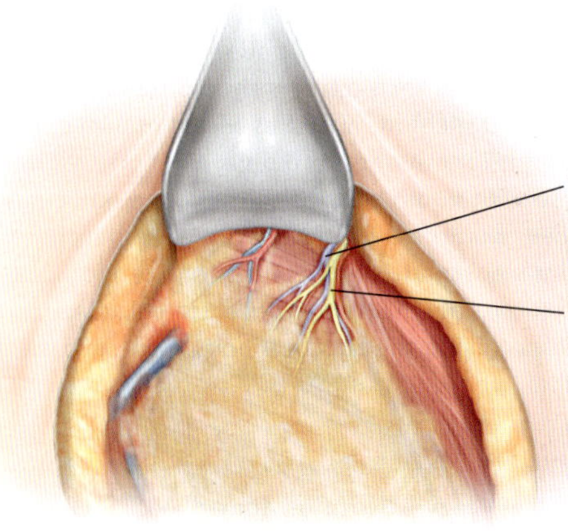

FIG 6 ● The medial pectoral nerve.

- For patients undergoing an ALND for a positive SLN, the pectoralis minor can be preserved. The lateral edge of the pectoralis minor muscle is freed by dividing the axillary fascia (**FIG 7**). The axillary fascia is an extension of the clavipectoral fascia that divides the subcutaneous fat from the axillary fat. Upon dividing the fascia, you will notice the protrusion of a more yellow, globular fat. This is the lymph node–bearing tissue that needs to be excised.
- The axillary contents are now swept laterally and the pectoralis minor muscle exposed along its length. Once this is done, the Thompson retractor can be repositioned so that both the pectoralis major and minor can be retracted anteriorly.
- If there is bulky adenopathy and exposure of the upper axillary lymph nodes is difficult, it may be necessary to divide the pectoralis minor muscle, and this is described subsequently.

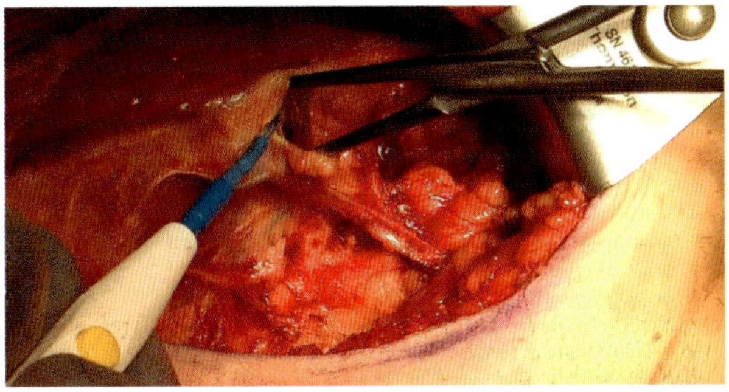

FIG 7 • The axillary (clavipectoral) fascia is divided with cautery, revealing the axillary fat underneath.

IDENTIFICATION OF THE AXILLARY VEIN

- The vein often becomes visible medially during the elevation of the pectoralis musculature. If not, its general location can be anticipated by identifying the underarm dimple at the inferior aspect of the upper arm and tracing it toward the chest wall (**FIG 8**). Dissection down to the vein should not be performed directly with cautery to avoid an inadvertent injury, but rather, a careful dissection is recommended (**FIG 9**). Small venous branches and lymphatics should be clipped or suture ligated. It is also important not to find yourself superior to the vein, as the axillary artery and brachial plexus can be injured. Once the vein has been identified, the inferior margin should be cleared. It is not necessary to skeletonize the vein.

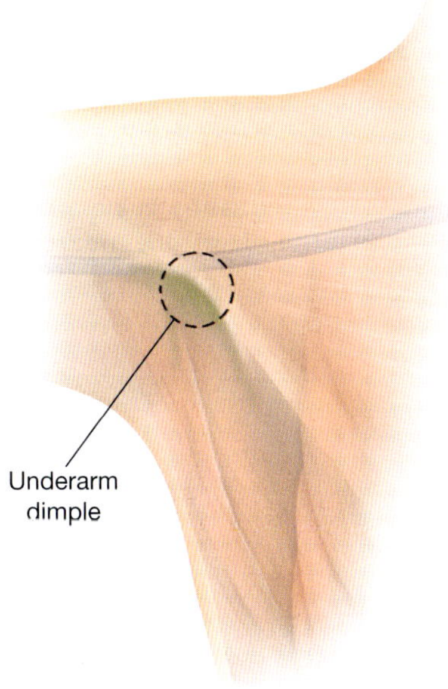

FIG 8 • The position of the axillary vein in the axilla can be estimated by locating the underarm dimple and tracing this back toward the chest wall.

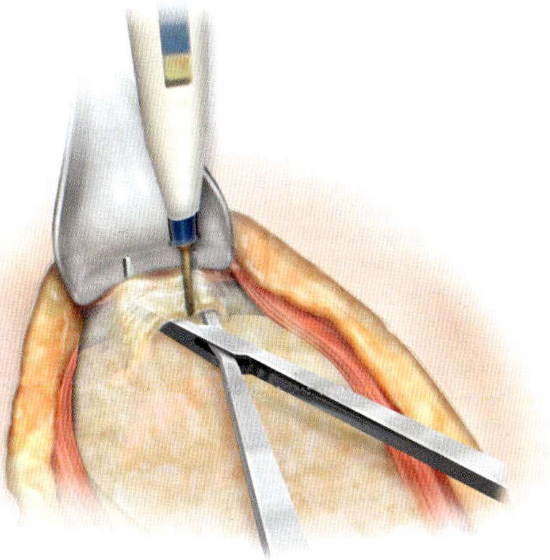

FIG 9 • Exposure of the axillary vein is accomplished by careful dissection with a right angle and cautery.

THE LATISSIMUS DORSI MUSCLE

- The final boundary to identify is the latissimus dorsi muscle. Again, this is often seen during the elevation of the inferior flap. If not, the lateral skin should be retracted laterally using skin hooks or sharp rakes, and the axillary contents retracted medially. Dissection down through the subcutaneous fat will identify the muscle (**FIG 10**). In obese patients, be careful not to overestimate how lateral the muscle is, as you may dissect past it and raise an unnecessary posterolateral flap. Likewise, being too medial puts the thoracodorsal bundle at risk. Once identified, it should be cleared by staying on the anterior surface of the muscle.

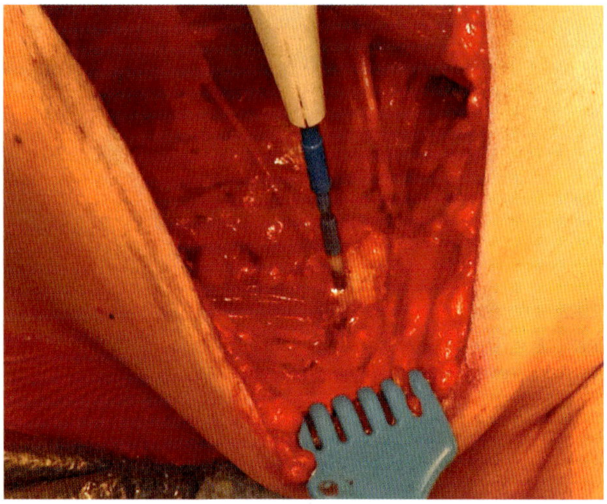

FIG 10 ● With lateral traction on the skin, the latissimus dorsi muscle is exposed and cleared on its anterior surface.

- In a small percentage of cases (approximately 5% to 7%), you may identify a more superficial muscle extending from the latissimus dorsi muscle to the pectoralis muscle, over the axillary vein. This is a muscular–tendinous structure known as a Langer's arch (**FIG 11**). This can often be disorienting, so it is important you be aware of this possibility and continue to dissect laterally to identify the latissimus dorsi. The Langer's arch, if present, will need to be divided and excised with the specimen.
- The latissimus muscle should be cleared up to the point where the tendinous insertion is reached beneath the axillary vein.

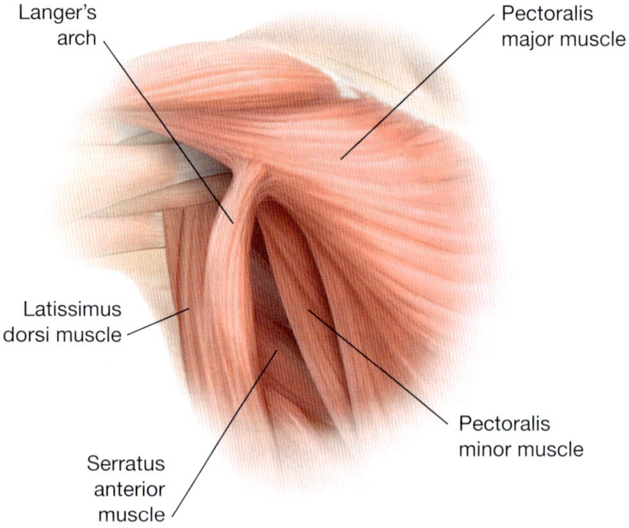

FIG 11 ● Anatomy of a Langer's arch.

THE THORACODORSAL NEUROVASCULAR BUNDLE

- Once the intersection between the vein and the latissimus is identified, the axillary contents are freed from lateral to medial. Lymphatics should be clipped rather than cauterized. The intercostobrachial nerve will be in this tissue, extending toward the arm and is commonly sacrificed during this operation. It is important to note that the intercostobrachial nerve does not need to be sacrificed. It can be dissected free by bivalving the specimen and freeing the nerve. However, this is not commonly done when an ALND is being performed for known cancer.
- It is important not to divide the axillary tissue to identify the thoracodorsal vein, but rather, make sure all the tissue between the latissimus dorsi and thoracodorsal bundle is dissected and included with the specimen. Failure to do this, for example, making the thoracodorsal bundle the lateral margin, will leave behind several lymph nodes. As these nodes primarily drain the arm, this is particularly important in melanoma.
- As the axillary vein is cleared medially, the thoracodorsal vein can be identified. The thoracodorsal vein comes off the posterior aspect of the vein. The other large tributary off the axillary vein is the lateral thoracic vein, but this comes off inferiorly, which serves as an important clue that it is not the thoracodorsal vein (**FIG 12**). Although the lateral thoracic vein will need to be ligated, this should not be done until the thoracodorsal vein is clearly identified. The thoracodorsal nerve may be directly behind the lateral thoracic vein, so take care when ligating it.
- Once the thoracodorsal vein is visualized, the artery can usually be seen pulsating in close proximity. The nerve, however, at this level, does not run next to the

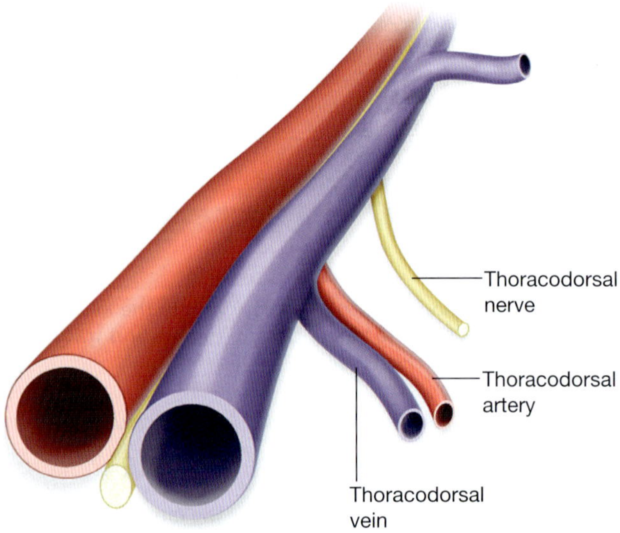

FIG 12 ● Whereas the lateral thoracic nerve enters the axillary vein on the inferior surface, the thoracodorsal vein tends to enter more posteriorly. This can be an important clue as to which vein you are looking at.

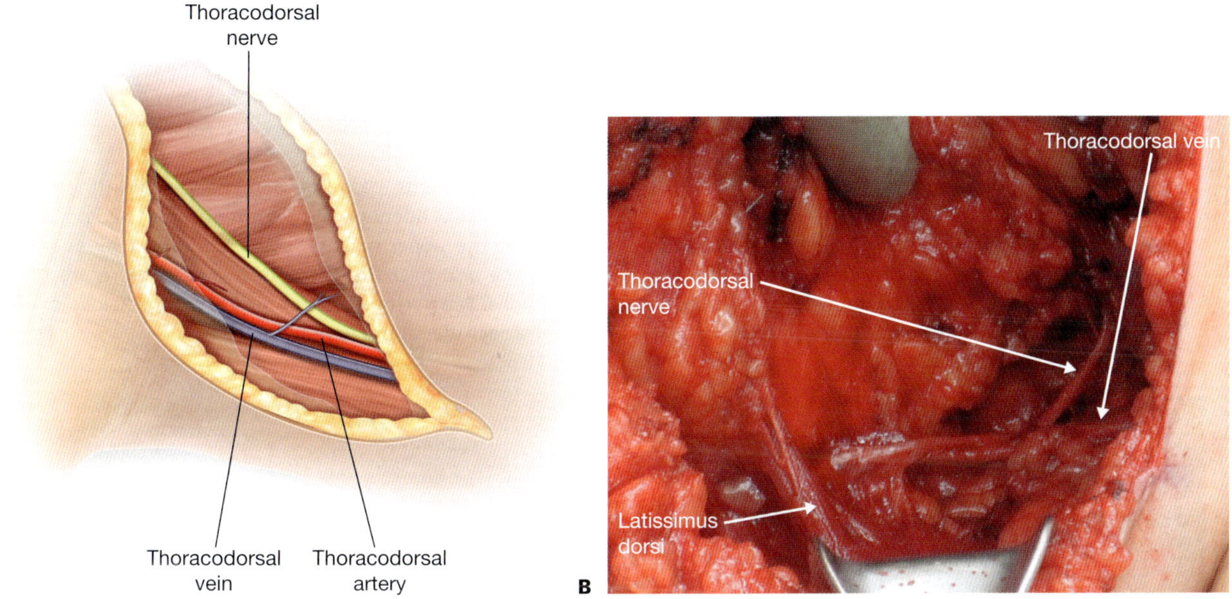

FIG 13 ● **A.** Relationship of the thoracodorsal nerve to the artery and vein. **B.** Intraoperative photo showing the nerve medial to the vein and artery and then joining the bundle inferiorly.

vein but is usually seated more medial, joining the vein and artery 1 to 2 cm inferiorly (**FIG 13A,B**). The nerve can easily be damaged by assuming it is next to the vein and dividing the more medial tissue. Careful dissection, avoiding the electrocautery, should be used to identify the nerve and trace it inferiorly until it joins the bundle.

- Although these anatomic relationships are generally true, the anatomy can be distorted by both bulky adenopathy and prior surgery. These can distort the relative positions of these structures, and this should be considered when having difficulty identifying them.
- Once the thoracodorsal nerve, artery, and vein are identified, they can be traced and dissected free down to their insertion into the latissimus dorsi. This can be facilitated by retracting the axillary contents anteromedially (which can sometimes be done with the long blade of the Thompson retractor). Although this step can be completed later, we prefer to free the entire bundle now, when visibility is optimized (**FIG 14**). There will be branches off of the thoracodorsal toward the specimen that will need to be clipped or ligated.

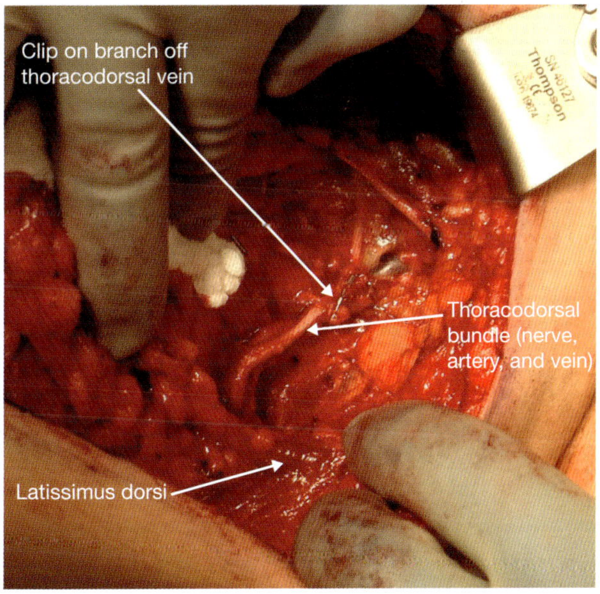

FIG 14 ● With the axillary contents swept medially from the latissimus dorsi, the entire bundle is visualized.

DISSECTION OF THE LEVEL II AND LEVEL III NODES

- Once the thoracodorsal is free, the axillary contents are released and the pectoralis major and minor once again retracted medially and anteriorly. The serratus anterior is identified and you will notice the yellow axillary fat extending up along the serratus, under the pectoralis minor, and along the axillary vein, like the top of a pyramid. This tissue bears the level II and III nodes. The axillary contents are dissected off of the serratus anterior. There is often a large vein that will need to be ligated.
- The intercostobrachial nerve can be seen exiting from the serratus anterior. Although this was likely ligated laterally, it needs to be divided again. The nerve should be cut with scissors flush with the muscle. This minimizes the chance of a neuroma and postoperative neuropathic pain, which is more likely if the nerve is divided with cautery or clips.
- The axillary fat is dissected off of the axillary vein. If you haven't already, you will note the axillary fat extending

superior to the vein, overlying the brachial plexus. This fat should be included with the specimen. There is a plane of tissue between the fat and the brachial plexus that allows this fat to be retracted inferiorly and can be easily dissected free, dividing only some loose areolar tissue (**FIG 15A,B**). Excessive cautery near the brachial plexus is strongly discouraged, and care is taken to clip or suture ligate any small vessels.

- Dissection of the upper axillary lymph nodes is facilitated by adducting the arm over the chest and held by an assistant. This allows the surgeon to reposition the Thompson retractor and gain more medial-anterior retraction, opening the axilla. The level II, and in some patients, the level III nodes, can be accessed this way and dissected from the thoracic inlet off the chest wall. It is important to carefully ligate the specimen and any small vessels, as this is a difficult area to return to in the case of bleeding.
- In many patients, based on body habitus or in the presence of bulky adenopathy, it is not possible to completely dissect the upper axillary lymph nodes just by adducting the arm over the chest. In this case, there are two options. The pectoralis minor muscle can be divided or an infraclavicular approach can be taken.

A

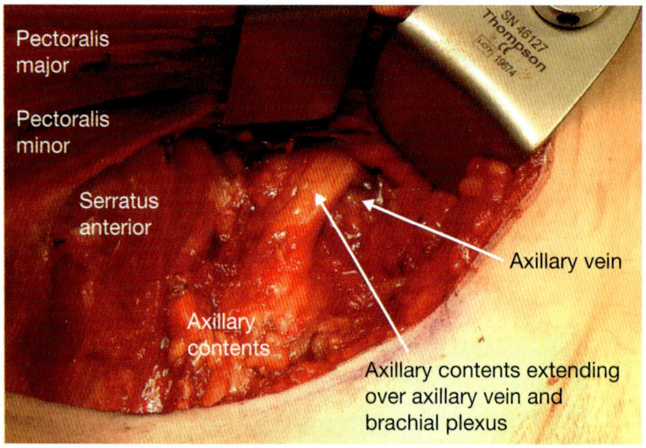

B

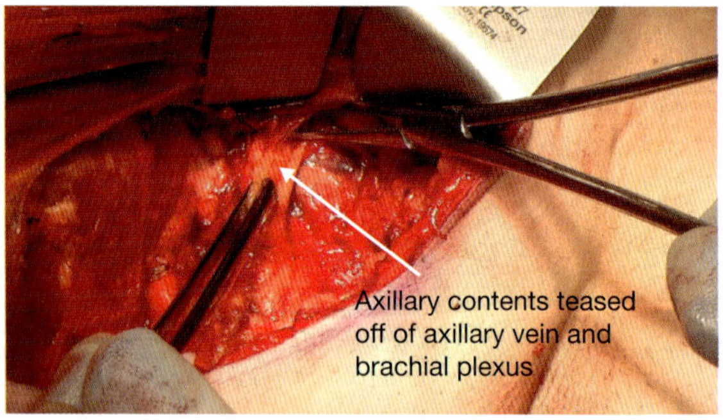

FIG 15 • **A.** Axillary contents extending superiorly over the vein and brachial plexus. **B.** This is teased down with a forceps and included with the specimen.

DIVISION OF THE PECTORALIS MINOR MUSCLE (PATEY PROCEDURE)

- In some cases, there may be direct involvement of the pectoralis minor muscle by tumor. In this case, the pectoralis minor should be resected en bloc with the axillary contents, dividing the muscle at the insertion point on the coracoid process and dividing it off the chest wall inferiorly (**FIG 16**). This greatly facilitates the removal of the level III lymph nodes.

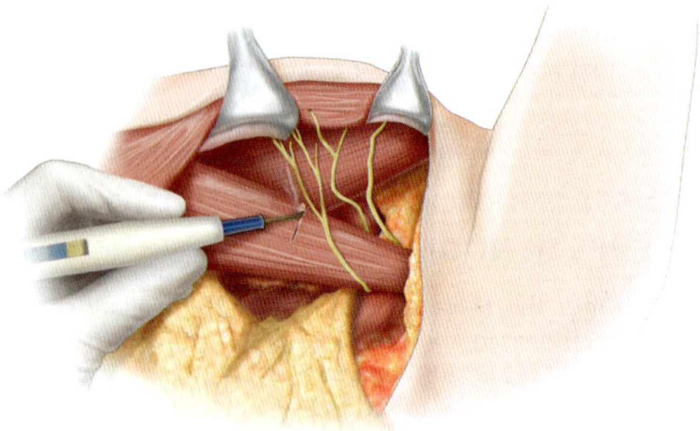

FIG 16 • The pectoralis minor muscle is divided to obtain easier access to the level III lymph nodes, taking care not to injure the pectoral nerves.

INFRACLAVICULAR APPROACH

- An alternate approach is to make a second transverse incision, approximately 2 cm below the clavicle, and then separating the clavicular from the sternal heads of the pectoralis major (**FIG 17**). The level III nodes can then be excised, taking care not to injure the neurovascular structures. Division of the pectoralis minor is adequate in the great majority of patients, but the infraclavicular approach can be extremely beneficial in patients with bulky adenopathy at the confluence of the cephalic and axillary veins and in patients who recur in level III after a prior level I and II ALND.

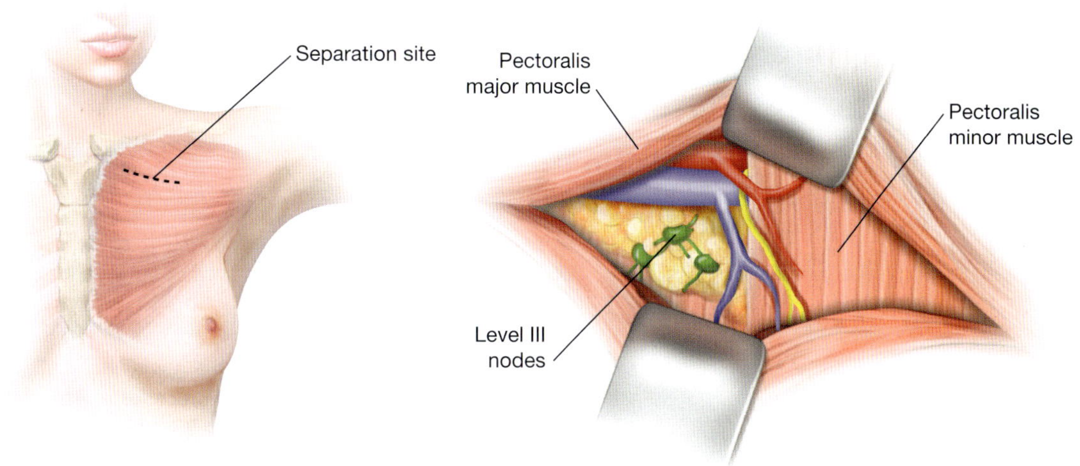

FIG 17 ● An alternate approach to the level III axillary nodes is to make an incision 2 cm below the clavicle and separate the clavicular and sternal heads of the pectoralis major.

EXPOSURE OF THE LONG THORACIC NERVE

- Once the level II and III nodes are free, they are brought laterally. The final structure to identify will be the long thoracic nerve. The nerve is commonly described as running along the serratus anterior, but this is incorrect. It is actually outside the fascia of the serratus, and this is exaggerated by the lateral retraction. Therefore, dissection directly on the serratus anterior will not identify the nerve and may lead to inadvertent injury. Dissection should be performed slightly laterally to the chest wall (**FIG 18**), and cautery should be used sparingly.
- Two anatomic landmarks can often help identify the nerve or estimate its position. First, the long thoracic and thoracodorsal nerve are roughly in the same anteroposterior (AP) plane. Therefore, by noting the location of the thoracodorsal nerve, you can estimate where you should be looking for the nerve. As before, this relationship can be altered by bulky disease or prior surgery. Second, the thoracodorsal vein often gives off a crossing branch toward the chest wall. This usually enters the chest wall at the level of the nerve.
- Once identified, the specimen is separated from the long thoracic nerve by carefully dissecting laterally to the nerve, allowing the nerve to move medially along the chest wall. This can often be done bluntly, but care should be taken not to stretch the nerve too much, as this can lead to injury and a temporary winged scapula.

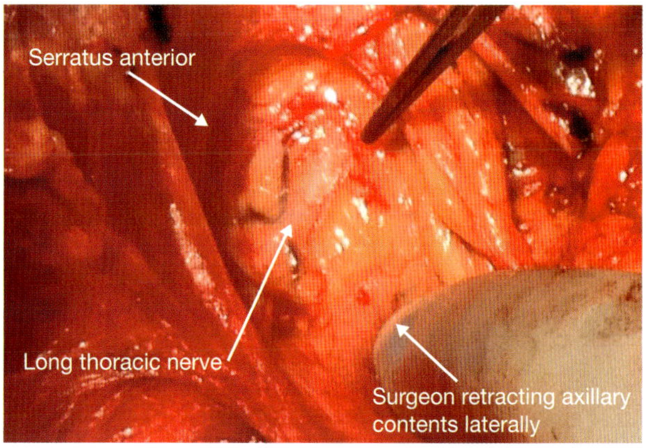

FIG 18 ● The long thoracic nerve is identified just lateral to the serratus anterior, which is emphasized by lateral retraction of the specimen.

REMOVAL OF THE SPECIMEN

- With both nerves free, the next step is to remove the tissue from between the nerves off of the underlying subscapularis muscle. At the level of the axillary vein, the fibrofatty tissue between the nerves should be clamped, taking care to be sure both nerves are free (**FIG 19**). The tissue is divided and tied off. This can be done in multiple steps. Once the subscapularis muscle is seen, the tissue can be easily divided off the muscle, constantly visualizing the nerves. Excessive lateral retraction can sometimes pull the serratus and the nerve, leading to accidental injury. This dissection should be carried inferiorly, past the point where both nerves enter their respective muscles. This can be facilitated by repositioning of the Thompson retractor.
- At this point, the specimen may still be attached inferiorly. Other than some veins going to the specimen, which can be suture ligated, this tissue can be divided with cautery, releasing the specimen, which is sent to pathology.

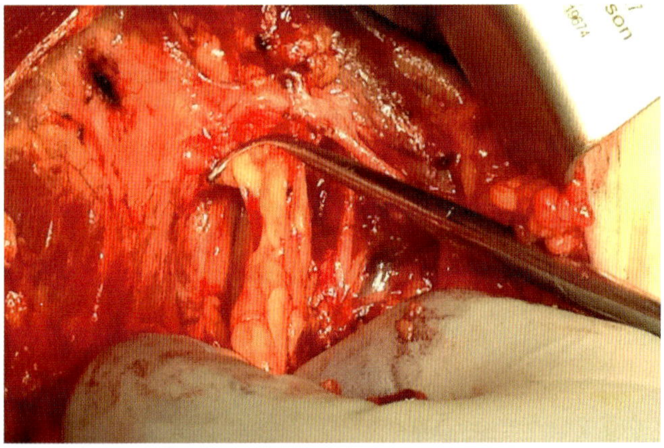

FIG 19 ● The axillary tissue below the vein and between the long thoracic and thoracodorsal nerve is clamped, being sure that both nerves are completely free. The tissue is divided and then taken off the subscapularis muscle.

DRAIN PLACEMENT AND INCISION CLOSURE

- The wound should be irrigated with saline or sterile water and thoroughly examined for hemostasis. This should include retraction of the pectoralis major and minor to explore this area. While assuring hemostasis, be careful not to use cautery near the long thoracic or thoracodorsal nerves.
- A single 10-mm flat channel drain is placed through a separate incision inferiorly and sutured to the skin. The drain should be cut so it just lies inferior to the axillary vein. The incision is closed using deep dermal 3-0 absorbable sutures and, for the typical closure, skin adhesive or absorbable monofilament suture. If a large amount of skin is needed to be excised, Nylon sutures may be appropriate.

PEARLS AND PITFALLS

Preoperative planning	■ A thorough neurovascular exam of the involved extremity is critical. Any suggestion of neurovascular involvement should prompt an MRI to assure resectability. ■ For patients who had prior axillary surgery, document any sensory or motor defects, as a nerve injury may have already occurred. ■ Be sure the patient is aware of what to expect postoperatively, including short-term and long-term lymphedema risk reduction and management.
Positioning	■ Having the arm prepped into the field so that it can be retracted over the chest is critical to performing a complete ALND.
Skin flaps	■ Avoid excessively thin flaps as this will lead to wound complications and a "sunken-in" appearance to the axilla. ■ Raise an adequate inferior flap early, as this allows better mobilization of the specimen and better exposure.
Elevating the pectoralis major and minor	■ Every attempt to preserve the medial pectoral nerve should be made. This requires care when mobilizing the pectoralis muscles.

Identifying the latissimus dorsi	■ Careful dissection should land you on the anterior surface of the latissimus dorsi. If you do not see it, slow down and use a right angle rather than continue to cauterize. If you are too medial, you could injure the thoracodorsal bundle. Be careful you are not too lateral (particularly in an obese patient).
Identifying the vein	■ Use the underarm dimple to estimate the location of the axillary vein. Being too far superior risks injury to the brachial plexus.
Thoracodorsal bundle	■ The thoracodorsal vein comes off the axillary vein posteriorly. If you find a vein coming off the inferior aspect of the axillary vein, it is probably the lateral thoracic, but do not ligate it until you have seen the thoracodorsal. ■ The nerve is usually medial to the vein at this level but not always. ■ If you can not locate the bundle, you can identify it at the level of the latissimus and trace it back toward the axillary vein.
Long thoracic nerve	■ Do not dissect directly on the serratus anterior—you will be medial to the nerve and mobilize it into your specimen. ■ Expect the long thoracic nerve in roughly the same AP plane as the thoracodorsal vein. ■ If you trace the thoracodorsal nerve along its length, a branch will head medially to the chest wall precisely where the long thoracic nerve lies.
Altered anatomy	■ Remember, bulky adenopathy or prior surgery (such as an SLN biopsy) can alter these relationships.

POSTOPERATIVE CARE

- The drain will remain in place until the output falls below 30 mL per 24 hours for 2 days in a row. The patient and their family should be shown how to care for the drain and record the drain output. A visiting nurse can be of assistance.
- Patients should be instructed to avoid repetitive activities with the arm or heavy lifting. Some surgeons also advise avoiding reaching over 90 degrees, particularly if the incision was excessively tight. However, patients should be encouraged to use the arm for normal activities and should be given exercises to maintain normal range of motion. Slings should not be given to patients.
- Once the drains are removed, physical therapy can be extremely helpful with returning to full range of motion.
- Patient education about the signs and symptoms of lymphedema and lymphedema prevention. Early recognition of lymphedema can improve the likelihood of management.
- Patients with stage III melanoma should be referred to medical oncology for a discussion of adjuvant therapies (high-dose interferon α-2b, biochemotherapy) or clinical trial. Patients with disease at high risk for relapse should also be considered for adjuvant radiation.

OUTCOMES

- For prospective trials, the adequacy of an ALND is often based on the number of lymph nodes identified within the axillary specimen. Morton et al.[6] in the MSLT-I trial recommended 15 or more nodes for an ALND, and this is a reasonable benchmark. However, this number will vary not only with surgical technique but also body habitus and the pathologist.
- For patients with AJCC stage IIIa disease, defined as having a nonulcerated primary with 1 to 3 nodes containing micrometastatic disease (diagnosed on SLN biopsy), the 5-year survival is approximately 78%, whereas the 10-year survival is 68%. For patients with AJCC stage IIIb disease, defined as either having an ulcerated primary with micrometastatic disease in 1 to 3 nodes or a nonulcerated primary with macrometastatic disease in 1 to 3 nodes, the 5-year survival is 59%, whereas the 10-year survival is 43%. For patients with AJCC stage IIIc disease, defined as an ulcerated primary with macrometastatic disease in 1 to 3 nodes, or any patient with 4 or more nodes, matted nodes, or in-transit disease and positive nodes, the 5-year survival is 40% and the 10-year survival is 24%. However, there can be considerable variability, as survival is impacted not only by the nodal status but also by age, gender, the Breslow thickness of the primary melanoma, the presence of ulceration, and the tumor mitotic rate.[7]
- Although data related specifically to ALNDs is limited, the reported regional recurrence rates after an ALND performed for a positive SLN biopsy are around 4% to 5%.[1,8,9]
- Regional recurrence after ALND is higher in patients with two or more positive axillary nodes, extracapsular extension, or any node greater than 3 cm in size. For patients with such high-risk features, axillary recurrence can be as high as 23% to 50%.[10–12] Although it does not appear to impact overall survival, the use of adjuvant radiation can reduce the risk of axillary recurrence by 50%.[13–15]

COMPLICATIONS

- Infection
- Hematoma
- Seroma
- Limited range of motion at the shoulder
- Axillary web syndrome
- Paresthesias of the axilla and upper inner arm
- Axillary vein thrombosis
- Lymphedema
- Winged scapula (injury to the long thoracic nerve)
- Latissimus dorsi paralysis (injury to the thoracodorsal nerve)
- Brachial plexus injury

REFERENCES

1. Namm JP, Chang AE, Cimmino VM, et al. Is a level III dissection necessary for a positive sentinel lymph node in melanoma? *J Surg Oncol.* 2012;105(3):225–258.
2. Nessim C, Law C, McConnell Y, et al. How often do level III nodes bear melanoma metastases and does it affect patient outcomes? *Ann Surg Oncol.* 2013;20(6):2056–2064.
3. Sabel MS, Wong SL. Review of evidence-based support for pretreatment imaging in melanoma. *J Natl Compr Canc Netw.* 2009;7(3):281–289.
4. Aloia TA, Gershenwald JE, Andtbacka RH, et al. Utility of computed tomography and magnetic resonance staging in patients with stage III melanoma diagnosed by sentinel lymphadenectomy. *J Clin Oncol.* 2006;24:2858–2865.
5. Bold RJ, Mansfield PF, Berger DH, et al. Prospective, randomized, double-blind study of prophylactic antibodies in axillary lymph node dissection. *Am J Surg.* 1998;176(3):239–243.
6. Morton DL, Cochran AJ, Thompson JF, et al. Sentinel node biopsy for early-stage melanoma: accuracy and morbidity in MSLT-I, an international multicenter trial. *Ann Surg.* 2005;242:302–313.
7. Balch CM, Gershenwald JE, Soong SJ, et al. Final version of 2009 AJCC melanoma staging and classification. *J Clin Oncol.* 2009;27:6199–6206.
8. Guggenheim MM, Hug U, Jung FJ, et al. Morbidity and recurrence after completion lymph node dissection following sentinel lymph node biopsy in cutaneous malignant melanoma. *Ann Surg.* 2008;247:687–693.
9. Veenstra HJ, van der Ploeg IM, Wouters MW, et al. Reevaluation of the locoregional recurrence rate in melanoma patients with a positive sentinel node compared to patients with palpable nodal involvement. *Ann Surg Oncol.* 2010;17:521–526.
10. Pidhorecky I, Lee RJ, Prouix G, et al. Risk factors for nodal recurrence after lymphadenectomy for melanoma. *Ann Surg Oncol.* 2001;8: 109–115.
11. Karakousis CP, Hena MA, Emrich LJ, et al. Axillary node dissection in malignant melanoma: results and complications. *Surgery.* 1990; 108:10–12.
12. Lee RJ, Gibbs JF, Prouix GM, et al. Nodal basin recurrence following lymph node dissection for melanoma: implications for adjuvant radiotherapy. *Int J Radiat Oncol Biol Phys.* 2000;46:467–474.
13. Burmeister BH, Mark Smithers B, Burmeister E, et al. A prospective phase II study of adjuvant postoperative radiation therapy following nodal surgery in malignant melanoma—Trans Tasman Radiation Oncology Group (TROG) study 96.06. *Radiother Oncol.* 2006;81: 136–142.
14. Beadle BM, Guadagnolo BA, Ballo MT, et al. Radiation therapy field extent for adjuvant treatment of axillary metastases from malignant melanoma. *Int J Radiat Oncol Biol Phys.* 2009;73(5):1376–1382.
15. Burmeister BH, Henderson MA, Anslie J, et al. Adjuvant radiotherapy versus observation alone for patients at risk of lymph-node field relapse after therapeutic lymphadenectomy for melanoma: a randomised trial. *Lancet Oncol.* 2012;13:589–597.

Chapter 29 Inguinal Lymph Node Dissection (Inguinofemoral and Ilioinguinal) for Metastatic Melanoma

Amod A. Sarnaik Vernon K. Sondak

DEFINITION

- Inguinofemoral lymphadenectomy (or superficial inguinal lymph node dissection) is defined as the en bloc removal of all lymphatic tissue contained within the femoral triangle, as well as the node-bearing tissue superior to the inguinal ligament but superficial to the external abdominal oblique aponeurosis, up to the level of the anterior superior iliac spine (ASIS).
- The procedure can be combined with a pelvic (also known as deep inguinal) node dissection, in which case it is designated as an ilioinguinal lymphadenectomy, that includes the separate removal of the obturator and external iliac lymph nodes at least up to the level of the iliac bifurcation.
- The procedure has been used for the management of inguinal metastasis from penile and vulvar carcinoma as well as cutaneous malignancies such as squamous cell, basal cell, adnexal, and Merkel cell carcinoma, but it is most commonly used for metastatic melanoma, the focus of this chapter.

DIFFERENTIAL DIAGNOSIS

- Patients who present with a palpable inguinal mass with a history of melanoma should be considered to have metastatic melanoma until proven otherwise.
- Patients who present with a palpable inguinal mass without a known history of melanoma should be investigated for a primary malignancy with complete skin/mucosal surface physical examination including the vulva, penis and perianal skin/anal canal, and a digital rectal examination to evaluate for melanoma, nonmelanoma skin cancer (squamous cell, basal cell, Merkel cell, or adnexal carcinoma), vulvar, penile, and anal cancer.
- For patients presenting with a palpable groin mass but without history or physical evidence of skin/mucosal surface cancers, the differential diagnoses include inguinal/femoral hernias, femoral aneurysm, reactive/infectious lymphadenopathy (cat-scratch fever or posttraumatic), lymphoma, or metastatic cancer of unknown primary origin (including melanoma).

PATIENT HISTORY AND PHYSICAL FINDINGS

- Prompt diagnosis of inguinal metastasis by the least invasive means when possible is a good start to minimize the morbidity of subsequent inguinal node dissection.
  - Patients with clinically occult inguinal disease can be diagnosed with sentinel lymph node biopsy. Inguinofemoral lymphadenectomy for microscopic nodal disease identified with sentinel lymph node biopsy appears to be associated with less morbidity compared to lymphadenectomy for macroscopic nodal disease.[1]
  - Patients with palpable groin masses not determined to be an aneurysm or hernia should be considered for a percutaneous fine needle or core needle biopsy to establish the diagnosis. If the mass is difficult to palpate or characterize, a diagnostic ultrasound with subsequent ultrasound-guided biopsy could be considered. Open biopsy should be reserved for when percutaneous biopsy is nondiagnostic, as the resulting scar and biopsy cavity from an open biopsy of a palpable mass render subsequent lymphadenectomy technically more difficult and can often result in wider skin flaps than what otherwise would be necessary.[2]
- Although currently considered to be the standard of care, the role of completion inguinofemoral lymphadenectomy in patients with micrometastatic melanoma found on sentinel lymph node biopsy is under investigation. Nodal observation as a potential alternative to immediate completion lymphadenectomy in melanoma patients with a positive sentinel node is being evaluated in the ongoing Multicenter Selective Lymphadenectomy Trial II. The trial randomizes patients with a positive sentinel lymph node to either immediate lymphadenectomy or observation with serial clinical examinations and ultrasonography. The patients randomized to observation may undergo a delayed completion lymphadenectomy if there is regional recurrence or may avoid the procedure and its associated morbidity if there is no evidence of regional disease during follow-up.
- Ilioinguinal lymphadenectomy is typically warranted for patients with radiographic evidence of metastatic disease in the pelvis. Other indications for an ilioinguinal lymph node dissection have not been definitively established and therefore are controversial. The clinical benefit of ilioinguinal lymphadenectomy for clinically occult metastatic disease when the pelvic nodes appear to be radiographically normal has not been demonstrated in a randomized, prospective trial to date. However, there are indications that are generally considered but not yet established.
  - Relative indications for ilioinguinal lymphadenectomy include any palpable inguinofemoral disease or four or more micrometastatic lymph nodes found at the setting of prior sentinel lymph node biopsy.
  - A possible but not yet established indication is any positive inguinofemoral sentinel lymph node biopsy result where the lymphoscintigraphy indicated evidence of "hot" nodes in the pelvis that were not removed in the sentinel lymph node procedure.
  - Some surgeons advocate for the positive status of the so-called "Cloquet's node" as an indication for ilioinguinal lymphadenectomy. However, there is a lack of uniform definition of Cloquet's node, as well as known examples

of lymphoscintigraphy performed for sentinel node biopsy where there is direct drainage from low or mid-inguinal nodes to pelvic nodes, bypassing all high inguinal nodes that would include Cloquet's node. Due to these factors, we do not rely on the status of Cloquet's node in any way.[2]

- Inguinofemoral or ilioinguinal lymph node dissections are performed under general anesthesia; therefore, the patient should be assessed for perioperative cardiac risk factors and referred for preoperative testing including cardiac stress test when clinically warranted.
- Patients should be clinically assessed for any preoperative lymphedema and typically are referred for fitted gradient compression stocking measurements to be used in the postoperative period. Although proof of the value of compression therapy is lacking, it is thought that early institution of compression therapy might minimize the risk of lymphedema in the early postoperative period.

IMAGING AND OTHER DIAGNOSTIC STUDIES

- Prior to lymphadenectomy, patients who are diagnosed with palpable inguinal metastatic melanoma typically are recommended to undergo whole body imaging (positron emission tomography–computed tomography [PET/CT] plus brain magnetic resonance imaging [MRI] or equivalent). Surgery is typically pursued in the absence of biopsy-proven distant disease, whereas systemic therapy is typically pursued if biopsy-proven distant disease is found.
- Patients who are diagnosed with micrometastatic inguinal melanoma by sentinel lymph node biopsy are not routinely recommended to undergo imaging due to the relatively low frequency of findings that are truly positive.

SURGICAL MANAGEMENT

Preoperative Planning

- Preoperative planning for a complete lymphadenectomy starts with careful consideration of the diagnostic procedures required to establish the diagnosis of metastatic disease. Percutaneous needle biopsy where feasible should be considered for palpable disease as discussed above. Orientation of the sentinel node incision should be planned to facilitate a potential inguinal lymph node dissection that will include resection of the sentinel node biopsy scar and cavity.
  - When the sentinel node is mapped below the inguinal ligament, the sentinel node incision should ideally be vertically oriented and at least 0.5 cm distal to the groin crease (**FIG 1A**).
  - When the sentinel node is mapped to above the inguinal ligament (typically with a flank primary melanoma), the sentinel node incision should ideally be obliquely or transversely oriented and at least 0.5 cm proximal to the groin crease (**FIG 1B**).
- For planning the completion lymphadenectomy, the operative side and site should be identified with the agreement of the patient and/or the representative of the patient in the preoperative holding area.
- Patients with a prior history of deep vein thrombosis (DVT) or known genetic predisposition to thrombosis are given a prophylactic dose of low-molecular-weight heparin preoperatively.
- A first-generation cephalosporin such as cefazolin (or equivalent if allergic to cephalosporins or penicillin) are routinely given intravenously within 30–60 minutes of the creation of the skin incision.

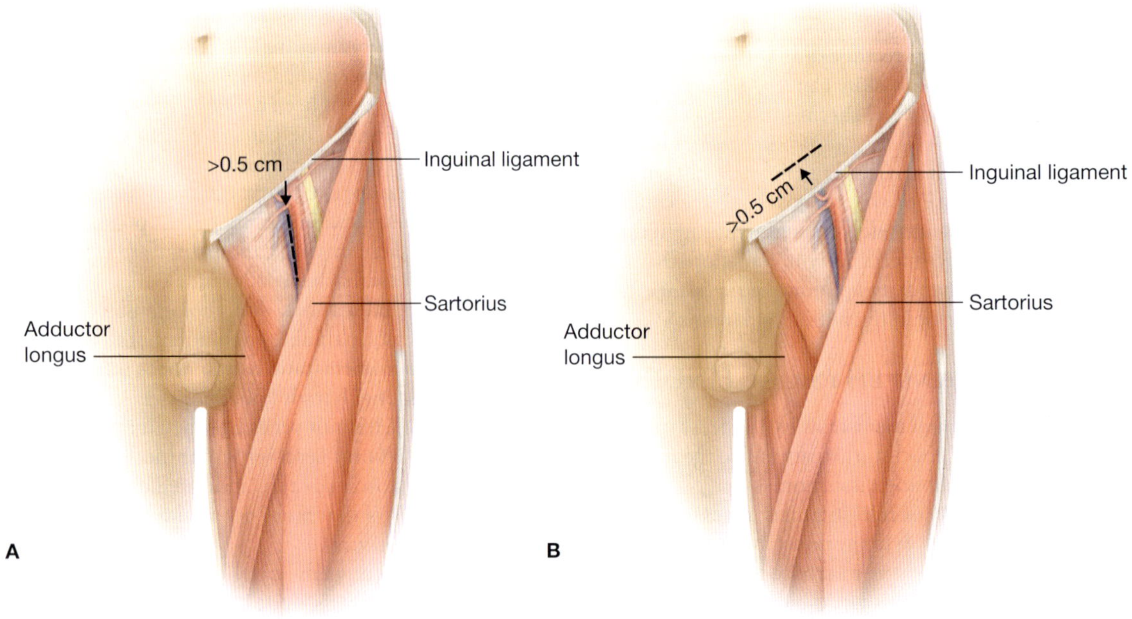

FIG 1 • **A.** The recommended orientation for sentinel node biopsy incision when the draining nodes map to the region inferior to the groin crease. **B.** The recommended orientation for sentinel node biopsy incision when the draining nodes map to the region superior to the groin crease.

Positioning

- The patient is placed in the supine position on a standard operating table. A sequential compression device (SCD) (knee length ipsilateral and thigh length contralateral) should be placed for DVT prophylaxis prior to induction of anesthesia. General anesthesia is required using either a laryngeal mask or endotracheal tube for inguinofemoral lymphadenectomy, but endotracheal tube is preferred for ilioinguinal dissections. Long-acting paralytic agents at induction are often avoided to allow for motor nerve stimulation to be evident during the course of the procedure. A urinary catheter is inserted for ilioinguinal dissections but may potentially be omitted for inguinofemoral dissections at the discretion of the surgeon. The patient is placed in a slight frog-leg position with all pressure points padded. The operative field should be prepared from the abdominal wall at the level of the umbilicus to the level of the knee. A groin towel secured with a sterile adhesive drape can be used to cover and exclude the genitalia from the field.

INGUINOFEMORAL (OR SUPERFICIAL) LYMPHADENECTOMY

Skin Incision and Raising of Flaps

- As stated previously, a well-placed node biopsy incision, or avoiding the creation of a preexisting incision by percutaneous instead of open biopsy of palpable metastasis, is important to minimize the area of required skin flaps.
- For a positive sentinel node where the sentinel node scar is below the inguinal crease, a curvilinear incision is made in a vertical orientation with an ellipse of skin to facilitate excision of the previous cavity of dissection (**FIG 2A**). For a positive sentinel node where the sentinel node scar is above the inguinal crease, a transversely or obliquely oriented incision is made to excise the previous cavity of dissection. A second counterincision can be made below the inguinal crease to reach the remaining femoral nodes (**FIG 2B**). In thin individuals, retraction can frequently allow for the extirpation of the femoral nodes distal to the inguinal crease without the need for the second incision.
- For palpable disease without a pre-existing biopsy scar, a skin incision is configured in a lazy "S" fashion (**FIG 2C**). If the tumor is close to the skin, an ellipse of skin overlying the palpable tumor should be included. The incision should also include any scar from prior node biopsy procedure if applicable. This incision can be extended in a cranial direction if needed for an ilioinguinal lymphadenectomy.
- Skin flaps are raised in order to clear the anticipated boundaries of the dissection (below) without being so thin to cause postoperative skin necrosis. Limiting the extent of the flaps to the borders of the femoral triangle avoids an unnecessarily wide field of dissection and therefore may be associated with a reduction in morbidity.
- The dissection is continued to the level of the muscular fascia with the following boundaries (**FIG 2D**):
  - Anterior superior iliac spine (ASIS) superolaterally
  - Pubic tubercle superomedially
  - The superior extent of dissection should encompass the tissue from the ASIS to the pubic tubercle resulting in approximately 3–5-cm clearance above inguinal ligament while leaving external oblique fascia intact.
  - Sartorius muscle laterally, incising the fascia
  - Adductor longus medially, incising the fascia
  - Crossing of the sartorius and adductor longus distally (the so-called apex of the femoral triangle)
- It should be noted that while there have been isolated reports suggesting that incising the fascia of the sartorius and adductor longus may increase lymphedema, this has not been established in large series and most surgeons incise the muscle fasciae as described earlier.
- During the course of the dissection, tissue that potentially contains lymphatic vessels should be clipped, tied, or sealed with harmonic shears.[3]
- A key point of the upper extent of the dissection on the abdominal wall is that the lymphadenectomy clears the subcutaneous and node-bearing tissue down to the external oblique fascia from the boundary of the ASIS to the pubic tubercle proximally and down to the inguinal ligament distally (**FIG 3**). The dissection can typically preserve the spermatic cord in males, but the round ligament can be divided, if necessary due to the presence of disease, in females.

Dissection of the Saphenous Vein Distally

- The distal portion of the saphenous vein is encountered along the medial boundary of the dissection approximately 3–5 cm proximal to the apex of the femoral triangle. In most cases, the saphenous vein is tied off distally with 2-0 silk and divided. The saphenous vein can potentially be preserved in select cases where the procedure is performed for micrometastatic disease, when and if any existing seroma cavity and scar tissue is separate from the vein.[1,4] Although saphenous vein preservation might theoretically reduce the likelihood of postoperative DVT and lymphedema, this maneuver has never been definitively shown to reduce postoperative complications in any prospective, randomized study. Therefore, saphenous preservation should only be considered in select cases performed for micrometastatic disease, where the vein is not involved with scar or seroma cavity, and the maneuver should never compromise the extent of dissection.

Dissection of the Femoral Vessels

- The superficial femoral artery is identified at the distal aspect of the dissection at the apex of the femoral triangle. At this level, the femoral artery lies anterior to the femoral vein. As the dissection proceeds distal to proximal, the femoral artery courses laterally while the femoral vein courses medially. The anterior surfaces of the femoral vessels are skeletonized, and the dissection is extended laterally at the same depth as the vessels to avoid injury to the femoral nerve, which is generally not directly visualized. The relationship of the femoral vessels to the boundaries of the femoral triangle is shown in **FIG 4**.

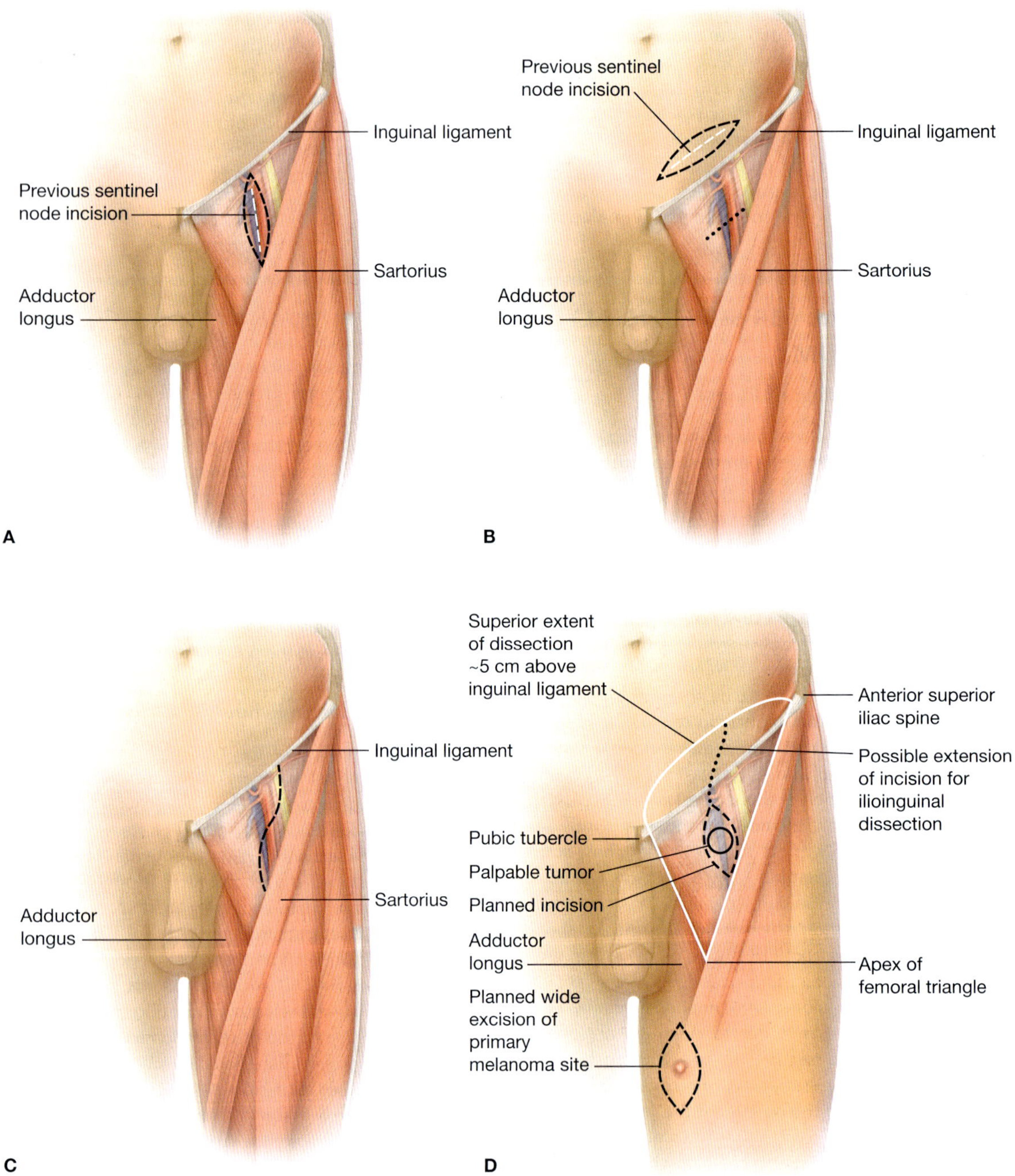

FIG 2 • **A.** The recommended orientation of a curvilinear incision for the indication of a positive sentinel node that mapped to the region inferior to the groin crease. **B.** The recommended orientation of an elliptical incision above the groin crease combined if necessary with a linear incision inferior to the groin crease. **C.** The recommended orientation of a lazy S incision that can include an ellipse of skin overlying palpable disease. Of note, to facilitate exposure for an ilioinguinal lymphadenectomy, it may be required for the incision to cross the groin crease. **D.** The operative field with denoted boundaries of the extent of inguinofemoral lymphadenectomy (white line) in a patient with an intact primary melanoma and clinically evident nodal disease. Note that the planned incision includes the palpable metastasis and that the incision can be optionally extended onto the abdominal wall for an ilioinguinal lymphadenectomy.

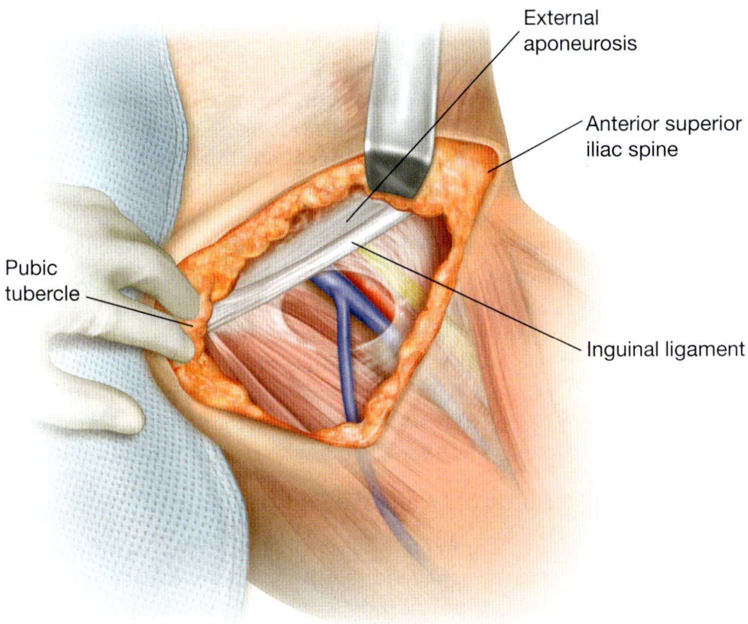

FIG 3 ● The superior extent of dissection clears all subcutaneous tissue 3–5 cm proximal to the inguinal ligament to a depth bounded by the underlying external oblique aponeurosis.

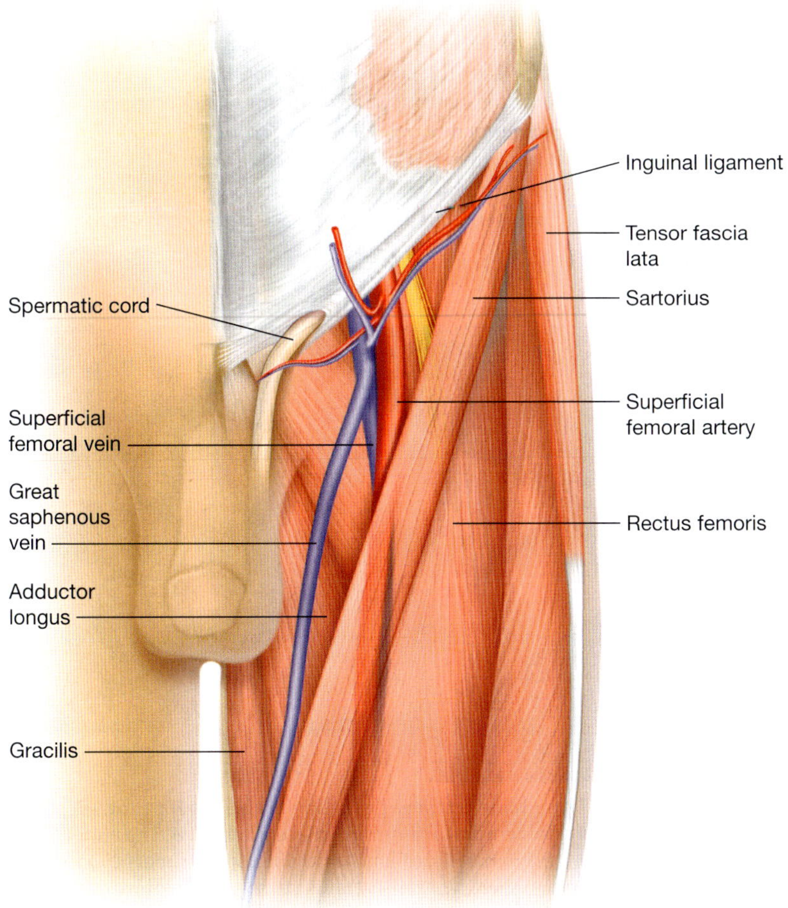

FIG 4 ● The relationship of the femoral artery and vein to the boundaries of the femoral triangle. Note at the distal apex of the femoral triangle, the femoral artery lies superficial to the femoral vein.

Completion of the Dissection and Ligation of the Saphenofemoral Junction

- The dissection continues in a distal to proximal direction up to the level of the saphenofemoral junction. If the saphenous vein is to be preserved, it is fully freed from the specimen; generally, several small- to medium-sized tributaries draining the specimen need to be divided and ligated individually. Otherwise, the entirety of the saphenous vein is included in the specimen and the remaining soft tissue is circumferentially dissected so that the specimen remains adherent only by the saphenofemoral junction (**FIG 5A**).
- The saphenous vein is doubly ligated at the level of the saphenofemoral junction, usually with a 3-0 silk suture ligature and a 2-0 silk tie, taking care not to narrow the femoral vein (**FIG 5B**). A formal closure of the stump with vascular suture is not routinely required but may be necessary if the saphenofemoral junction is very broad or if palpable tumor extends in close proximity to the femoral vein itself.

Sartorius Muscle Transposition Flap

- Sartorius muscle transposition is used to cover the exposed femoral vessels in the groin whenever there is concern about the integrity of the overlying skin flap closure. Some surgeons routinely perform this in all cases, whereas others do it selectively or not at all.[1,5] We use it in most cases but routinely omit it when the incision is placed high in the groin (i.e., not directly overlying the exposed vessels) and in selected younger patients, including children, especially athletes or other very active individuals.
- The tendinous portion of the sartorius muscle is taken off its point of origin at the ASIS with electrocautery. It is important to divide the muscle as high as possible to maximize the length of muscle available for the flap. It is critical to obtain meticulous hemostasis at the cut muscle edge, as there is little or no tissue at that level to tamponade bleeding and a small ooze can continue for hours postoperatively. To mobilize the muscle for the transposition flap without tension, a few lateral feeding vessels generally need to be tied off, and the lateral fascia is incised well down the length of the muscle. The muscle is transposed over the femoral vessels and secured in place to the external abdominal oblique aponeurosis/inguinal ligament with three or four interrupted, horizontal mattress 2-0 non-absorbable, braided polyester sutures oriented so that the knots are pushed down onto the sartorius muscle. The sutures are placed in a staggered fashion to avoid being placed at the same level in the ligament, which would otherwise weaken the fascia (**FIG 6**).

Placement of Drain and Closure

- If a concomitant pelvic dissection (i.e., superficial and deep lymphadenectomy) is planned, see the following text and closure is deferred until completion of that portion of the procedure.
- A flat or round closed-suction drain is routinely placed in the bed of dissection and brought out through a separate stab incision relatively close to the wound but away from the thinnest parts of the skin flaps. The incision is closed with interrupted 3-0 absorbable, polygalactin sutures for the subcutaneous tissue and a running suture of 4-0 absorbable, monofilament suture for the subcuticular skin layer. Cyanoacrylate adhesive (or equivalent) is used over the subcuticular closure for extra protection. The leg is wrapped with an Ace wrap from the level of the metatarsals to mid-thigh, and a thigh-length SCD is placed over the Ace and on the contralateral extremity. The urinary catheter, if used, is left in place at the end of the case.

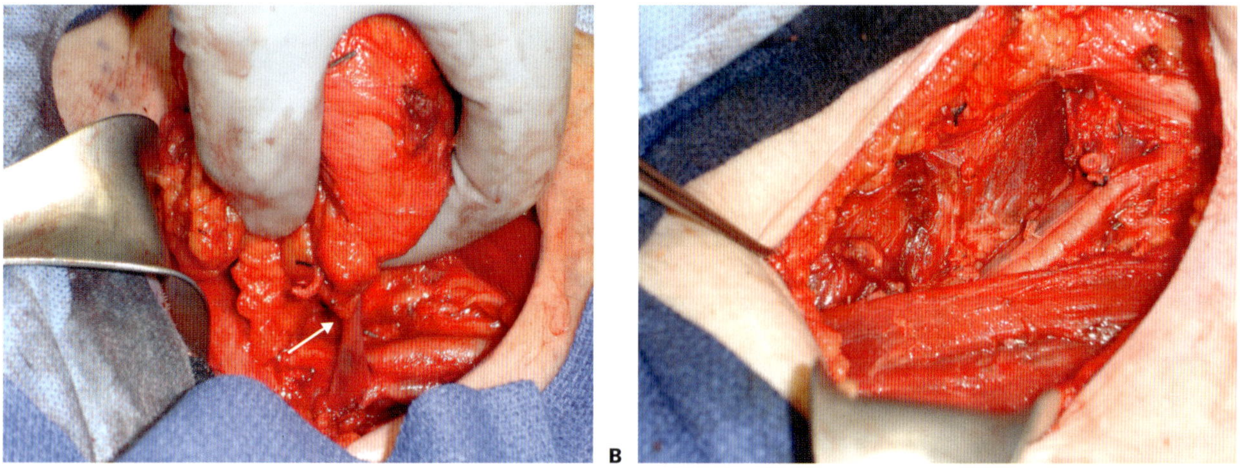

A B

FIG 5 ● **A.** The appearance of the completed left inguinofemoral lymphadenectomy dissection with a view of the specimen attached only by the saphenofemoral junction *(arrow)* with the superficial femoral artery immediately lateral. **B.** The appearance of the ligated saphenofemoral junction *(arrow)* after removal of the specimen without any narrowing of the superficial femoral vein, and a view of the superficial femoral artery lateral to the vein as well as the sartorius muscle that forms the lateral boundary of the dissection.

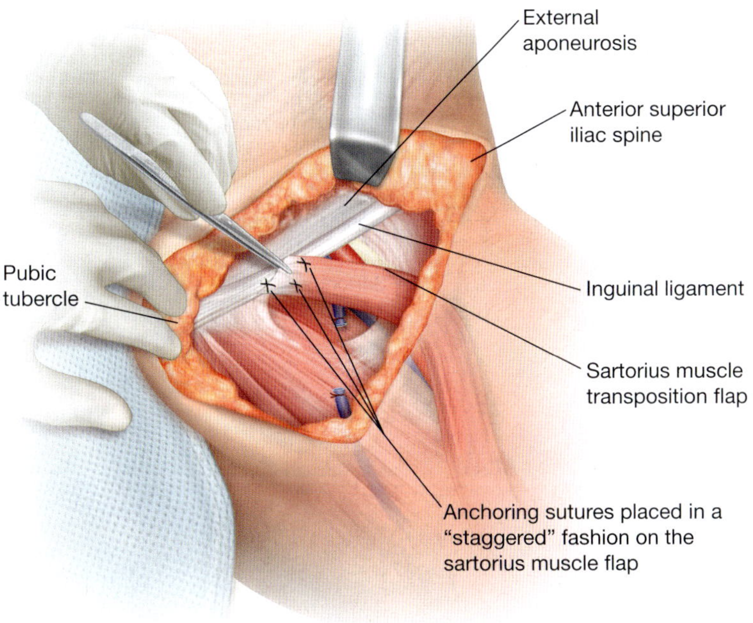

FIG 6 ● Sutures that anchor the sartorius muscle transposition flap are placed in a staggered fashion instead of being placed on a single plane in order to avoid weakening the fascia.

ILIOINGUINAL LYMPHADENECTOMY

Division of the Abdominal Wall and Retroperitoneal Exposure of the Pelvis

- When conducted as a portion of a combined ilioinguinal lymphadenectomy, the pelvic portion of the lymphadenectomy occurs through the same incision. The incision may need to be lengthened sufficiently above the inguinal crease to ensure adequate visualization (**FIG 2D**).
- The pelvic portion of the ilioinguinal lymphadenectomy involves the removal of the obturator and iliac nodes up to the bifurcation of the iliac vessels through a retroperitoneal approach. In some individuals, the common iliac nodes can be removed if grossly involved by extending the fascial incision cephalad, but para-aortic nodes are considered beyond the scope of the dissection and are rarely accessible through the retroperitoneal approach.
- Through the same skin incision used for the inguinofemoral dissection, the external and internal abdominal oblique aponeuroses are incised parallel to the direction of the fibers of the respective muscles (**FIG 7A**). The peritoneum is retracted superiorly and medially, which typically mobilizes the ureter out of the field. Retraction of the peritoneal contents superiorly and medially exposes the external iliac artery and vein with associated node-bearing tissue (**FIG 7B**).

Retrieval of Iliac Nodal Tissue

- The external iliac vessels are skeletonized over their anterior aspect. All fibrofatty and lymphatic tissue overlying the iliac vessels is retrieved from the bifurcation proximally to the posterior aspect of the inguinal ligament distally.

Retrieval of Obturator Nodal Tissue

- The external iliac vein is retracted laterally to expose the obturator space medially. Fibrofatty and lymphatic tissue is removed down to the level of the obturator nerve (**FIG 8**). Caution should be taken when dissecting medially as the obturator vessels and tributaries are difficult to visualize and can be difficult to control if injured.
- The obturator foramen and the pubic rami should be carefully inspected and palpated to ensure that nodes are not left behind in those locations.

Placement of Drain and Closure

- While not absolutely required, a second closed-suction drain can be deployed into the bed of the dissection and brought through the divided abdominal muscle fibers distally, exiting the skin through a separate stab incision. The internal and external abdominal oblique fasciae are closed with absorbable monofilament sutures. Closure then proceeds as described earlier in the inguinofemoral dissection.

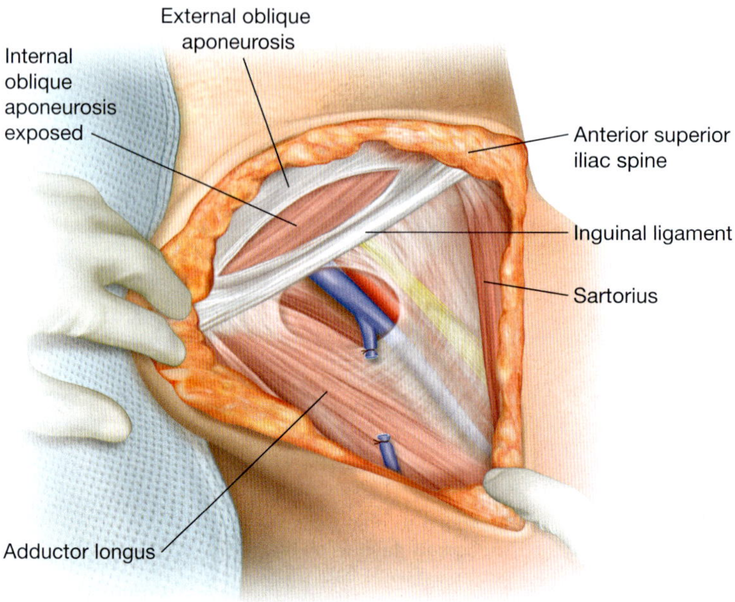

A

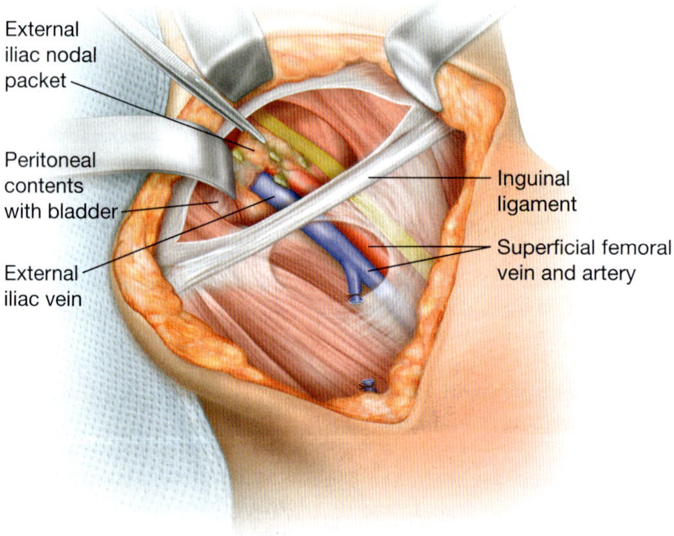

B

FIG 7 ● **A.** The external oblique aponeurosis has been incised in a direction parallel to its fibers, exposing the underlying internal oblique aponeurosis. **B.** Anterior view of the external iliac artery and vein with delivery of the external iliac nodal packet.

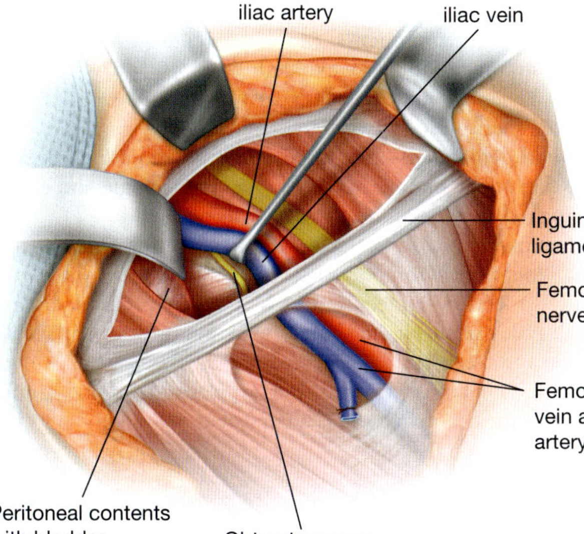

FIG 8 ● Appearance of the completed ilioinguinal dissected field with the obturator nerve exposed deep and medial to the external iliac vessels.

PEARLS AND PITFALLS

Indications	■ The diagnosis of inguinal metastasis should be made using the least invasive method possible. ■ Palpable disease should be evaluated by percutaneous fine needle aspiration or core needle biopsy rather than open biopsy whenever possible. ■ Sentinel node biopsy incisions should be fashioned while being mindful of the possibility that inguinal lymphadenectomy may be required in the future. ■ Sentinel node biopsy incisions directly in the inguinal crease are not advised due to the difficulty with the subsequent lymphadenectomy incision if necessary. ■ In cases where there is nodal disease without a known primary, a careful physical examination to identify a primary cancer is warranted, including examination of the skin of the lower body, digital rectal examination, and examination of the penis/vulva.
Placement of incision	■ Incisions should be fashioned to avoid crossing the inguinal crease where feasible.

Extent of resection	■ Saphenous vein preservation may be considered for cases being performed for micrometastatic disease and when the vein is not involved with scar or the seroma/biopsy cavity.
	■ Indications for inclusion of pelvic lymphadenectomy in the absence of clear-cut pelvic involvement have not been definitively established; but typically, scenarios for which ilioinguinal lymphadenectomy is potentially considered are the following:
	  ■ Macroscopic inguinofemoral disease
	  ■ Four or more positive nodes identified at sentinel lymphadenectomy
	  ■ Pelvic drainage observed at the time of lymphoscintigraphy with a positive inguinofemoral sentinel node

Key postoperative care	■ Patients are typically placed on bedrest overnight. ■ DVT prophylaxis is typically instituted on the evening of the procedure and continued while the patient is in the hospital unless there is clinical concern for hemorrhage. ■ Lymphedema precautions include compression with Ace wraps or fitted compression garments with aggressive institution of lymphedema therapy at the first clinical sign of lymphedema.

POSTOPERATIVE CARE

- The patient is typically kept on bedrest overnight with the urinary catheter, if used, in place, and affected extremity raised to above the level of the heart. The affected extremity is kept wrapped with an Ace from the metatarsals to mid thigh, with thigh-length SCDs in place on the contralateral extremity and over the Ace on the ipsilateral extremity.
- If the patient's physical examination and the drain output are not concerning for postoperative bleeding, prophylactic subcutaneous low-molecular-weight heparin is administered on the evening of the procedure and continued daily while the patient is hospitalized.
- On the first postoperative day, the urinary catheter, if present, is removed and the patient is encouraged to ambulate.

- After an inguinofemoral lymphadenectomy, patients are discharged after 1 or 2 nights when pain is controlled with oral analgesics.
- After ilioinguinal lymphadenectomy, patients are kept nil per os for the first night. If there is no sign of ileus, the diet can be advanced on postoperative day 1. Patients typically remain in the hospital for at least 2 nights and are discharged when pain is controlled with oral analgesics and are tolerating a diet.
- On discharge, patients are encouraged to ambulate to minimize risk of DVT, wear Ace or fitted gradient compression stockings during the day, and to elevate the operated leg above the level of the heart at night.
- At the first clinical sign of lymphedema, lymphedema therapy is ordered and verification of compliance with the fitted compression stockings is done.

OUTCOMES

- Five-year overall survival rates for melanoma metastatic to regional lymph nodes are listed below[6]:
  - Stage IIIA melanoma—1 to 3 nodes involved with microscopic disease and nonulcerated primary tumor—78%
  - Stage IIIB melanoma—1 to 3 nodes involved with microscopic disease and an ulcerated primary tumor or 1 to 3 nodes involved with macroscopic disease and a nonulcerated primary tumor—59%
  - Stage IIIC melanoma—4+ nodes involved, 1 to 3 nodes involved with macroscopic disease and an ulcerated primary tumor, matted lymphadenopathy, or disease that includes in-transit and nodal metastasis—40%

COMPLICATIONS AND RELEVANT MANAGEMENT

- Seroma—if symptomatic can be percutaneously drained; open drainage should be avoided
- Lymphedema—managed with early compression and lymphedema therapy
- Wound dehiscence—risk is minimized by confining area of the flap to the boundaries of the femoral triangle and can be managed with a wound vac device as needed
- Infection—typically managed with oral antibiotics
- DVT/pulmonary embolism—risk is minimized by the routine use of low-molecular-weight heparin prophylaxis and high index of suspicion should be maintained for early diagnosis and treatment
- Sensory deficit is common but typically does not require management unless there is a persistent neuralgia
- Recurrence

REFERENCES

1. Sabel MS, Griffith KA, Arora A, et al. Inguinal node dissection for melanoma in the era of sentinel lymph node biopsy. *Surgery*. 2007;141:728–735.
2. Sarnaik AA, Puleo CA, Zager S, et al. Limiting the morbidity of inguinal lymphadenectomy for metastatic melanoma. *Cancer Control*. 2009;16:240–247.
3. Janetschek G, Hobisch A, Peschel R, et al. Laparoscopic retroperitoneal lymph node dissection. *Urology*. 2000;55:136–140.
4. Dardarian TS, Gray HJ, Morgan MA, et al. Saphenous vein sparing during inguinal lymphadenectomy to reduce morbidity in patients with vulvar carcinoma. *Gynecol Oncol*. 2006;101:140–142.
5. Judson PL, Jonson AL, Paley PJ, et al. A prospective, randomized study analyzing sartorius transposition following inguinal-femoral lymphadenectomy. *Gynecol Oncol*. 2004;95:226–230.
6. Balch CM, Gershenwald JE, Soong SJ, et al. Final version of 2009 AJCC melanoma staging and classification. *J Clin Oncol*. 2009;27:6199–6206.

Chapter **30**

Minimally Invasive Inguinal Lymph Node Dissection for Melanoma

James W. Jakub

DEFINITION

- Minimally invasive inguinal lymph node dissection (MILND) is defined as an inguinal lymph node dissection performed through trocar ports. Many names have been coined for this videoscopic approach, and unfortunately, minimally invasive has also been used by some to describe an open technique using smaller incisions.
- The terminology surrounding the inguinal node dissection can be confusing. Urologic groin dissections separate the superficial inguinal basin as anterior to the cribriform fascia and the "deep" inguinal nodes as those nodes along the femoral vessels deep to this fascial layer. Melanoma surgeons have historically referred to both of these basins as a "superficial inguinal lymph node dissection" or "inguinalofemoral" and the pelvic or external iliac/obturator lymph nodes are referred to as a "deep inguinal lymph node dissection" or "ilioinguinal." In this chapter, when we describe an inguinal lymph node dissection, it will refer to all the nodes in the groin distal to the inguinal ligament and superficial to the external oblique aponeurosis, superficial and deep to the cribriform fascia. The deep or ilioinguinal dissection is discussed in Chapter 29.

ANATOMY

- The anatomy critical to the MILND is identical to that for the conventional open operative approach and is depicted in **FIGS 1A,B** and **2**. The superficial and deep inguinal lymph nodes are separated by the cribriform fascia, which is violated at the fossa ovalis. There are approximately 10 lymph nodes in the superficial basin and five in the deep.
- The borders of the femoral triangle are graphically depicted in **FIG 2**.

NATURAL HISTORY

- Complete inguinal lymph node dissection is advised for any patient with melanoma metastatic to the inguinal lymph nodes in the absence of distant metastases. Microscopic and macroscopic subclassifications of stage III disease are distinguished as clinical and not pathologic entities.[1] If disease is detected by physical exam, this is considered macroscopic, whereas a positive sentinel lymph node (SLN) represents microscopic disease regardless of the tumor burden identified pathologically. Stage III melanoma patients represent a very heterogeneous cohort and prognosis varies greatly based on the number of positive lymph nodes, nodal burden in the lymph nodes, and presence or absence of synchronous in-transit metastasis. Five-year overall survival for this group of patients is approximately 50%, but based on the specific subcategory varies widely from 25% to 75%.

PATIENT HISTORY AND PHYSICAL FINDINGS

- An MILND is indicated in most cases that would be considered for traditional inguinal nodal dissection including melanoma; cutaneous squamous cell carcinoma (SCC); and some urologic (penile), gynecologic (vulvar), anal, or low-lying rectal cancers.
- Physical examination should not only evaluate the inguinal nodal basin but also identify in-transit disease between the primary and inguinal nodal basin, particularly in the case of melanoma. Radiographic or gross nodal disease can be found cephalad to the inguinal ligament and superficial to the external oblique aponeurosis, especially in cases of a truncal primary.
- For lower extremity disease, the popliteal nodal basin should be evaluated; and for disease of the trunk, consideration for contralateral inguinal or axillary drainage needs to be considered based on location of the primary.
- Physical examination should also evaluate for prior scars in the field (sentinel lymph node biopsy [SLNB] or saphenous vein harvest from prior coronary artery bypass graft [CABG]) and skin changes suggestive of cutaneous involvement. This can be direct extension with overlying cutaneous hyperemia and fixation of disease or nodularity/ulceration that is often seen in SCC. For penile primaries, the genitals and base of penis should be inspected for cutaneous involvement.
- Most frequently, an MILND will be performed for microscopic disease following a positive SLNB. In this setting, waiting a minimum of 6 weeks from the SLNB to the MILND allows time for the acute operative inflammatory changes to resolve. An MILND may be considered in selected cases of macroscopic disease. Caution and sound clinical judgment should be used to avoid violating the specimen, assuring an en bloc resection and for radiographic disease, that the identified disease to be resected will indeed be contained inside the contents of dissection.
- MILND is contraindicated in the setting of cutaneous involvement or a prior lymphadenectomy in the same field. MILND may be considered in a prior radiated field, but again, caution should be stressed.

IMAGING AND OTHER DIAGNOSTIC STUDIES

- Positive SLNB for microscopic disease
  - In general, this is a delayed diagnosis and MILND is offered as a staged procedure, as typically, frozen section is not performed on SLNs for melanoma. Even in institutions where frozen section is performed on SLNs (such as

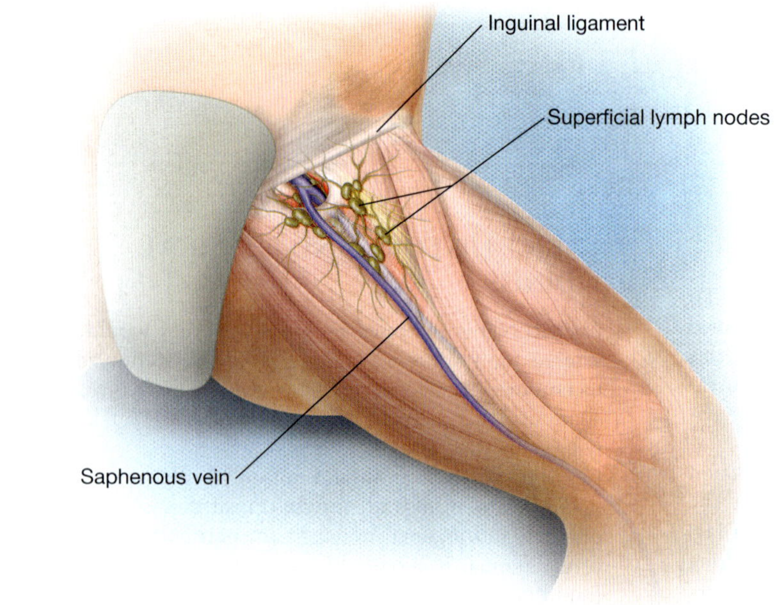

A

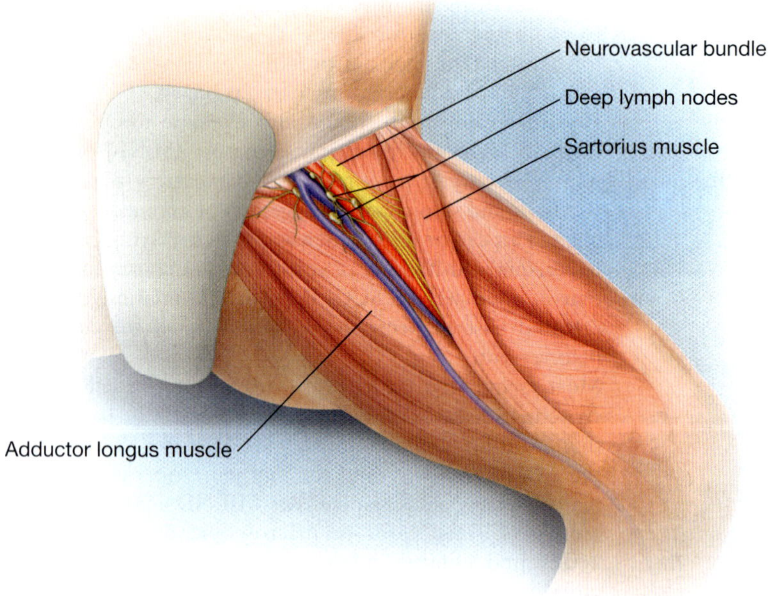

B

FIG 1 • **A,B.** Anatomy of the superficial and deep inguinal basin.

our own), there is no need to freeze the SLNs of the groin if MILND may be offered at a later date.

- The yield of systemic imaging to find clinically occult stage IV disease after a positive SLN is less than 5% and typically not warranted prior to MILND.[2–4]
- Deep pelvic (external iliac/obturator) node dissection is typically not required.

- Clinical inguinal regional nodal disease
  - In the setting of a palpable inguinal lymph node, a fine needle aspiration (FNA) to confirm the clinical diagnosis is frequently appropriate prior to embarking on an inguinal node dissection.
  - A search for systemic disease with whole-body imaging (computed tomography [CT] scan or positron emission tomography [PET]/CT) is reasonable prior to MILND as the true positive rate is above 10%.[5,6]
  - The decision to embrace a routine, selective or nihilistic, and hence, almost never approach to the pelvic basin will not be covered in this section. In general, for clinically apparent disease, I strongly consider a combined deep pelvic node dissection at the same setting.
  - There is limited data on minimally invasive approach to the pelvic lymph nodes for melanoma. Technically, it can be performed as clearly shown in clinical practice with gynecologic and urologic procedures. However, the role in melanoma is not defined. Basic questions such as, "Should an extraperitoneal versus an intraperitoneal approach be used?" and "Is converting an extraperitoneal

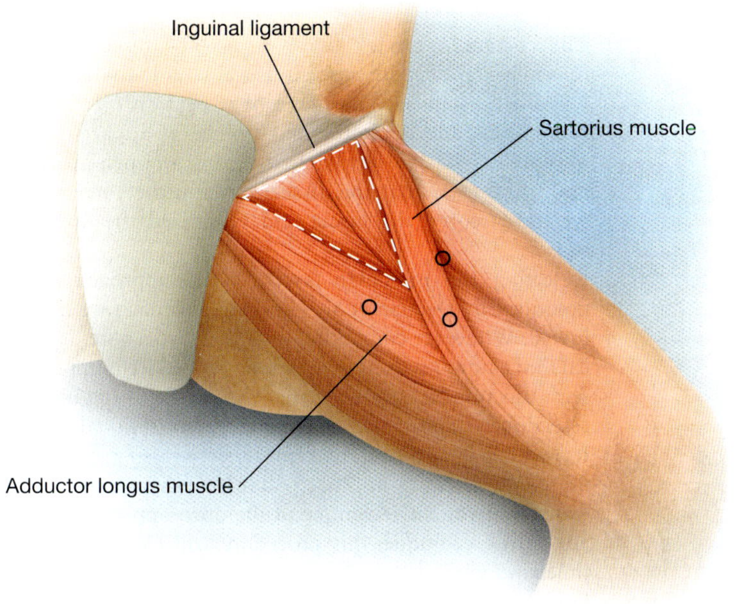

FIG 2 • Borders of the femoral triangle as well as trocar placement for MILND.

disease to an intraperitoneal operation sound?" have not been established. At the time of this writing, when performing a combined inguinal and a pelvic node dissection, I personally perform this as an open approach.

NONOPERATIVE MANAGEMENT

- The current standard, off protocol, is for a regional node dissection for all cases of a positive SLN, including immunohistochemical disease only.
- At the time of this publication, the Multicenter Selective Lymphadenectomy Trial II (MSLT II) randomizing patients with a positive SLNB to observation of the basin or standard lymph node dissection, just closed to accrual.

SURGICAL MANAGEMENT

- A word of caution: Data on short- and long-term morbidity are limited at the time of this publication.[7,8] Seromas are common and can be prolonged; wound complications requiring more than outpatient oral antibiotics are rare. Randomized single institution (Delman, personal communication, February 2013) and single-arm multi-institutional surgical trials (NCT01500304) are actively ongoing to define the short-term morbidity and surgical learning curve for this procedure. One measure of oncologic adequacy of the procedure is lymph node yield and this appears to be similar.[7,9] There is no data to date regarding oncologic outcomes and patients need to be clearly made aware, that as of the time of this publication, it is unknown if the regional control and cure rates with this approach are worse, better, or equivalent to a standard open approach. This candid discussion is necessary as part of the informed consent process (at the time of this printing one manuscript has been published).[9]

Preoperative Planning

- Preoperative baseline bilateral limb volumes should be considered.
- Brief with anesthesia and the operating room (OR) team prior to the start of the procedure:
  - Hypercarbia is to be expected. Unlike laparoscopy performed in an intraperitoneal location, this entire dissection is performed in the subcutaneous plane and much higher levels of carbon dioxide (CO_2) will be systemically absorbed. Anesthesia team needs to be aware and appropriate ventilatory modifications made to avoid the need for conversion.
  - Ensure you have towers in correct position, patient position is rehearsed, and desired equipment, including dissector and laparoscopic supplies, are in the room.
- Prophylactic antibiotics are provided.
- Mechanical venous thromboembolism (VTE) prophylaxis in the form of sequential compression devices are placed on the contralateral leg. Chemical VTE prophylaxis in the form of subcutaneous heparin is provided prior to incision and ideally prior to induction of general anesthesia.
- A Foley catheter is placed sterilely on the prepped field and sealed out of the dissection field with the genitalia by a sterile towel and Ioban.

Positioning

- In the typical setup, the patient is positioned supine with the legs split either on a split-leg table (my preference) or in the synchronous position with Yellofin gel stirrups. The operative leg is abducted and slightly flexed at the knee (**FIG 3**). If the leg is left straight, the surgeon will almost inevitably perform the dissection too lateral. The surgeon and the assistant stand so one is between the legs and the other stands lateral to the operative leg. The surgeon and the assistant may change positions during certain portions of the procedure if desired. The surgical technician stands on the opposite side of the patient's body.
- Video towers are placed at the head of the table, one above each shoulder (**FIG 3**). Minimal operative instrumentation is needed on the Mayo stand. If there is a need to emergently convert, appropriate instruments should be immediately available.

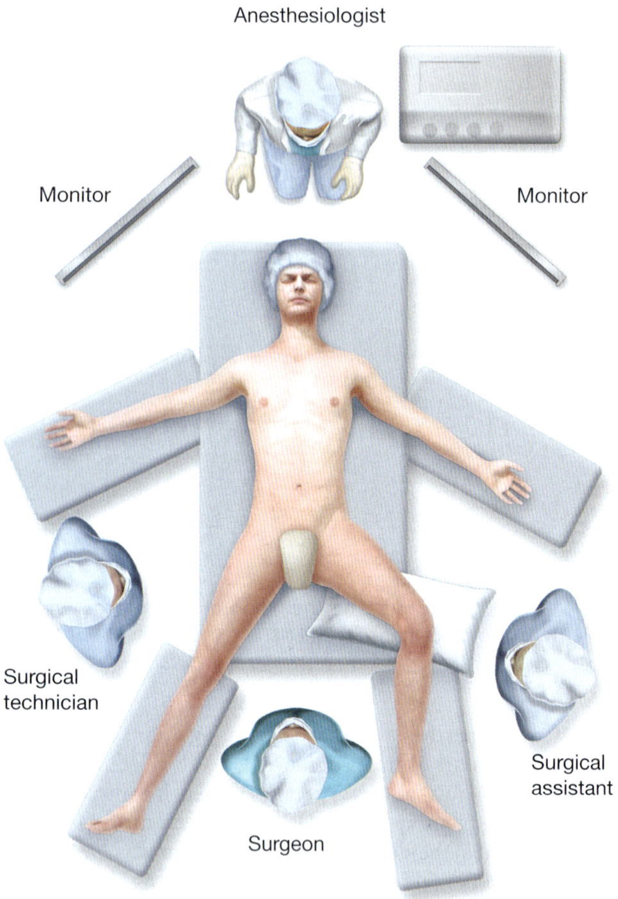

FIG 3 • Operating theater setup and patient position.

Approach

- The current approach involves en bloc resection of the muscular fascia and saphenous vein with the lymphadenectomy specimen. The plane of dissection off the sartorius muscle and adductor may not be as apparent with a minimally invasive approach as during an open procedure, and to be clear that the dissection is in the correct plane, we have scored the fascia and visualized the underlying muscle.
- Resecting the muscular fascia is the approach initially described by Delman et al.[10] and the approach we have followed. Whenever embarking on a new procedure, it is critical that caution is exercised and the procedure is approached with this mindset, assuring that the extent of the oncologic resection is at least as complete as the traditional standard for which it is meant to replace. It is also true that the minimally invasive approach should, as much as possible, exactly mirror the technique of the open approach. As with any novel technique, this procedure will likely evolve with time, and with experience, it may be shown that a muscular fascia and saphenous vein preserving approach is as safe and oncologically sound.
- We do not excise the SLNB scar if present. We also do not make an open incision to confirm the adequacy of dissection because the videoscopic view should make this obvious. If there is any question of inadequate resection, a small proximal incision can be made and the extent of the oncologic operation should not be jeopardized because of a perceived feeling of inadequacy or failure by "converting."

MINIMALLY INVASIVE INGUINAL LYMPH NODE DISSECTION

Operating Room Setup

- In the typical setup, the patient is positioned supine with the legs split either on a split-leg table (my strong personal preference) or in the synchronous position with Yellofin gel stirrups. The operative leg is abducted and slightly flexed at the knee (**FIG 3**). The surgeon and the assistant stand so one is between the legs and the other stands lateral to the operative leg. The surgeon and the assistant may change positions during certain portions of the procedure if desired. The surgical technician stands on the opposite side of the patient's body.
- Video towers are placed at the head of the table, one above each shoulder (**FIG 3**). Minimal operative instrumentation is needed on the Mayo stand. If there is a need to emergently convert, appropriate instruments should be immediately available.
- The anatomy critical to the MILND is identical to that for the conventional open operative approach and is depicted in **FIGS 1** and **2**. The superficial and deep inguinal lymph nodes are separated by the cribriform fascia, which is violated at the fossa ovalis. There are approximately 10 lymph nodes in the superficial basin and five in the deep.
- The borders of the femoral triangle are graphically depicted in **FIG 2**.
- External landmarks are identified. Palpation is performed to identify the medial border of dissection, which is the adductor longus muscle. This is marked with a marking pen. Next, similar palpation is performed to identify the sartorius muscle and identify its medial border, which will mark the lateral boundary of the dissection. The convergents of these lines occur at the distal border of dissection, which is the apex of the femoral triangle. Proximal dissection extends 3 to 5 cm cephalad to the inguinal ligament and it includes the soft tissues superficial to the external oblique in this location.
- Next, the three trocar sites are marked. The distal most incision is marked 3 cm from the apex of the femoral triangle. The other two trocars are placed proximal to this, each 5 cm apart, one medial and one lateral (see **FIG 5A,B**). Through one of the trocar sites, blunt dissection is performed with the index finger separating along the natural avascular plain between the subcutaneous fat and underlying soft tissue. Three 10/12 mm trocars are next introduced. As a

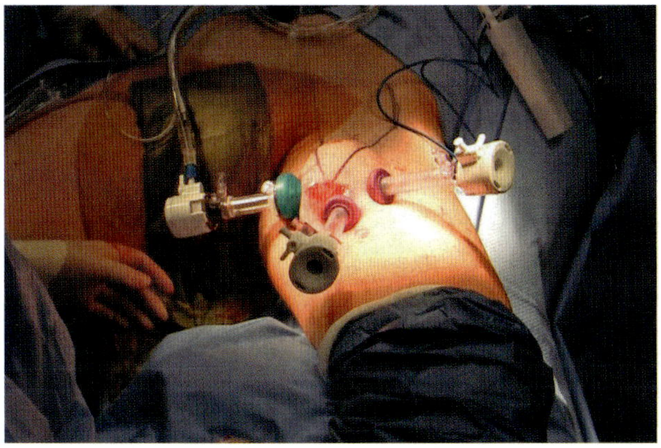

FIG 4 ● Photo depicting trocar placement and initial CO_2 insufflation at beginning of case (image © Mayo Clinic, 2014).

result of the thin subcutaneous tissue, a leak around the trocar may be encountered. As a result, the incision should be kept to a minimum and only one trocar site should be used for the initial blunt dissection. Short trocars are ideal, and bariatric instruments should be available in order to reach the proximal most dissection. Using trocars with balloons to minimize the leak are ideal.

- CO_2 insufflation is performed. Initially, 25 mmHg for 10 minutes and then decreased to 15 mmHg for the remainder of the procedure (**FIG 4**).

Superficial Dissection

- I perform the entire dissection with an ultrasonic dissector (personal preference) or LiqaSure® device, except when freeing the tissue from the external oblique aponeurosis where I use a hook cautery.
- Camper's fascia is preserved. Dissection is performed superficial to Scarpa's fascia.
- Initial dissection starts in a space created by the digital dissection and CO_2 insufflation. The dissection is begun distally and continued proximally. The initial dissection is performed in order to create a working space between the subcutaneous tissue and underlying regional contents.
- Dissection is performed fairly superficially, superficial to Scarpa's fascia. This can be appreciated with an external view showing the transillumination of the light source through the skin (**FIGS 5A,B**). Dissection can be assisted by external palpation over the previously marked boundaries of the triangle. Running a finger up and down the previously drawn landmarks while viewing internally assists one in defining the borders and extent of the superficial dissection. As dissection is completed more proximally, the loose areolar tissue overlying the external oblique aponeurosis can be appreciated. The entire anterior dissection within the externally marked triangle should be completed.

Sartorius Exposure

- The next portion of the procedure is the lateral dissection to identify the sartorius muscle. Dissection is performed through the fatty tissue until the sartorius fascia is identified.

A

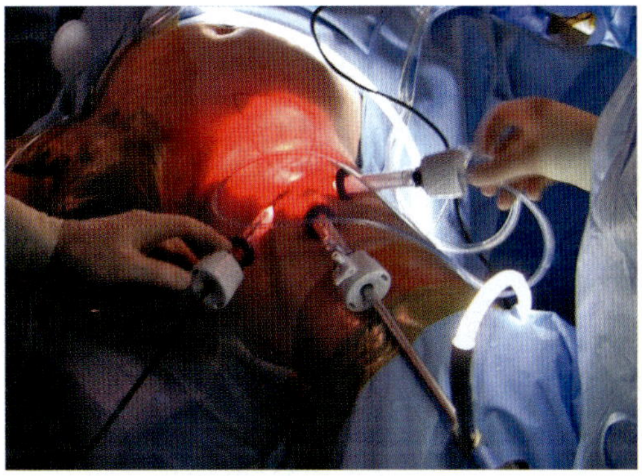

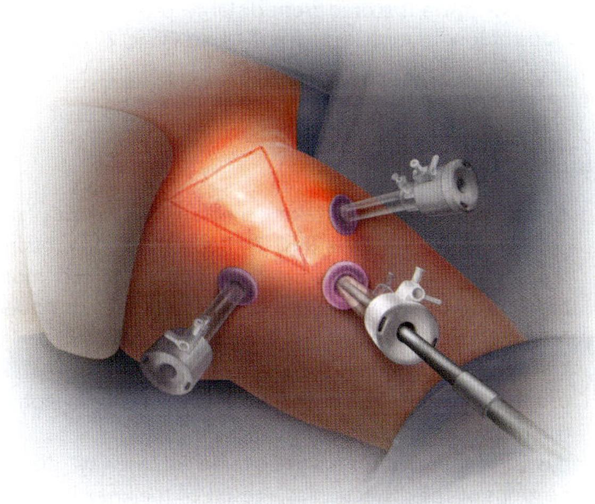

B

FIG 5 ● **A,B.** Photo and image demonstrating trocar placement, flap thickness, and drain placement. Dissection is quite superficial and this is demonstrated in these images showing how well the light transilluminates through the skin flaps (Fig. 5a © Mayo Clinic, 2014).

The fascia is divided, identifying the underlying muscular fibers of the sartorius. This is initiated distally, and once identified, you simply march proximally up this layer. The fascia is continually scored from distal to proximal as shown in **FIG 6**. This is continued up toward the inguinal ligament.

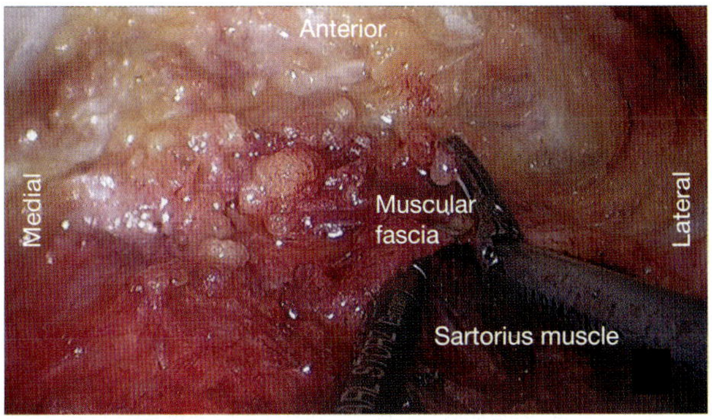

FIG 6 ● The lateral border of the deep dissection is shown here. The muscular fascia is scored from distal to proximal exposing the sartorius muscle (image © Mayo Clinic, 2014).

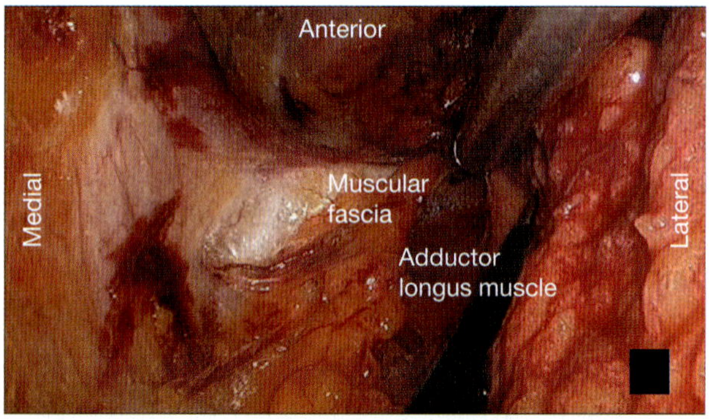

FIG 7 ● The medial border of the deep dissection is shown here. The muscular fascia is scored from distal to proximal exposing the adductor longus muscle (image © Mayo Clinic, 2014).

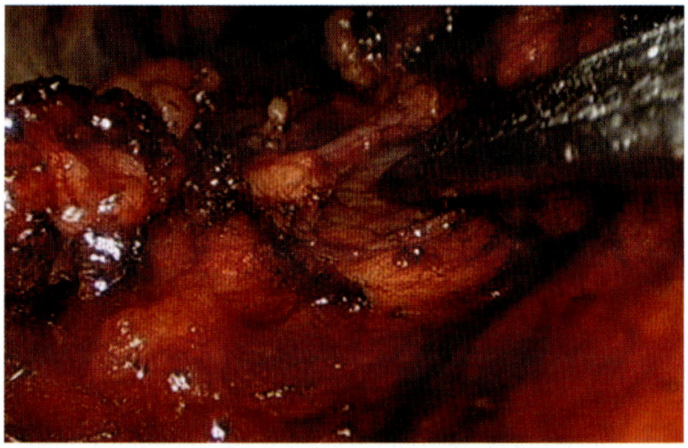

FIG 9 ● The distal saphenous vein is being divided as it crosses the adductor longus muscle (image © Mayo Clinic, 2014).

Adductor Longus Exposure

- A similar approach is taken medially to identify the adductor longus muscle (**FIG 7**). Because of the crossing saphenous vein, the medial dissection is started more proximal in this location. This dissection is also continued proximally to the inguinal ligament.
- The specimen is rolled laterally off the adductor. As we progress medially, the deep border of dissection becomes the pectineus muscle (**FIG 8**).
- It is fairly common for the knee to be "in the way" during portions of the dissection as a result of the knee bumped and the leg position. I find that I am not infrequently operating with the handle of the dissection device turned upside down to accommodate this reality.

Exposure and Division of Distal Saphenous Vein

- The next step is to identify and divide the saphenous vein distally. At this point, the dissection is begun more proximally on the adductor longus.
- The saphenous vein is identified and circumferentially dissected out. It is located two-thirds of the distance from the inguinal ligament to the apex of the triangle as the vein crosses the adductor muscle.
- The vein can be divided with an endovascular stapler, LigaSure® or ultrasonic dissector per surgeon preference and vessel caliber (**FIG 9**).

Apex Dissection

- Next, the apex dissection is completed. This is the remaining soft tissue between the sartorius and the adductor at the distal most aspect of the dissection.
- The contents are grasped and elevated under tension with traction in both the superficial and cephalad direction (**FIG 10**). This tissue is controlled with the nondominant hand, as the dissection of the remaining tissue over the apex is completed.

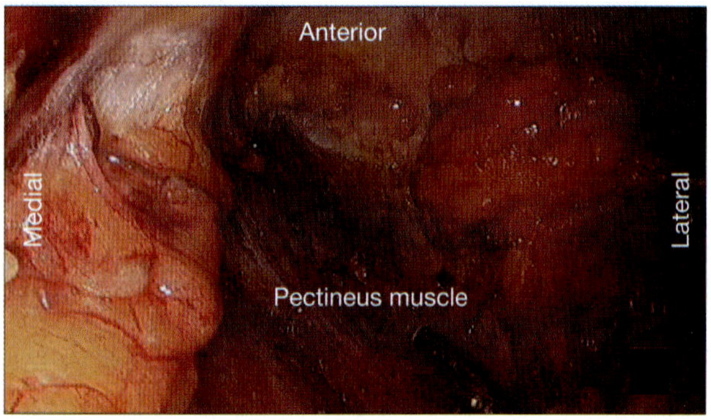

FIG 8 ● The pectineus muscle is exposed as the proximal portion of the specimen is rolled from medial to lateral off the adductor (image © Mayo Clinic, 2014).

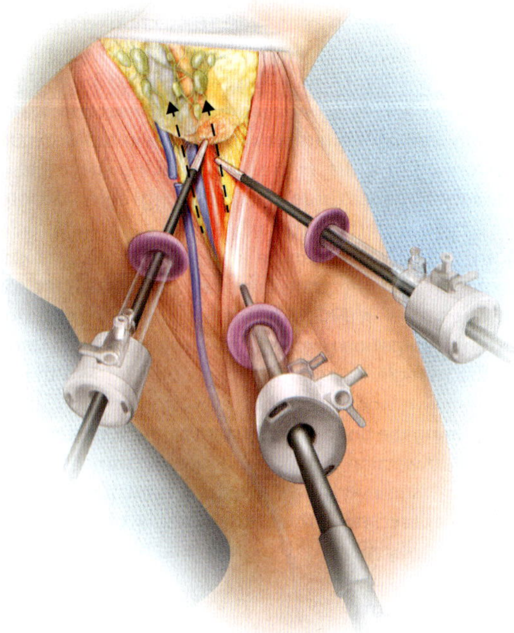

FIG 10 ● At the apex of the femoral triangle, the contents are grasped and retracted under tension by pushing the specimen anterior and cephalad.

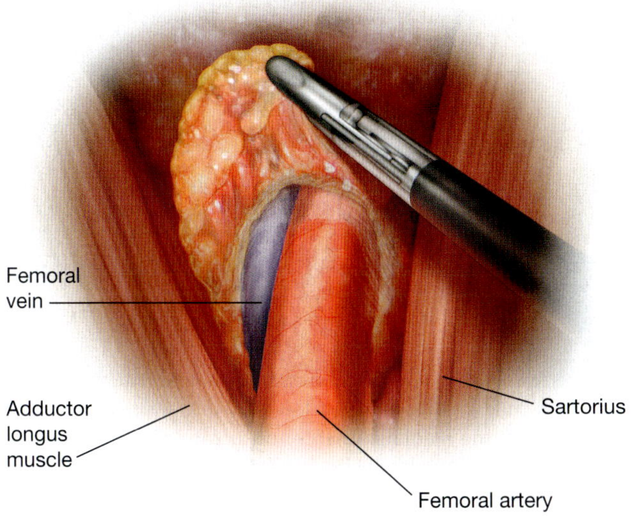

FIG 11 ● As the dissection at the apex continues deep from distal to proximal, the femoral vessels will come into view with the artery the first to be encountered.

- At this point, the dissection is performed by walking up the medial aspect of the sartorius from distal to proximal and rotating the contents medially. Because the femoral nerve lies in this location, a thin rim of fat is left on top of the nerve.
- As this process is repeated and continued, beginning at the apex and dissecting proximally, the femoral vasculature will be identified at this location (**FIG 11**).
- Because of the position of the lower extremity in abduction and flexion, the femoral artery lays directly anterior to the femoral vein. The femoral vein is deep and medial, and as we dissect proximally, the vessels will spiral and the two vessels will ultimately become parallel with each other lying in the same plain. Dissection should stay directly on the adventitia of the femoral vessels. Some prefer to use a laparoscopic Kittner for this dissection. I mainly use the dissection shears. The anterior half of the vessels are completely exposed.
- **FIG 12A,B** show the relative position change of vessels in relation to each other as we proceed from distal to proximal; this is accentuated by the leg being in a position of abduction.
- The deep inguinal lymph nodes are resected en bloc with this procedure. Our deep dissection plain is deep to the cribriform fascia. The cribriform fascia is an extension of the fascial lata. It separates the superficial inguinal lymph nodes from the deep inguinal lymph nodes. The cribriform fascia is penetrated by the saphenous vein at the fossa ovalis. The plane of dissection is depicted in **FIG 12A,B**.
- The femoral vein is appreciated deep and medial to the artery, just proximal to the apex. This is dissected out in a similar fashion. The anterior as well as the medial and lateral aspect of the vessels are skeletonized. There is no need to circumferentially dissect out these structures (**FIG 13A,B**).

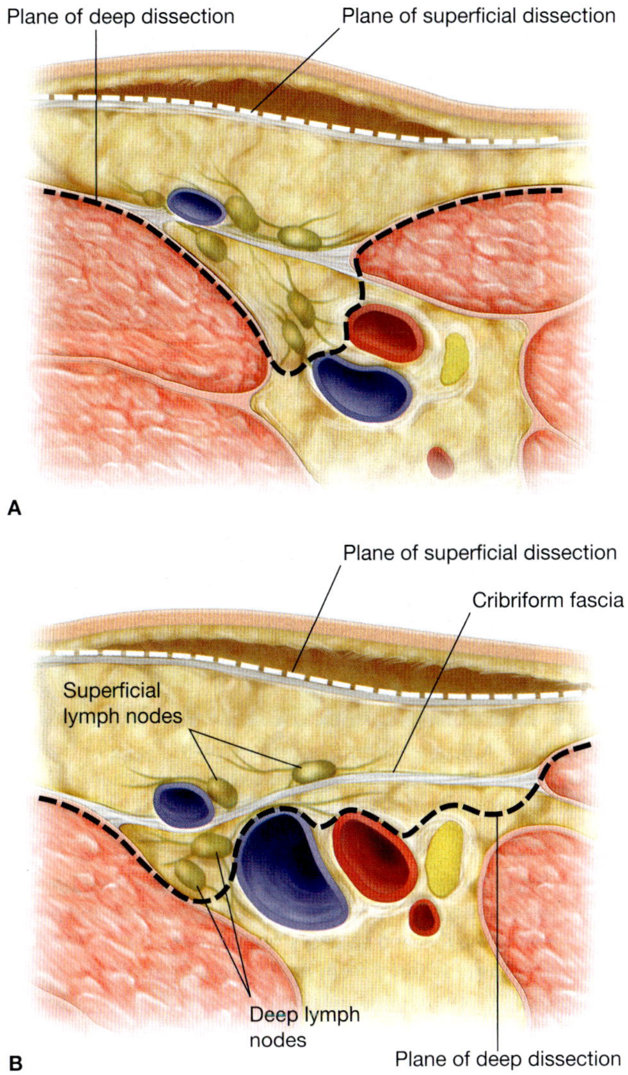

FIG 12 ● **A,B.** The superficial and deep dissection planes are graphically depicted here. These figures also demonstrate the relative position change of vessels in relation to each other as we proceed from distal to proximal, respectively.

- The femoral vein will be somewhat collapsed because of the CO_2 insufflation in this closed space. Its caliber will also be seen to fluctuate with ventilation.
- The medial dissection is completed off the adductor as we progress more proximally. As we continue our dissection, we simply walk up the adductor from distal to proximal. Continued anterior traction is applied to the specimen as we expose the vessels heading toward the inguinal ligament.

Proximal Dissection of Saphenous Vein at the Fossa Ovalis

- The medial and anterior surface of the femoral vein is skeletonized and we continue along medial aspect of this vessel under the inguinal ligament. Based on how far proximal you prefer to dissect here, Cloquet's lymph node can be removed en bloc with the specimen. If desired, a suture can be placed to mark Cloquet's node.

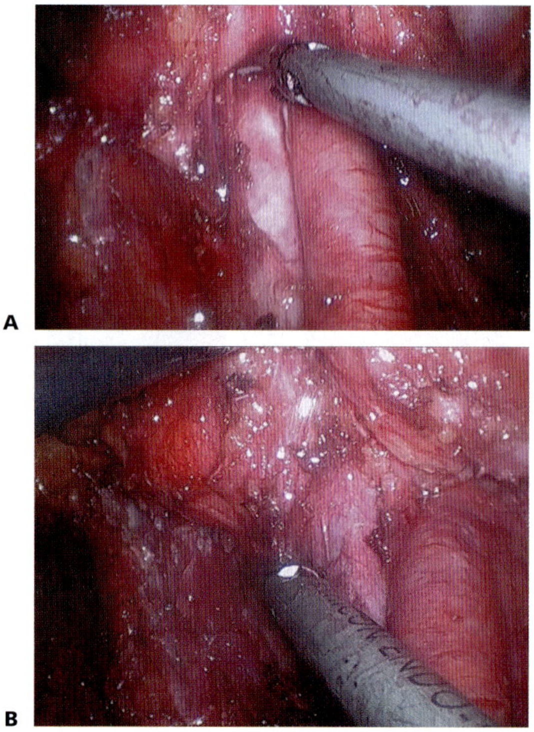

FIG 13 ● **A,B.** Intraoperative photos of the relationship of the vessels to each other and relative position change from distal to proximal, respectively (images © Mayo Clinic, 2014).

- The pectineus muscle can be seen here as the deep boundary of dissection. At this point, dissection is deep and proximal to the shelving edge of the inguinal ligament (**FIG 14**).
- The tissue is freed from medial to lateral off the previously exposed inguinal ligament.
- At this point, the saphenofemoral junction is identified, coming directly anterior off the femoral vein, approximately 3 cm distal to the inguinal ligament as the saphenous vein penetrates the cribriform fascia at the fossa ovalis. This will be identified as you dissect from distal to proximal along the medial surface of the femoral vein (**FIG 15**).

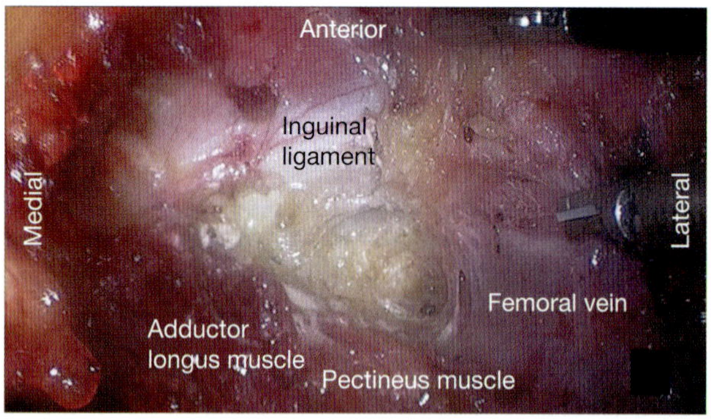

FIG 14 ● This image shows the empty space created deep to the inguinal ligament at the proximal/medial aspect of the dissection. The medial aspect of the femoral vein is skeletonized. One can choose to extend proximal to include Cloquet's lymph node with the specimen (image © Mayo Clinic, 2014).

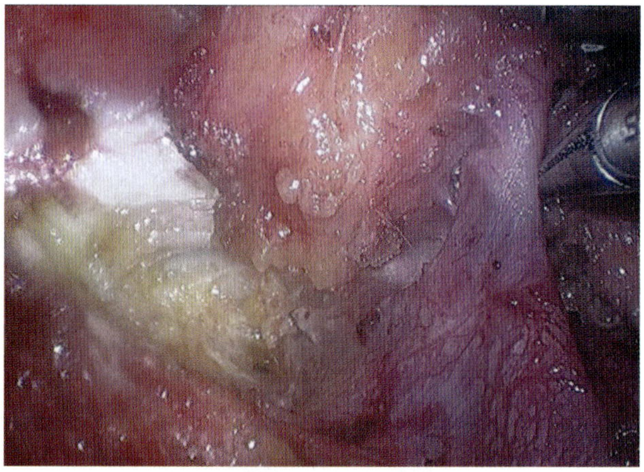

FIG 15 ● The saphenofemoral junction is identified as the dissection off the medial and anterior surface of the femoral vein is continued proximally (image © Mayo Clinic, 2014).

- The saphenofemoral junction is cleared and divided with a linear endovascular stapler (**FIG 16**). The proximal/medial tissue must first be freed off the femoral vein before this can be accomplished. It is better to complete this dissection proximal and medial to the saphenofemoral junction and make this window wider than you expect before attempting to introduce the stapler.
- The remaining proximal dissection of the femoral vessels (mostly cephalad and lateral) is then completed, removing the inguinal contents off of the remaining attachments with the femoral vessels. Short trocars and long instruments have been necessary in my experience in order to reach this proximal most dissection.
- If not already done so, any remaining soft tissue cephalad to the inguinal ligament is to be included (3 to 5 cm). This is easily peeled down off the external oblique aponeurosis, using hook cautery if desired, and included en bloc with the specimen. The remaining attachments with the inguinal ligament and external oblique aponeurosis are completed.

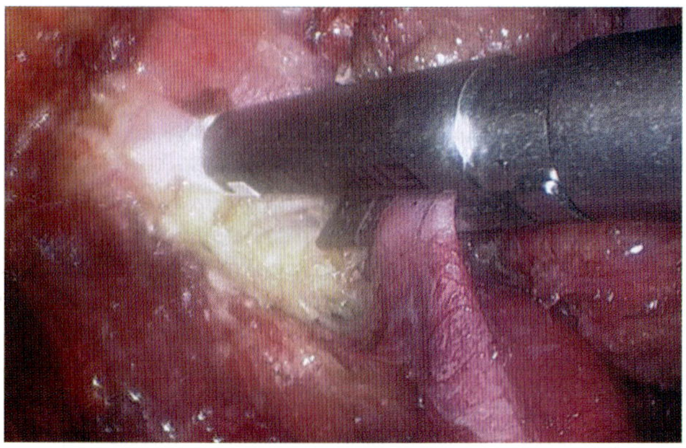

FIG 16 ● The intraoperative photo shows the proximal saphenous vein being divided with an endovascular stapler (image © Mayo Clinic, 2014).

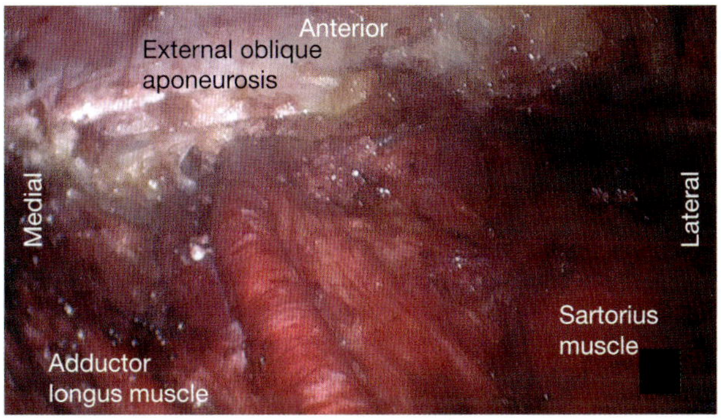

FIG 17 ● Intraoperative photo at the completion of the operation showing the musculature of the femoral triangle exposed, including the fascia overlying the external oblique aponeurosis, proximal to the inguinal ligament, and skeletonization of the anterior half of the femoral vessels (image © Mayo Clinic, 2014).

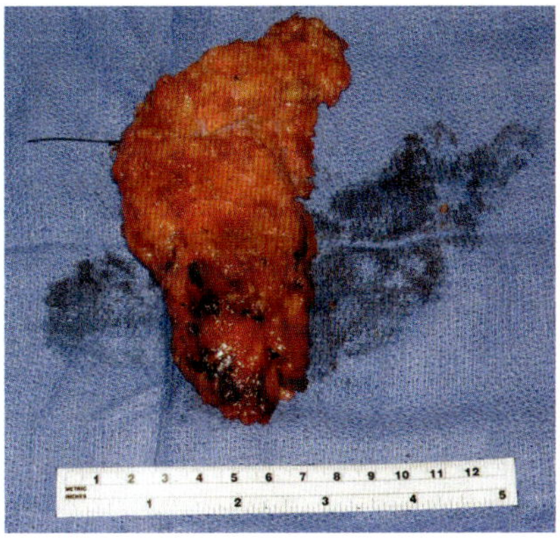

FIG 18 ● Photo of the inguinal contents after en bloc resection using the minimally invasive approach (image © Mayo Clinic, 2014).

- In a similar fashion, any remaining lateral attachments are freed off the sartorius followed by the final attachments off the inguinal ligament.

Specimen Removal

- Once the specimen is free, the contents are placed in an endobag.
- The anatomic boundaries are clearly delineated and you can visualize the soft tissue removed cephalad overlying the external oblique aponeurosis (**FIG 17**).
- Once completed, the drain is passed through the lateral trocar sites.
- The extracted specimen is depicted in **FIG 18**.
- A photo taken 1 week postoperatively is shown (**FIG 19**). It should be noted that the proximal longitudinal scar is from the original SLNB and not part of the MILND.
- At the end of the case, the genitals will be edematous from the CO_2 dissection. This is not a concern; the Foley can be removed at the end of the case and this should resolve by morning rounds. Crepitance up to the chest has been reported in some cases but has never been of clinical significance in my experience and to my knowledge. A chest strap during the operation can serve avoid this.

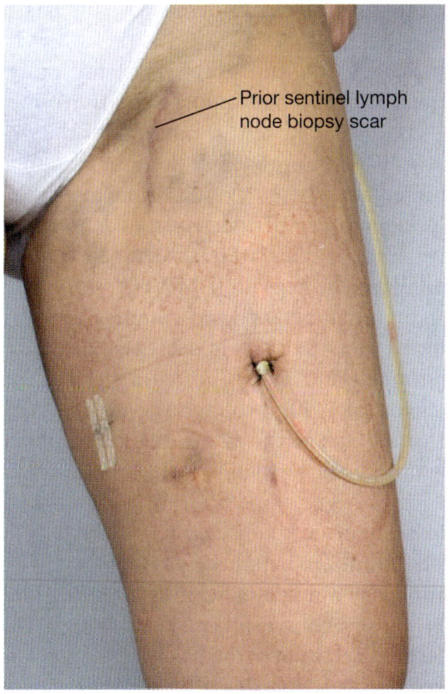

FIG 19 ● Photo of operative leg at the first postoperative visit.

PEARLS AND PITFALLS

High conversion rate	■ Embarking on this procedure without adequate training ■ Frustration and lack of patience ■ As with any new minimally invasive procedure, this should be scheduled at a date and time when there are limited other external pressures.
Unable to reach proximal dissection	■ Placing trocars too distal or instruments too short
Dissection too lateral	■ Typically, this is a result of not placing the leg in adequate abduction and external rotation prior to the start of the procedure.

Inadequate lymphadenectomy	▪ Not staying within defined anatomic boundaries ▪ Not dissecting anterior to Scarpa's fascia ▪ Not dissecting the deep inguinal lymph nodes by staying on the adventitia of the femoral vessels (not dissecting deep to the cribriform fascia) ▪ Not dissecting the tissue cephalad to the inguinal ligament
Conversion secondary to hypercarbia	▪ Not briefing with anesthesia team and making appropriate minute ventilation adjustments
Constant leak during case	▪ Finger dissection of more than one port site at start of case and making incisions too large
Drain not holding suction	▪ Not sealing incision closed tightly around drain at end of case. There is no subcutaneous fat between trocar site and cavity, unlike an abdominal procedure or open nodal dissections in which the drain is passed through a subcutaneous tunnel, so this remains very unforgiving.
Seroma/prolonged drain days	▪ See section regarding Postoperative Care

POSTOPERATIVE CARE

- Patient is admitted as an outpatient overnight and discharged within 23 hours. Drain care is reviewed in detail. Same-day discharge could be considered as pain has not been an issue.
- Regarding seromas, activity, and drain days, my practice continues to evolve. I went from limited activity to one of minimal activity and near bed rest at home until the drain comes out, and my current approach at the time of publication is back to limited activity. As a result of the malignancy, the immediate perioperative period, restricted activity to almost one of bedrest, patients were discharged home on daily low-molecular-weight heparin (LMWH), prophylactic VTE dosing. This minimal activity and compression of the surgical site did not appear to result in decreased drain days, so I have since stopped and allow limited activity. If considering home chemical VTE prophylaxis with LMWH, there is no need for a home health or visiting nurse; patients can be taught while in the hospital to self-administer this medication.
- The patients are seen prior to discharge by the physical medicine and rehabilitation lymphedema therapist. Compressive leg wrapping is applied as well as compression to the operative field (compressive biker shorts with a foam insert or sock placed directly over the basin). I have no data this decreases seroma or lymphedema or allows for earlier drain removal. Patients and family are educated on dressing changes and follow-up is arranged for the 1-week postoperative visit.
- Ensure the drain is holding suction prior to discharge.
- Redness and minor bruising of the flap is typical and noted on postoperative day 1 and on the first postoperative visit. These findings do not represent cellulitis and antibiotics are generally not indicated.
- There are two approaches to the drain removal. This is a balance between an increased risk of infection as the drain days increase versus accepting a higher seroma rate. The verdict is not out on the best approach here:
    - Remove drain at 2 to 3 weeks regardless of output and accept a seroma. Observation of the seroma is reasonable, if asymptomatic. Patients need to be educated preoperatively that a fluid collection will develop in their groin and not to be concerned.
    - Leave drain until output is less than 30 to 40 mL a day for 2 consecutive days. This often means keeping the drain up to 7 weeks.
    - As a result of the expected prolonged number of drain days (NOT flushing up the drain, just rinsing the bulb and emptying), our drain care regimen consists of rinsing the bulb with dilute Dakin's solution three times a day and placing a chlorhexidine Biopatch around the drain exit site and sealing it with a Tegaderm. The chlorhexidine disc is changed every third day and the drain site is cleaned with an alcohol wipe with each dressing change. This practice is based on Dr. Degnim's work in breast surgery and I only use for groin dissection because of the prolonged drain days.[11]

OUTCOMES

- The outcome data is limited[7,8] and frank discussion with the patient must be held explaining that this operation is being performed for malignancy, but it remains unknown if this is as oncologically sound as an open approach. The extent of resection should never be jeopardized to accomplish the procedure with the smallest incision possible. Seromas and prolonged drain days appear to be the Achilles heel thus far; we are exploring ways to combat this. Based on the limited experience worldwide, wound complications including breakdown and infections appear to be much less of an issue compared to the open approach (no big incision, no big wound problem). If lymphedema rates will be decreased is unknown at present. Major neurovascular structures are in the field and at risk. Flap necrosis can occur, but despite very thin flaps, I have not personally seen this.

COMPLICATIONS

- Seroma
- Hematoma
- Wound dehiscence
- Flap necrosis
- Major vascular injury
- Femoral nerve injury
- Drain not holding suction
- Recurrence
- Lymphedema
- Infection
- Anesthesia risks
- Hypercarbia
- Inadequate lymphadenectomy

ACKNOWLEDGMENTS

The figures and content were funded in part by the Fraternal Order of Eagles Cancer Research Fund Fellowship Program.

REFERENCES

1. Balch CM, Gershenwald JE, Atkins MB, et al. Melanoma of the skin. In: Edge SB, Compton CC, Fritz AG, et al, eds. *AJCC Cancer Staging Manual*. New York, NY: Springer; 2010:325–344.
2. Miranda EP, Gertner M, Wall J, et al. Routine imaging of asymptomatic melanoma patients with metastasis to sentinel lymph nodes rarely identifies systemic disease. *Arch Surg*. 2004;139(8):831–836; discussion 836–837.
3. Aloia TA, Gershenwald JE, Andtbacka RH, et al. Utility of computed tomography and magnetic resonance imaging staging before completion lymphadenectomy in patients with sentinel lymph node-positive melanoma. *J Clin Oncol*. 2006;24(18):2858–2865.
4. Gold JS, Jaques DP, Busam KJ, et al. Yield and predictors of radiologic studies for identifying distant metastases in melanoma patients with a positive sentinel lymph node biopsy. *Ann Surg Oncol*. 2007;14(7): 2133–2140.
5. Brady MS, Akhurst T, Spanknebel K, et al. Utility of preoperative [(18)]f fluorodeoxyglucose-positron emission tomography scanning in high-risk melanoma patients. *Ann Surg Oncol*. 2006;13(4):525–532.
6. Tyler DS, Onaitis M, Kherani A, et al. Positron emission tomography scanning in malignant melanoma. *Cancer*. 2000;89(5);1019–1025.
7. Abbott AM, Grotz TE, Rueth NM, et al. Minimally invasive inguinal lymph node dissection (MILND) for melanoma: experience from two academic centers. *Ann Surg Oncol*. 2013;20(1):340–355.
8. Delman KA, Kooby DA, Rizzo M, et al. Initial experience with videoscopic inguinal lymphadenectomy. *Ann Surg Oncol*. 2011;18(4): 977–982.
9. Martin BM, Etra JW, Russell MC, et al. Oncologic outcomes of patients undergoing videoscopic inguinal lymphadenectomy for metastatic melanoma. *J Am Coll Surg*. 2014;218(4):620–626. doi:10.1016/j.jamcollsurg.2013.12.016.
10. Delman KA, Kooby DA, Ogan K, et al. Feasibility of a novel approach to inguinal lymphadenectomy: minimally invasive groin dissection for melanoma. *Ann Surg Oncol*. 2010;17(3):731–737.
11. Degnim AC, Scow JS, Hoskin TL, et al. Randomized controlled trial to reduce bacterial colonization of surgical drains after breast and axillary operations. *Ann Surg*. 2013;258(2):240–247.

Chapter **31**

Selective Neck Dissection for Melanoma

Vasu Divi

DEFINITION

- The goal of a selective neck dissection for melanoma is the complete removal of the lymph nodes and lymphatics that drain a specific region of skin in the head and neck.
- This procedure is performed for patients presenting with clinically evident regional metastasis as well as for patients with a positive sentinel lymph node.

PATIENT HISTORY AND PHYSICAL FINDINGS

- All patients with melanoma of the head and neck should undergo palpation of the regional lymphatics, including the parotid glands and cervical levels 1 to 5.
- Melanomas at the junction of the neck and the chest, back, or shoulder should also include palpation of the axillary lymph nodes.
- All patients with melanoma, particularly those with proven regional metastases, should have a focused review of symptoms, looking for symptoms concerning for metastatic disease.
- All patients with melanoma should also have a complete skin exam, looking for second primary cutaneous malignancies.

IMAGING AND OTHER DIAGNOSTIC STUDIES

- Preoperative imaging of the neck is not necessary in patients without clinically evident neck disease.
- In patients with palpable adenopathy
  - Imaging by contrast-enhanced computed tomography (CT) scan is generally recommended to evaluate the extent of disease.
  - Fine needle aspiration is used to obtain pathologic diagnosis of the enlarged lymph node.
- In cases of distant metastatic disease, the need for selective neck dissection is balanced against the life expectancy of the patient. In many cases, achievement of regional control in the neck is preferred, given the complications of untreated disease in the head and neck.

SURGICAL MANAGEMENT

Preoperative Planning

- Determination of the type of neck dissection to be performed is based on the location of the primary tumor and location of neck disease.
- The relevant lymphatic basins of the head and neck include the parotid lymph nodes, levels 1 to 5, and the postauricular lymph nodes (**FIG 1**).
- This serves as a rough guide to when different lymphatic basins should be addressed; ultimately, the clinician should dissect all lymphatic basins that could potentially be harboring clinical disease based on an understanding of lymphatic drainage patterns.
  - The removal of the superficial lobe of the parotid gland is performed for any primary cutaneous tumor anterior to the external auditory canal and above the angle of the mandible.

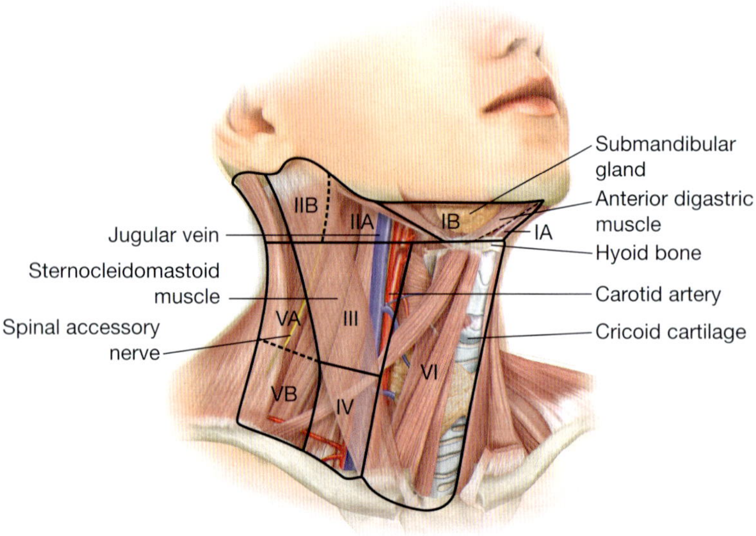

FIG 1 • Levels of the neck. Level 1 includes all nodes between the contralateral anterior belly of the digastric, ipsilateral posterior belly of the digastric, and the inferior edge of the mandible. Level 2 includes the nodes below the skull base between the posterior belly of the digastric, posterior edge of the SCM, and above the level of the hyoid. Level 3 includes all nodes between the hyoid bone and cricoid cartilage arch, between the lateral and the internal carotid artery, and the posterior edge of the SCM. Level 4 includes all nodes between the cricoid cartilage arch and clavicle, between the lateral and the internal carotid artery, and the posterior edge of the SCM. Level 5 includes all nodes from the skull base down to the posterior border of the sternocleidomastoid muscle to the clavicle, anterior to the trapezius muscle.

- Levels 1 to 4 are dissected with any lesion involving the scalp anterior to the plane of the external auditory canal, facial skin, or anterior neck skin.
- Levels 2 to 5 are dissected with any lesion involving the scalp posterior to the plane of the external auditory canal or posterior neck skin.
- If the primary lesion is in the scalp and located very close to the plane of the external auditory canal, dissection should include levels 1 to 5.

Positioning

- Patients are placed supine with the top of the head at the edge of the surgical bed.
- A bump is placed underneath the shoulder blades to allow for extension of the neck, being careful to maintain support of the head on the operating room (OR) table.

SELECTIVE NECK DISSECTION LEVELS 1 TO 4

- A curvilinear incision is made midway between the angle of the mandible and the clavicle; the incision travels within a neck crease, extending a few centimeters from the mastoid tip toward the approximate midpoint of the thyroid cartilage (**FIG 2**).
- Skin is incised down through the subcutaneous tissue and platysma.
- Subplatysmal skin flaps are elevated to expose the deeper contents overlying levels 1 to 4 of the neck; this will extend to the mentum, along the strap musculature in the midline, to the posterior border of the sternocleidomastoid muscle (SCM), and down to the level of the clavicle (**FIG 3**).
- The marginal mandibular nerve is identified in the superficial layer of the cervical fascia near the angle of the mandible and is identified using nerve stimulation. The nerve is dissected free and elevated over the plane of the mandible (**FIG 4**).

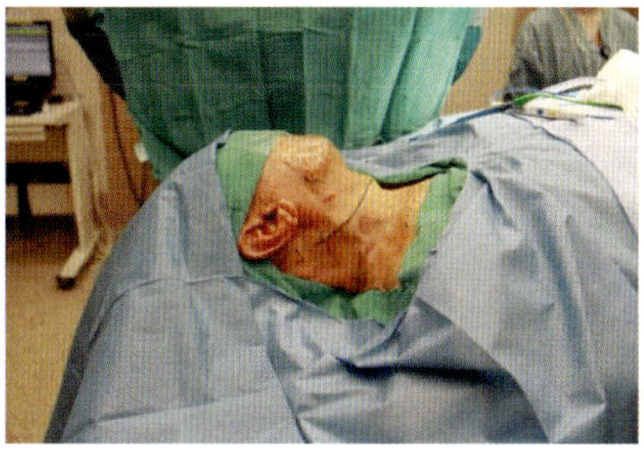

FIG 2 ● The neck incision is marked out between the mandible and clavicle.

- The facial artery and vein are identified and ligated as they cross over the plane of the mandible.
- The tissue over the mandible is then incised from the mentum to the angle of the mandible, taking care not to injure the previously dissected marginal mandibular nerve. This tissue is pulled inferiorly, taking care to remove the perifacial lymph nodes located near the facial vessels. During this

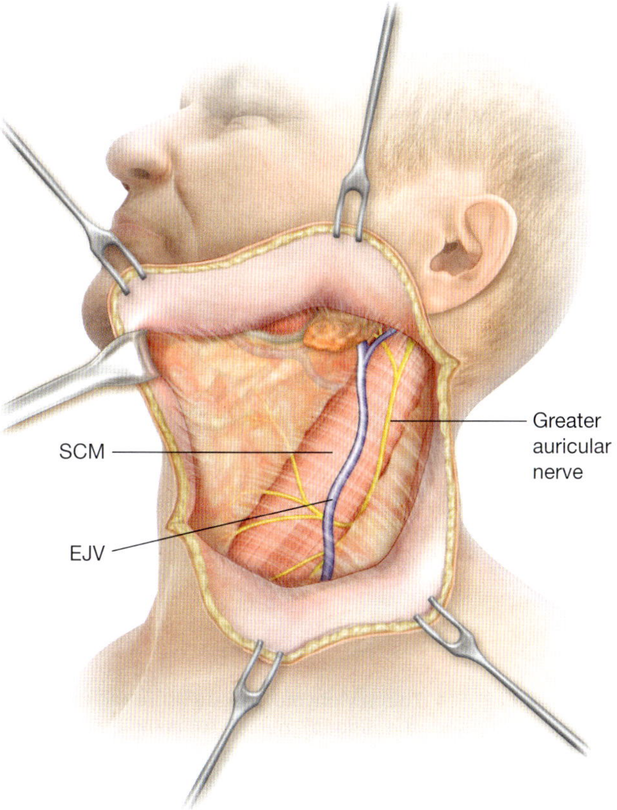

FIG 3 ● The neck incision is completed with subplatysmal flaps elevated superiorly and inferiorly.

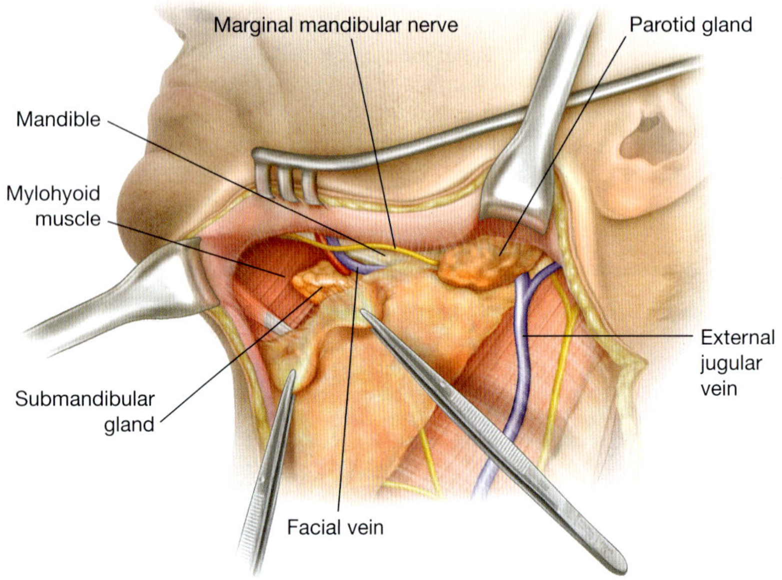

FIG 4 • The marginal mandibular nerve is elevated over the mandible and the contents of level 1A are dissected posteriorly. Division of the facial artery and vein would occur at this point or earlier in the dissection.

dissection, the retromandibular vein may be identified and ligated as it travels through the tail of the parotid gland.

- Incise soft tissue over contralateral anterior belly of the digastric muscle from mentum down to hyoid bone.
- Begin elevating contents of level 1A by pulling tissue laterally off the mylohyoid muscle toward the ipsilateral anterior belly of the digastric muscle; this will require division of tissue along the hyoid bone inferiorly.
- Bring packet of tissue over ipsilateral digastric and back onto mylohyoid until the edge of the mylohyoid is reached see **FIG 4**.
- Retract the mylohyoid muscle medially to allow for exposure of the contents deep to the submandibular gland. This may require some blunt dissection in this area. Identify the hypoglossal nerve, lingual nerve, and submandibular duct (**FIG 5**).
- Divide the submandibular duct, taking care not to cause excessive bleeding from the nearby veins (**FIG 6**).
- Divide the submandibular ganglion and allow the lingual nerve to retract superiorly.
- Pull the submandibular gland and packet of tissue laterally, carefully dividing the tissue over the posterior belly of the digastric (**FIG 7**).
- Approximately halfway up the posterior belly, the facial artery is again seen travelling under the digastric and into the submandibular gland; divide the artery a second time.
- Trace the posterior belly superiorly, dividing the overlying tissue until the SCM is reached. If it has not already

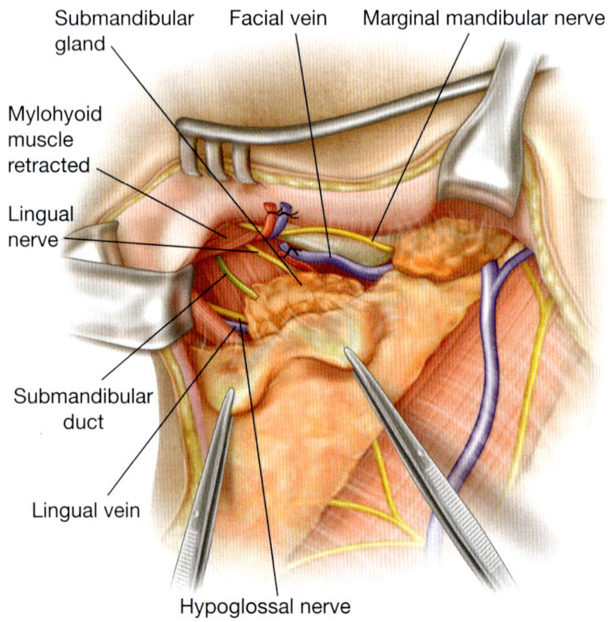

FIG 5 • The mylohyoid muscle is retracted anteriorly exposing the lingual nerve, submandibular duct, and hypoglossal nerve. The hypoglossal nerve is in a deeper plane than the lingual nerve and is only exposed after dividing the overlying fascia.

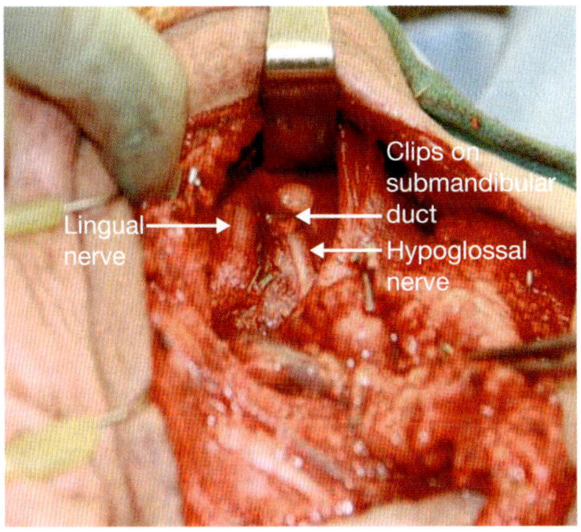

FIG 6 ● View of the right neck level 1B with the submandibular gland removed and the mylohyoid muscle retracted anteriorly. Clips are seen on the submandibular duct remnant.

been divided, the retromandibular vein is usually encountered as it exits the parotid gland near the angle of the mandible—carefully divide the vein.

- The SCM is then "unwrapped." At the posterior edge of the SCM, incise the fascia over the muscle. This will require division of the cutaneous nerves that course over the muscle; the great auricular branch to the ear as well as the external jugular can sometimes be traced out and saved.
- Pull the fascia medially to unwrap the SCM; be careful to take all tissue over the muscle because lymph nodes associated with the external jugular vein must be removed.

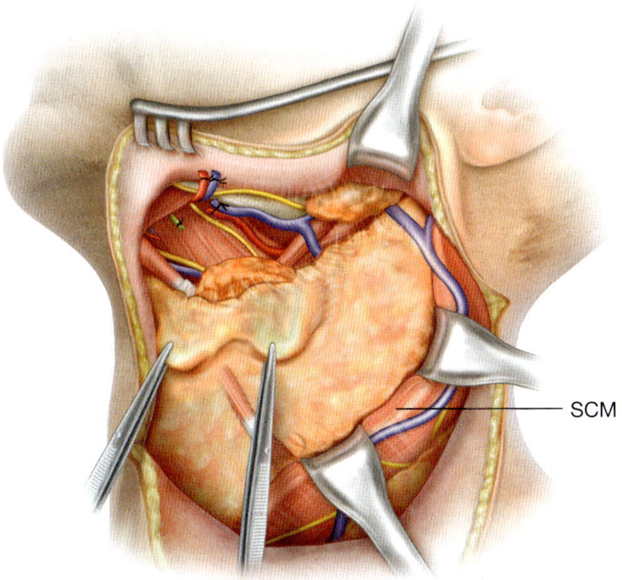

FIG 7 ● The contents of level 1B are pulled over the posterior belly of digastric. The facial artery could be dissected free from the gland (as shown) or divided a second time as it crosses under the digastric.

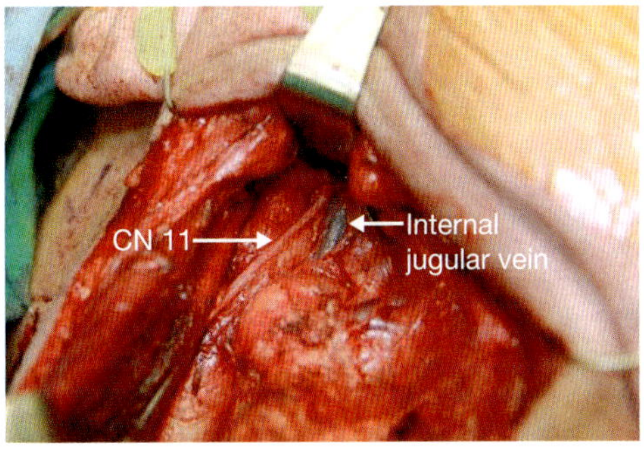

FIG 8 ● The contents of the right-sided level 2 are exposed with CN 11 in clear view as it courses over the internal jugular. The posterior belly of digastric is retracted superiorly.

- After the anterior surface of the SCM is wrapped, carefully roll the muscle outward to start unwrapping the deep surface; at the junction of the upper one-third and lower two-thirds, the cranial nerve (CN) XI (the spinal accessory nerve) will be encountered as it enters the muscle.
- Continue to unwrap and elevate the muscle of the floor of the neck until the posterior edge is reached, taking care to not stretch or injure CN XI.
- At this point, the posterior belly of the digastric should be traced underneath the SCM and then mobilized so it can be pulled superiorly.
- At the hyoid bone, the omohyoid muscle is identified and traced low into the neck to the posterior edge of the SCM. It is mobilized as well so it can be pulled inferiorly.
- Next, the posterior belly of the digastric is pulled superiorly while CN XI is traced underneath the muscle by dividing the overlying tissue until it courses over the internal jugular (IJ) vein; the nerve usually passes superficial to the vein (80%) but can also pass deep to it (20%) (**FIG 8**).
- The spinal accessory nerve is elevated off the deep neck and is circumferentially dissected up to the IJ; the wall of the IJ vein is then skeletonized (**FIG 9**).
- The transverse process of C1 is palpated on the floor of the neck. This will serve as the superior limit of dissection.
- Lymphatic tissue of level 2B is mobilized by dividing the tissue between the IJ and the posterior edge of the SCM down to the level of the floor of the neck (levator scapulae muscle). Superiorly, the contents of level 2B will need to be pulled underneath the CN XI (**FIG 9**).
- The posterior edge of dissection parallels the posterior border of the SCM. This tissue is incised down to the floor of the neck as well, taking care to not divide the cervical rootlets (**FIG 10**).
- The inferior margin of dissection is approximately at the clavicle. The omohyoid muscle can be retracted inferiorly or divided to access this area.
- Start by identifying the IJ low in neck and skeletonizing the wall. Next, divide the tissue adjacent to the IJ down to the floor of the neck. This tissue needs to be carefully ligated with sutures or clips due to the presence of the thoracic duct. The tissue is divided between the IJ and the posterior edge of the SCM.

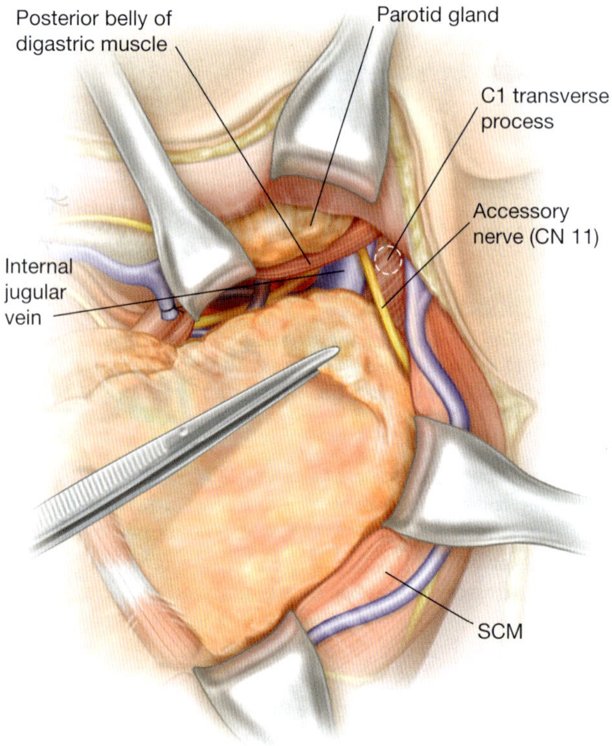

FIG 9 • The contents of level 2B are dissected and passed underneath CN 11. The transverse process of C1 is palpable beneath the muscle.

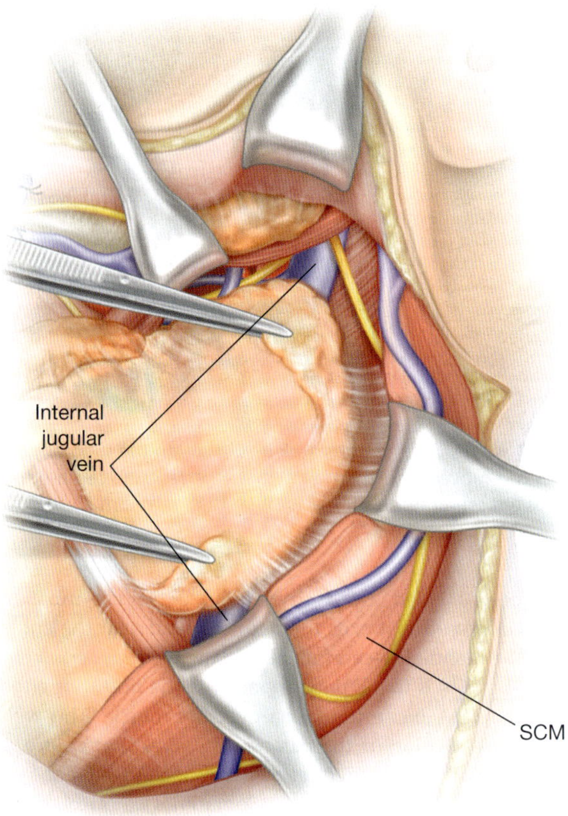

FIG 11 • The inferior dissection at the level of the clavicle is complete, allowing the lymphatic tissue of levels 2, 3, and 4 to be elevated off the floor of the neck.

- The tissue is then brought forward off the floor of the neck onto the IJ vein (**FIG 11**). Follow the fascia of the floor without violating the fascia covering the deep neck muscles.
- The package of tissue is then brought over the IJ by entering the fascia of the carotid sheath; as the tissue is dissected off the IJ, the branches of the IJ are ligated (**FIG 12**). Once the IJ is nearly circumferentially dissected, the carotid artery is in view (**FIG 13**).
- The hypoglossal nerve is identified underneath the digastric. This is traced posteriorly, dividing the overlying tissue and veins until the nerve travels between the carotid and IJ (**FIG 14**).
- The package is brought over the carotid until the superior thyroid artery is seen; at this point, transition is made to the fascia of the visceral space (**FIG 15**).
- The package of tissue is then truncated at the lateral border of the strap musculature.

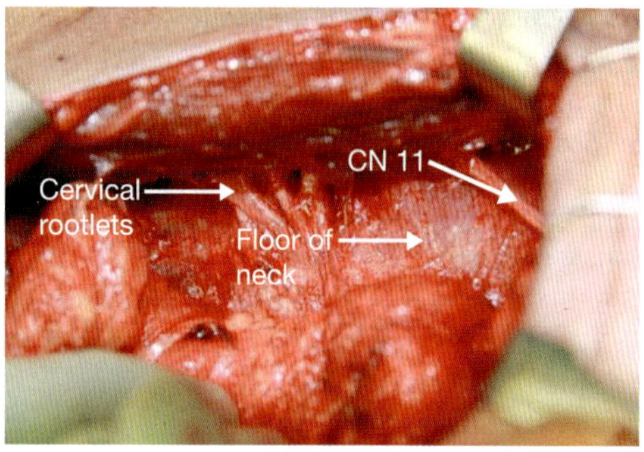

FIG 10 • With the SCM retracted in the right neck, the contents are elevated off the floor of the neck. CN 11 is seen on the right side of the picture, and in the middle of the picture, the cervical rootlets are seen piecing the floor of the neck and wrapped around the posterior SCM.

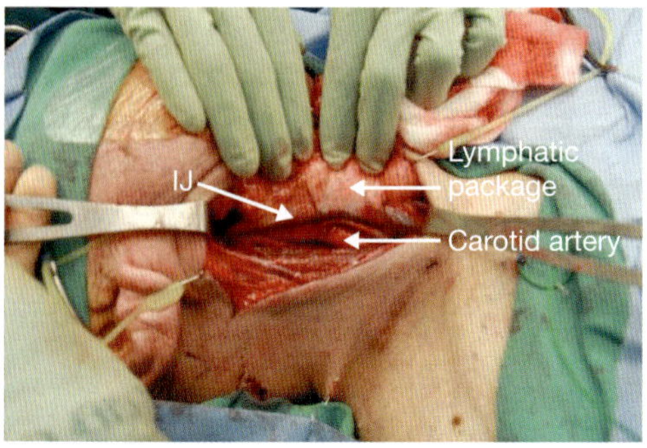

FIG 12 • The lymphatic package is pulled medially in the right neck, still attached to the internal jugular. The package will be taken off of the IJ and onto the visceral space.

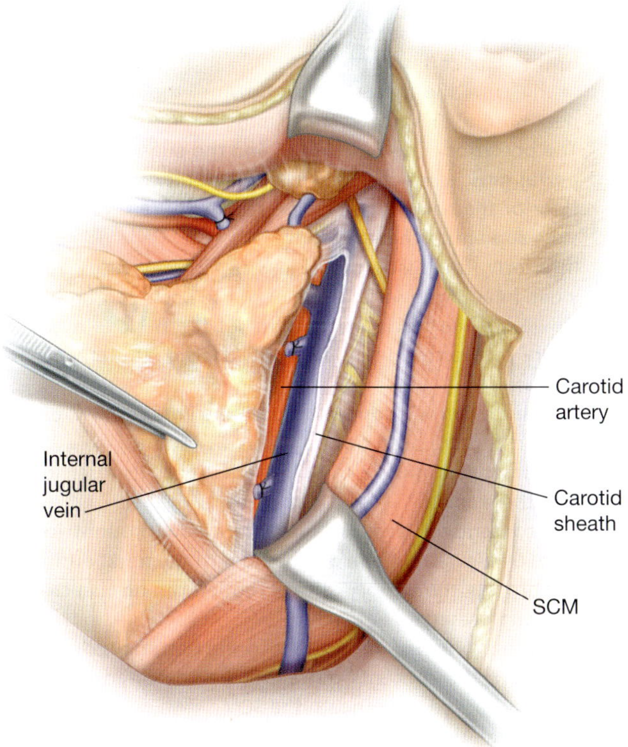

FIG 13 ● The carotid sheath is entered and the branches of the IJ are divided allowing the packet to be transitioned onto the carotid artery.

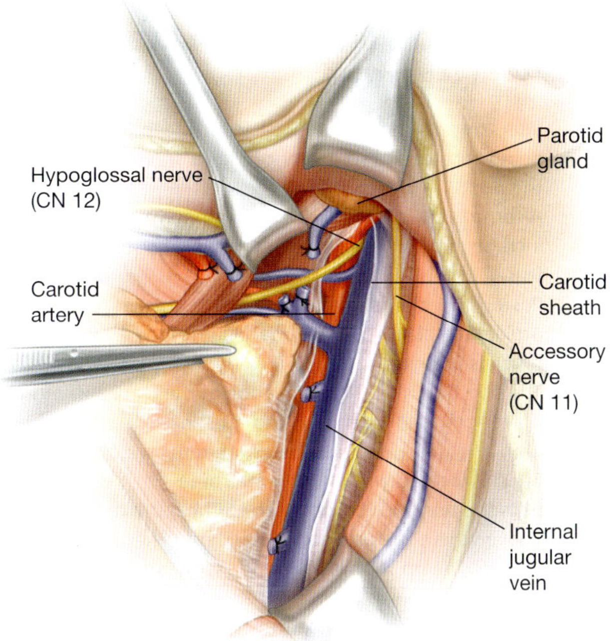

FIG 14 ● The hypoglossal nerve is traced out from where it crosses the digastric until it courses between the carotid and the IJ. The overlying veins are delicate and must be divided carefully to avoid significant bleeding which could obstruct the view of the vein.

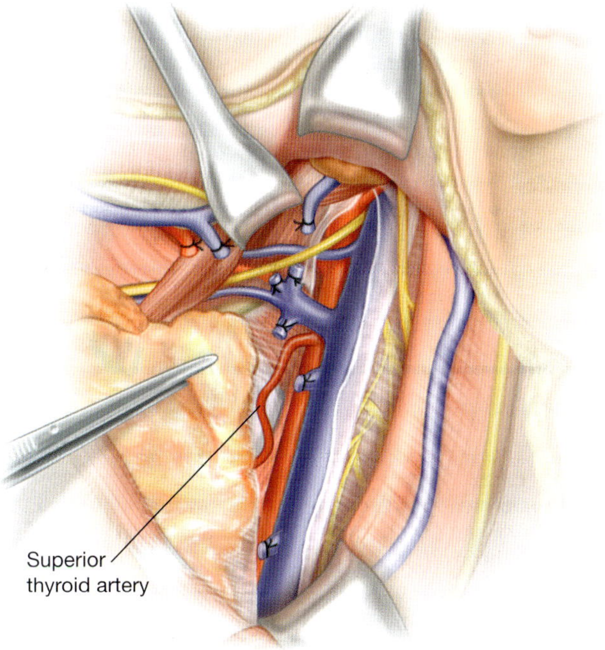

FIG 15 ● The packet is transitioned off the carotid space and onto the visceral space carefully preserving the superior thyroid artery.

SELECTIVE NECK DISSECTION LEVELS 2 TO 5 (POSTERIOR-LATERAL NECK DISSECTION)

- The skin incision is modified from the prior procedure being located more posteriorly and travelling lower in the neck.
- Alternatively, a "limb" can be dropped down from the incision to give access to the area over the supraclavicular fossa.
- Posteriorly, the platysma is absent; therefore, the approximate plane of the superficial layer of the cervical fascia is followed.
- The skin flap is raised to the edge of the trapezius muscle posteriorly and inferiorly; the muscle edge is often not seen and therefore must be estimated.
- CN XI is located within the level 5 area. The nerve usually exits the posterior border of the SCM approximately 2 cm above where the great auricular nerve wraps around the muscle. The position is confirmed with nerve stimulation.
- Once the nerve is identified, it is traced from the posterior edge of the SCM until it travels underneath the trapezius muscle; as the nerve approaches the trapezius, it often splits into more than one branch, each of which should be preserved.
- The nerve is then mobilized and elevated from the level 5 contents.
- Next, the posterior superior edge of the SCM is skeletonized.
- This dissection is carried out to the level of the mastoid tip, where the dissection turns posteriorly until the edge of the trapezius is identified.
- In this area, the tissues are cut down to the floor of the neck until the levator scapulae muscle is identified.
- The posterior edge of the SCM and the edge of the trapezius muscle are dissected in their entirety down to the floor of the neck; care is taken to not injure CN XI as it exits and enters these muscles.
- Inferiorly, the tissue at the level of the clavicle is divided heading toward the floor of the neck; careful not to violate the fascia of the floor of the neck to avoid injury to the transverse cervical vessels or the brachial plexus.
- This dissection will connect to both the anterior SCM dissection and the posterior trapezius dissection.
- The omohyoid muscle can be divided near its insertion into the scapula.
- The contents of level 5A and 5B are now brought forward by elevating them off the floor of the neck; during this process, the sensory cervical rootlets can be dissected free and preserved or divided.
- Once the contents are brought to the posterior edge of the SCM, the contents can either be truncated at this point or tucked underneath the SCM.
- The remainder of the levels 2 to 4 neck dissection proceeds as described above; begin by identifying the posterior belly of the digastric muscle and tracing it up to the SCM.

UNIQUE SCENARIOS

- Skin involvement
  - Involvement of the skin can happen from metastatic disease in the neck or from a primary lesion in the neck.
  - Extent of involvement should be determined based on CT scan and palpation with careful attention to the platysma and dermis.
  - Mark at least 1 cm around areas of subcutaneous or dermal involvement; closure is assisted by using elliptical-shaped excisions and paying close attention to resulting skin flaps for rotation or advancement.
  - At the time of skin incision, these areas should incised down through the level of the platysma.
  - Subplatysmal skin flaps are elevated around the area of involvement, leaving the skin overlying the tumor pedicled on the tumor.
- Involvement of structures
  - Necessity for resection of the SCM, CN XI, IJ, or additional structures is based on involvement seen on imaging studies or at the time of surgery.
  - Tumor should never be violated to preserve any of these structures.

PEARLS AND PITFALLS

Communication with anesthesia	■ It is essential that the patient is not paralyzed for the operation to allow for monitoring of the marginal mandibular nerve, CN XI, and CN XII. Short-acting paralytics used for induction generally wear off by the time the incision is made.
Placement of incision	■ The incision should be about two fingerbreadths below the edge of the mandible to avoid injuring the marginal mandibular nerve during skin flap incision and elevation.
Identification of structures	■ The fascial planes provide excellent boundaries for dissection and should almost always be followed during the neck dissection.
Excision	■ If grossly positive lymph nodes are encountered, take a cuff of normal tissue to surround the node. This can involve removing a portion of the SCM or sacrificing the IJ.

Division of specimen	▪ The specimen is typically divided into the corresponding levels of the neck dissection to allow pathology to separately report which levels contained positive lymph nodes.
Prior to closure	▪ The level 4 area of the neck is checked for a chyle leak with a sustained Valsalva maneuver. Any evidence of clear or milky fluid should be treated by sewing over or clipping the area.

POSTOPERATIVE CARE

- Following surgery, patients are admitted to the general inpatient unit.
- Postoperative antibiotics are continued for 24 hours.
- Postoperative subcutaneous heparin is used immediately following surgery.
- Closed suction drains are used until output is less than 30 mL per day.
- Patients with extensive CN XI dissection are seen by physical therapy for arm mobilization and strengthening exercises.

OUTCOMES

- The rate of regional recurrence after selective neck dissection for melanoma depends on the extent of cervical disease at the time of resection. It is as low as 15% for micrometastatic disease and as high as 50% for macroscopic disease with extracapsular extension.
- Postoperative radiation therapy is considered for patients with extracapsular extension, a single node greater than 4 cm, three or more positive nodes, or for neck dissections following a regional recurrence.
- Recurrent neck disease after neck dissection must be carefully evaluated to determine resectability.

COMPLICATIONS

- Hematoma
- Chyle leak
- CN XI injury
- Hypoglossal injury
- Marginal mandibular weakness
- Stroke

SUGGESTED READINGS

1. Janfaza P, ed. *Surgical Anatomy of the Head and Neck*. Cambridge, MA: Harvard University Press; 2011.
2. Silver CE, Rubin JS. *Atlas of Head and Neck Surgery*. New York, NY: Churchill Livingstone; 1999.
3. Lucioni M. *Practical Guide to Neck Dissection: Focusing on the Larynx*. Berlin, Germany: Springer-Verlag; 2013.

Chapter **32** Popliteal Dissection

Glenda G. Callender   Kelly M. McMasters

DEFINITION

- Popliteal dissection, or popliteal lymphadenectomy, is the removal of all lymph node–bearing tissue from the popliteal fossa. This procedure is most commonly performed for melanoma but may rarely be performed for other cutaneous cancers or for the limited number of sarcomas that have a propensity to metastasize to lymph nodes.
- Popliteal dissection is indicated in patients with no evidence of distant metastatic disease who are found to have the following:
  - Positive popliteal sentinel lymph node biopsy (microscopic nodal disease)
  - Clinically positive popliteal lymph nodes (macroscopic nodal disease)
- Boundaries of the popliteal fossa (**FIG 1**)
  - Superomedial: semitendinosus and semimembranosus muscles
  - Superolateral: biceps femoris muscle
  - Inferomedial: medial head of the gastrocnemius muscle
  - Inferolateral: lateral head of the gastrocnemius muscle and plantaris muscle
  - Roof: skin, superficial fascia, deep (popliteal) fascia
  - Floor: popliteal surface of femur, capsule of knee joint, oblique popliteal ligament, fascia overlying popliteus muscle

PATIENT HISTORY AND PHYSICAL FINDINGS

- A thorough history should be elicited prior to treatment, including a detailed past medical and surgical history, present medications and allergies, and a personal and family history of cancer. A complete head-to-toe skin examination should be performed. All lymph node basins (cervical, supraclavicular, axillary, epitrochlear, inguinal, popliteal) should be evaluated for clinically positive lymph nodes.
- Clinically positive lymph nodes typically present as a palpable mass. However, enlarged lymph nodes in the popliteal fossa may not be easily palpable because of the thick overlying fascia. Therefore, a careful examination of the popliteal fossa is essential.
- Most patients undergo popliteal dissection because of a positive sentinel lymph node biopsy. Sentinel lymph node biopsy has now become the standard of care for evaluating regional lymph node basins in patients with cutaneous melanoma greater than 1 mm in Breslow thickness who have no evidence of distant metastatic disease (see Chapter 27). Current standard of care for patients with positive sentinel lymph nodes includes completion lymphadenectomy of the involved lymph node basin; observation alone should be performed in the context of a clinical trial. Approximately 50% of patients with a positive popliteal sentinel lymph node biopsy will also have documented inguinal disease; therefore, popliteal and inguinal dissections are often performed concomitantly.[1,2]

IMAGING AND OTHER DIAGNOSTIC STUDIES

- A clinically positive lymph node should be evaluated using fine needle aspiration biopsy. Popliteal dissection is performed for a positive biopsy.
- For patients with clinically negative lymph nodes, preoperative lymphoscintigraphy should be performed at the time of the initial sentinel lymph node biopsy even if the primary melanoma is located on an extremity. Lymphoscintigraphy will demonstrate drainage to popliteal lymph nodes in 1% to 9% of patients with distal lower extremity melanoma (i.e., below the knee; **FIG 2**).[1–5] By far, the most common locations for primary melanomas that drain to the popliteal fossa are the posterolateral foot and posterior lower leg; however, primary melanomas of the anterior lower leg or

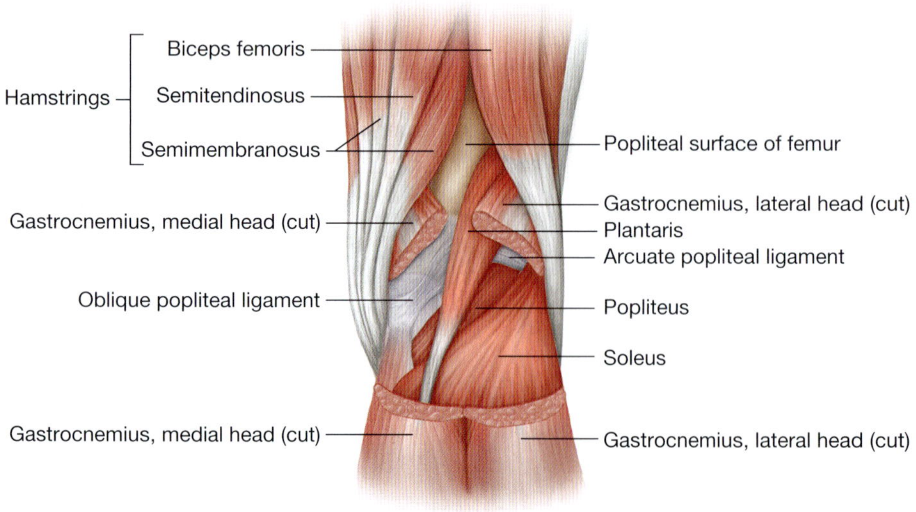

FIG 1 • Boundaries of the popliteal fossa (right leg).

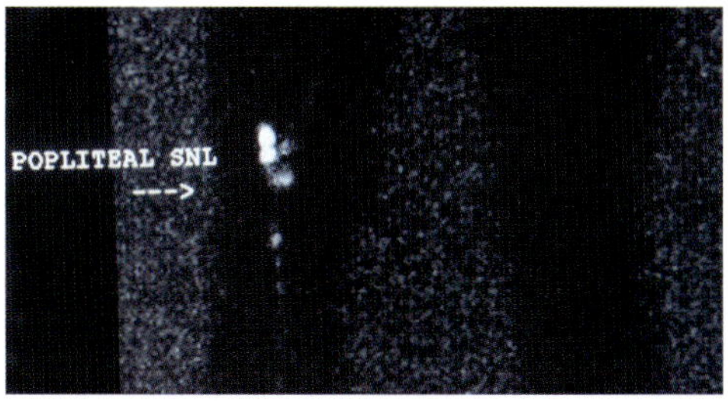

FIG 2 ● Lymphoscintigraphy demonstrating lymphatic drainage to the popliteal fossa from a primary melanoma of the distal right foot.

anteromedial aspect of the foot will also occasionally drain to the popliteal fossa.[1–4] The overall incidence of a positive popliteal lymph node is 0.3% to 2.8%.[1–3,5]

SURGICAL MANAGEMENT

Preoperative Planning

- In the preoperative area, a focused history and physical examination should be repeated, and the patient's prior pathology and imaging studies should be reviewed.
- The patient should be marked to confirm laterality.
- Although there are no data that specifically address the wound infection rate in popliteal dissection, we favor the administration of a dose of preoperative antibiotics, particularly if concomitant inguinal dissection is planned.

Positioning

- The patient is placed prone, with pressure points padded, and the operative knee slightly flexed (**FIG 3**). The operative leg should be prepped circumferentially from above the midthigh to below the midcalf.
- If a concomitant inguinal dissection is planned, the popliteal dissection is usually performed first.

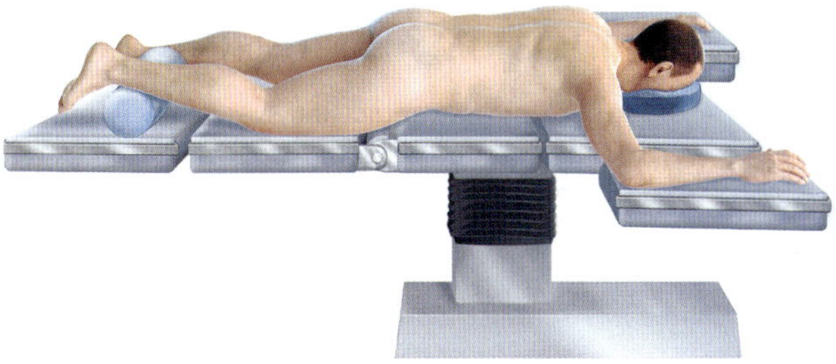

FIG 3 ● Patient position for popliteal dissection. Note that the operative leg (right) is slightly flexed.

PLACEMENT OF INCISION

- There are two options for the incision for popliteal dissection (**FIG 4**). The incision should be planned such that a prior incision for sentinel lymph node biopsy can be excised.
- The S-shaped incision was described by Karakousis[6] in his initial report of the technique of popliteal dissection. This incision typically extends from approximately 10 cm proximal to the joint crease along the lateral thigh overlying the biceps femoris

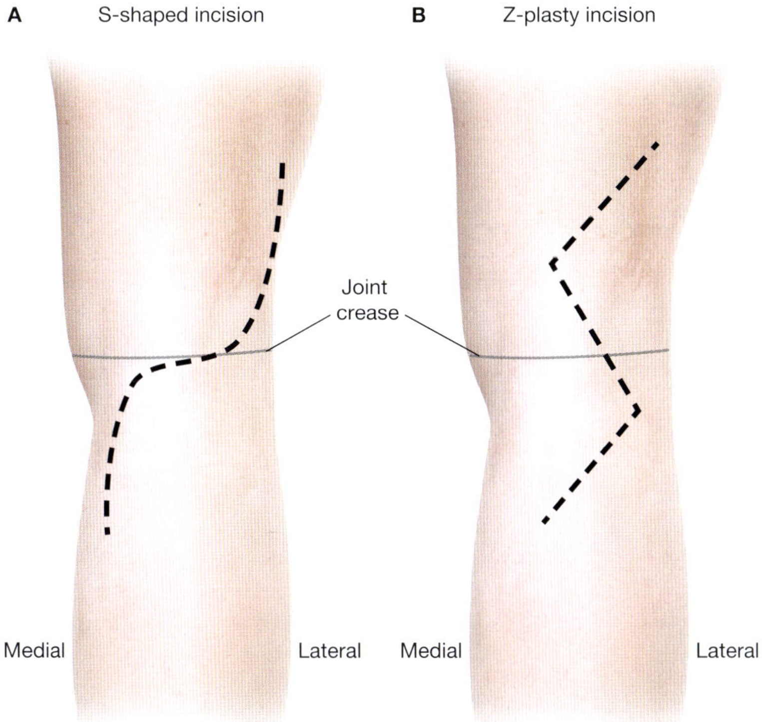

FIG 4 ● Incisions for popliteal dissection (right leg). **A.** S-shaped incision. **B.** Z-plasty incision.

muscle, crosses the joint transversely, and extends approximately 10 cm distal to the joint crease along the medial calf overlying the medial aspect of the gastrocnemius muscle (**FIG 4A**). A mirror image of this incision, extending from the medial thigh to the lateral calf, is also acceptable and may be preferable depending on the orientation of the incision used to perform the sentinel lymph node biopsy.

- We prefer a Z-plasty incision that allows for optimal exposure and heals without joint contracture.[7] Again, the orientation is typically superolateral to inferomedial. The width and length of the Z is relative to the size of the lower thigh, usually with an interior angle ranging from 100 to 120 degrees (**FIG 4B**).

SKIN INCISION AND RAISING OF FLAPS

- The incision is created and dissection is carried down through the subcutaneous tissue. Medial and lateral flaps are raised while traction is maintained with skin hooks. The flaps should expose all of the boundaries of the popliteal fossa, remaining above the deep fascia.
- The lesser saphenous vein is exposed inferiorly; it should be ligated and divided (**FIG 5**).

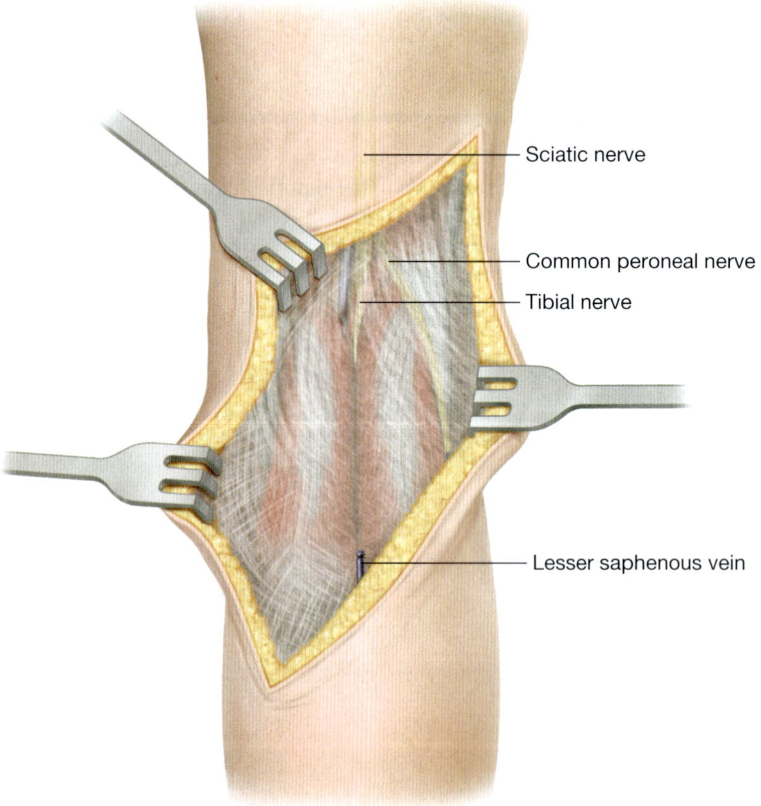

FIG 5 • Medial and lateral skin flaps are raised, and the lesser saphenous vein is divided (right leg).

INCISION OF THE DEEP FASCIA AND IDENTIFICATION OF STRUCTURES TO BE PRESERVED

- The deep fascia is incised vertically with great care not to injure underlying structures; the nerves are very superficial (**FIG 6**).
- The common peroneal nerve runs laterally in the field, just medial to the biceps femoris muscle. The lateral sural nerve branches medially from it and eventually connects inferiorly with the medial sural nerve to form the sural nerve. The lateral sural nerve may be sacrificed if necessary; no significant deficit is appreciated as long as the medial sural nerve remains intact.
- The tibial nerve is the most superficial midline structure. It lies lateral to the popliteal vessels at the superior aspect of the popliteal fossa then courses anterior to the vessels and lies medial to them at the inferior aspect of the popliteal fossa. The medial sural nerve branches off of the tibial nerve and descends in the groove between the heads of the gastrocnemius muscle to where it connects inferiorly with the lateral sural nerve. The medial sural nerve should be preserved if possible; however, it can be divided if greater access to deeper structures is needed. The patient will experience sensory loss along the lateral aspect of the ankle and foot.
- The popliteal vessels are ensheathed; upon opening the sheath, the popliteal artery will be located slightly medial and deep to the popliteal vein (**FIG 7**). The popliteal vein has several small tributaries below the level of the lesser saphenous vein branch, which can cause bothersome bleeding.

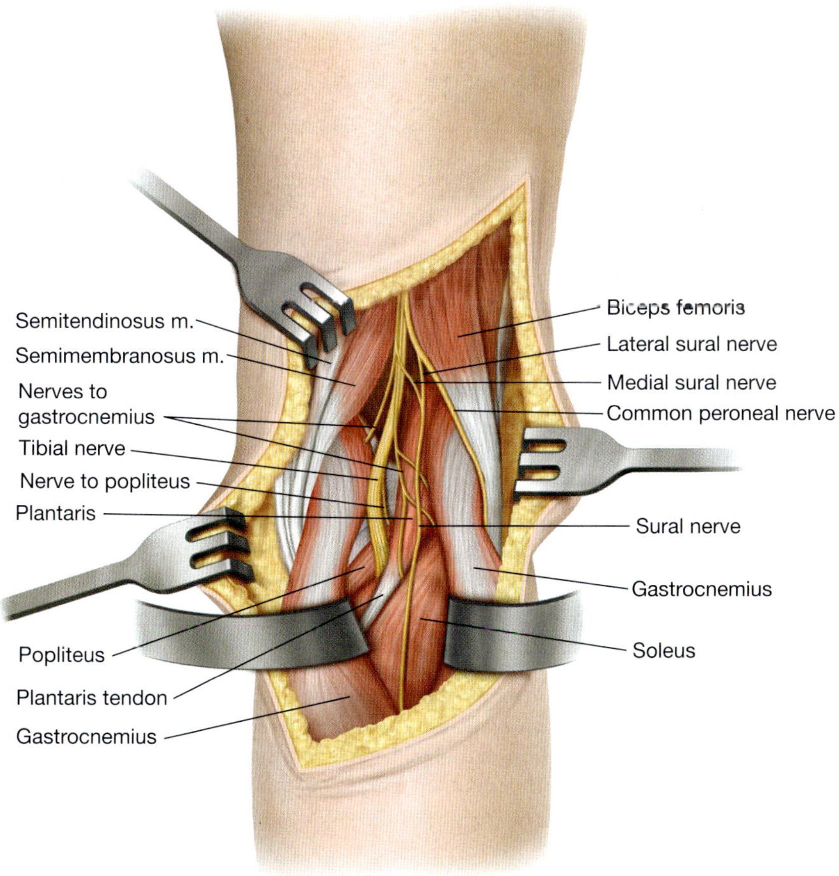

FIG 6 • Upon opening the deep fascia and entering the popliteal fossa, the nerves are exposed (right leg).

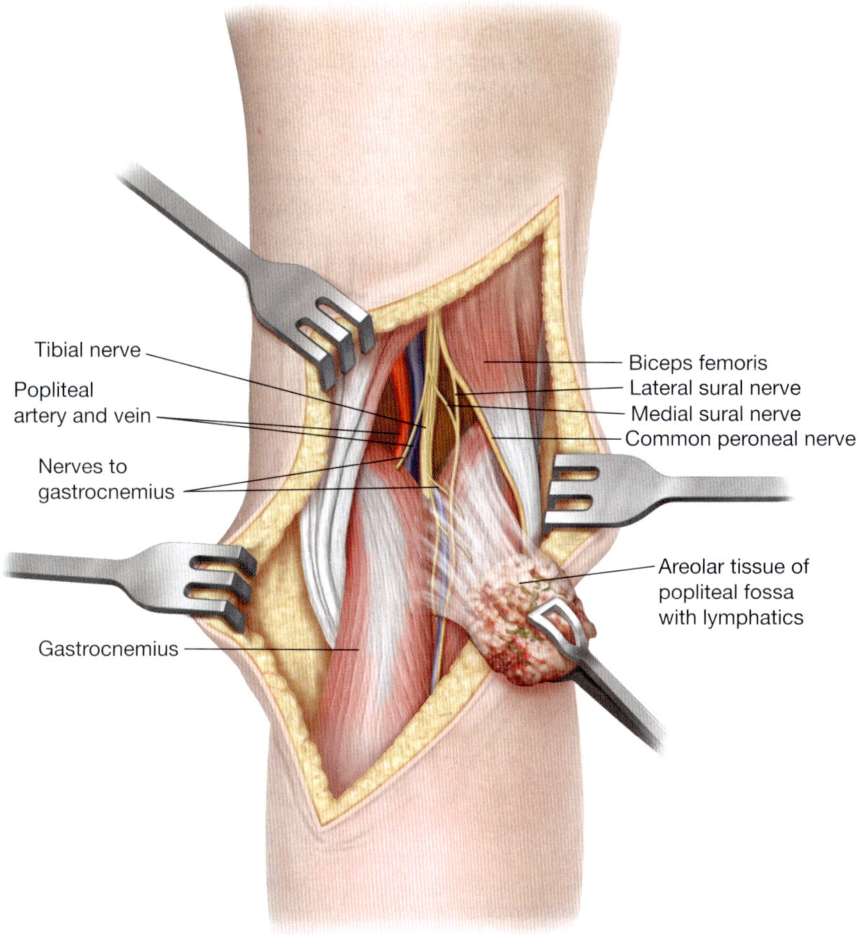

FIG 7 • The nodal specimen is swept away from the nerves and vessels (right leg). Careful attention must be made to the space between the popliteal vessels and the knee joint (anterior/deep to the vessels) as one to two lymph nodes are commonly located here and are easily overlooked.

DISSECTION OF FIBROFATTY NODE–BEARING TISSUE AWAY FROM NERVES AND VESSELS

- The fibrofatty node–bearing tissue is dissected sharply away from the nerves and vessels and is removed in continuity, with care to preserve all important structures (**FIGS 7** and **8**).
- It is important to recognize that one or two lymph nodes are frequently located in the space between the popliteal artery and the knee joint (i.e., anterior to the popliteal artery from the anatomic perspective or deep to the popliteal artery from the perspective of the operating surgeon). These lymph nodes are often overlooked; this space should be carefully dissected so as to not leave lymphatic tissue behind.
- After removal of the specimen, the popliteal fossa should be evaluated thoroughly by inspection and palpation to ensure that all lymphatic tissue has been resected.
- The specimen is sent to pathology for permanent section.

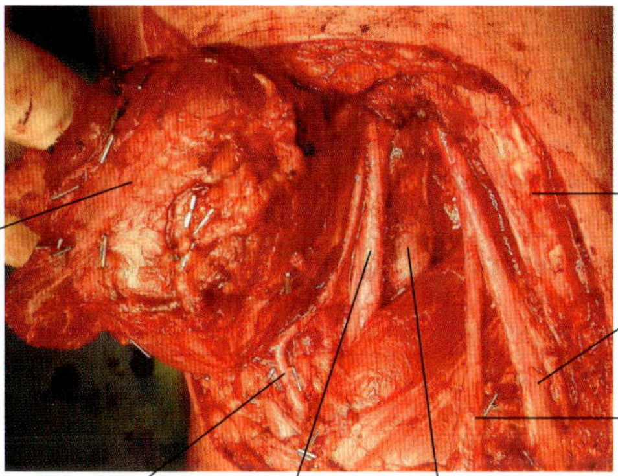

FIG 8 ● Photograph depicting resection of bulky disease in the popliteal fossa (right leg). Skin and subcutaneous tissue were resected en bloc with the specimen, and plastic surgical reconstruction was required for closure.

CLOSURE

- Hemostasis is achieved. The wound is irrigated copiously with saline.
- A 15-Fr round fluted, closed suction drain is placed into the wound and brought out through a separate stab incision (usually inferiorly; **FIG 9**).
- The incision is closed using absorbable suture for the deep dermis and a subcuticular stitch for the skin. A sterile dressing is applied.

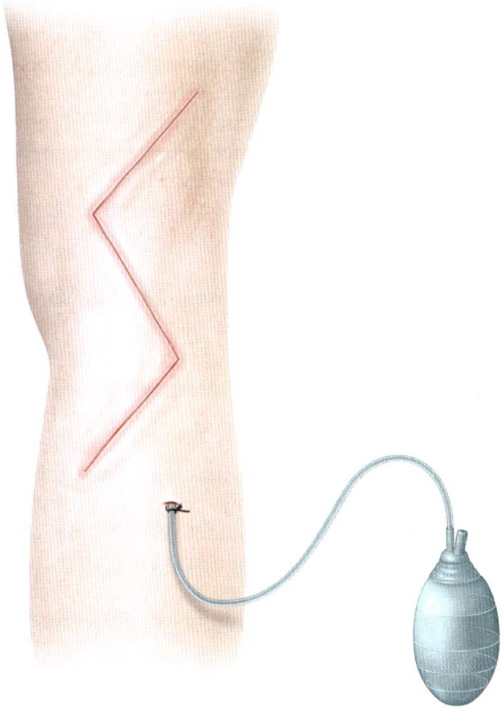

FIG 9 ● The drain is brought out through a separate stab wound inferiorly (right leg).

PEARLS AND PITFALLS

Indications	■ Clinically palpable lymph nodes may be difficult to appreciate in the popliteal fossa because of thick overlying fascia. ■ Most patients undergo popliteal dissection because of a positive sentinel lymph node biopsy.
Incision	■ Options are S-shaped and Z-plasty to preserve joint function. ■ Orient incision so that prior sentinel lymph node biopsy scar is excised (usually superolateral to inferomedial).

Raising of medial and lateral flaps	■ Extend flaps to boundaries of popliteal fossa. ■ Ligate and divide lesser saphenous vein inferiorly.
Incision of the deep fascia and identification of structures to be preserved	■ Take care as fascia is incised; important structures lie directly beneath it. ■ Identify common peroneal nerve, tibial nerve, medial sural nerve, lateral sural nerve, popliteal artery, and popliteal vein. ■ Division of lateral sural nerve alone results in no significant deficit. ■ Division of medial sural nerve results in sensory loss.
Dissection of fibrofatty node–bearing tissue away from nerves and vessels	■ Remember to dissect the space between the popliteal artery and the knee joint (i.e., anterior or deep to the artery), as one or two lymph nodes are frequently identified in this location and are easily overlooked.
Closure	■ Place a drain.

POSTOPERATIVE CARE

- The patient remains hospitalized at least overnight, but perhaps for several days, depending on the extent of other lymphadenectomies that may have been performed during the same operation. A posterior knee splint (knee immobilizer) is used for the first few postoperative days to allow for wound healing prior to returning to full mobility. Ambulation is often initially difficult; physical therapy is useful. The drain may be removed when output falls below 30 mL per day; typically, this is a relatively short interval compared with drain times for axillary or inguinal dissections.

OUTCOMES

- Lymphedema is rare after popliteal dissection, and the functional outcome of the knee is usually excellent.
- The popliteal fossa is historically reported to contain 6 to 7 lymph nodes.[6] However, contemporary experience suggests that finding far fewer nodes is more common.[7] In a recent study of 15 patients who underwent popliteal sentinel lymph node biopsy, the mean number of popliteal lymph nodes harvested was 1.4 (range was 1 to 3); however, in 6 patients who subsequently underwent completion popliteal dissection, the mean number of lymph nodes in the popliteal dissection specimen was 0.3, with 4 of the 6 patients' specimens yielding no additional (nonsentinel) lymph nodes.[2]
- Overall, the 5-year survival for patients with stage III melanoma (lymph node–positive disease) ranges widely (14% to 85%), with the 5-year survival of a patient with a single microscopically positive lymph node approximating 70%.[8–10] It is difficult to determine whether the presence of a positive popliteal lymph node carries a different prognosis when compared with the presence of a positive lymph node in one of the more commonly involved regional lymph node basins (i.e., axillary, inguinal, cervical). Because popliteal disease is overall quite rare, the literature contains only case reports and small case series, most of which include both patients with micrometastatic disease and patients with clinically palpable disease.[1,3] A relatively large contemporary study in the literature reports on 15 patients who underwent popliteal sentinel lymph node biopsy; 8 patients had a positive sentinel lymph node. At an average follow-up of 64 months, 3 (37.5%) patients had died of melanoma, 1 (12.5%) was alive with disease, and 4 (50%) had no evidence of disease.[2] Given the very small numbers, these statistics are likely similar to overall 5-year survival rates for patients with positive nodes in the more commonly involved regional lymph node basins.

COMPLICATIONS

- Common complications of popliteal dissection include wound infection (cellulitis or abscess), seroma, and hematoma.
- Injury to the common peroneal nerve results in postoperative foot drop and sensory loss or paresthesias over the dorsum of the foot (including the space between the great and second toes) and lateral shin.
- Injury to the tibial nerve results in postoperative loss of plantar flexion of the foot, loss of flexion of the toes, weakened inversion of the foot, and sensory loss or paresthesias over the posterior aspect of the leg and the sole of the foot.

REFERENCES

1. Thompson JF, Hunt JA, Culjak G, et al. Popliteal lymph node metastasis from primary cutaneous melanoma. *Eur J Surg Oncol.* 2000;26:172–176.
2. Steen ST, Kargozaran H, Moran CJ, et al. Management of popliteal sentinel nodes in melanoma. *J Am Coll Surg.* 2011;213:180–187.
3. Menes TS, Schachter J, Steinmetz AP, et al. Lymphatic drainage to the popliteal basin in distal lower extremity malignant melanoma. *Arch Surg.* 2004;139:1002–1006.
4. Uren RF, Howman-Giles R, Thompson JF. Patterns of lymphatic drainage from the skin in patients with melanoma. *J Nucl Med.* 2003;44:570–582.
5. Marone U, Caraco C, Chiofalo MG, et al. Resection in the popliteal fossa for metastatic melanoma. *World J Surg Oncol.* 2007;5:8.
6. Karakousis CP. The technique of popliteal node dissection. *Surg Gynecol Obstet.* 1980;151:420–423.
7. Sholar A, Martin RCG II, McMasters KM. Popliteal lymph node dissection. *Ann Surg Oncol.* 2005;12:189–193.
8. Balch CM, Gershenwald JE, Soong SJ, et al. Multivariate analysis of prognostic factors among 2,313 patients with stage III melanoma: comparison of nodal micrometastases versus macrometastases. *J Clin Oncol.* 2010;28:2452–2459.
9. McMasters KM, Ross MI, Reintgen DS, et al. Final results of the Sunbelt Melanoma Trial [abstract 9003]. *J Clin Oncol.* 2008;26:15s.
10. Morton DL, Thompson JF, Cochran AJ, et al. Sentinel-node biopsy or nodal observation in melanoma. *N Engl J Med.* 2006;355:1307–1317.

Chapter 33 Isolated Limb Infusion

Jeffrey J. Sussman Joseph S. Giglia

DEFINITION

- *Isolated limb infusion* is the term that is commonly used to indicate a minimally invasive, low flow rate, nonoxygenated perfusion of an extremity with chemotherapy to effect control of a cancer within that extremity[1] (**FIG 1**). It is a more recent modification of a more traditional technique commonly referred to as *isolated limb perfusion* (see Chapter 34), which uses higher flow rates and an oxygenated circuit to perfuse the chemotherapy through the extremity where vascular control is obtained during an open procedure and is often combined with a formal node dissection. Comparatively, isolated limb infusion is a shorter, better tolerated, less complex procedure, not requiring a perfusionist, an oxygenator, nor blood products to prime the extracorporeal circuit.[2,3] Proponents of limb perfusion claim a higher response rate, particularly in bulky disease; however, the techniques have not been compared in a randomized fashion.

PATIENT HISTORY AND PHYSICAL FINDINGS

- The most common indication for this procedure is a patient with in-transit melanoma restricted to an extremity whose lesions are too numerous or recurrent to be amenable to simple excision. It should be thought of as a limb salvage technique to treat regionally advanced disease and has no proven systemic benefit. Therefore, it is not commonly used in the face of distant metastasis unless regional control/palliation is the central goal.
- Common malignancies treated in this manner include melanoma and Merkel cell carcinoma. Other histologies treated less commonly include squamous cell carcinoma and sarcoma.
- A through history and physical should be performed with attention to documenting location and extent of extremity disease, limb function, edema, vascular exam, and evaluation of draining nodal basins.
- Limb volume is estimated by water displacement.
  - Sequential circumferential measurements or computed tomography (CT) volumetric measurements have been described as alternatives.
  - The contralateral limb should be measured if the involved limb is edematous.
  - The limb is submerged in a water tank up to level anticipated to be at bottom of tourniquet. The water level is marked and then after removal of the limb, the tank is filled with a measured amount of water to reach the marked level.
- Patients should have nonoccluded arterial and venous systems to allow catheter placement and chemotherapy infusion.

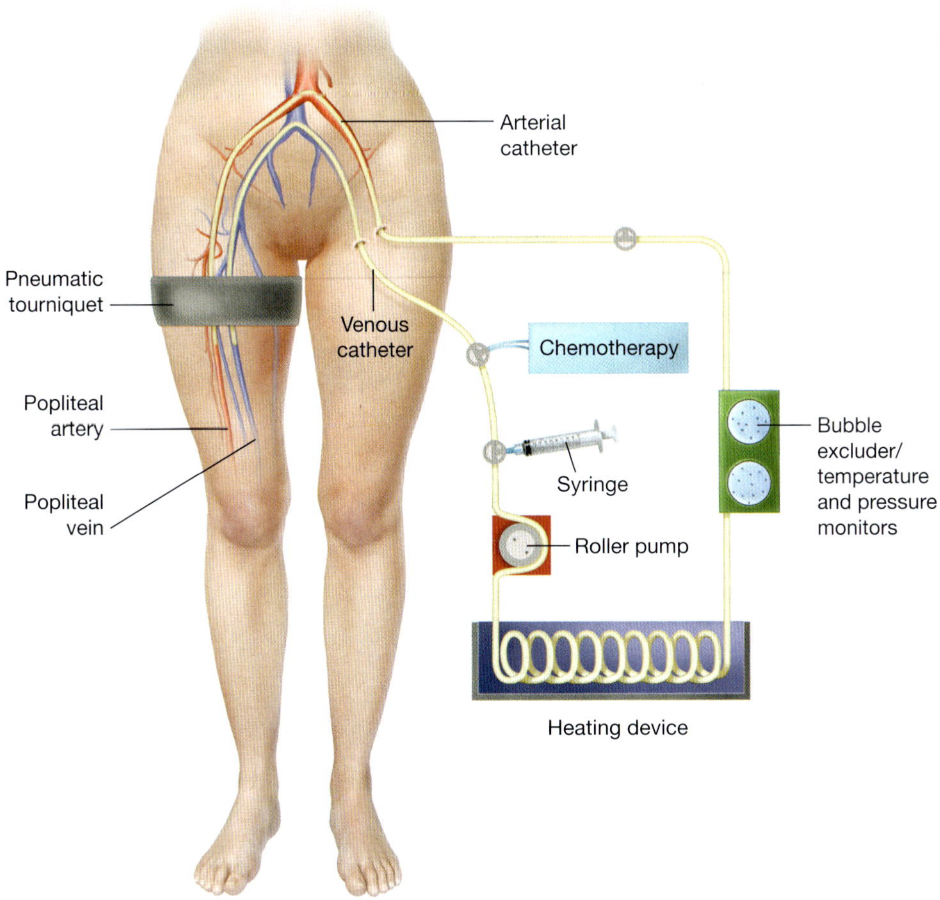

FIG 1 • Schematic of circuit used for isolated limb infusion. Roller pump is optional.

- The extent of disease needs to be distal enough in the extremity to be able to place a tourniquet proximally.
  - In selected cases, this may require resection of limited more proximal disease combined with infusion of greater distal disease burden distally.
  - Isolated limb infusion can be combined with a lymph node dissection with direct placement of the catheters in the exposed vessels.

IMAGING AND OTHER DIAGNOSTIC STUDIES

- Arterial and venous duplex ultrasound to establish arterial and venous patency. With adequate collaterals, limb infusion has been described even when superficial vessels are occluded.
- Imaging to evaluate limb disease burden if lesions are deep seated and difficult to quantitate on exam
- Imaging to evaluate for distant disease including brain magnetic resonance imaging (MRI); whole body positron emission tomography (PET)/CT; and/or chest, abdomen, pelvis contrast-enhanced CT scans

SURGICAL MANAGEMENT

- Patients should be discussed in multidisciplinary fashion to consider alternatives to isolated infusion including isolated limb perfusion; intralesional therapy; simple excision; radical excision, including circumferential excision and grafting or amputation; radiation; or systemic cytotoxic, immunotherapeutic, and other biologic therapies as well as clinical trial eligibility.

Preoperative Planning

- Who and where vascular access is to be obtained should be determined preoperatively and may be institution specific. Possible methods include the following:
  - Interventional radiology. Vascular access can be performed in the interventional radiology suite, with the patient then transported to the operating room (OR) with the arterial and venous catheters in place.
  - Vascular surgery. Some vascular surgeons have the training, experience, and interest to perform the vascular access as an alternative to the interventional radiologist. Access can be obtained in the OR directly if appropriately equipped with fluoroscopic capabilities. Although additional OR time is required if done in the OR, the catheters can more easily be manipulated later, as needed. Moreover, access can be obtained under general anesthesia and risk of dislodgement during transport/bed transfer is eliminated.
  - Chemotherapy. Melphalan and dactinomycin are prepared just prior to the procedure. The calculated drug dosage is often reduced if the patient's actual body weight exceeds ideal body weight by multiplying the calculated drug dose by the ratio of ideal to actual body weight.
  - Melphalan dose is 7.5 mg/L volume for lower extremity infusions (maximum dose of 100 mg) or 10 mg/L volume for the upper extremity (maximum dose 50 mg).
  - Dactinomycin dose is 1% of the melphalan dose (maximum 0.5 mg).
  - The drugs are mixed together in 400-mL normal saline lower extremity (200 mL upper extremity) and delivered to OR for administration.

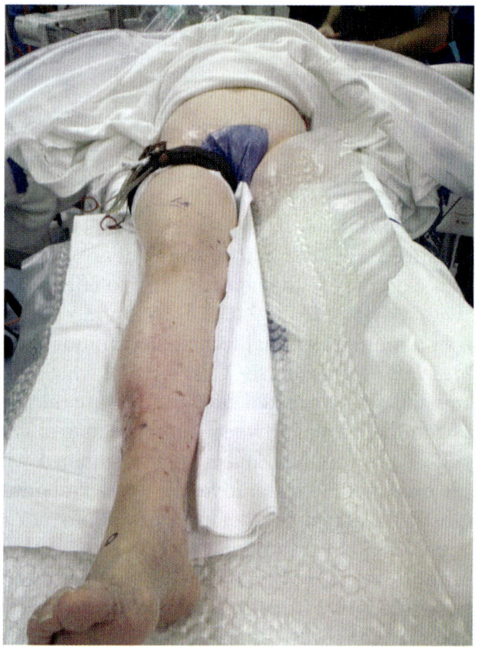

FIG 2 • Exposed affected limb with tourniquet proximally.

Positioning

- The patient is positioned supine on a fluoroscopy-capable OR bed for vascular access or in case catheter manipulation is needed.
- The room should be prewarmed.
- A heated circulating water blanket is placed around the affected extremity or an external radiant heater utilized (**FIGS 2** and **3**).

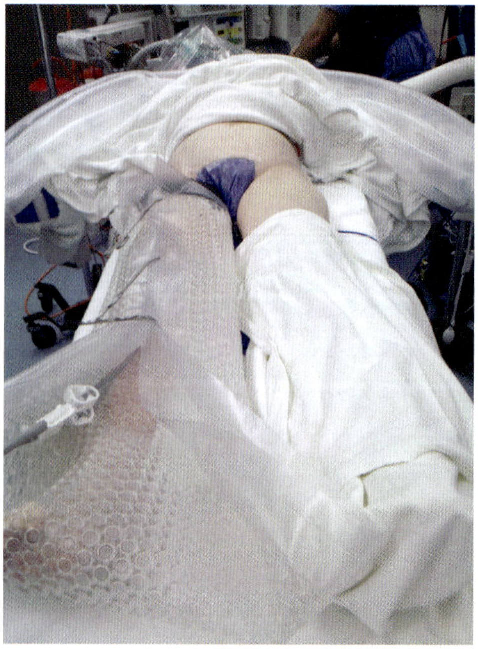

FIG 3 • Affected limb wrapped in water blanket.

- Heated air blankets are placed on the patient's trunk and head or an external radiant heater is used.
- A pneumatic tourniquet is placed on the proximal aspect of the extremity with the lower edge marked with a radiopaque hemostat. For distal-only infusions, the tourniquet can be placed lower.
- Needle temperature probes are inserted into deep and superficial locations within the proximal and distal limb locations.
- Baseline activated clotting time (ACT) is obtained.

VASCULAR ACCESS

- Venous and arterial access is obtained in the uninvolved lower limb using the Seldinger technique with ultrasound and fluoroscopic guidance.
- After placing a vascular access sheath, a 5- or 6-Fr 100-cm catheter is introduced into the external iliac artery retrograde and manipulated across the iliac bifurcation and down the index limb arterial system to a point beyond the lower edge of the tourniquet. Similarly, a 7- to 8-Fr catheter is placed thru the venous system and positioned below the tourniquet (**FIG 4**).
- The patient is heparinized at 200 to 300 units/kg to obtain an ACT of 400.

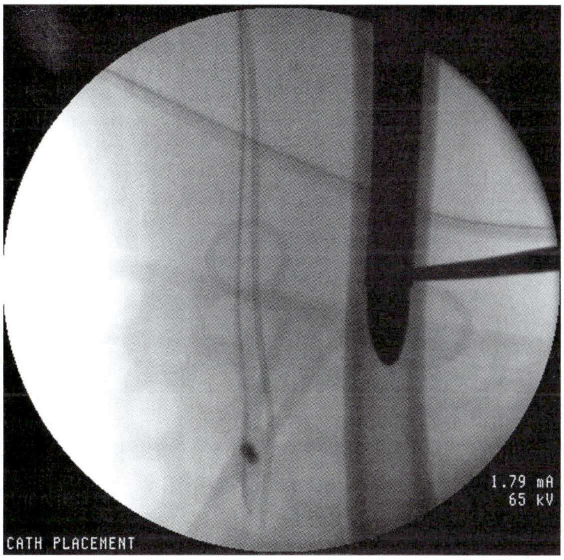

FIG 4 ● Radiograph of extremity with catheters in place below lower edge of pneumatic tourniquet. Note, wire in arterial catheter will be removed prior to infusion.

INFUSION CIRCUIT

- The catheters are connected to sterile ¼″ pump tubing with high-flow stopcock connectors and a 20-mL syringe as a hand pump or thru a single roller pump (**FIGS 5** and **6**).
- The circuit then passes through a heat exchange unit or heated water bath set to heat the fluid to 41°C followed by a bubble excluder before connecting to the arterial catheter. The circuit is primed with saline.
- Inflate the tourniquet to 250 to 300 mmHg.
- Adequate flow is obtained by hand pumping the syringe and using the three-way stopcock to pull from the venous catheter and infuse toward the arterial catheter. Alternatively, a roller pump can be used at rate approximately 100 mL per minute.

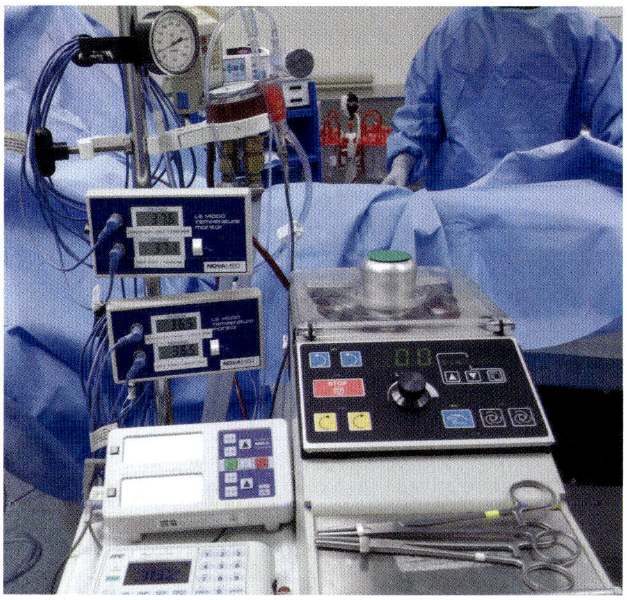

FIG 5 ● Photograph of roller pump workstation with temperature monitors, heat exchanger (water bath not depicted), ACT monitor, pressure gauge, and patient in background.

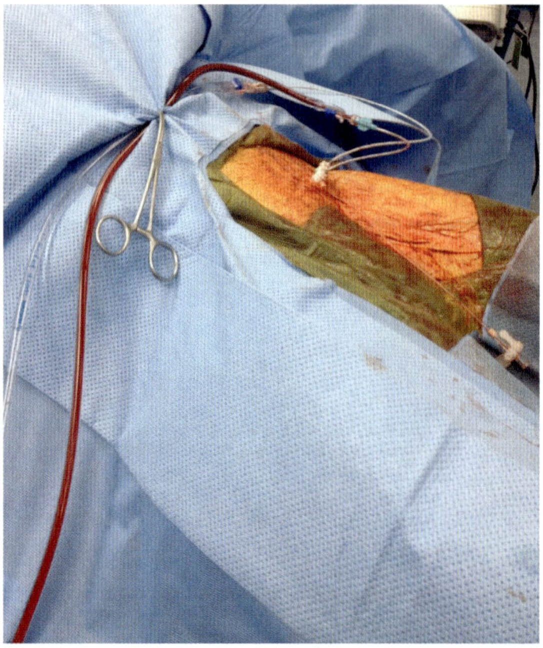

FIG 6 ● Contralateral groin with catheters in place connected to infusion circuit.

CHEMOTHERAPY INFUSION

- If the hand or foot is not to be perfused, an Esmarch bandage is tightly wrapped around the hand or foot to exclude the chemotherapy.
- Papaverine (60 mg for the lower extremity, 30 mg for the upper extremity) is infused into the circuit.
- The chemotherapy drug and dosage is double checked and then infused into circuit.
- Chemotherapy and blood are circulated for 30 minutes by hand pump syringe or roller pump method.
- Temperature, flow rate, pressure, and extremity are monitored. Blood gas and ACT are checked at 10- to 15-minute intervals.

CHEMOTHERAPY WASHOUT

- The venous tubing is disconnected from circuit and allowed to gravity drain blood into a waste container.
- One liter of lactated Ringer's solution (500 mL upper extremity) is infused into the arterial circuit.

CONCLUSION

- The tourniquet is released after notification to anesthesiologist of possible electrolyte and volume changes.
- The catheters are removed while leaving sheaths in place. Esmarch bandage, if used, is removed.
- Vascular exam of infused extremity is assessed and, if baseline, protamine is given to reverse the heparin.
- Once ACT is corrected, the sheaths are removed with pressure applied for hemostasis at the vascular puncture sites.

PEARLS AND PITFALLS

Drug dosing	■ If no ideal body weight correction, overall response rate may be increased; however, toxicity is also increased without clear improvement in complete response rate.
Poor venous return	■ Catheter may be up against valve, vein sidewall, or pulled back under tourniquet. ■ With heating, limb may vasodilate leading to relative intravascular volume loss. Infusing an extra 500-mL saline into limb through arterial circuit may help.
Proximal disease	■ An Esmarch bandage can be used as a tourniquet high on the limb to allow for greater volume of leg infused.

Limb temperature	■ Pumping heated blood through circuit prior to chemotherapy administration can heat up limb internally to greater than 37°C in 5 to 15 minutes.
Antiemetics	■ Steroids should not be used as antiemetics during or after anesthesia as they have an unknown effect on response rate.
Residual melanin pigmentation	■ Response may continue over several months. In-transit lesions may flatten but retain pigment. Biopsy may indicate melanin-laden macrophages without viable tumor.

POSTOPERATIVE CARE

- The patient is routinely extubated and admitted to an appropriate care unit capable of frequent neurovascular extremity monitoring for first 24 hours. Baseline serum creatinine phosphokinase (CPK), complete blood count (CBC), and chemistry panel are obtained.
- The extremity should be elevated when in bed, but the patient is allowed to get out of bed after 24 hours if extremity toxicity is not evident.
- Twice-daily physician examination should be performed, checking for vascular access complications, vascular and neurologic exam, and for compartment syndrome. Daily CPK is obtained, as muscle injury will routinely occur to some extent.
- CPK levels are expected to rise, peaking on postoperative days 4 and 5. Once levels begin to decrease and the extremity is stable, then the patient may be discharged. If the patient is reliable and has immediate health care access, it may be possible to discharge patient sooner with careful outpatient follow-up and instructions as the inpatient care after the first day is for toxicity monitoring.
- If the CPK levels rapidly rise sooner than day 4 and/or exceed 1,000 IU/L, then the patient is in danger of developing a compartment syndrome and potential limb loss. Steroids can ameliorate associated inflammation and decrease risk of requiring operative intervention. Dexamethasone can be given at 4 mg every 6 hours with rapid taper when the CPK drops below 1,000 IU/L.

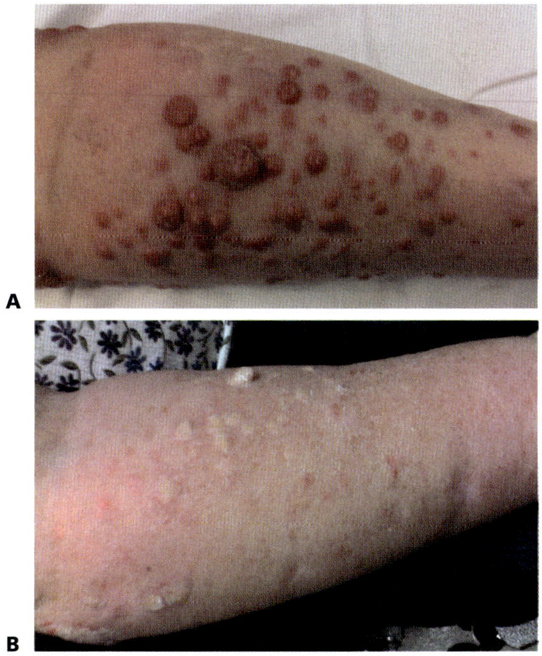

FIG 7 • **A.** Photograph of limb with in-transit disease. **B.** Photograph of same limb 4 weeks following isolated limb infusion.

OUTCOMES

- A complete clinical response is seen in 30% to 40% of patients after a single isolated limb infusion with another 30% to 50% of patients experiencing a partial response.[4–7] Complete responses are often durable, whereas partial responses are usually not (**FIGS 7A,B**). Response may take 2 to 6 weeks to be seen clinically. Limb salvage is obtained in the vast majority of patients, whereas 5-year overall survival is approximately 30% due to distant disease progression. Nearly all patients will develop some side effects from the procedure including skin erythema and lymphedema. Approximately half of patients will report return to baseline limb function by 3 months and the remainder by a year.
- Isolated limb infusion is better tolerated with less toxicity as compared to isolated limb perfusion, is technically easier to perform, and appears to have similar response rates.

COMPLICATIONS

- Potential complications related to vascular access include hematoma, pseudoaneurysm, dissection, and embolization. Stroke can be a complication of upper extremity arterial access.
- Toxicity from the isolated limb infusion of chemotherapy into the extremity skin and soft tissue are classified by the Wieberdink grading scale (Table 1).[8] Grade V or limb loss occurs in less than 1% of cases.
- Systemic toxicity from the chemotherapy should be rare but might include nausea and bone marrow suppression.

Table 1: Wieberdink Extremity Toxicity Scale

Grade I	No reaction
Grade II	Slight erythema and/or edema
Grade III	Considerate erythema and/or edema with some blistering; slightly disturbed motility permissible
Grade IV	Extensive epidermolysis and/or obvious damage to the deep tissues, causing definite functional disturbances; threatening or manifest compartmental syndromes
Grade V	Reaction that may necessitate amputation

From Wieberdink J, Benckhuysen C, Braat RP, et al. Dosimetry in isolated perfusion of the limbs by assessment of perfused tissue volume and grading of toxic tissue reactions. Eur J Cancer Clin Oncol. *1982;18(10):905–910.*

REFERENCES

1. Thompson JF, Waugh RC, Saw RPM, et al. Isolated limb infusion with melphalan for recurrent limb melanoma: a simple alternative to isolated limb perfusion. *Reg Cancer Treat*. 1994;7:188–192.
2. Testori A, Verhoef C, Kroon HM, et al. Treatment of melanoma metastases in a limb by isolated limb perfusion and isolated limb infusion. *J Surg Oncol*. 2011;104:397–404.
3. Thompson JF, Kam PC, Lindner P, et al. Isolated limb infusion. In: Balch CM, Houghton AN, Sober AJ, et al, eds. *Cutaneous Melanoma*. 4th ed. St. Louis, MO: Quality Medical Publishing; 2003:495–507.
4. Beasley GM, Peterson RP, Yoo J, et al. Isolated limb infusion for in-transit malignant melanoma of the extremity: a well tolerated but less effective alternative to hyperthermic isolated limb perfusion. *Ann Surg Oncol*. 2008;15(8):2195–2205.
5. Beasley GM, Caudle A, Petersen RP, et al. A multi-institutional experience of isolated limb infusion: defining response and toxicity in the US. *J Am Coll Surg*. 2009;208(5):706–715.
6. Kroon HM, Moncrieff M, Kam PC, et al. Outcomes following isolated limb infusion for melanoma. A 14-year experience. *Ann Surg Oncol*. 2008;15(11):3003–3013.
7. McClaine RJ, Giglia JS, Ahmad SA, et al. Quality of life outcomes following isolated limb infusion. *Ann Surg Oncol*. 2012;19(5):1373–1378.
8. Wieberdink J, Benckhuysen C, Braat RP, et al. Dosimetry in isolated perfusion of the limbs by assessment of perfused tissue volume and grading of toxic tissue reactions. *Eur J Cancer Clin Oncol*. 1982;18(10):905–910.

Chapter 34 Isolated Limb Perfusion

Omgo E. Nieweg Oscar E. Imhof Bin B.R. Kroon

DEFINITION

- Compared to other cancer types, melanoma has a particular biology in various respects. In-transit dissemination is typical of this disease and occurs in a few percentage of patients. In-transit metastases grow from tumor cells that are stuck in a lymph vessel in the skin or in the subcutaneous tissue. Such metastases are preferably excised but they tend to recur in larger numbers (**FIG 1**). Isolated perfusion can be considered when they are situated on a limb and their number is too great or they recur too frequently.
- Isolated limb perfusion (ILP) enables treatment of an arm or leg with a high dose of chemotherapy without exposing the remainder of the body to the drug(s). This is accomplished by isolating the limb from the body's circulation and creating a separate oxygenated blood circuit. This is in contrast to isolated limb infusion (ILI), a low-flow, nonoxygenated perfusion that is described in Chapter 33. ILP and ILI are therapeutic options for patients with locally or regionally advanced melanoma that would otherwise require a more debilitating operation, for example, amputation.

PATIENT HISTORY AND PHYSICAL FINDINGS

- After treatment of their primary melanoma, patients are instructed to regularly examine the scar of the excision for local recurrence and to check the skin and subcutaneous tissue around this area up to the regional lymph node basin for visible or palpable satellite and in-transit metastases. The physician who follows the patient inquires about new regional lesions. Patients themselves detect about half of the recurrences, but at an early stage, they can look quite innocuous. The detection of the more subtle ones requires the expertise and suspicious mind of an experienced surgeon.
- A detailed history should be obtained to assess the general condition of the patient and to be informed about other relevant ailments, allergies, and medication.
- Physical examination of melanoma patients is aimed at detecting a local recurrence, satellite metastases, in-transit metastases, regional lymph node involvement, and a subsequent primary melanoma. A detailed examination of the skin, the regional subcutaneous tissue, and the regional node field is warranted.
- The vascular situation of the limb is assessed. The presence of peripheral arterial pulsations needs to be sufficient to allow for ILP.

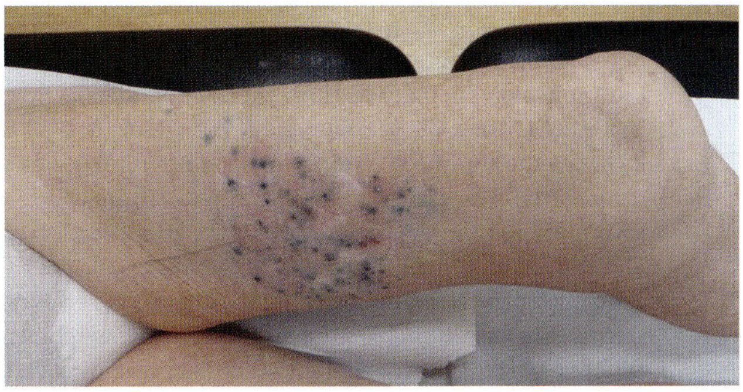

FIG 1 • Extensive in-transit metastases on the left thigh.

IMAGING AND OTHER DIAGNOSTIC STUDIES

- The presence of advanced melanoma in the extremity should be confirmed by biopsy.
- In addition to the routine preoperative tests, screening for metastases elsewhere is appropriate as their presence may change the treatment plan. Whole body positron emission tomography (PET) or computed tomography (CT) and magnetic resonance imaging (MRI) of the brain are frequently recommended for this purpose.
- Arteriography is indicated if the arterial blood supply is questionable. A complete obstruction in the target artery or a major impediment downstream renders perfusion impossible. Extensive arterial calcification per se is not a contraindication.
- An elevated tumor marker such as the TA90 glycoprotein antigen or the S100 protein provides an opportunity to monitor the course of the disease.

SURGICAL MANAGEMENT

Rationale and Contraindications

- Extensive involvement limited to a certain region is typical for melanoma.
- The rationale for ILP is that melanoma is sensitive to cytotoxic drugs but effective treatment requires a higher dosage compared to various other cancer types. In contrast to the vital organs, the normal tissues in the extremities tolerate such a high dose. ILP with cytotoxic medication may improve regional tumor control while limiting the systemic side effects.
- The procedure makes it possible to vary physiologic conditions such as blood flow, temperature, and oxygenation.
- Prophylactic ILP is not indicated in patients with excised high-risk primary melanoma without evidence of regional metastases.[1]
- The contraindications are listed in Table 1. A major vascular obstruction may prevent access to the artery and precludes the operation.
- Diabetes mellitus with severe peripheral vascular disease is a contraindication.
- ILP should not be performed in children as it may damage the epiphyseal plates.
- Previous radiotherapy is a relative contraindication as perfusion may cause necrosis of prior irradiated skin.
- A large superficial tumor with major tendon involvement is a relative contraindication.

Table 1: Absolute and Relative Contraindications to Isolated Limb Perfusion

Absolute contraindications
Obstruction of major artery
Diabetes with serious peripheral vascular disease
Child with open epiphyseal plates
Relative contraindications
Previous radiotherapy
Large superficial tumor with major tendon involvement
Brain metastases
Infected wound or ulcer

- Brain metastases tend to bleed and their presence is a relative contraindication.
- An infected wound or ulcer is another relative contraindication.
- ILP can be carried out safely at an advanced age.[2] The presence of regional node involvement is not a contraindication, as this procedure can be combined with a regional node dissection. In the presence of distant metastases, systemic therapy is a reasonable first option, but perfusion can provide good regional palliation in the presence of refractory blood-borne metastases.

Anatomy

- For advanced disease of the leg, ILP can be performed at the femoral or iliac level. The arm can be treated at the brachial level or through the axilla.

Preoperative Planning

- ILP requires cooperation of the surgeon, the perfusionist, and the nuclear medicine worker in addition to the customary operating room team.
- Melphalan is the standard drug used in current practice. The dosage of the drug is adjusted to the need of the individual patient. The volume of the extremity is an often used parameter to calculate the required melphalan dose. The volume can be determined using a water reservoir (FIG 2). Adjustments to the dosage can be made based on risk factors for regional toxicity like female gender and obesity.

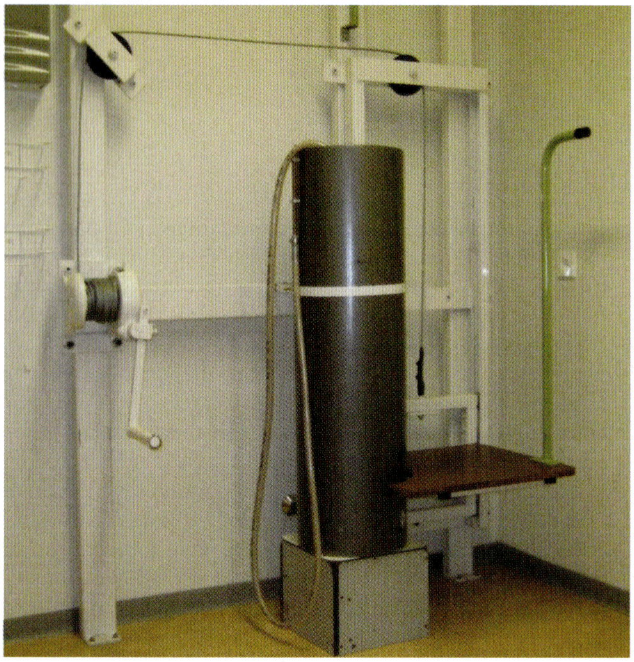

FIG 2 • Water reservoir for measuring the volume of a limb. On the right is the elevator to bring the patient up to the required height. The elevator handle is on the left.

- ILP requires sophisticated technology. The surgeon should verify the availability of the required drug(s) and make sure that the necessary equipment and materials are present and in good working order.
- General anesthesia is required. Epidural anesthesia is to be avoided as it induces vasodilation and predisposes to leakage of blood from the systemic circulation to the perfusion circuit.
- Preoperative antibiotics are not necessary.

TECHNIQUES

ISOLATED FEMORAL PERFUSION

Positioning

- The patient is placed on the operating table in a supine position. The leg may be slightly exorotated.
- The leg is prepped and draped in a sterile fashion in its entirety.
- A pneumatic tourniquet is positioned around the upper thigh, but it is not inflated yet.
- A heating blanket is wrapped around the knee and the lower leg.
- A cotton doughnut is positioned underneath the heel to prevent decubitus.
- The operating table is tilted toward the surgeon.

Incision

- A longitudinal incision of approximately 10 cm is made starting just below the pneumatic tourniquet (FIG 3). The incision runs over the sartorius muscle. The skin and the subcutaneous tissue are divided and, subsequently, the fascia. Adson retractors are placed (FIG 4).

Access to the Superficial Femoral Vessels and Cannulation

- The external femoral vessels run behind the sartorius muscle. The vessels are reached either medially or laterally from the muscle. The thin fascia covering the vessels (FIG 5) is incised, exposing the superficial femoral artery. The artery is mobilized over the exposed length (FIG 6). Small arteries branching from the superficial femoral artery are ligated and divided. A vessel loop facilitates the dissection. The accompanying vein is identified when the artery is pulled aside (FIG 7). The vein is mobilized over the exposed length. Attributing branches are ligated at the confluence and divided.
  - Heparin is administered in a quantity of 150 units/kg body weight.

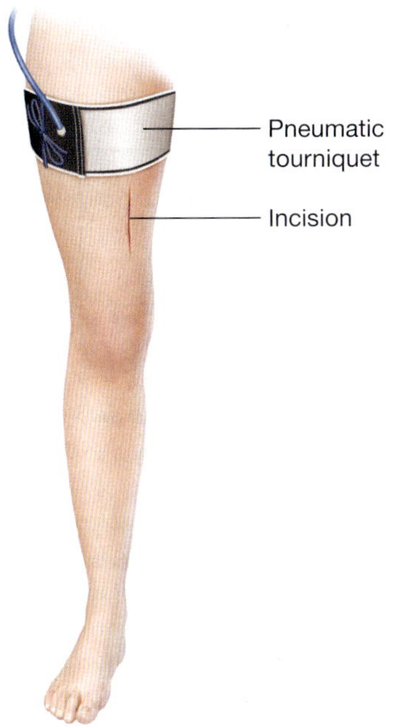

FIG 3 ● The incision is made over the inner thigh just below the pneumatic tourniquet.

- Open access to the saphenous vein at the level of the ankle is gained to measure the venous pressure. The venous pressure is monitored throughout the procedure and should not deviate more than 10 mm H_2O from the initial assessment. An increase is associated with postoperative morbidity.
- The appropriate diameter of arterial and venous cannulae for the perfusion is determined. The cannulae are tunneled subcutaneously underneath the tourniquet to the open wound to prevent kinking.
- The vein is clamped cranially and caudally. A transverse venotomy of a few millimeters is performed.

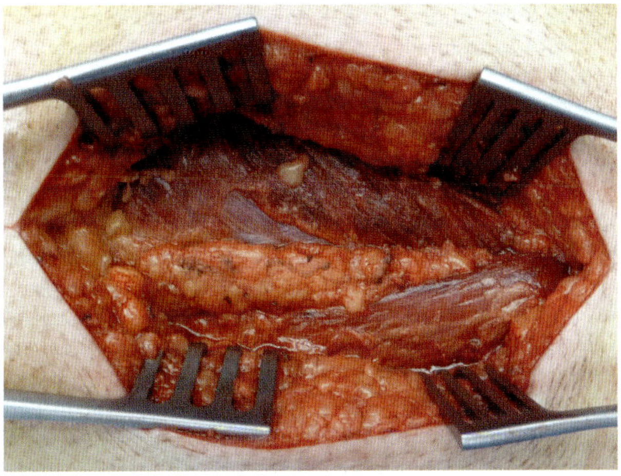

FIG 4 ● The long adductor muscle **(above)** and the sartorius muscle **(below)** are exposed. The superficial femoral vessels lie behind the sartorius muscle.

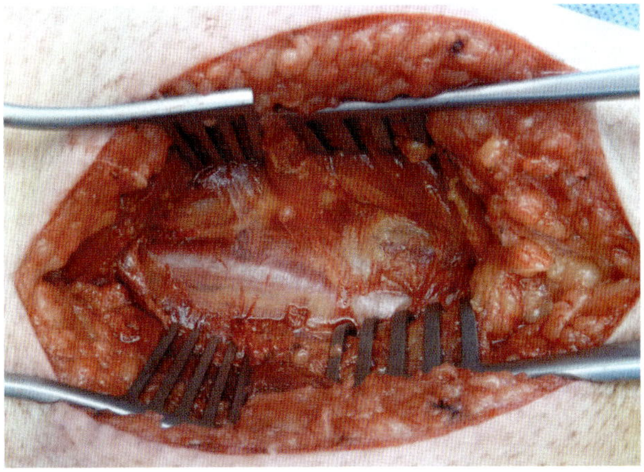

FIG 5 ● The superficial femoral artery can be seen through the thin fascia that covers the vessels.

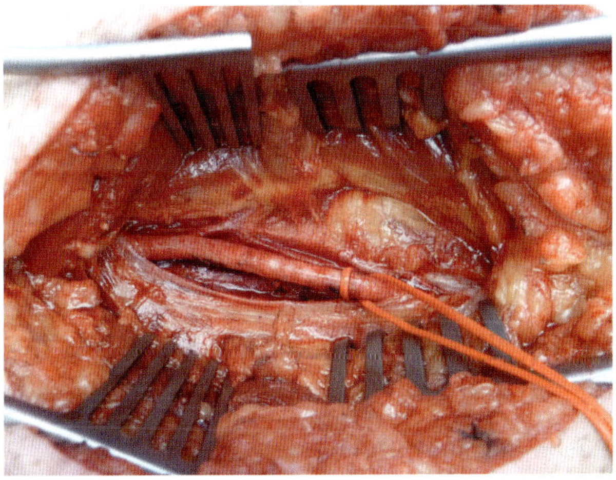

FIG 6 ● The superficial femoral artery is mobilized.

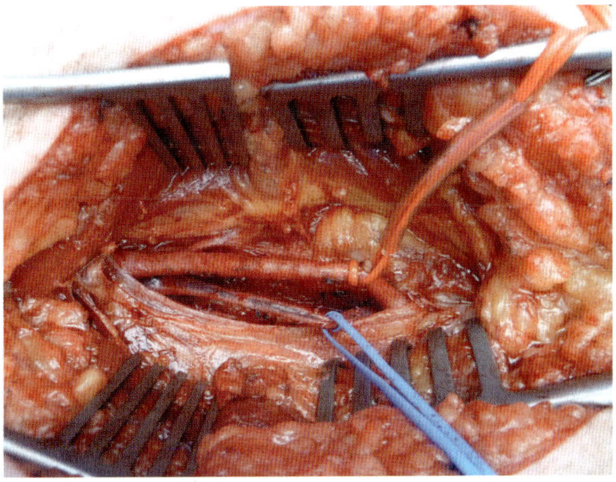

FIG 7 ● The superficial femoral artery is pulled aside (red vessel loop) and the accompanying vein is identified and dissected (blue vessel loop).

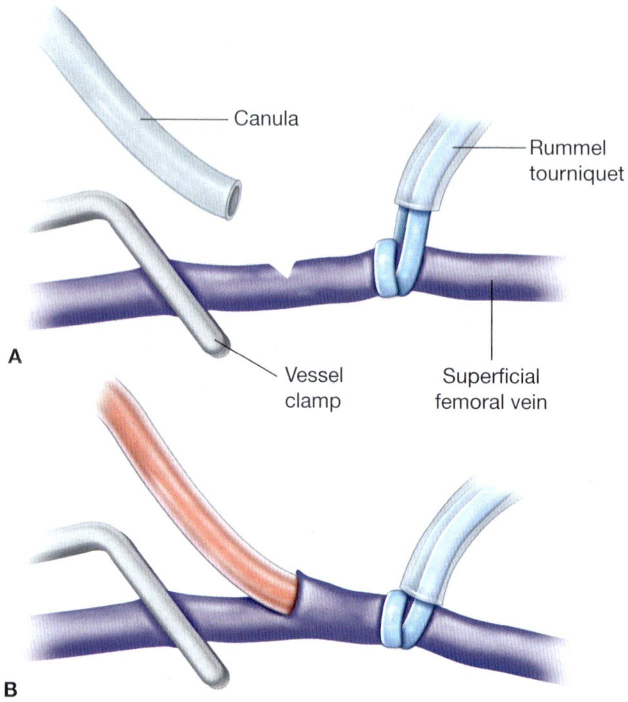

FIG 8 ● **A,B.** Insertion of cannula in superficial femoral vein.

The cannula is inserted caudally and secured with the vessel loop (**FIG 8A,B**). The cannula is hooked up to the extracorporeal circuit and 300 mL of blood is tapped for the perfusion circuit. Subsequently, the arteriotomy is performed in a similar fashion and the arterial cannula is introduced and secured, and the circuit is completed (**FIG 9**).

Establishing the Perfusion

- The perfusion device consists of a reservoir to collect the venous blood, an oxygenator, a heat exchanger and a roller pump (**FIG 10**). In addition to the patient's

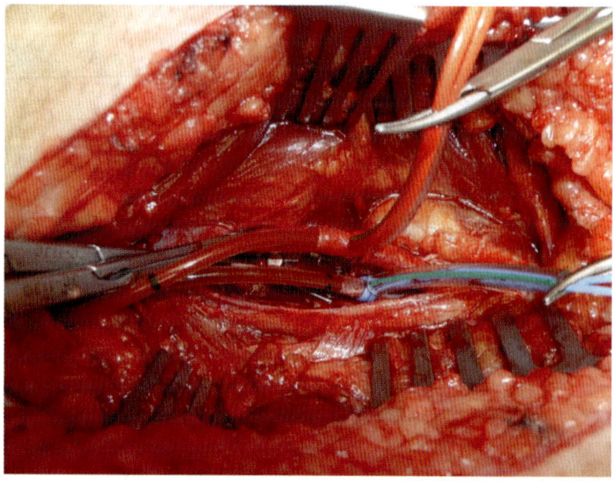

FIG 9 ● The cannulae in the superficial femoral artery and vein are secured with vessel loops tightened through Rummel tourniquets.

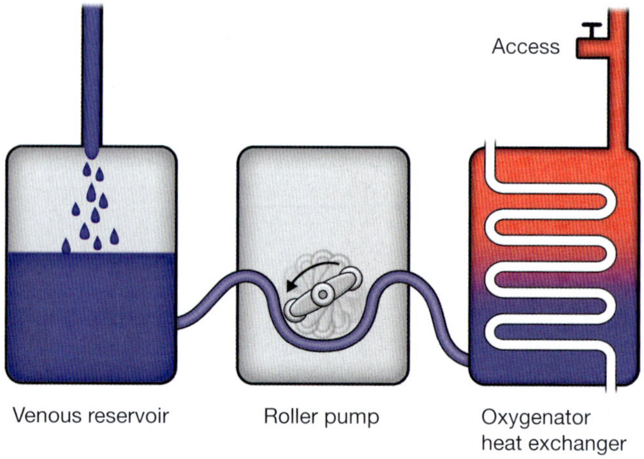

FIG 10 ● The perfusion device contains a venous inflow reservoir, a roller pump, an oxygenator annex heat exchanger, and access to the circuit for tapping blood and administration of drugs.

own blood, the perfusion fluid consists of 100 mL of a crystalloid solution (lactated Ringer's solution), 200 mL 6% hydroxyethyl starch solution (HES) and 2,500 units of heparin. The hematocrit is approximately 30%. The flow should be generous, but it should not increase the venous pressure in the limb. The flow is typically 30 to 60 mL/L lower extremity volume/min. The venous blood is recollected by gravity.
- Thermistor probes are inserted in the subcutaneous tissue and a muscle compartment of the lower leg and the thigh. At this point, the leg is found to be around 34°C.
- The heating blanket is another tool to attain the desired temperature of 37°C.
- The tourniquet is inflated to a pressure of 350 mmHg, if necessary higher. This occludes the collateral vessels to and from the systemic circulation in the skin, the subcutaneous tissue and muscles. **FIG 11** shows the setup at this point.
- Escape of the drug(s) from the limb to the main circulation is to be avoided. Leakage can be monitored continuously by administering a small dose of a radiopharmaceutical such as technetium 99m-labeled serum human albumin to the perfusion circuit.[3] An even smaller background dose is administered intravenously into the systemic circulation. A gamma-ray detector is placed over the heart (**FIG 12**). The percentage of leakage can be calculated when the number of counts increases after correction for the physical half-life of the radionuclide (**FIG 13**).
- Substantial leakage either way can also be detected by assessing the fluid level in the venous return reservoir.
- The drug is administered when the flow and venous pressure are stable, when the tissue temperatures are around 37°C, and there is no leakage. Melphalan has always been the drug of choice. The dosage is 10 mg/L of perfused volume with adjustments based on risk factors for morbidity. The dose should not exceed 150 mg.
- The limb is exposed to the melphalan for 1 hour.
- The temperature in the various tissues is kept between 37°C and 38°C.

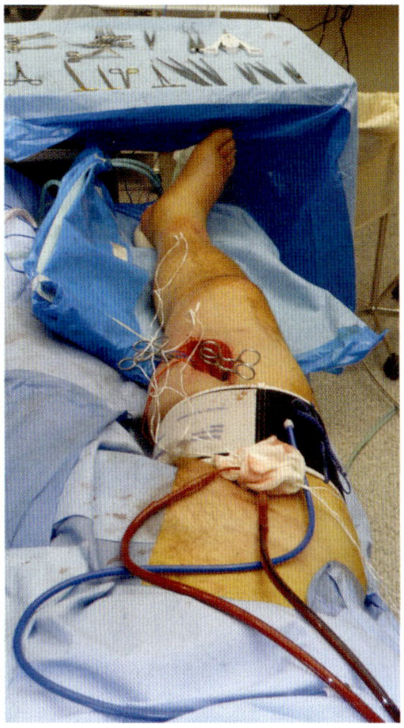

FIG 11 • From top to bottom, note the cotton doughnut under the heel to prevent decubitus, the thermistors with the white cords to monitor the tissue temperatures, the blue warming blanket that is folded open for the picture, the open wound that would normally be covered with a wet gauze to prevent the vessels from drying out, the pneumatic tourniquet around the root of the thigh, and the arterial **(left)** and venous cannulae tunneled subcutaneously underneath the tourniquet.

- Tumor necrosis factor-α induces apoptosis of tumor endothelial cells and is beneficial in patients with bulky tumor nodules.[4] It causes thrombosis and increased melphalan penetration. A dose of 3 mg is given 30 minutes preceding the melphalan administration. When tumor necrosis factor is used, the temperature of the leg is increased from 37°C to 39°C to 40°C in the last half hour. At this time, most of the melphalan has been accumulated in the tissues, which limits potential heat-induced toxicity.
- Parameters to monitor are flow, venous and arterial blood gas values, venous and arterial pressure in the perfusion circuit, leakage to or from the systemic circulation, and venous pressure and tissue temperature in the limb.
- There is considerable variation in the perfusion technique between institutions. Some surgeons use body weight (0.5 to 1.5 mg/kg) or another parameter to calculate the melphalan dose instead of the volume of the leg. Some surgeons use other drugs than the ones described here, such as dactinomycin or cisplatin. Tumor necrosis factor is not registered throughout the world. If available, the dosage used ranges between 0.5 and 4 mg. Despite its obvious advantages, few surgeons use autologous blood for the perfusion circuit. Temperatures up to 43°C have been used for the leg, but these higher temperatures tend to severely increase the postoperative morbidity. The venous pressure is not always measured to guide the flow. The duration of the perfusion in different institutions ranges from 45 to 90 minutes. Judging by the published response rates, one technique is not necessarily better than another.

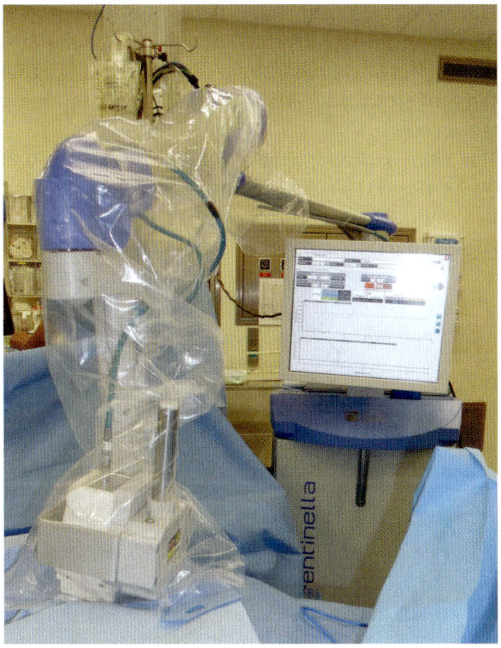

FIG 12 • Mobile gamma-ray detector with screen to assess leakage.

Terminating the Perfusion

- After the leg has been exposed to the drug for the intended duration, the perfusate is washed from the leg using a colloid or a similar fluid followed by a lactated Ringer's solution. Massaging the leg helps to clear the less well-perfused tissues. The leg will be seen to turn pale.
- Meanwhile, the temperature probes and the venous pressure cannula are removed. The saphenous vein is ligated.

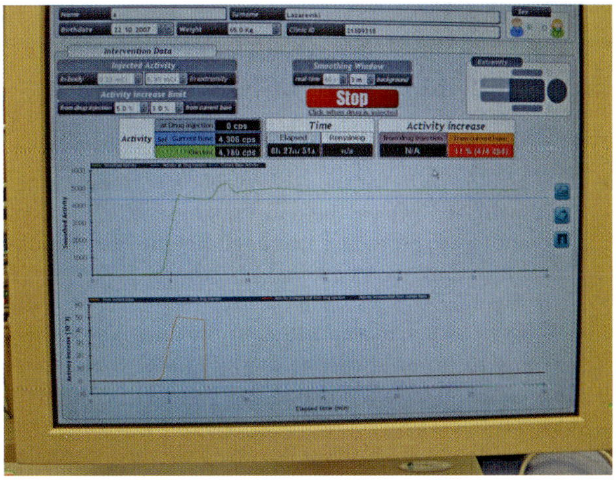

FIG 13 • The *green* curve reflects the leakage. Note steep increase when background radiopharmaceutical is administered to the systemic circulation and subsequent two bumps up when the main dose initially passes through the perfusion circuit. The curve is flat thereafter, indicating adequate isolation during the perfusion.

- The flushing is terminated when the fluid that comes back from the leg is clear. The tourniquet is deflated and taken off. The cannulae are removed from the superficial femoral artery and vein and the distal vessel clamps are reapplied.
- The vein is closed with a running Prolene 6-0 suture (**FIG 14**) and the clamps are removed. The artery is closed with horizontal mattress sutures using double-armed Prolene 6-0 (**FIG 15**).

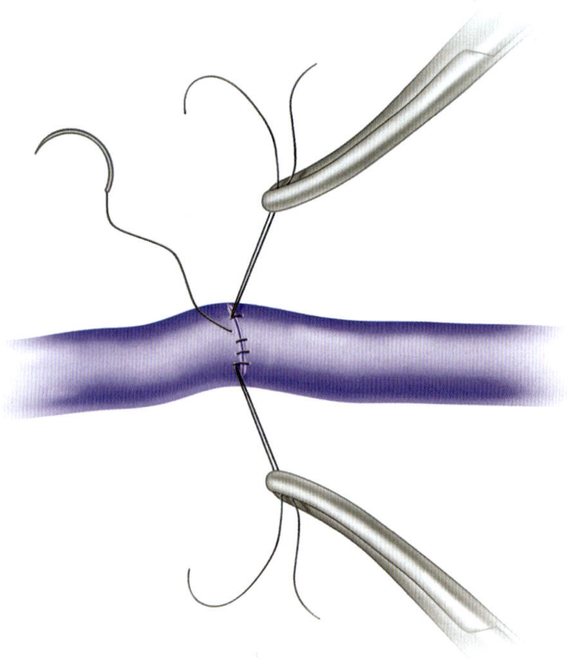

FIG 14 • The vein is closed with a running Prolene 6-0 suture.

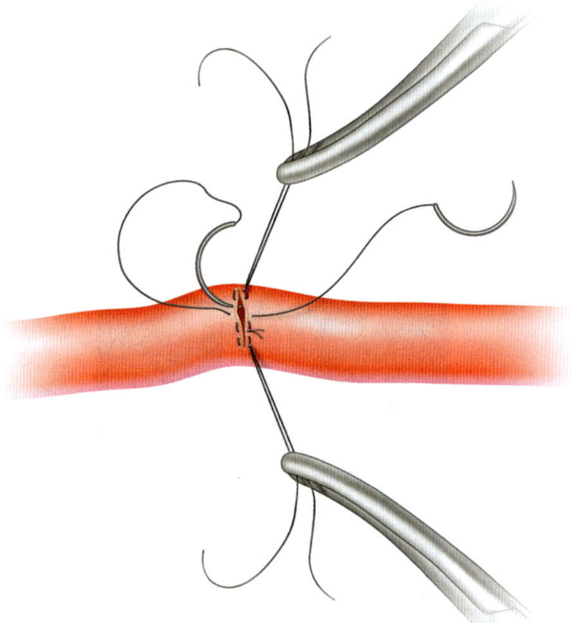

FIG 15 • The artery is closed with double-armed Prolene 6-0. Horizontal mattress sutures evert the edges of the arterial wound in order to appose the endothelium layers.

- The clamps from the artery are removed and the leg assumes a pinkish hue. The nuclear medicine worker will now see an upward turn in his curve and the leakage, which typically is 0% during the perfusion, ends up being 2% or 3%.
- A vacuum drain is inserted and the wound is closed in layers.
- Protamine administration to counter the heparin is optional.

ISOLATED ILIAC PERFUSION

Aspects Specific to Isolated Iliac Perfusion

- Isolated perfusion at the external iliac level is performed if the disease involves the upper thigh. Specific points inherent to this procedure that are different from femoral perfusion are described here.
- The approach to the external iliac vessels is extraperitoneal. The Bookwalter retractor provides an excellent exposure. An external iliac and obturator lymph node dissection is carried out first (see Chapter 29, Inguinal Lymph Node Dissection). These nodes may contain metastasis, but even if this is not the case, their dissection is worthwhile because they can become involved later on and a retroperitoneal approach is challenging after perfusion. Also, an iliac and obturator node dissection results in little morbidity.
- Arterial branches and venous tributaries of the external iliac vessels are ligated and divided. The obturator artery and vein are ligated and also other vessels that connect to the thigh. The internal iliac vessels may be clamped temporarily.
- The tips of the cannulae are positioned in the common femoral vessels.
- Because the diameter of the iliac vein is generous, a longitudinal venotomy can be performed without fear of stenosis after suturing.
- Occlusion of collateral vessels is obtained by wrapping an Esmarch rubber bandage around the thigh through the groin, anchored by a Steinmann pin in the iliac crest. The Steinmann pin is inserted before the heparin is administered.
- Prolene 5-0 is used for closing the vessels.

ISOLATED BRACHIAL PERFUSION

Aspects Specific to Isolated Brachial Perfusion

- Isolated perfusion at the brachial level is performed if the disease is limited to the forearm. Some specific points inherent to this procedure are described here.
- The patient is placed on the operating table in a supine position. The arm is placed in 90% abduction.
- A pneumatic tourniquet is wrapped around the proximal upper arm.
- An 8-cm longitudinal incision is made over the medial aspect of the upper arm, caudally from the tourniquet.
- Microvascular instruments are used.
- The cannulae are led through a subcutaneous tunnel underneath the tourniquet to avoid kinking.
- Both veins may be cannulated if the venous return from a single one is insufficient.
- The quantity of autologous blood needed to prime the extracorporeal circuit is 200 mL.
- Venous pressure measurement is performed using the cephalic vein at the wrist (**FIG 16**).
- The tourniquet is inflated to a pressure of 250 mmHg.
- The dosage of melphalan is 13 mg/L of perfused volume if the volume of the arm exceeds 3.5 L, with adjustments based on risk factors for morbidity. Otherwise, 10 mg/L of perfused volume is given. The dosage of tumor necrosis factor is 2 mg.
- Prolene 6-0 sutures are used for closing the vessels. Alternatively, the vein(s) may be ligated because there is sufficient collateral circulation.

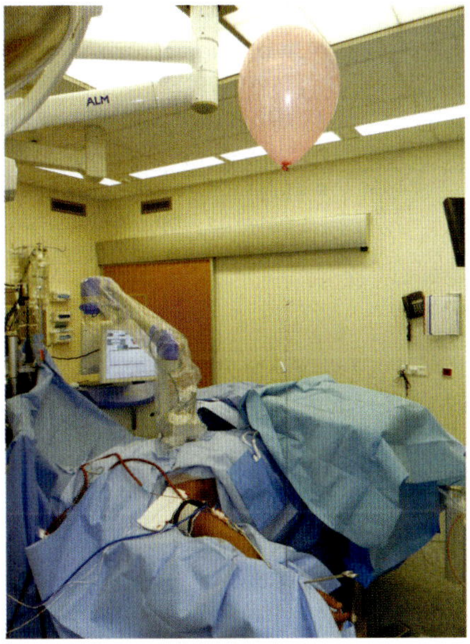

FIG 16 • Helium-filled balloon keeping up the venous pressure line in a brachial perfusion.

ISOLATED AXILLARY PERFUSION

Aspects Specific to Isolated Axillary Perfusion

- Isolated perfusion at the level of the axilla is performed if the disease involves the upper arm. Some specific points inherent to this procedure and differing from the brachial perfusion are described here.
- The axilla is approached via an incision along the lateral margin of the major pectoral muscle. Axillary lymph node dissection is optional (see Chapter 28, Axillary Lymph Node Dissection for Melanoma).
- The axillary vein is exposed and dissected. The axillary artery lies amidst the brachial plexus and is mobilized. Branches are ligated and divided.
- Occlusion of collateral vessels is obtained by wrapping an Esmarch rubber bandage around the upper arm through the axilla anchored by a Steinmann pin in the humeral head. A cotton pad underneath the bandage protects the brachial plexus from undue pressure.[5]

PEARLS AND PITFALLS

Volume measurement	■ If the limb is edematous, the volume of the contralateral limb—if normal—should be measured to guide the melphalan dosage.
Drug dosage	■ A sufficient dose for the desired effect is warranted but an excessive dose can be associated with limb-threatening morbidity. The surgeon threads a thin line and this implies a careful calculation of the drug dose and attention to the details of the procedure.
Prevention of systemic side effects	■ Extremely high doses of cytotoxic drugs are used and the toxicity in case of leakage of the drugs to the systemic circulation can be life threatening. Therefore, painstaking occlusion of collateral vessels and meticulous measuring of leakage are of the essence.
Insertion of the cannula in the femoral vein	■ Valves in the femoral vein may prevent accurate positioning of the venous cannula. A high arterial inflow and temporary clamping of the vein create a generous outflow, which opens the valves and facilitates advancing the cannula. Alternatives are abduction of the leg or cannula insertion over a Fogarty catheter.

Perfusion	▪ The hand and foot are particularly sensitive to the side effects of melphalan. Their exposure to the drug can be limited by temporarily excluding them from the perfusion circuit. This can be accomplished by wrapping the hand or foot in a tight Esmarch rubber bandage for the first 30 minutes of the melphalan perfusion.
Major tendon involvement is a contraindication	▪ A large superficial tumor mass with substantial tendon involvement intuitively appears as an appropriate indication for perfusion. However, a complete response will lead to necrotic tendons that may necessitate amputation.
Autologous blood	▪ Most surgeons use allogeneic blood, but autologous blood obtained at the beginning of the procedure is cheaper and safer.
Elderly patients	▪ In contrast to what is often suggested in the literature, advanced age is not a contraindication, as ILP is effective and quite safe in elderly patients.[2]
Palliation	▪ In the presence of refractory blood-borne metastases, ILP can provide valuable palliation for patients with otherwise unmanageable limb disease that is bothersome because of pain, recurrent bleeding, or fungating infection.

POSTOPERATIVE CARE

- Overnight monitoring of the distal arterial pulsations is obligatory as arterial occlusion at the level of the sutured arteriotomy is a complication that is threatening in the first few hours.
- Postoperatively, the leg is kept elevated on a Braun frame to limit development of edema. The vacuum drain is removed the next day. Patients experience surprisingly little pain. Muscle-setting exercises are performed, but bed rest is maintained until the inflammatory signs subside.
- Creatine phosphokinase is checked daily. An increase in the first few days is normal but an excessive level may indicate muscle necrosis due to a compartment syndrome.
- An anticoagulant is given for the duration of 3 months.
- Responding dermal in-transit metastases may be seen to wrinkle, shrink, and develop a crust. Subcutaneous metastases typically soften and show fluctuation on physical examination.
- The patient is mobilized when the inflammatory signs subside. The patient is discharged when fully mobilized, usually after 7 to 10 days.

OUTCOMES

- There appears to be no relationship between limb toxicity and tumor response to the treatment.[6]
- A response may become evident as early as on the operating table but may also take up to 9 months. Remaining lesions can be excised later in case of a partial response. ILP results in a complete response in 54% of the patients.[7] The complete response is durable in half of them. In an additional 30% of patients, a partial response is obtained. The complete response rate when tumor necrosis factor is used is around 70%,[8] but the end result is not better than with melphalan alone. Ten-year survival in patients with a complete response is 49%.[9]
- Long-term survivors have a better quality of life than comparable control individuals.[10]
- The Wieberdink classification is used to quantify the limb morbidity (Table 2).[11]
- Acute regional toxicity determines long-term morbidity. One year after treatment, 44% of the patients show some degree of morbidity: recurrent infections, 3%; neuropathy, 4%; pain, 8%; muscle atrophy or fibrosis, 11%; limb malfunction, 15%; or lymphedema, 28%.[12] The lymphedema can be attributed to concomitant lymph node dissection.
- Postoperative toxicity necessitates amputation in 0.9% of the patients.[13] Amputation for intractable recurrence is required in 2.4% of the patients.[14]

COMPLICATIONS

- Perioperative mortality is less than 1%.[13,15]
- If tumor necrosis factor is used, some of the drug inevitably remains in the body and may cause a slight fever immediately after the operation.
- Serious postoperative complications associated with ILP are rare but they demand urgent intervention. Arterial thrombosis looms in the first few hours and requires thrombectomy. A venous patch is often necessary to ensure a sufficient flow.
- Excessive swelling of the muscles in the limb compresses the vessels, which may decrease the blood supply and lead to a compartmental syndrome. Excruciating pain suggests this diagnosis and it can be confirmed by measuring the intracompartmental pressure. Timely fasciotomy of the involved muscle compartments prevents permanent damage.
- In the first few days, an inflammatory response typically develops and the leg becomes red, warm, and slightly edematous.
- Over a period of 2 to 3 weeks, the edema and redness subside and give way to a tan discoloration that gradually disappears over the course of several months.

Table 2: Wieberdink Classification of Postoperative Limb Morbidity

1	No skin reaction
2	Redness, edema
3	Blisters
4	Superficial necrosis, damage to deep tissues causing functional disturbance, threatening or manifest compartmental syndrome
5	Necrosis requiring amputation

Wieberdink J, Benckhuysen C, Braat RP, et al. Dosimetry in isolation perfusion of the limbs by assessment of perfused tissue volume and grading of toxic tissue reactions. Eur J Cancer Clin Oncol. *1982;18:905–910.*

REFERENCES

1. Schraffordt Koops H, Vaglini M, Suciu S, et al. Prophylactic isolated limb perfusion for localized, high-risk limb melanoma: results of a multicenter randomized phase III trial. European Organization for Research and Treatment of Cancer Malignant Melanoma Cooperative Group Protocol 18832, the World Health Organization Melanoma Program Trial 15, and the North American Perfusion Group Southwest Oncology Group-8593. *J Clin Oncol*. 1998;169:2906–2912.
2. Noorda EM, Vrouenraets BC, Nieweg OE. Safety and efficacy of isolated limb perfusion in elderly melanoma patients. *Ann Surg Oncol*. 2002;9:968–974.
3. Klaase JM, Kroon BBR, van Geel AN, et al. Systemic leakage during isolated limb perfusion for melanoma. *Br J Surg*. 1993;80:1124–1126.
4. Deroose JP, Eggermont AM, van Geel AN, et al. Isolated limb perfusion for melanoma in-transit metastases: developments in recent years and the role of tumor necrosis factor alpha. *Curr Opin Oncol*. 2011;23:183–188.
5. Vrouenraets BC, Eggermont AM, Klaase JM, et al. Long-term neuropathy after regional isolated perfusion with melphalan for melanoma of the limbs. *Eur J Surg Oncol*. 1994;20:681–685.
6. Beasley GM, Tyler DS. Optimizing regional therapy for melanoma. *Ann Surg Oncol*. 2009;16:1095–1097.
7. Vrouenraets BC, Nieweg OE, Kroon BBR. Thirty-five years of isolated limb perfusion for melanoma: indications and results. *Br J Surg*. 1996;83:1319–1328.
8. Alexander HR, Fraker DL, Bartlett DL, et al. Analysis of factors influencing outcome in patients with in-transit malignant melanoma undergoing isolated limb perfusion using modern treatment parameters. *J Clin Oncol*. 2010;28:114–118.
9. Sanki A, Kam PC, Thompson JF. Long-term results of hyperthermic, isolated limb perfusion for melanoma: a reflection of tumor biology. *Ann Surg*. 2007;245:591–596.
10. Noorda EM, Van Kreij RHJ, Vrouenraets BC, et al. The health-related quality of life of long-term survivors of melanoma treated with isolated limb perfusion. *Eur J Surg Oncol*. 2007;33:776–782.
11. Wieberdink J, Benckhuysen C, Braat RP, et al. Dosimetry in isolation perfusion of the limbs by assessment of perfused tissue volume and grading of toxic tissue reactions. *Eur J Cancer Clin Oncol*. 1982;18:905–910.
12. Vrouenraets BC, Klaase JM, Kroon BBR, et al. Long-term morbidity after regional isolated perfusion with melphalan for melanoma of the limbs. The influence of acute regional toxic reactions. *Arch Surg*. 1995;130:43–47.
13. Cavaliere R, Di Filippo F, Giannarelli D, et al. Hyperthermic antiblastic perfusion in the treatment of local recurrence or "in-transit" metastases of limb melanoma. *Semin Surg Oncol*. 1992;8:374–380.
14. Kapma MR, Vrouenraets BC, Nieweg OE, et al. Major amputation for intractable extremity melanoma after failure of isolated limb perfusion. *Eur J Surg Oncol*. 2005;31:95–99.
15. Sonneveld EJ, Vrouenraets BC, Van Geel AN, et al. Systemic toxicity after isolated limb perfusion with melphalan for melanoma. *Eur J Surg Oncol*. 1996;22:521–527.

Chapter 35 Thyroid Lobectomy

Amy C. Fox Paul G. Gauger

DEFINITION

- Total thyroid lobectomy is defined as the surgical removal of an entire thyroid lobe and isthmus. It can be used as a diagnostic or a therapeutic procedure.
- Thyroid disease requiring a lobectomy is most often due to the presence of a thyroid nodule. Palpable thyroid nodules are common and occur in 4% to 7% of the general population with an increased incidence with advanced age.[1]
- The most common indications for a thyroid lobectomy are the following:
  - A thyroid nodule with diagnostic uncertainty
  - A symptomatic thyroid nodule (e.g., compressive unilateral goiter or autonomous toxic nodule)

DIFFERENTIAL DIAGNOSIS

- Benign thyroid nodule
- Toxic adenoma
- Thyroid cancer
- Intrathyroidal parathyroid adenoma
- Lymph node

PATIENT HISTORY AND PHYSICAL FINDINGS

- Although thyroid nodules are common, the vast majority of them are benign. A thorough patient history can assist the clinician in determining which thyroid nodules may require surgical management. Previous radiation to the neck, a rapidly growing mass, hoarseness, associated lymphadenopathy, or a family history of cancer may raise the suspicion of malignancy. Dysphagia, choking, or intolerance to things around the neck may suggest local compressive symptoms from a large thyroid nodule.
- The physical exam should focus on characteristics of the thyroid such as size, firmness, and the presence of nodules. The neck should be palpated for associated lymphadenopathy.

IMAGING AND OTHER DIAGNOSTIC STUDIES

- **Thyroid function studies.** A thyroid-stimulating hormone (TSH) can assess the biochemical status of the patient's thyroid. A TSH should be obtained prior to any fine needle aspiration to ensure the patient is not hyperthyroid.
- **Ultrasonography.** Neck ultrasound is a user dependent but highly sensitive adjunct in the evaluation of the thyroid and cervical lymphadenopathy. It can also assist in fine needle aspiration of thyroid nodules. A high-frequency probe of 7.5 MHz to 10 MHz is required.
- **Biopsy.** Fine needle aspiration can help determine benign from potentially malignant nodules. It is often done using ultrasound guidance. The cytopathology results can be categorized according to the Bethesda system.[2] These categories are associated with varying risks of malignancy allowing for different proposals for clinical management (Table 1).[3]
- **Computed tomography (CT).** A preoperative neck or chest CT is usually not necessary except in specific situations:
  - Malignancy—A neck CT may suggest local invasion of the thyroid into surrounding structures such as the carotid artery, internal jugular vein, or trachea which could potentially modify the operative approach. A CT scan of the neck can also provide a detailed map of cervical lymphadenopathy. A chest CT can evaluate for metastatic disease.
  - Large goiters—A neck and chest CT scan can help determine the degree of tracheal obstruction or substernal extension of large goiters. Patients with clinical evidence of airway obstruction should have a CT to provide anatomic information to help manage a potentially difficult airway.
- **Laryngoscopy.** Flexible laryngoscopy should be performed on all patients with hoarseness or a previous history of neck surgery. This provides a current assessment and baseline evaluation of bilateral vocal cords prior to surgery.

SURGICAL MANAGEMENT

- Thyroid lobectomy is therapeutic for patients with a unilateral goiter or a solitary toxic nodule which is symptomatic.
- Thyroid lobectomy is diagnostic and can potentially be therapeutic for patients with indeterminate thyroid nodules such as those categorized as "follicular lesions of undetermined significance," "follicular neoplasms," or "suspicious for malignancy."
- Although thyroid malignancy often warrants surgical intervention, thyroid lobectomy is typically not the standard of care. Total thyroidectomy is recommended for most thyroid malignancies greater than a centimeter in size. A thyroid lobectomy may sometimes be appropriate for very small (less than a centimeter) well-differentiated thyroid cancers in select patients.
- In any thyroid lobectomy, the patient and surgeon should be prepared for the conversion to a total thyroidectomy if intraoperative findings dictate this need. If the patient was

Table 1: Thyroid Fine Needle Aspiration Classification Scheme and Clinical Management

Category	Risk of Malignancy	Suggested Management
Nondiagnostic		Repeat FNA under ultrasound
Benign	<1%	Monitor
Follicular lesion of undetermined significance (e.g., atypia)	5%–10%	Repeat FNA or thyroid lobectomy
Follicular neoplasm	20%–30%	Thyroid lobectomy
Suspicion for malignancy	50%–75%	Thyroid lobectomy or total thyroidectomy
Malignant	100%	Total thyroidectomy

FNA, fine needle aspiration.
From Cibas ES, Ali SZ. The Bethesda system for reporting thyroid cytopathology. Thyroid. *2009;19(11):1159–1165; Baloch ZW, Cibas ES, Clark DP, et al. The National Cancer Institute thyroid fine needle aspiration state of the science conference: a summation.* Cytojournal. *2008;5:6.*

not counseled of this possibility, the surgeon should complete the lobectomy and defer definitive management until appropriate consent from the patient.

Preoperative Planning

- Thyroid lobectomy is performed under a general anesthesia, but locoregional anesthetic with sedation may be adequate for lobectomy in select patients.
- Routine use of preoperative antibiotics is not common as wound infections after thyroid lobectomy are rare.[4]

Positioning

- The patient is placed in the supine position with the arms padded and tucked at the side (**FIG 1**). A roll can be placed under the shoulders to help extend the neck; however, extreme extension should be avoided as this can cause postoperative discomfort.

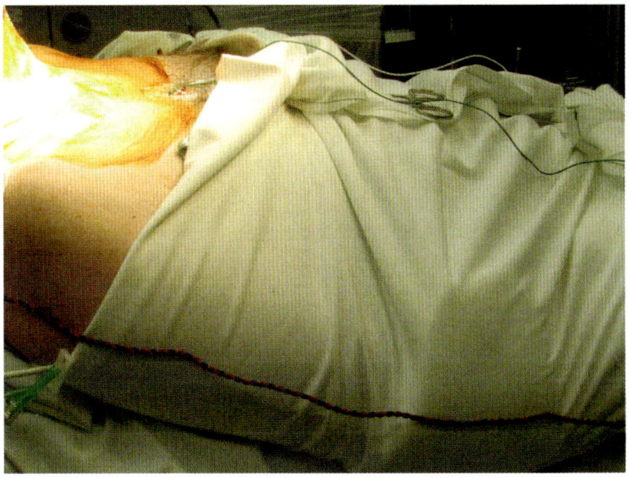

FIG 1 • Patient positioning. The arms should be padded and can be tucked to the side with a sheet using a towel clip.

SKIN INCISION AND FLAP CREATION

- A low collar incision is placed symmetrically across the neck despite only removing a lobe. The incision is ideally located about two fingerbreadths above the sternal notch or 1 cm below the cricoid cartilage (**FIG 2**). This location provides good exposure to the entire thyroid gland and particularly the superior pole.
- Placing the incision in a skin crease can provide excellent cosmetic results. If no skin crease is appropriate, Langer's lines provide an adequate guide.

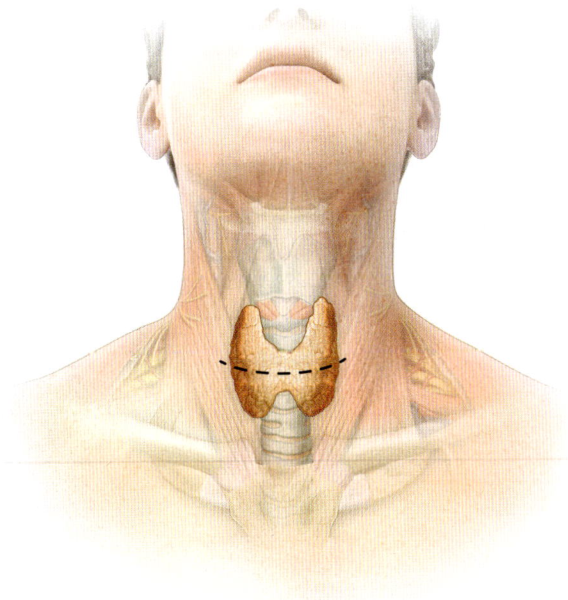

FIG 2 • Incision anatomy. The sternal notch and cricoid cartilage are palpated to help determine the incision site.

GLAND EXPOSURE

- The incision is carried through the subcutaneous tissue and platysma. Subplatysmal flaps are created to enhance mobility from the incision (**FIG 3**). These flaps should extend to the thyroid cartilage superiorly and the suprasternal notch inferiorly. The assistant should retract the skin to help create the plane of dissection. The anterior jugular veins will remain down on the strap muscles if the correct plane is dissected.
- The midline raphe between the strap muscles is opened and dissection extends down to the level of the isthmus (**FIG 4**).
- The sternohyoid and, subsequently, the sternothyroid muscles are dissected off the thyroid and reflected laterally.
- The thyroid lobe is then retracted medially with a finger or hemostatic clamp. The space between the thyroid and the carotid sheath is opened bluntly until the prevertebral fascia is encountered (**FIG 5**). During this portion of

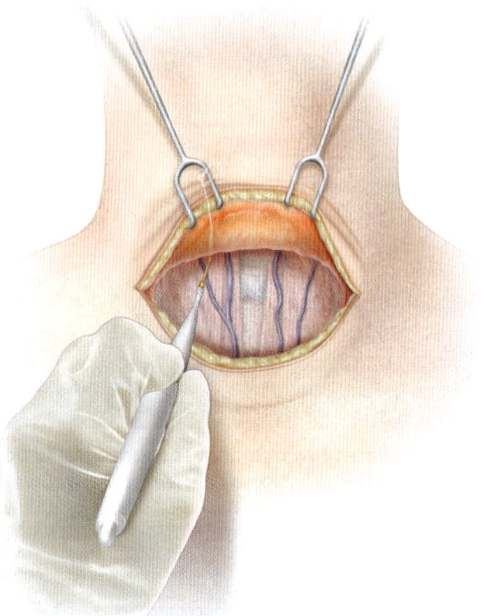

FIG 3 ● Creation of subplatysmal flaps. Adequate retraction helps creation of the subplatysmal flaps and prevents buttonholing the skin.

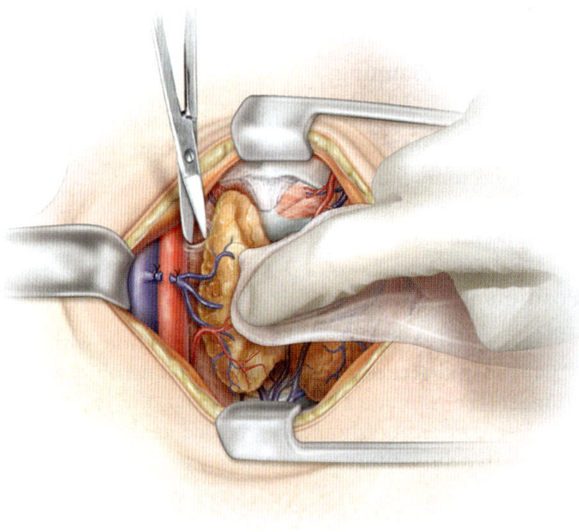

FIG 5 ● Exposure of the posterior thyroid. The thyroid is retracted toward the midline and the middle thyroid vein is divided. The areolar tissue behind the thyroid can be bluntly dissected with scissors.

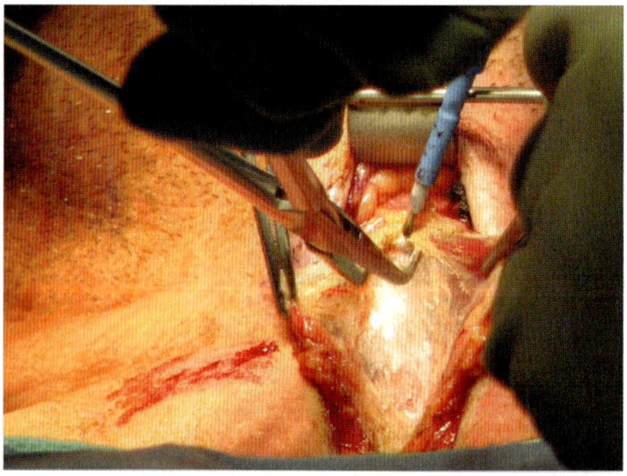

FIG 4 ● Exposure of the thyroid. The midline raphe between the strap muscles is avascular and provides access to the thyroid when opened.

the dissection, the middle thyroid vein should be controlled and ligated.

- Dissection of the isthmus can help mobilize the thyroid gland. The superior suspensory ligament and associated vessels at the superior border of the isthmus should be divided. A pyramidal lobe can be dissected and divided if present.
- The inferior vessels and attachments to the trachea along the inferior border of the isthmus should also be divided.
- The contralateral thyroid lobe can be palpated to ensure no abnormalities; however, formal dissection on the contralateral side should be avoided to prevent scar formation.

SUPERIOR POLE DISSECTION

- The cricothyroid space is an avascular space between the cricothyroid muscle and thyroid gland. This space can be bluntly opened all the way to the prevertebral fascia. Retraction of the superior pole of the thyroid in the inferior and lateral directions can facilitate this dissection (**FIG 6**).
- The external branch of the superior laryngeal nerve may be identified during this dissection and should be preserved. The nerve is vulnerable to injury as it crosses the vessels close to the superior pole of the thyroid prior to its insertion into the muscle. The anatomic variations of the nerve in relation to the superior thyroid vessels are best described by Cernea et al.[5] (**FIG 7**).
- The superior pole vessels are divided at the level of the thyroid capsule to prevent injury of the nerve (**FIG 6**). This dissection should proceed from medial to lateral.
- A superior parathyroid gland may be identified in this area and should be dissected off the gland.

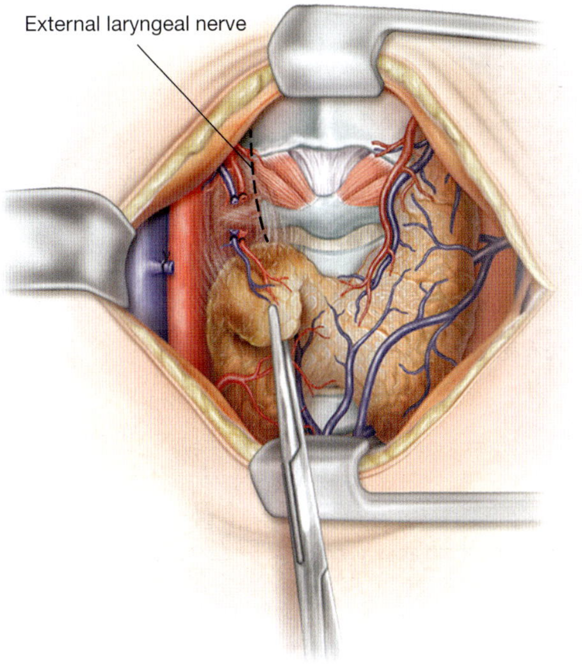

FIG 6 ● Exposure of the superior pole. The cricothyroid space is opened up bluntly. Retraction of the superior pole in a lateral and inferior direction helps to minimize the risk of injury to the external branch of the superior laryngeal nerve *(dotted line)*.

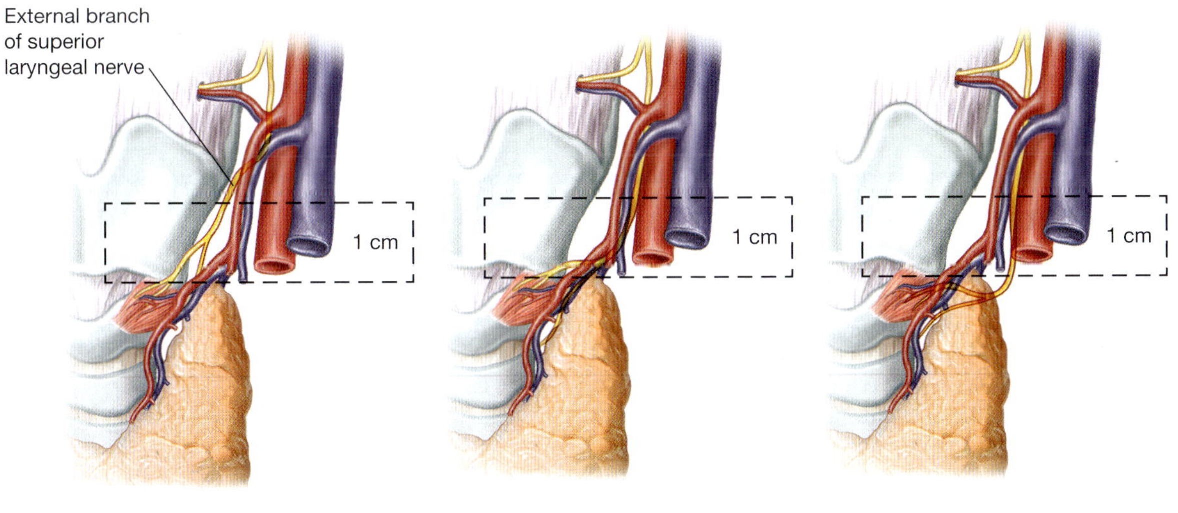

FIG 7 ● Anatomic variations of the external branch of the superior laryngeal nerve. The nerve crosses the vessels greater than a centimeter from the superior pole in type 1 anatomy. Type 2 anatomy places the nerve at higher risk of injury during dissection because it crossed less than a centimeter from the superior pole (type 2a) or even below it (type 2b). (From Cernea CR, Ferraz AR, Nishio S, et al. Surgical anatomy of the external branch of the superior laryngeal nerve. *Head Neck*. 1992;14:380–383.)

LATERAL LOBE DISSECTION

- Once the superior pole is mobilized, the lateral and inferior aspect of the thyroid can be dissected. The thyroid lobe should be retracted medially or elevated out of the wound. An assistant should retract the carotid sheath laterally to open up the lateral space.
- The identification and preservation of the recurrent laryngeal nerve is critical to the dissection. The nerve should be identified early and can often be found where it passes inferior to the inferior thyroid artery. Once the nerve is found, the dissection proceeds along the course of the nerve up to its cricothyroid insertion. The nerve is most vulnerable in this area.

- The tertiary vessels of the inferior thyroid artery are divided at the level of the thyroid capsule (**FIG 8**). This capsular dissection helps decrease the risk of nerve injury and devascularization of the parathyroid glands.
- The attachments of the thyroid to the trachea are freed by dividing the ligament of Berry.

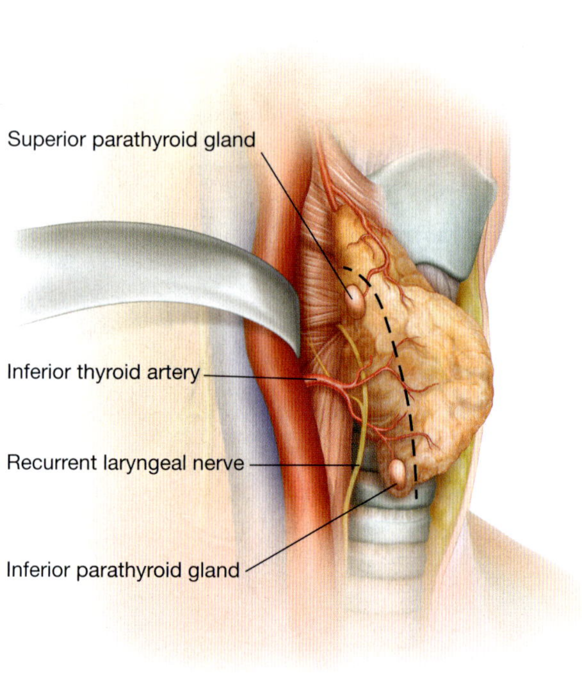

FIG 8 • Division of the inferior thyroid artery. The tertiary branches of the inferior thyroid artery are ligated at the thyroid capsule to prevent injury to the recurrent laryngeal nerve and the blood supply to the parathyroid glands. The *dotted line* denotes the area of dissection.

PARATHYROID PRESERVATION

- The inferior and superior parathyroid glands should be identified and preserved. This is accomplished by careful dissection and reflection of them in a posterolateral direction away from the thyroid. The main trunk of the inferior thyroid artery should not be ligated as it typically provides the blood supply to both parathyroid glands.

TRANSECTION OF THE THYROID

- A thyroid lobectomy requires transection of the thyroid at the junction of the isthmus and contralateral lobe. If this junction is small, a Harmonic scalpel can transect this area while providing good hemostasis. If the area is bulky or a Harmonic scalpel is not available, a clamp can be placed across the area of transection. A knife is then used to transect the thyroid and the specimen is removed (**FIG 9**). A running absorbable suture can be placed as a hemostatic stitch underneath the clamp.

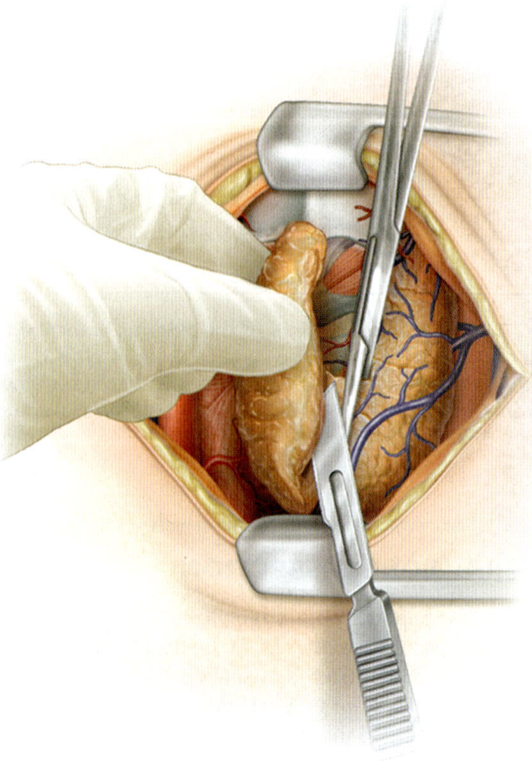

FIG 9 • Transection of the thyroid. The junction between the isthmus and contralateral lobe is transected to remove the specimen.

CLOSURE

- Prior to closure, the surgical field is meticulously evaluated for hemostasis. Small occult bleeding can lead to clinically significant neck hematomas if not controlled.
- The parathyroid glands are evaluated once more for viability. Additionally, the lobectomy specimen should be examined for the inadvertent removal of a normal parathyroid gland. If either situation arises, the parathyroid gland should be minced up and implanted into the ipsilateral sternocleidomastoid.
- The recurrent laryngeal nerve is examined with visual inspection or nerve monitoring to ensure an intact circuit.
- After adequate hemostasis and inspection, the strap muscles are reapproximated with absorbable interrupted sutures (**FIG 10**). Placement of these sutures requires care to avoid injury to the anterior jugular veins.
- The platysma is reapproximated with buried interrupted sutures.
- The skin can be closed in a variety of ways. If the wound appears to be under tension during closure, removal of the shoulder roll can help. Our practice is to close the skin with a knotless running subcuticular Prolene stitch followed by the placement of skin glue. Once the glue dries, the Prolene is removed and Steri-Strips are placed as a dry dressing over the incision. Other alternatives to reapproximate the skin include the use of a running absorbable suture or the use of skin glue exclusively.

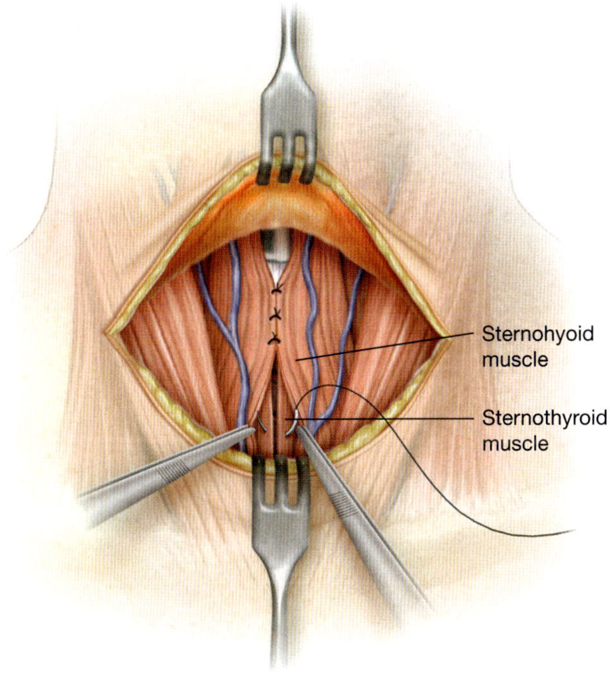

FIG 10 ● Closing the strap muscles. The strap muscles are reapproximated with interrupted sutures.

PEARLS AND PITFALLS

Incision aesthetics	■ A natural skin crease should be used if present. ■ An incision too cephalad is very noticeable with normal clothing. ■ An incision too caudal can increase the risk of keloid formation.
Parathyroid preservation	■ If a parathyroid gland cannot be preserved, it should be placed into cold saline for preservation. ■ A small portion of the parathyroid gland should be sent for frozen section to confirm normal parathyroid tissue. ■ The gland should then be minced into small pieces and implanted into the ipsilateral sternocleidomastoid. ■ A clip or permanent suture can mark the autograft sites.
Hemostasis	■ Hemostasis can be evaluated under Valsalva maneuver to look for occult bleeding. ■ Drains are rarely needed and are never a substitute for adequate hemostasis. ■ Electrocautery should be avoided in the area of the recurrent laryngeal nerve.
Large substernal goiter	■ Most substernal goiters located above the brachiocephalic vein can be removed through a cervical incision. ■ Dissection of the superior pole and early transection of the isthmus can provide added mobility needed to pull up a goiter from behind the sternum. ■ The patient should be counseled and the chest prepped in case a mini-sternotomy is needed.

POSTOPERATIVE CARE

- The patient should be monitored in the postoperative area for a few hours to ensure no significant hematoma develops.
- An ice pack may be placed over the neck to assist with pain and swelling. Once the patient is sufficiently awake, the diet may be advanced as tolerated.
- After a period of monitoring, most patients may be safely discharged home after a thyroid lobectomy. Patients should expect to resume their normal activities within a few days of surgery.
- Most patients will not require thyroid hormone replacement after a lobectomy if the remaining lobe is normal. Thyroid hormone levels should be checked about 2 months after surgery to ensure the other lobe is adequately functioning.

COMPLICATIONS

- Hematoma
- Hypocalcemia
- Hoarseness
- Vocal cord paralysis
- Wound infection

REFERENCES

1. Hegedüs L. Clinical practice. The thyroid nodule. *N Engl J Med*. 2004;351(17):1764–1771.
2. Cibas ES, Ali SZ. The Bethesda system for reporting thyroid cytopathology. *Thyroid*. 2009;19(11):1159–1165.
3. Baloch ZW, Cibas ES, Clark DP, et al. The National Cancer Institute thyroid fine needle aspiration state of the science conference: a summation. *Cytojournal*. 2008;5:6.
4. Moalem J, Ruan DT, Farkas RL, et al. Patterns of antibiotic prophylaxis use for thyroidectomy and parathyroidectomy: results of an international survey of endocrine surgeons. *J Am Coll Surg*. 2010;210(6):949–956.
5. Cernea CR, Ferraz AR, Nishio S, et al. Surgical anatomy of the external branch of the superior laryngeal nerve. *Head Neck*. 1992;14:380–383.

Chapter 36 Total Thyroidectomy

Saïd C. Azoury Martha A. Zeiger

DEFINITION

- Total thyroidectomy involves removal of all thyroid tissue, including both lobes and isthmus, while preserving the parathyroid glands, the recurrent laryngeal nerve (RLN), and the external branch of the superior laryngeal nerve.

ANATOMY

- The thyroid gland typically weighs 20 g and has a right and left lobe bridged by a narrow isthmus.
- The thyroid gland is located in the central compartment of the anterior neck below the thyroid cartilage.
- The thyroid cartilage forms the laryngeal prominence or the "Adam's apple."
- The thyroid lobes lie medial to the carotid sheaths and sternocleidomastoid muscles.
- The anterolateral surface of the gland is covered by the sternothyroid and sternohyoid muscles (**FIG 1**).
- The "thyroid sheath" is a connective tissue expansion of the pretracheal fascia and envelops the thyroid, condensing posteromedially into the ligament of Berry.
- The thyroid gland receives its blood supply from the superior and inferior thyroid arteries.
- The superior thyroid artery arises from the ipsilateral external carotid artery and the superior thyroid vein runs with the artery.
- The middle thyroid vein drains into the ipsilateral internal jugular. The inferior thyroid artery originates from the thyrocervical trunk. The left RLN arises from the vagus at the level of the aortic arch and loops around the ligamentum arteriosum; the right RLN loops around the right subclavian artery (**FIG 2**).

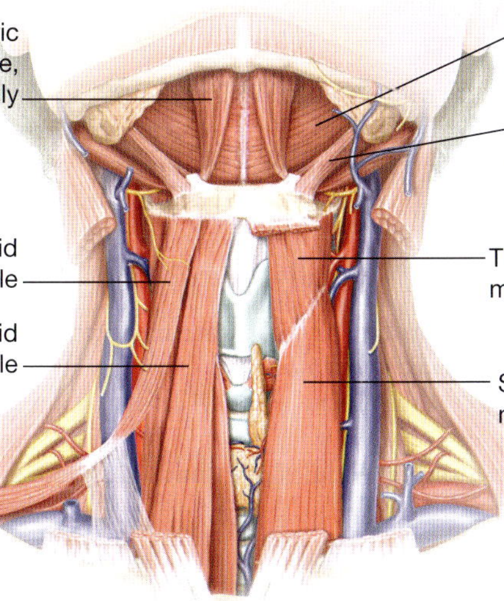

FIG 1 • Strap muscles of the neck.

- The right RLN may be nonrecurrent in 0.5% to 1% of individuals.
- The RLN innervates all the intrinsic muscles of the larynx except the cricothyroid muscles.
- The internal branch of the superior laryngeal nerve is the sensory nerve for the supraglottic larynx. The external branch of the superior laryngeal nerve lies on the inferior pharyngeal constrictor muscle and descends alongside the superior thyroid vessels before innervating the cricothyroid muscle.
- The superior parathyroid glands are generally located posterior to the superior thyroid lobe and the RLN. The inferior parathyroid locations are more variable but oftentimes are located anterior to the inferior thyroid lobes and RLN or on the inferolateral aspect of the lobes.

INDICATIONS FOR TOTAL THYROIDECTOMY

Graves' Disease[1–3]

Thyroid Cancer

- In general, total thyroidectomy is indicated for follicular or papillary thyroid cancer.[4–6] Patients may also need a concomitant central lymph node dissection.[4–6] Total thyroidectomy with central lymph node dissection is typically indicated for medullary thyroid cancer.[7]

Multinodular Goiter

- Total thyroidectomy is indicated for symptomatic multinodular goiter (MNG) or for patients who have suspicious or indeterminate thyroid nodules on fine needle aspiration biopsy (FNAB).[8–10]

PATIENT HISTORY AND PHYSICAL FINDINGS

History

- Thyroid cancer is more common in extremes of age, younger than 20 or older than 60 years.
- Most thyroid nodules are asymptomatic, and most patients are euthyroid.
- Thyroid nodules are more common in females, but there is a greater risk of malignancy in males.
- One must inquire about a history of radiation therapy and family history of thyroid cancer: Nearly 90% of radiation-associated thyroid cancers are papillary.
- Personal or family history of other endocrine disorders such as a history of thyroid cancer, primary hyperparathyroidism, pancreatic islet cell tumors, pituitary tumors, or adrenal tumors is essential to understand a patient's risk.
- Medullary thyroid cancer is a known component of multiple endocrine neoplasia 2 (MEN2).
- Weight gain, fatigue, depression, constipation, dry skin, and brittle nails are symptoms of hypothyroidism; weight loss, weakness, anxiety, palpitations, and diarrhea are symptoms of hyperthyroidism; both are key elements of the review of systems portion of a history.

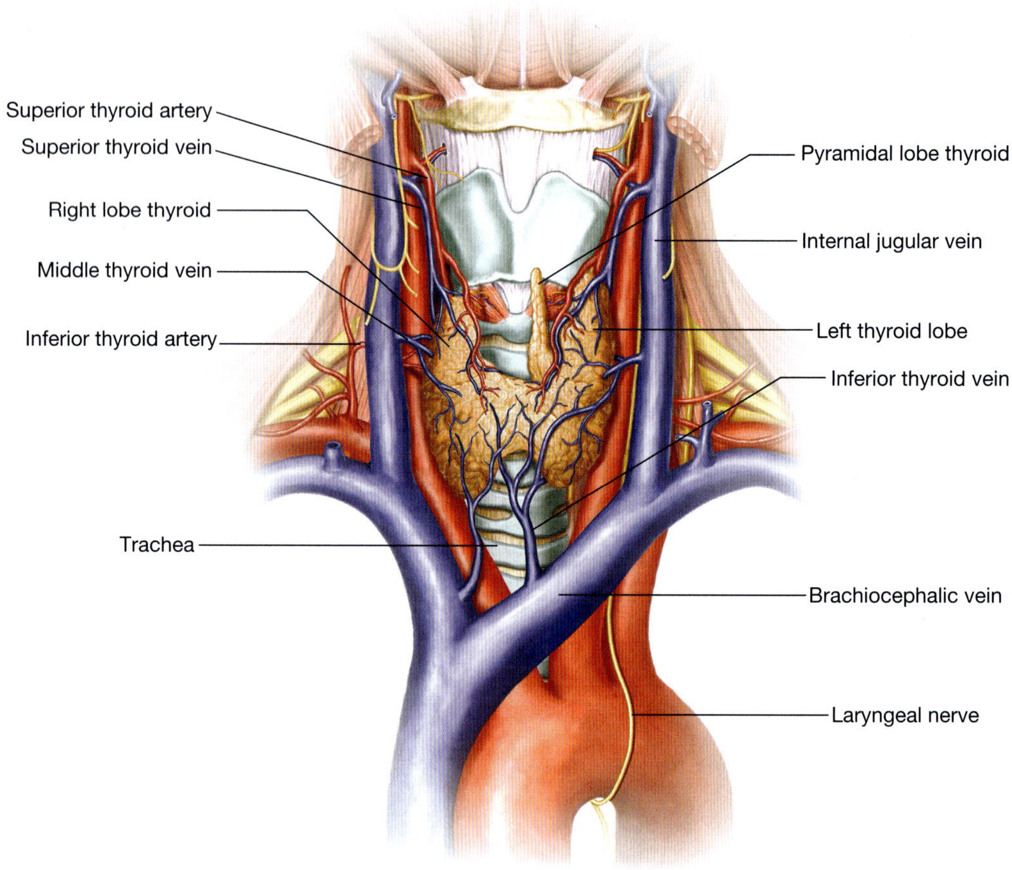

FIG 2 • Anatomic location of thyroid gland and vascular anatomy.

- One should inquire about symptoms of dysphagia, dyspnea, voice change, cough, or trouble breathing.

Physical Exam

- Size of thyroid nodules, firmness of the nodules, and the presence of substernal extension are important to assess.
- Findings suggestive of cancer include nodule fixation, hard texture, and associated cervical lymphadenopathy.
- Important eye signs include stare, lid lag, dryness, diplopia, or exophthalmos (**FIG 3**); all of which can suggest Graves' disease.

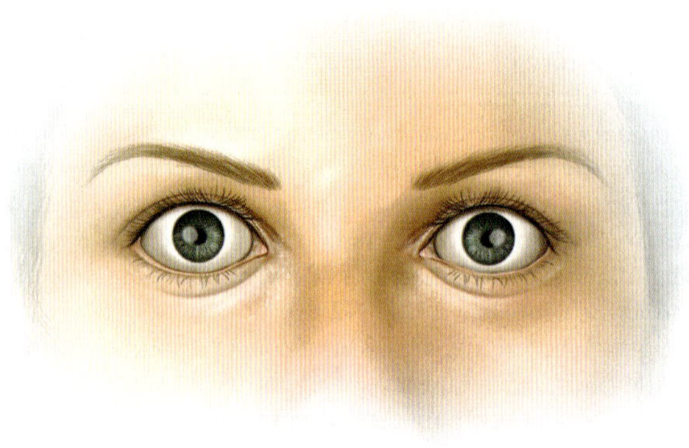

FIG 3 • Graves' ophthalmopathy: prominent stare.

- Extremities should be examined for pretibial myxedema (waxy, discolored induration, and swelling) that can be associated with severe hypothyroidism.

IMAGING AND OTHER DIAGNOSTIC STUDIES

Thyroid-Stimulating Hormone (Normally 0.5 to 5 μU/mL)

- A serum thyroid-stimulating hormone (TSH) should be measured to determine if the patient is hypo-, hyper-, or euthyroid. There is an inverse relationship between the free thyroxine (T4) level and the TSH concentration.

Free Thyroxine (Normally 12 to 28 pmol/L)

- Free T4 is a sensitive and accurate measurement of biologically active thyroid hormone.
- In early hyperthyroidism, total T4 levels are normal but free T4 levels are elevated.
- Hyperfunctioning nodules are much less likely to harbor malignancy.

Serum Thyroglobulin

- Thyroglobulin is primarily used to detect recurrent thyroid cancer.

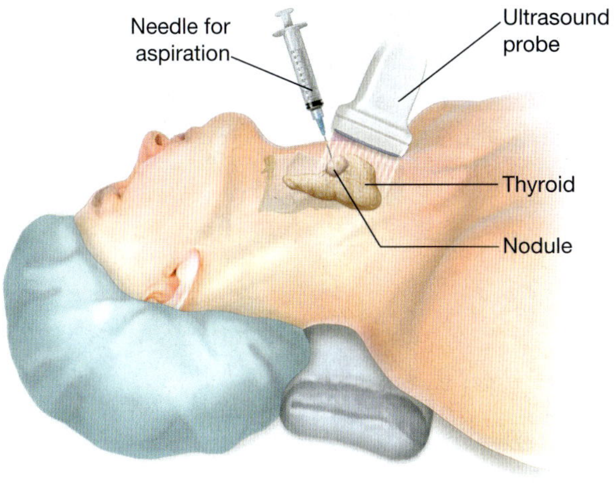

FIG 4 • FNA of thyroid nodule.

Fine Needle Aspiration Biopsy

- Ultrasound-guided needle aspiration is performed using 23- to 27-gauge needles and a 10-mL syringe (**FIG 4**).
- FNAB specimens are classified as malignant, benign, indeterminate (atypical cells of undetermined significance, suspicious for follicular or Hürthle cell neoplasm, or suspicious for malignancy), or insufficient for diagnosis.
- Overall sensitivity of FNAB is 95% to 98%.[7]

Iodine Scintigraphy

- Elevated iodine uptake with diffuse uptake and enlargement is consistent with Graves' disease.
- The risk of malignancy in "hot" lesions is extremely low. Iodine scintigraphy should only be used if the patient is hyperthyroid and has nodular disease to determine if a nodule is responsible for the hyperthyroidism.

Antithyroglobulin and Antithyroid Peroxidase Antibodies

- Anti-thyroid peroxidase (anti-TPO) antibodies are associated with Hashimoto's thyroiditis. Antithyroglobulin (anti-Tg), if present, makes following patients with thyroid cancer for Tg elevation unreliable.

High-Resolution Ultrasonography

- Ultrasound is recommended to determine the number, size, and characteristics of the thyroid nodules.
- Increased intranodular vascularity, irregular margins, the so-called "halo sign" or anechoic rim, microcalcifications, and hypoechogenicity are generally associated with a malignancy.
- Cervical ultrasound to assess for lymphadenopathy is recommended for suspicious or malignant thyroid nodules.

Computed Tomography

- Computed tomography (CT) imaging is indicated for substernal goiters or if a cancer is large or appears fixed to surrounding anatomic structures.

NONOPERATIVE MANAGEMENT

Antithyroid Drugs: Propylthiouracil and Methimazole

- When used for Graves' Disease, generally, propylthiouracil (PTU) (100 to 300 mg three times daily) or methimazole (10 to 30 mg three times daily) are the antithyroid drugs of choice.
- Both drugs inhibit the organic binding of iodine and thyroperoxidase coupling of iodotyrosines. PTU also inhibits the peripheral conversion of T4 to triiodothyronine (T3).

Radioactive Iodine Therapy

- Radioiodine therapy has been the preferred treatment for most patients with Graves' disease.
- Radioiodine therapy is indicated postoperatively for patients with thyroid cancer who have a high risk of recurrence.

Close Follow-up

- Patients with asymptomatic and benign thyroid nodules should be followed with serial neck ultrasounds and repeat fine needle aspiration (FNA) as needed.
- Patients may need longitudinal neck ultrasounds and repeat FNA.

SURGICAL MANAGEMENT

- The use of total thyroidectomy for benign disease has increased over the last 15 years in the United States from 17.6% (1993–1997) to 39.6% (2003–2007) compared with 82.4% and 60.4% for partial thyroidectomy over the same periods.[11]
- Total thyroidectomy for Graves' is the gold standard advocated by endocrine surgeons.
- In one study of patients with Graves' disease, reasons for having thyroid surgery were persistent disease despite medical therapy (46.6%), patient preference (24.1%), MNG/cold nodules (20.3%), failed radioactive iodine (RAI) treatment (16%), and ophthalmopathy (12.1%).[12]
- In general, the indication for total thyroidectomy should be considered in cases of suspicious or definite malignant nodules; the presence of thyroid nodules; and a history of head and neck irradiation, Graves' disease, large or substernal goiter, or symptomatic goiter (dysphagia, pressure, dyspnea).
- The most important goals of surgery for MNG are to prevent recurrence after surgery and to definitively diagnose thyroid nodules that were indeterminate or suspicious preoperatively.
- The advantage of total thyroidectomy, compared to subtotal thyroidectomy, for treatment of Graves' is the avoidance of recurrent hyperthyroidism, which has been reported to be as high as 22% following subtotal thyroidectomy.[7,13,14]
- Advantages of total thyroidectomy over thyroid lobectomy for well-differentiated thyroid carcinoma (WDTC) include the fact that papillary thyroid cancer can be multifocal, facilitation of radioiodine imaging and ablation for residual metastatic disease, and the use of serum thyroglobulin for postoperative disease surveillance.
- Surgery is often recommended for patients with severe ophthalmopathy; this condition can be worsened by RAI.
- Surgery is appropriate in children and in pregnant women with Graves' disease.[15]
- Surgery is indicated for a substernal goiter because these are usually symptomatic and substernal nodules cannot be assessed by FNA.

Preoperative Planning

- Thyroid scintigraphy is only indicated in a subset of patients with hyperthyroidism.
- FNA under ultrasound guidance is the gold standard when there is a suspicion for thyroid cancer and should be performed if a nodule is found to be greater than 1 cm and/or if the nodule has suspicious ultrasound characteristics.[7] FNA provides quick and specific information that helps to guide definitive surgical management.
- High-resolution ultrasound of the neck can be used to evaluate for cervical lymphadenopathy.
- Laryngoscopy is often used before surgery whether for benign or malignant disease, especially for patients with voice changes, to determine the extent and any involvement of surrounding structures including the RLN.

Intraoperative Positioning of the Patient

- Patient is placed in supine position with arms tucked at the sides.
- A soft roll is placed lengthwise beneath the shoulders to extend the neck, and a soft foam "donut-shaped" rest is used to stabilize the head.
- Patient is further placed in a *semi-Fowler's position*, with the head of the bed at approximately 30 degrees (**FIG 5**).

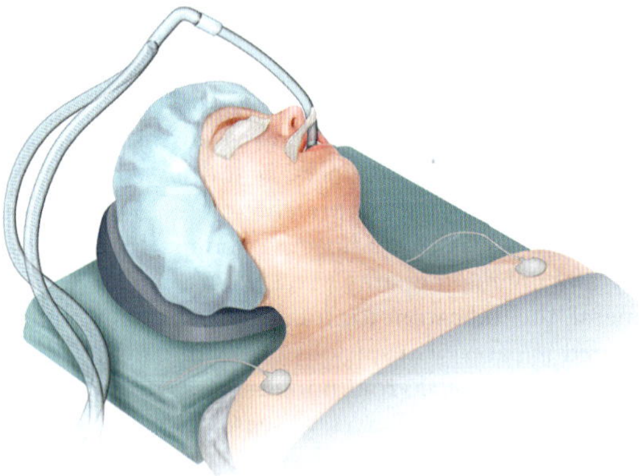

FIG 5 • Semi-Fowler's position.

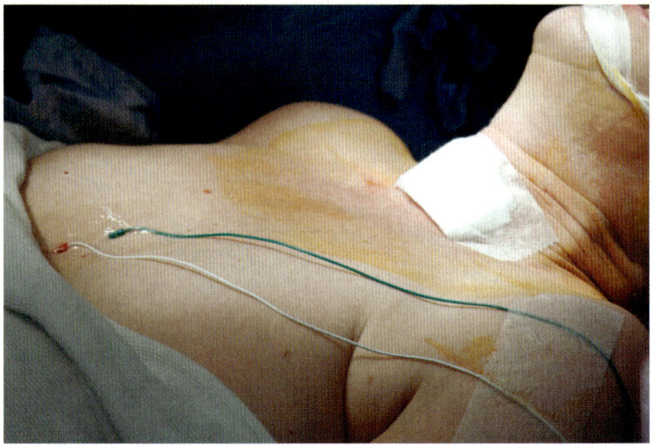

FIG 6 • RLN nerve monitoring wires anchored to the patient's shoulder, out of the way of the neck and the sterile operating field.

- The RLN nerve monitoring wires are anchored to the patient's shoulder, out of the way of the neck and the sterile operating field (**FIG 6**).

Approach

- During surgery, great care should be taken to identify the recurrent and superior laryngeal nerves, the parathyroid glands, and their vascular supply. Parathyroid glands can be distinguished from surrounding structures by their fine surface vascular pattern and brown hue.
- Intraoperative nerve monitoring with electrode attached to endotracheal tube allows for stimulation and detection of the RLN and superior laryngeal nerves.
- Due to the vascularity of the thyroid gland, many surgeons use LigaSure rather than bipolar cautery, ties, or clips.[16] The duration of the procedure with the use of the LigaSure is significantly shorter, and there are fewer complications compared to the classic "tie and knot" technique.[16]
- There is no statistical difference noted in the literature when comparing suture tying and Harmonic scalpel complications.[17,18]
- Clips can also be used for hemostasis on the specimen side.

TOTAL THYROIDECTOMY

- With the patient lying supine in a semi-Fowler's position with the arms tucked at the sides, the anterior surface of the neck is prepped and draped, exposing the anterior neck from the sternal notch to the chin and from both anterior borders of the sternocleidomastoid muscles (**FIG 7**).
- Transverse curvilinear collar incision is made approximately two fingerbreadths above the sternal notch, along a normal skin crease. The length of the incision varies depending on the patient's body habitus and the size of the thyroid gland (**FIG 8**).
- The subcutaneous tissue and platysma are divided, and skin flaps are raised in a subplatysmal plane from the sternal notch inferiorly to the level of the thyroid cartilage superiorly and the sternocleidomastoid muscles laterally. Skin hooks aid with the exposure and flap elevations (**FIG 9**).
- Strap muscles are separated in the midline from the thyroid cartilage to the sternal notch and are reflected laterally (**FIG 10**).

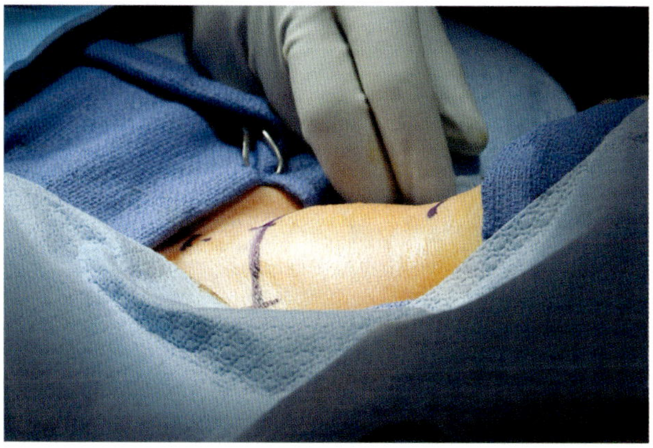

FIG 7 ● Patient prepped and draped, with thyroid cartilage and sternal notch anatomic landmarks marked out as well as the proposed incision.

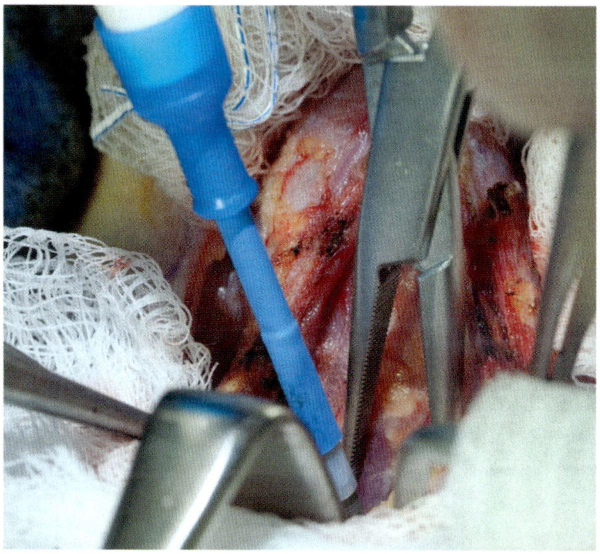

FIG 10 ● Strap muscles are separated in the midline from thyroid cartilage to the sternal notch using electrocautery.

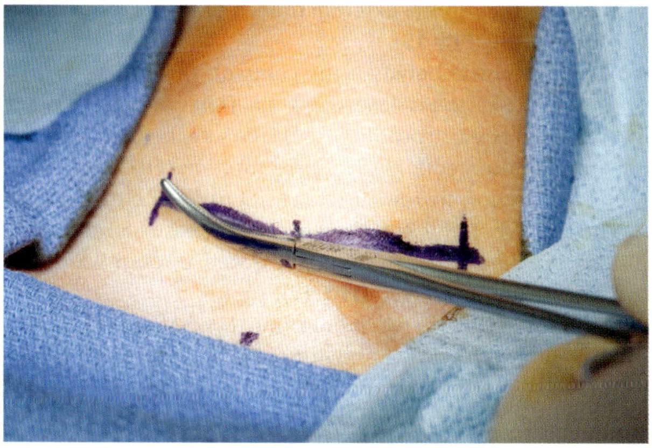

FIG 8 ● Incision marking.

- Horizontal division of the sternohyoid and sternothyroid muscles may be necessary to fully expose a large thyroid gland (FIG 11).
- If the pyramidal lobe is easily identified during this phase of the operation, it can be dissected free from its attachments and ligated to allow for greater mobility of the gland (FIG 12).
- Typically, the middle thyroid veins are the first vessels identified in the dissection and are ligated and divided (FIG 13).
- Superior pole vessels are then identified by exerting traction on the upper pole of the gland, oftentimes using a Babcock clamp to aid with the retraction. The superior thyroid vessels are individually ligated, and we typically use the LigaSure for this (FIG 14).

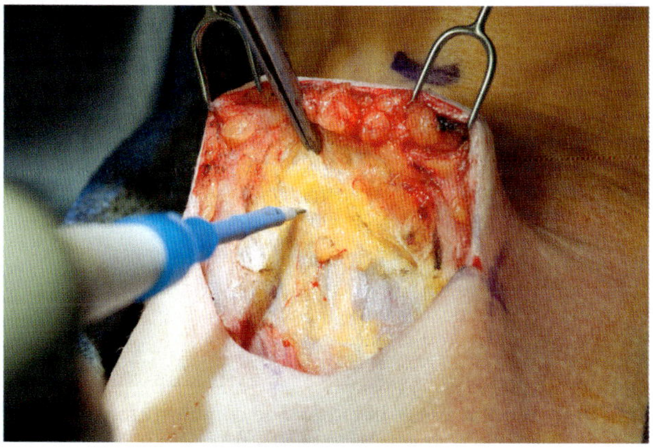

FIG 9 ● Skin hooks aiding with the exposure and flap elevations to allow for subplatysmal dissection.

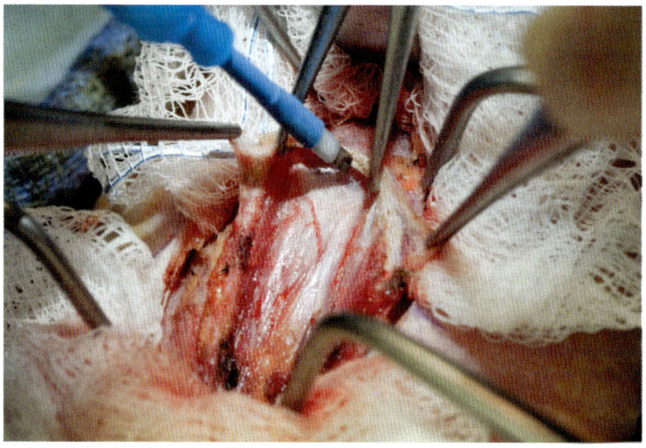

FIG 11 ● Division of sternothyroid muscles helps to fully expose the thyroid gland.

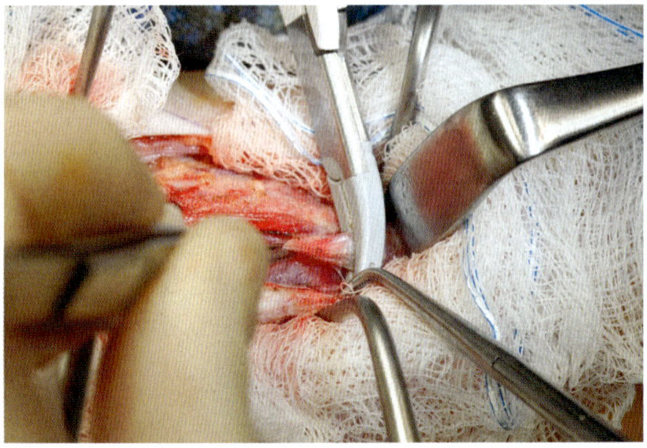

FIG 12 • Dissection and mobilization of the pyramidal lobe and ligation of its attachments.

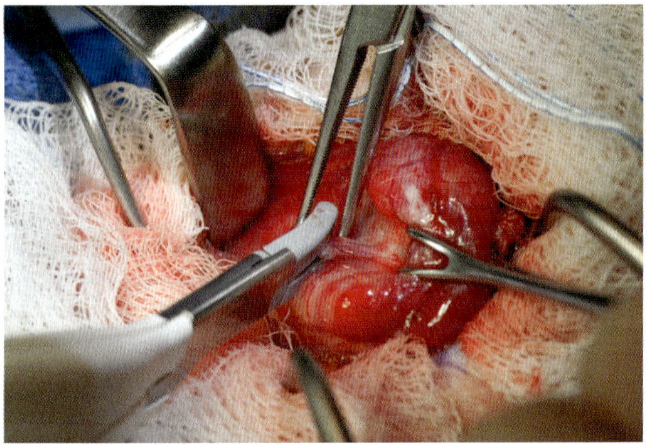

FIG 13 • Ligation of the middle thyroid vein.

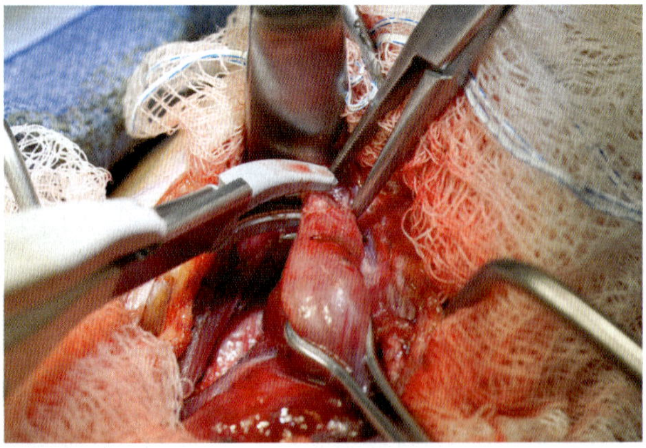

FIG 14 • Superior pole vessels are identified and individually ligated.

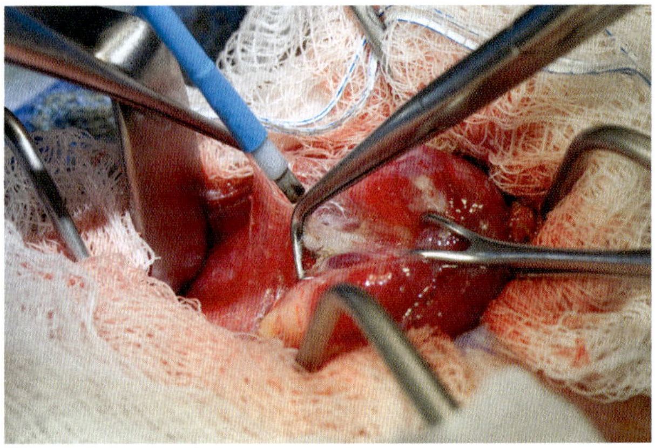

FIG 15 • Subcapsular dissection is carried close to thyroid gland to avoid injury to the external branch of the superior laryngeal nerve.

- Subcapsular dissection is carried close to thyroid gland to avoid injury to the external branch of the superior laryngeal nerve (**FIG 15**).
- Areolar tissue between the common carotid artery and the thyroid lobe is dissected using a combination of blunt dissection, electrocautery, and LigaSure, helping to facilitate anteromedial thyroid lobe rotation (**FIG 16**).
- The inferior thyroid artery is identified, and its close proximity to the RLN then allows for easy identification of the nerve. The RLN is then traced through its entire course and preserved (**FIG 17**).
- Intraoperative nerve monitoring is often used to help confirm the location and integrity of the nerve (**FIG 18**).
- The inferior pole of the thyroid gland is mobilized once the RLN is identified, and this is done by ligating the branches of the arteries and veins close to the thyroid

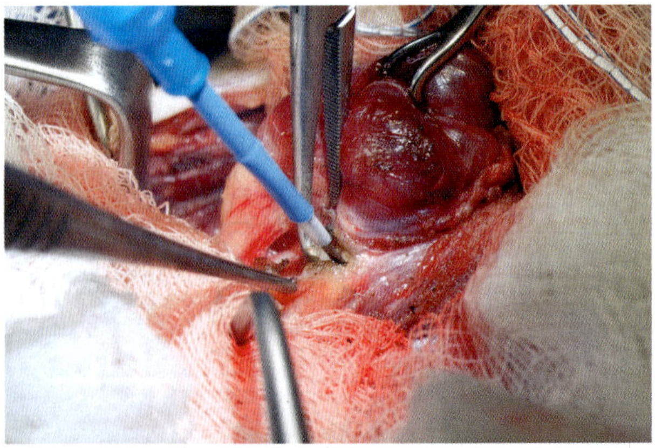

FIG 16 • Areolar tissue between the common carotid artery and thyroid lobe is dissected with electrocautery.

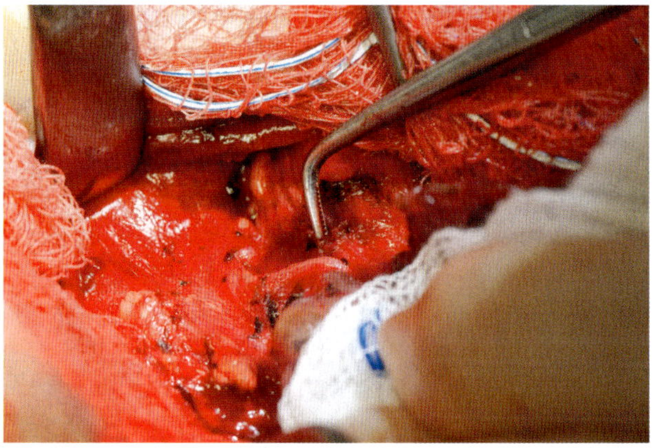

FIG 17 • The thyroid gland is rotated anteromedially, and the recurrent laryngeal nerve is traced along its entire course. Note the RLN at the tip of the right angle.

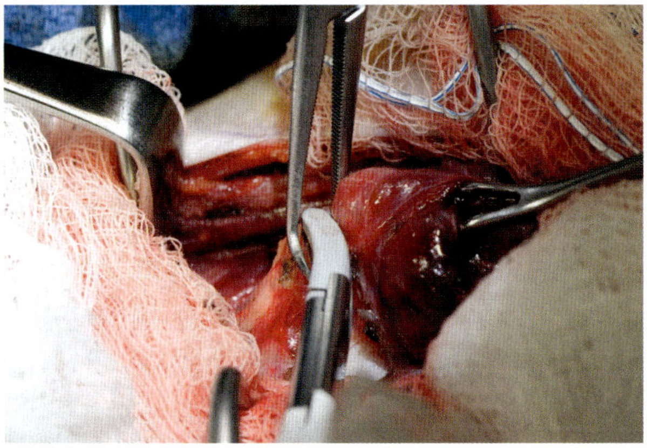

FIG 19 • Ligation of the inferior thyroid vessels close to the gland.

gland. By ligating the vessels close to the gland, the blood supply to the inferior parathyroid gland is therefore preserved (**FIG 19**).

- The anterior surface of the trachea is then exposed (**FIG 20**), and simultaneous anteromedial retraction of the superior and inferior poles of the thyroid enhances the exposure of the RLN (**FIG 21**).
- The remaining branches of the inferior thyroid artery are ligated and divided close to the thyroid parenchyma using various techniques including surgical clip and tie or LigaSure (**FIG 22**).
- The remaining thyroid lobe and ligament of Berry are separated from the RLN, preserving the blood supply to the superior parathyroid gland (**FIG 23**).
- Once the lobe of the thyroid gland has been separated from the RLN, the remainder of the ligament of Berry can be divided, separating the isthmus form the trachea (**FIG 24**).

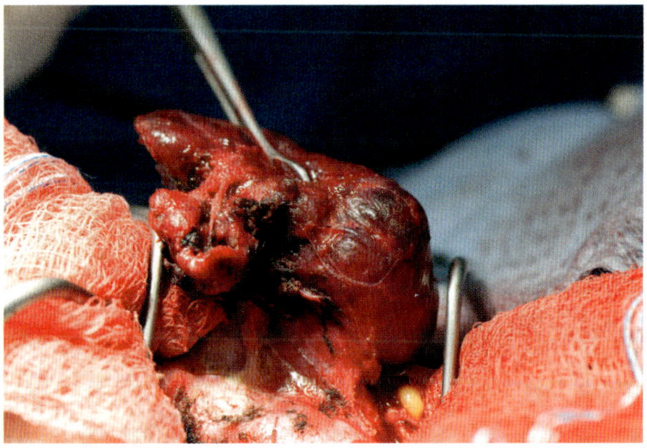

FIG 20 • Anterior surface of the trachea exposed.

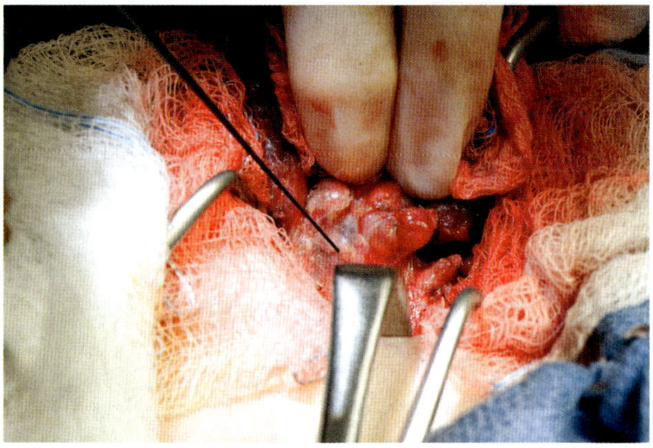

FIG 18 • Intraoperative nerve monitoring being used to help with identifying the RLN and confirming its integrity.

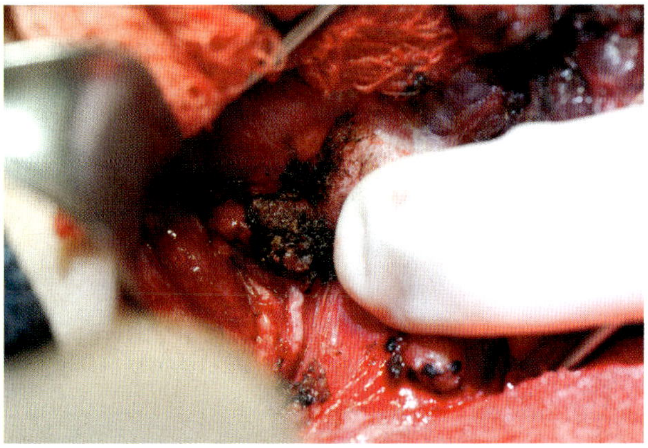

FIG 21 • RLN exposed, with the gland anteromedially retracted and countertraction applied to the trachea.

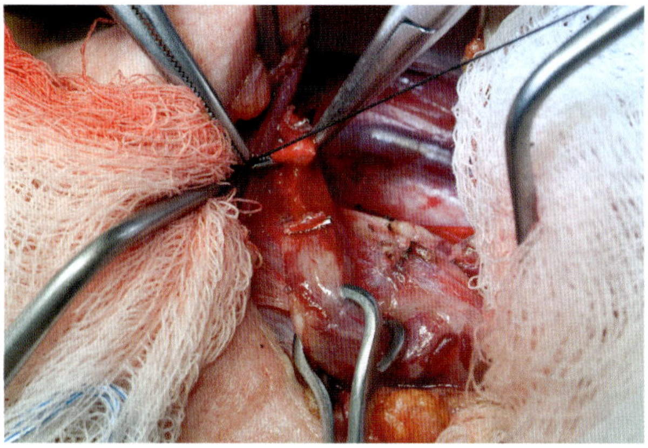

FIG 22 ● Inferior thyroid pole vessels are ligated and divided close to the thyroid gland, with careful attention paid to the blood supply of the parathyroid glands.

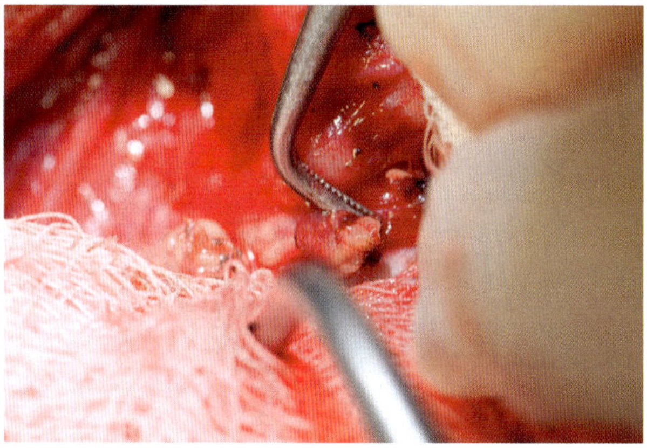

FIG 23 ● Parathyroid gland dissected free and preserved with its blood supply seen at the tip of the right angle.

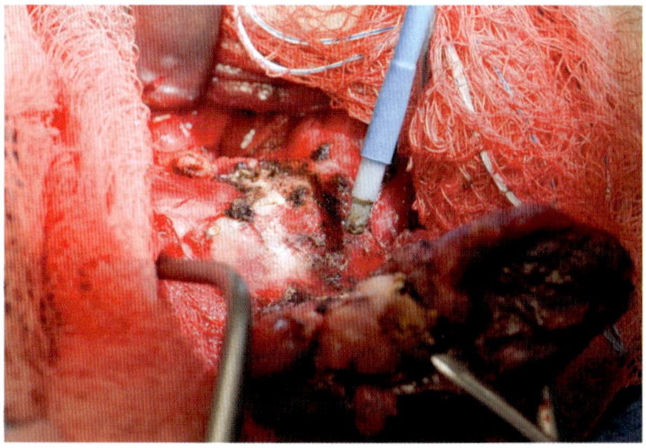

FIG 24 ● Traction placed on the thyroid gland as the ligament of berry is divided, thereby releasing the gland from its tracheal attachment.

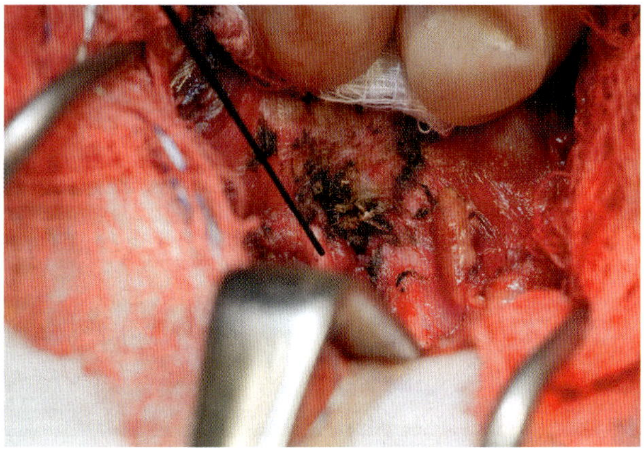

FIG 25 ● Integrity of the RLN is confirmed, both by visual inspection and with the nerve probe.

- The contralateral lobe is resected in an identical fashion, and after complete removal, the integrity of the RLN is confirmed, both by visual inspection and with the nerve probe (**FIG 25**).
- The trachea is left exposed and hemostasis is then attained, followed by irrigation with normal saline (**FIG 26**).
- The sternohyoid muscles are reapproximated in the midline using a running or locking suture, through only fascia and not muscle. The inferior aspect is left open over a distance of 1 to 2 cm to allow blood to decompress into the subcutaneous space if bleeding develops (**FIG 27**).
- The platysmal muscle layer is then reapproximated using simple interrupted suture (**FIG 28**).
- A subcuticular running suture technique, with a free knotless tail left on either end of the incision, is used to closely reapproximate the skin. Careful attention is paid to the cosmesis of the closure (**FIG 29**).
- A single Steri-Strip is placed horizontally in the direction of the incision, and a suture tail is left free on either end of the incision (**FIG 30**).

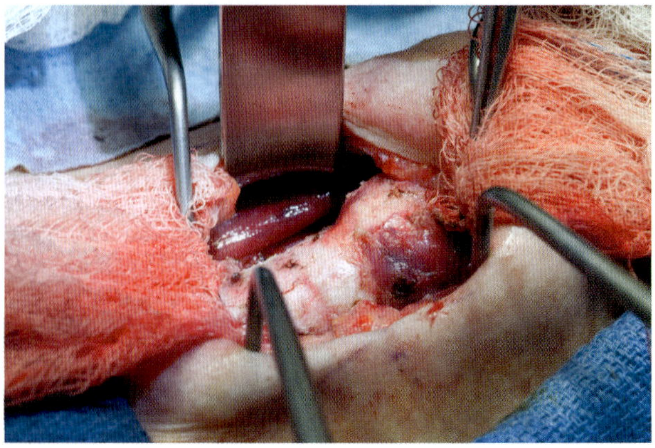

FIG 26 ● The trachea is left exposed and hemostasis is then attained, followed by irrigation with normal saline.

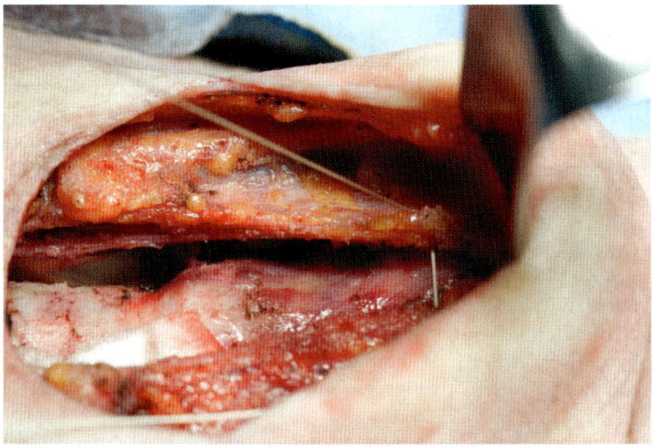

FIG 27 ● Sternohyoid muscles reapproximated in midline with inferior margin left open.

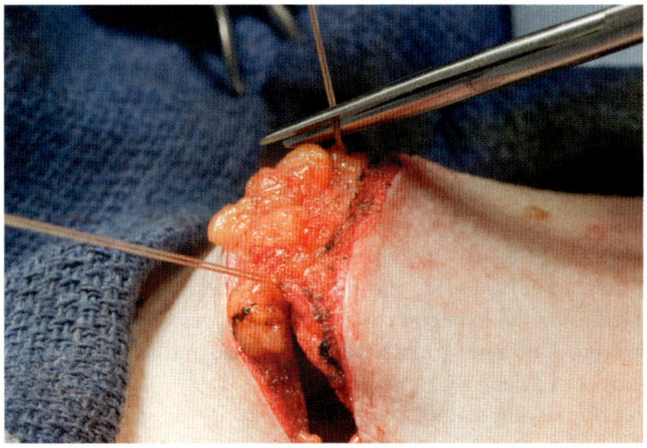

FIG 28 ● Platysmal muscle layer reapproximated in the midline with simple interrupted suture.

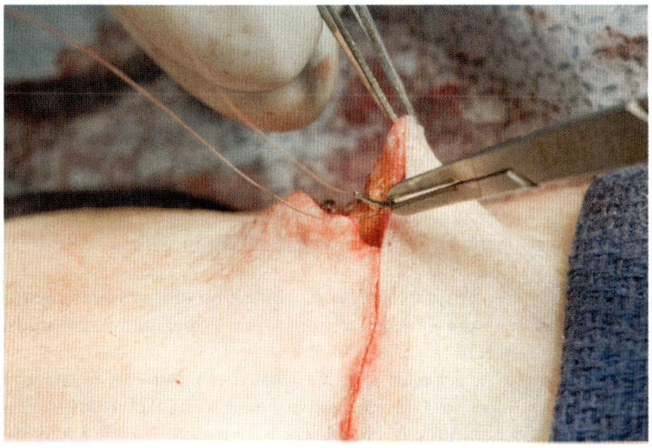

FIG 29 ● Subcuticular running suture technique.

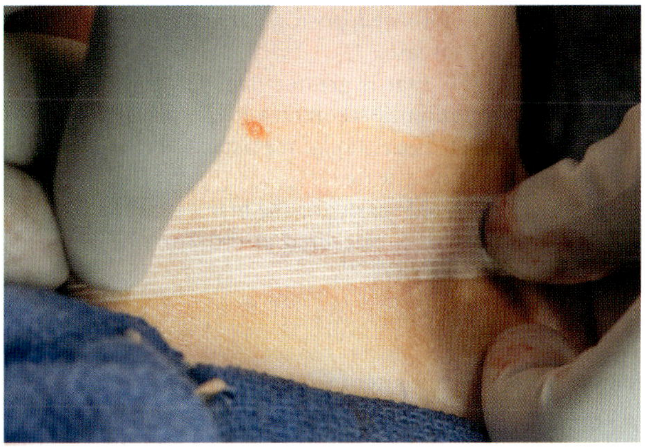

FIG 30 ● Steri-Strip applied along the length of the incision.

PEARLS AND PITFALLS

Subcapsular dissection	■ A subcapsular dissection, in close proximity to the thyroid capsule, is the approach of choice, taking meticulous care to preserve blood flow to parathyroid glands, and identify the RLNs, protecting them all the way to their insertion in the cricopharyngeus muscle. This approach helps minimize the risk of postoperative hypocalcemia and nerve injury.
Gentle retraction	■ This simple subtlety of surgeon's technique helps to avoid nerve injury and preserve vascular supply to the parathyroid glands.
Intraoperative nerve monitoring	■ Easy to setup and aids with the identification of the RLN, oftentimes before visualization. It allows for functional assessment of an anatomically intact RLN and also permits vagal nerve identification to confirm RLN function when visual identification is difficult. Pitfall of this is that it is expensive, requires a learning curve, and may be associated with false-positive or false-negative nerve signals if not properly interpreted.
Vessel ligation	■ The Harmonic scalpel and LigaSure have been shown to result in decrease length of operation.
Closure of strap muscles	■ Strap muscles are approximated in the midline with a running, locking suture, and 1 to 2 cm is left open at its inferior margin. This will allow blood to escape into the subcutaneous space in the event of a postoperative hemorrhage, so that pressure against the airway is minimized. Platysmal muscles are reapproximated using a simple interrupted technique; again, in the event of a hematoma, the individual sutures can be cut to allow for simple evacuation.
Use of a neck drain	■ Drains are almost never used.
Skin closure	■ A 4-0 subcuticular stitch is used. A suture tail is left at the corner of each end of the skin incision, and piece of Steri-Strip is applied horizontally along the incision. If the wound needs to be redressed, the original dressing is removed, and the two ends of the sutures can be used to produce countertraction on either end of the incision and a new Steri-Strip can then be neatly applied.

POSTOPERATIVE CARE

- Total or ionized calcium are checked on the morning of postoperative day 1, as some reports have shown that nearly one-third of patients will have mild temporary hypocalcemia within the first 1 to 2 days after surgery.[9]
- Calcium supplementation is administered based on how low the postoperative calcium level is and as needed for any numbness or tingling.
- Levothyroxine (1.6 µg/kg/day) is prescribed and started 3 days after surgery, unless the patient is already on supplementation or is hyperthyroid; TSH suppression with levothyroxine is thought to improve recurrence and survival rates in cancer patients.
- Laryngoscopy is indicated postoperatively if the patient complains of hoarseness or for any voice changes in order to assess for RLN or vocal cord damage.
- For those with locally advanced disease or with macroscopic residual tumor, radioactive ^{131}I therapy is given adjuvantly. Serum thyroglobulin is followed postoperatively to detect persistent or metastatic disease.
- For patients with WDTC that is greater than 1.5 cm, RAI remnant ablation is oftentimes recommended, especially if there is residual remnant tissue, nodal metastasis, extrathyroidal extension, or distant disease.
- Ultrasonography is indicated yearly for the first 2 years after treatment; thyroid function is measured directly by free T4 and indirectly by TSH.

OUTCOMES

- MNG is more likely to recur after bilateral subtotal thyroidectomy than after total or near-total thyroidectomy, with relapse rates after subtotal thyroidectomy reported to be as high as 9% to 43%; and the risk of malignancy in remaining thyroid tissue, 4% to 17%.[9]
- It is important to emphasize that reoperative thyroid surgery is associated with more risk of complications that the first operation.

COMPLICATIONS

- Transient or permanent RLN injury
- Bilateral RLN injury
- Transient or permanent hypoparathyroidism
- Injury to the external branch of the superior laryngeal nerve
- Postoperative neck hematoma
- Surgical site infection

REFERENCES

1. Järhult J, Andersson PO, Duncker L. Alternating from subtotal thyroid resection to total thyroidectomy in the treatment of Graves' disease prevents recurrences but increases the frequency of permanent hypoparathyroidism. *Langenbecks Arch Surg*. 2012;397:407–412.
2. Barczyński M, Konturek A, Stopa M, et al. Total thyroidectomy for benign thyroid disease: is it really worthwhile? *Ann Surg*. 2011;254(5):724–730.
3. Stålberg P, Svensson A, Hessman O, et al. Surgical treatment of Graves' disease: evidence-based approach. *World J Surg*. 2008;32(7):1269–1277.
4. Burns WR, Zeiger MA. Differentiated thyroid cancer. *Semin Oncol*. 2010;37(6):557–566.
5. Byrd JK, Yawn RJ, Wilhoit CS, et al. Well differentiated thyroid carcinoma: current treatment. *Curr Treat Options Oncol*. 2012;13:47–57.
6. Suliburk J, Delbridge L. Surgical management of well-differentiated thyroid cancer: state of the art. *Surg Clin North Am*. 2009:89(5):1171–1191.
7. McHenry CR, Lin J. Management of thyroid cancer. In: Cameron JC, Cameron AM, eds. *Current Surgical Therapy*. 10th ed. Philadelphia, PA: Elsevier Saunders; 2011:608–610.
8. Yang W, Shao T, Ding J, et al. The feasibility of total or near-total bilateral thyroidectomy for the treatment of bilateral multinodular goiter. *J Invest Surg*. 2009;22:195–200.
9. Ozbas S, Kocak S, Aydintug S, et al. Comparison of the complications of subtotal, near total and total thyroidectomy in the surgical management of multinodular goiter. *Endocr J*. 2005;52:199–205.
10. Dogan L, Karaman N, Yilmaz KB, et al. Total thyroidectomy for the surgical treatment of multinodular goiter. *Surg Today*. 2011;41:323–327.
11. Ho TW, Shaheen AA, Dixon E, et al. Utilization of thyroidectomy for benign disease in the United States: a 15-year population-based study. *Am J Surg*. 2011;201(5):570–574.
12. Liu J, Bargren A, Schaefer S, et al. Total thyroidectomy: a safe and effective treatment for Graves' disease. *J Surg Res*. 2011;168:1–4.
13. Barczyński M, Konturek A, Hubalewska-Dydejczyk A, et al. Randomized clinical trial of bilateral subtotal thyroidectomy versus total thyroidectomy for Graves' disease with a 5-year follow-up. *Br J Surg*. 2012;99:515–522.
14. Sugino K, Ito K, Nagahama M, et al. Surgical management of Graves' disease -10-year prospective trial at a single institution. *Endocr J*. 2008;55(1):161–7.
15. Accetta P, Accetta I, Accetta AC, et al. Total thyroidectomy for benign thyroid diseases. *Rev Col Bras Cir*. 2011;38(4):223–226.
16. Ignjatović M, Kostić Z. Thyroidectomy with LigaSure. *Surg Today*. 2011;41:767–773.
17. Gentileschi P, D'Ugo S, Iaculli E, et al. Harmonic Focus™ versus "knot tying" during total thyroidectomy: a randomized trial. *Updates Surg*. 2011;63:277–281.
18. He Q, Zhuang D, Zheng L, et al. Harmonic focus in total thyroidectomy plus level III-IV and VI dissection: a prospective randomized study. *World J Surg Oncol*. 2011;9:141.

Chapter 37 Thyroidectomy for Substernal Goiters

Andrew G. Shuman Ashok R. Shaha

DEFINITION

- A goiter refers to any abnormal thyroid enlargement secondary to nutritional deficiency, endocrine disease, or neoplasm. In general terms, substernal goiter applies to conditions in which the majority of the thyroid volume lies below the thoracic inlet.

PATIENT HISTORY AND PHYSICAL FINDINGS

- A comprehensive medical history is obligatory, including assessment of the indications for surgery, consideration of medical comorbidities, and ensuring that patients are medically optimized and risk-stratified for surgery. Any prior operative records and pathology reports should be reviewed in advance.
- A detailed physical examination is mandatory, including consideration of upper airway patency and visualization of the larynx to assess vocal fold mobility.
- Flexible fiberoptic laryngoscopy is helpful in evaluating glottic function and assessing the airway.

IMAGING AND OTHER DIAGNOSTIC STUDIES

- Cross-sectional imaging (usually computerized tomography) is invaluable in defining the intrathoracic anatomic extent of the mass and its relationship to critical cervical and intrathoracic structures.[1]
- Intravenous contrast may delay the ability to use radioactive iodine but should be used whenever anatomic considerations may affect the surgical planning or technique.
- Ultrasound may also be employed but is of limited use in assessing the intrathoracic extent of disease.
- A thoughtful approach to the airway is necessary. In addition to history, physical examination, and imaging studies, exclusion of cardiopulmonary factors affecting respiration is important.
- Spirometry and flow-volume loops are useful adjuncts in order to understand the underlying respiratory physiology. However, surgical decisions are made based on functional and anatomic considerations rather than strictly physiologic tests.
- Preoperative laboratory studies should include thyroid function testing and thyroglobulin.
- In the case of a thyroid mass or nodule, fine needle aspiration (preferably image-guided) with cytologic evaluation should be attempted prior to surgery.

SURGICAL MANAGEMENT

- Consideration for removal of substernal goiters is multifactorial.[2]
- Indications for an operation may relate to the need to make a diagnosis, extirpate malignancy, ameliorate compression of the upper aerodigestive tract, or relieve venous outflow obstruction (superior vena cava syndrome).
- In most patients meeting criteria for surgery, medical options other than watchful waiting are limited.
- Given that most goiter operations are elective, prudent and deliberate preoperative planning and counseling are essential. The indications, risks, benefits, and alternatives of surgery versus expectant management should be discussed.

Preoperative Planning

- Preoperative communication with anesthesia is critical. Although most patients can be readily intubated, airway compression or deviation must be considered. Atraumatic intubation is necessary.[3]
- The endotracheal tube cuff should be well below the vocal folds to avoid both glottic trauma and inadvertent extubation, as the endotracheal tube has a tendency to be displaced with movement during surgery.
- Thoracic surgeons should provide preoperative input and be available to assist in cases in which their presence may be needed.
- Options such as small endotracheal tubes, endotracheal tubes facilitating nerve monitoring, and/or fiberoptic bronchoscopy/intubation should be discussed prior to induction with anesthesia.
- Fiberoptic intubation is rarely necessary, although adjunctive technologies, such as the GlideScope®, may be useful.

Positioning

- The patient is positioned supine with gentle neck extension. Effort should be made to prepare and drape in a manner that facilitates some movement of the head and neck while preserving the sterile field.
- Overextension of the neck may put the recurrent laryngeal nerves (RLNs) under tension and make them more difficult to identify.
- Even if sternotomy is not planned, the chest should be prepped for access in case of either an emergency or the inability to free the gland transcervically.

Anatomy

- The tuberculum of Zuckerkandl is a posterolateral prominence of thyroid tissue that frequently approximates the location of the RLN.[4]
- Berry's ligament is a condensation of the pretracheal fascia that attaches the thyroid to the airway. Small vessels run along the ligament, and it may be in close proximity to the RLN, requiring careful attention in order to ensure preservation of the nerve when the thyroid is being mobilized.
- In general, the substernal component of the thyroid gland originates from one lobe. Left substernal goiters are anteriorly displaced by the aortic arch. Right substernal goiters are frequently nestled between the superior vena cava and the prevertebral muscles (**FIG 1**).
- Posterior mediastinal goiters are rare, but when present, the RLN may be anteriorly displaced.
- In rare cases, substernal goiters may not be contiguous with the cervical thyroid gland.

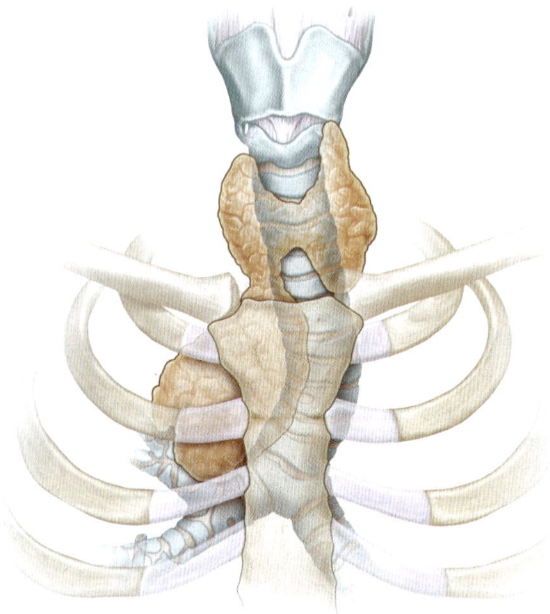

FIG 1 ● Anatomy of substernal goiter. The substernal component of the thyroid gland usually originates from one lobe. Left substernal goiters are anteriorly displaced by the aortic arch. Right substernal goiters (pictured) are frequently nestled between the superior vena cava and the prevertebral muscles.

Approach

- The cervical vascular supply, anterior position, and rarity of bilateral intrathoracic extension typically facilitate complete removal of substernal goiters transcervically.[5]
- Less than 10% of substernal goiters require sternotomy or thoracotomy.
- Relative indications for sternotomy include the following:
  - Prior mediastinal surgery
  - Retroesophageal/posterior mediastinal location
  - Goiter abutting the carina
  - Intrathoracic malignancy with extrathyroidal extension
  - Intimate association with the great vessels
  - Massive substernal goiters that physically cannot be removed through the neck
- When sternotomy is indicated, a "T" incision is frequently preferred.
- Transcervical dissection and ligation of vessels occur prior to opening the chest. However, in cases with venous obstruction, sternotomy precedes vessel ligation in order to limit intrathoracic venous distension.
- The sternotomy may be partial or complete.
- Care is necessary in order to identify and manage aberrant mediastinal vascular tributaries supplying the thyroid gland.
- The intrathoracic trajectory of the RLNs can be identified and preserved under direct vision.
- Lateral thoracotomy typically provides suboptimal visualization of critical structures but may be preferred in specific cases.
- Video-assisted thoracic surgery may also be considered.

INCISION AND EXPOSURE

- Exposure is critical, as satisfactory access facilitates appropriate visualization. Thus, a generous transverse neck incision is planned within an existing neck crease, approximating the level of the cricoid cartilage.
- The strap muscles are identified and divided along the midline raphe. In order to obtain sufficient access, the strap muscles are transected at least on the side of intrathoracic extension (**FIG 2**).

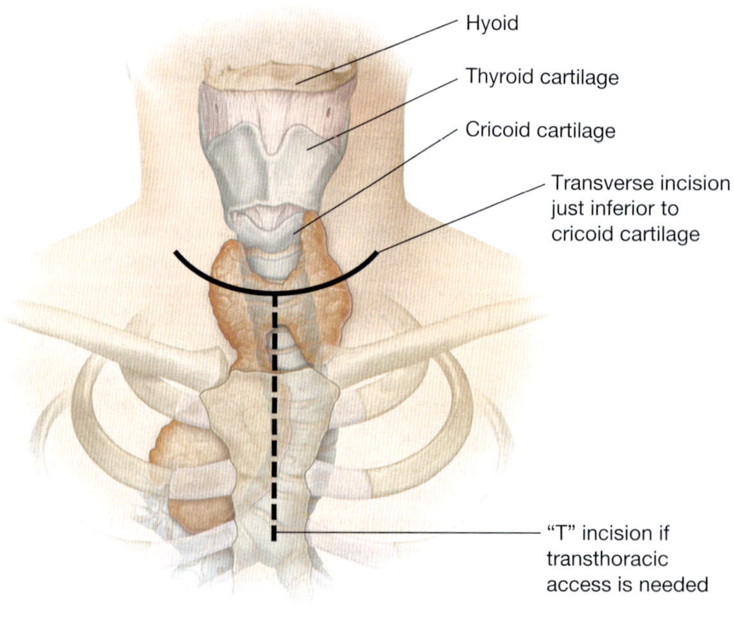

FIG 2 ● Incision and exposure. The patient is positioned supine with gentle neck extension. A generous transverse neck incision is planned within an existing neck crease, approximating the level of the cricoid cartilage. The chest should be prepped within the field. When sternotomy is indicated, a "T" incision is preferred.

MOBILIZATION OF THYROID GLAND

- As the thyroid is gently and bluntly freed from surrounding areolar tissue, meticulous attention is necessary to ensure extracapsular dissection in order to maintain a bloodless field.
- The middle thyroid vein is isolated and divided.
- The superior parathyroid gland is identified and preserved, given that the inferior glands are at higher risk for injury during dissection of the substernal extent of the thyroid gland.
- When necessary, devascularized or excised parathyroid glands may be autotransplanted into the sternocleidomastoid muscle. Perform frozen section confirmation of histology prior to reimplantation.
- The superior thyroid pedicle is isolated and divided close to the superior pole, taking care not to injure the superior laryngeal nerve or superior parathyroid gland.

IDENTIFICATION OF RECURRENT LARYNGEAL NERVE

- The RLN is identified. The size and bulk of the thyroid gland may make this dissection difficult, and the nerve may be displaced from its standard anatomic position. In general, its entry into the larynx at the cricothyroid joint is the most consistent and reliable location for identification.
- The RLN is traced and exposed inferiorly. In cases in which the substernal goiter is posteriorly positioned, the nerve is likely to be displaced anteriorly, putting it at higher risk for injury.
- In some cases, the thyroid gland will need to be displaced in order to facilitate nerve dissection, which involves retrograde dissection of the RLN from the cricothyroid joint inferiorly while displacing the thyroid gland anteromedially ("toboggan approach") (**FIG 3**).
- The RLN may branch prior to its entry into the larynx, and such anatomic variations should be expected. Anterior divisions of the nerve are more likely to be motor branches.

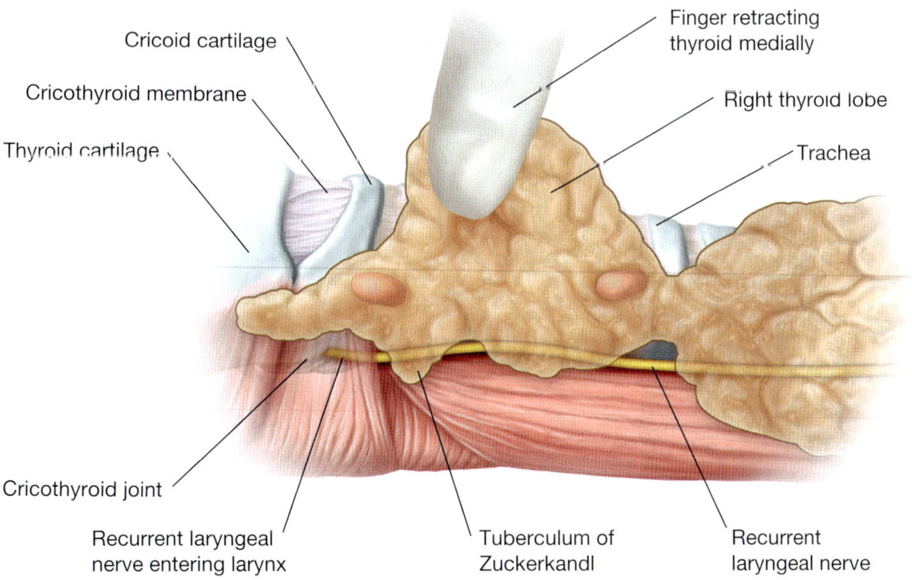

FIG 3 • Identification of RLN. The RLN's entry into the larynx at the cricothyroid joint is the most consistent and reliable location for identification. The RLN is traced and exposed inferiorly. In some cases, the thyroid gland will need to be displaced in order to facilitate nerve dissection, which involves retrograde dissection of the RLN from the cricothyroid joint inferiorly while displacing the thyroid gland anteromedially ("toboggan approach").

LIGATION OF THE INFERIOR PEDICLE AND MOBILIZATION

- The inferior thyroid vessels are isolated and divided meticulously. Damage to these vessels during mobilization can cause intrathoracic hemorrhage not amenable to transcervical hemostasis.
- Gentle, blunt substernal dissection should commence laterally, under the sternocleidomastoid muscle, and progress medially. It may be useful to divide the sternal head of this muscle to improve access. Small venous tributaries are frequently encountered and divided.
- Hemoclips, LigaSure™, or other hemostatic adjunctive devices may be employed at the surgeon's discretion (**FIGS 4** and **5**).

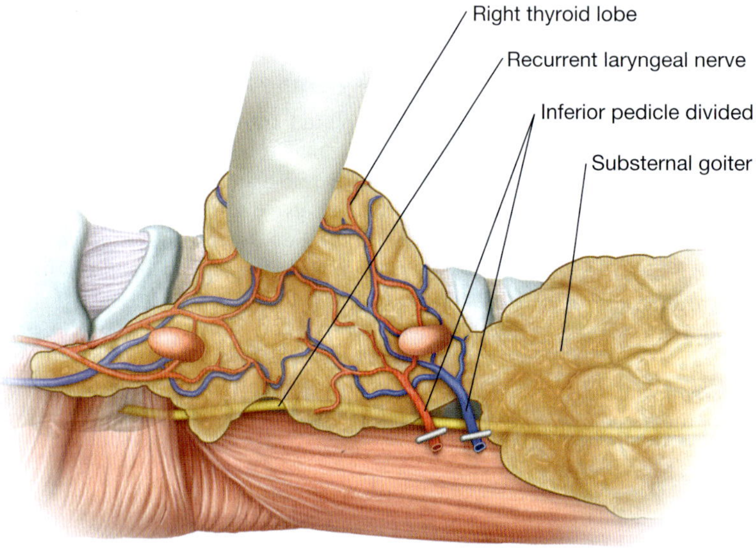

FIG 4 ● Ligation of the inferior pedicle. The inferior thyroid vessels are isolated and divided meticulously. Damage to these vessels during mobilization can cause intrathoracic hemorrhage not amenable to transcervical hemostasis. It may be difficult to visualize and preserve the ipsilateral inferior parathyroid gland.

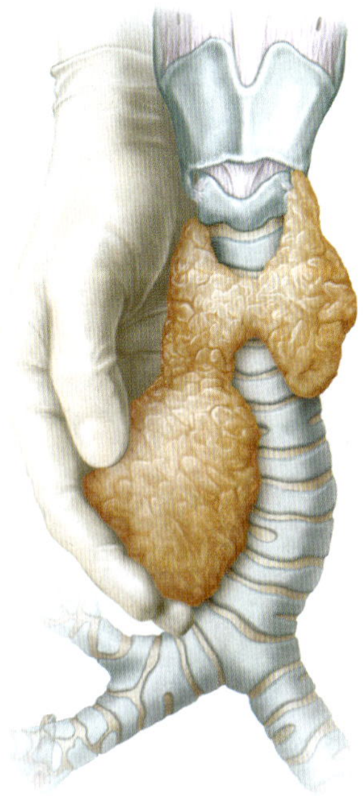

FIG 5 ● Mobilization of substernal goiter. Gentle, blunt substernal finger dissection should commence laterally, under the sternocleidomastoid muscle, and progress medially.

CONTRALATERAL DISSECTION

- The procedure is repeated on the other thyroid lobe.
- Typically, the lobe with substernal extension is removed first in order to ensure that the RLN is preserved prior to contralateral dissection. If the nerve monitor is being used, it is appropriate to test the dissected nerve's integrity prior to contralateral surgery.
- Care should be taken when freeing the gland off of the cricothyroid joint and Berry's ligament, as small vessels can cause bleeding that obscures visualization of the RLN.

CLOSURE

- Closed suction drain placement is frequently indicated due to the large potential space created by expansive substernal goiters.
- Wound closure is performed in the standard manner, taking care to reapproximate divided muscles (sternocleidomastoid and straps). The midline raphe between the strap muscles should be loosely approximated to facilitate egress of blood and transudate and to mitigate airway compression in the case of an expansile hematoma.
- The method of skin closure is at the discretion of the surgeon (**FIG 6**).
- Smooth extubation and anesthetic emergence is important in order to limit sudden increases in intrathoracic pressure. If airway concerns are present, delayed extubation can be considered.

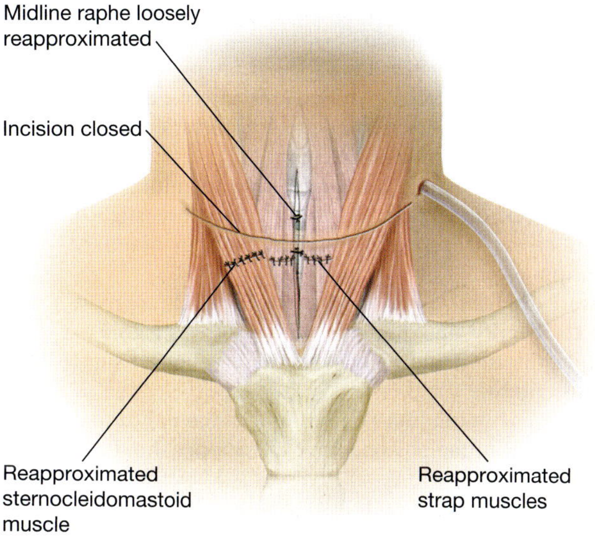

FIG 6 ● Closure. Take care to reapproximate divided muscles (sternocleidomastoid and straps). The midline raphe between the strap muscles should be loosely approximated to facilitate egress of blood and transudate. Closed suction drain placement is frequently indicated.

PEARLS AND PITFALLS

Indications	■ Given that most goiter operations are elective, prudent and deliberate preoperative planning and counseling are essential.
Approach	■ Sternotomy is rarely necessary for removal of a substernal thyroid gland.
Positioning	■ The patient should be placed supine with gentle neck extension and draped in a manner that facilitates movement of the head and neck.
Airway	■ Although most patients can be readily intubated, airway compression or deviation must be considered. Because the endotracheal tube has a tendency to become displaced during surgical manipulation, confirm that the cuff is well below the vocal folds.
Exposure	■ Satisfactory access is critical for safety and visualization. Use a generous transverse neck incision and consider dividing strap muscles at least on the side of intrathoracic extension.
Plane of dissection	■ As the thyroid is mobilized, meticulous attention is necessary to ensure extracapsular dissection in order to maintain a bloodless field.
Management of parathyroid glands	■ The inferior glands are at higher risk for injury or devascularization during dissection of the substernal extent of the thyroid gland. Thus, make sure to identify and preserve the superior parathyroid glands.

POSTOPERATIVE CARE

- Check postoperative serum calcium levels. The use of intraoperative and/or postoperative parathyroid hormone levels is optional. Decisions regarding calcium supplementation and further laboratory studies should be based on individual circumstances, laboratory findings, and clinician preferences.
- Patients should be informed to call 911 if they develop any sudden difficulty breathing or neck swelling.
- Patients should be encouraged to ambulate early and perform pulmonary toilet, although they should restrict from strenuous physical activity and heavy lifting for a few weeks.

COMPLICATIONS

- Surgical site infection—In general, strict adherence to aseptic technique and maintenance of the sterile field assures that surgical site infections are uncommon in patients without underlying risk factors. Perioperative antibiotics should be administered in accordance with established guidelines.[6]
- Seroma—Some degree of seroma formation within the operative bed is inevitable. Intervention rarely becomes necessary.
- Intraoperative hemorrhage—Meticulous technique including limiting shearing/tearing vessels and maintaining an

intact thyroid capsule are critical. Rarely, uncontrolled intrathoracic hemorrhage will require emergent sternotomy and/or aggressive resuscitation.

- Hematoma—Approximately 1% to 3% of cases will develop a postoperative hematoma that requires intervention. All cases of expansile hematomas require consideration of airway compression and prompt attention.
- Nerve injury—The RLNs are susceptible to injury both within the neck and chest. Rates of injury are slightly higher in cases of substernal goiter than in standard thyroidectomies.
- Hypoparathyroidism—Inferior parathyroid glands are more difficult to identify and preserve with substernal goiters, making identification and meticulous preservation of superior glands critical.
- Hemothorax/pneumothorax—Intrathoracic complications are quite rare. Routine postoperative chest x-ray should be considered.
- Tracheomalacia—Despite frequent tracheal deviation and/or compression, clinically significant tracheomalacia is rare. The adult airway is quite resilient, and even long-standing compression will not often be problematic.

REFERENCES

1. Netterville JL, Coleman SC, Smith JC, et al. Management of substernal goiter. *Laryngoscope*. 1998;108:1611–1117.
2. Katlic MR, Wang C, Grillo HC. Substernal goiter. *Ann Thorac Surg*. 1985;39:391–399.
3. Newman E, Shaha AR. Substernal goiter. *J Surg Oncol*. 1995;60(3):207–212.
4. Mohebati A, Shaha AR. Anatomy of thyroid and parathyroid glands and neurovascular relations. *Clin Anat*. 2012;25(1):19–31.
5. Mack E. Management of patients with substernal goiters. *Surg Clin North Am*. 1995;75(3):377–394.
6. Ríos A, Rodríguez JM, Balsalobre MD, et al. The value of various definitions of intrathoracic goiter for predicting intra-operative and postoperative complications. *Surgery*. 2010;147(2):233–238.

Chapter **38**

Subtotal Thyroidectomy for Graves' Disease

Edwin L. Kaplan   Raymon H. Grogan

DEFINITION

- Subtotal thyroidectomy means the removal of most of both lobes of the thyroid, but some thyroid tissue is intentionally left on one or both sides of the neck.
  - Total thyroidectomy alone or with appropriate neck dissections is the procedure of choice for most thyroid cancers and is discussed in Chapter 36.
  - Thyroid lobectomy is used for some unilateral benign colloid nodules or goiters and for many indeterminate thyroid lesions; that is, when the fine needle aspirate demonstrates a possible follicular neoplasm or a follicular lesion of undetermined significance (FLUS) that requires operation (see Chapter 35).
  - Subtotal thyroidectomy is frequently used in the treatment of *benign* thyroid diseases such as nontoxic or toxic multinodular goiters, especially when the disease is bilateral and commonly in the treatment of Graves' disease, although near-total or total thyroidectomy may be more appropriate in some patients.
  - The purpose of subtotal thyroidectomy is to reduce the incidence of postoperative complications of total thyroidectomy—permanent hypoparathyroidism and recurrent laryngeal nerve injury—and to leave functional thyroid tissue in the neck of some patients. Although the rate of complications of total thyroidectomy is low in the hands of expert thyroid surgeons, most surgeons would agree and most studies have demonstrated a lower incidence of complications when subtotal thyroidectomy is performed.
  - This section will briefly discuss the diagnosis and preoperative assessment of patients with benign thyroid conditions and will illustrate the preoperative management and surgical technique when performing *a subtotal thyroidectomy for Graves' disease.*

PATIENT HISTORY AND PHYSICAL FINDINGS

- In order to differentiate these benign thyroid conditions, a careful history and physical examination are first necessary.
- History: Of greatest importance is a previous history of low-dose (or high-dose) radiation to the neck, which is associated with an increased risk of thyroid cancer. Also important are the metabolic status of the patient and whether or not there are symptoms of respiratory impairment, pressure on the trachea, or difficulty swallowing from an enlarged thyroid or from thyroid nodules.
  - Major symptoms of hypothyroidism
    - Severe fatigue, weight gain, dry skin, irregular menstrual periods, constipation, depression, hair loss, brittle nails, feeling cold, slowness of speech, and puffiness. In its most severe form, hypothyroid coma may rarely occur.
  - Major symptoms of hyperthyroidism (thyrotoxicosis)
    - Weight loss despite a normal or an increased appetite, rapid or irregular heartbeat, nervousness, anxiety, irritability, tremor, sweating, changes in menstrual pattern, increased sensitivity to heat, more frequent bowel movements, fatigue, muscle weakness, difficulty sleeping, and fine brittle hair. In its most severe form, thyroid storm might occur.
  - Respiratory and compressive changes and difficulty swallowing
    - Nodules of the thyroid or an enlarged thyroid (goiter) may cause pain and tenderness in the neck as well as trouble breathing. As the thyroid enlarges, the trachea can be compressed and narrowed and eventually respiratory impairment may occur resulting in coughing, shortness of breath, and stridorous breathing. Rarely, an enlarged goiter can result in recurrent laryngeal nerve impairment with hoarseness. Pressure from a goiter or from thyroid nodules can also result in trouble swallowing.
  - Physical findings
    - The physician should assess the size of the thyroid gland and the size, consistency, number, and position of any thyroid nodules; whether or not the trachea is deviated; and if any enlarged and abnormal lymph nodes are present in the central or lateral neck. Finally, the physician should assess whether there are any signs of thyrotoxicosis in general or evidence of manifestations of Graves' disease such as exophthalmos, pretibial myxedema, and a diffuse goiter with a bruit.

IMAGING AND OTHER DIAGNOSTIC STUDIES

- Thyroid function tests
  - Almost all patients with hypothyroidism have an elevated thyrotropin (TSH) level with low free thyroxine (FT4) and triiodothyroxine (T3) values.
  - Almost all thyrotoxic patients have a suppressed TSH with elevated FT4 and T3 values.
- Tests for autoimmunity
  - In Hashimoto's disease and Graves' disease, antibodies to thyroid peroxidase (anti-TPO antibodies) are found in up to 90% of patients, whereas antithyroglobulin (anti-TG) antibodies are found in approximately 50%. Elevated anti-TSH receptor antibodies (TSab) are also commonly detected in patients with Graves' disease and these thyroid-stimulating immunoglobulins (TSI) are the cause of the thyrotoxicosis of Graves' disease.
- Imaging and nuclear uptake scanning
  - The thyroid uptake of radioiodine or technetium isotopes is usually increased in toxic multinodular goiter, toxic adenoma, and Graves' disease.
  - Nuclear scans may help to differentiate each of these diseases.
    - With toxic multinodular goiter, an enlarged thyroid gland is noted with one or more "hot" areas usually among other "cold" areas.
    - Toxic adenoma. A single hot area is clearly seen which corresponds to the thyroid nodule. The remaining thyroid

tissue is suppressed and barely visualized on the scan.
    - Graves' disease. Both lobes of the thyroid demonstrate increased uptake of isotope on the scan.
  - Other imaging studies
    - Ultrasound examinations are commonly used to evaluate the thyroid for nodules and to identify abnormal lymph nodes and have replaced a nuclear scan unless a hot nodule is suspected.
    - Computerized tomography (CT) scan and magnetic resonance imaging (MRI) exams are helpful to evaluate the presence or absence of tracheal compression; abnormal lymph nodes; or the presence, size, and anatomic location of a substernal goiter. These are often reserved for goiters that extend below the clavicle or if significant tracheal narrowing is of concern.
    - The most important test to evaluate a thyroid nodule is a fine needle aspiration (FNA) with cytologic examination. This exam should be used liberally. Usually, it is performed under ultrasound guidance in order to be certain that the nodule in question has correctly been sampled.

DIFFERENTIAL DIAGNOSIS

- A short list of common benign thyroid conditions:
  - Thyroid abnormalities associated with normal thyroid function or hypothyroidism
    - Single colloid nodule or cyst
    - Single microfollicular or macrofollicular adenoma
    - Multinodular goiter
    - Hashimoto's thyroiditis
  - Thyroid abnormalities associated with thyrotoxicosis
    - Toxic adenoma
    - Toxic multinodular goiter
    - Graves' disease
      - Graves' disease is an autoimmune disease characterized by a goiter, thyrotoxicosis, and exophthalmic eye disease. Less commonly, pretibial myxedema is also present. It is closely related to Hashimoto's thyroiditis, which usually presents with hypothyroidism.
      - It was described first in the English language by Caleb Perry (1755–1822) but commonly bears the name of the Irish physician, Robert Graves. On the European continent, it is called Basedow's disease.
      - As an autoimmune thyroid disease, it exhibits both antibodies and cell-mediated immunity directed to thyroid peroxidase (TPO) and thyroglobulin (TG) as well as stimulating antibodies against the TSH receptor (called TSab, but formerly called long-acting thyroid stimulator [LATS]). Antibodies against eye muscle and fibroblasts are also found in the serum of same patients with severe Graves' ophthalmopathy.
      - Incidence of Graves' disease
        - Found in women 5 to 8 times more commonly than in men
        - Thirty cases per 108,000 population annually in Ohmstead County, Minnesota
        - Increases in incidence during each decade from adolescence to 60 years of age
        - Six percent of all Americans have autoimmune thyroid disease.

SURGICAL MANAGEMENT

- A thyroidectomy is usually indicated for the following reasons:
  - To treat thyroid malignancies and some benign thyroid nodules
  - To establish a definitive diagnosis when diagnosis by FNA is equivocal, nondiagnostic, or indeterminate
  - To alleviate pressure symptoms or respiratory difficulties associated with a malignant or a benign process
  - To remove a substernal goiter
  - To remove an unsightly goiter
  - As definitive therapy for individuals with thyrotoxicosis—selected patients with hot nodules, toxic multinodular goiter, and Graves' disease
- Preparation for surgery
  - Most patients undergoing a thyroid operation are euthyroid and require no specific preoperative preparation related to their thyroid gland. Determination of serum calcium and parathyroid hormone (PTH) levels may be helpful. Endoscopic or indirect laryngoscopy might be helpful for all patients preoperatively but definitely should be done in those who are hoarse or who have had a change in voice and in others who have had a prior thyroid, parathyroid, carotid, lateral neck, anterior cervical disc, or chest operation in order to detect the possibility of a recurrent laryngeal nerve injury.
- Hypothyroidism
  - Modest hypothyroidism is of little concern when treating a surgical patient; however, severe hypothyroidism can be a significant risk factor. Severe hypothyroidism can be diagnosed clinically by myxedema as well as by slowness of affect, speech, and reflexes. Circulating thyroxine and triiodothyronine values are low. The serum TSH level is high in all cases of hypothyroidism that are not caused by pituitary insufficiency. In the presence of *severe* hypothyroidism, both the morbidity and the mortality of surgery are increased as a result of the effects of both the anesthesia and the operation. Such patients have a higher incidence of perioperative hypotension, cardiovascular problems, gastrointestinal hypomotility, prolonged anesthetic recovery, and neuropsychiatric disturbances. They metabolize drugs slowly and are very sensitive to all medications. Therefore, when severe myxedema is present, it is preferable to defer elective surgery until a euthyroid state is achieved.
- Hyperthyroidism
  - Toxic multinodular goiter and a toxic adenoma are usually treated to a euthyroid state with an antithyroid medication such as methimazole (Tapazole) or propylthiouracil (PTU), and the possible use of a beta-adrenergic blocker such as propranolol. Radioiodine therapy may sometimes be used as definitive therapy.
  - Operative therapy for a toxic multinodular goiter is usually a subtotal or total thyroidectomy. For a toxic adenoma, enucleation of the nodule or a thyroid lobectomy is curative because a hot nodule is almost always benign. This can be confirmed preoperatively by FNA evaluation. Furthermore, because most of the thyroid tissue remains after enucleation, the majority of patients become euthyroid postoperatively without the need for thyroid hormone replacement.
- Treatment of patients with Graves' disease
  - In the United States, most patients with thyrotoxicosis have Graves' disease. Furthermore, in the United States,

over 90% of all patients with Graves' disease are treated with radioiodine therapy.

- Operative indications for Graves' disease may include very young patients, others with very large goiters, some pregnant women, and those with suspicious thyroid nodules or severe ophthalmopathy.
- For greatest safety, patients with Graves' disease should be treated preoperatively with PTU or methimazole and iodine drops to restore a euthyroid state and to prevent *thyroid storm*. Thyroid storm is the name for the most severe manifestations of thyrotoxicosis including a very rapid heart rate or cardiac arrhythmias, fever, disorientation, hypotension, coma, and even death. In the past, mortality of thyroid storm was very high, but now, with the use of beta-blockers, antithyroid medications, iodine, oxygen, glucose, possibly adrenocortical steroids, and intensive care measures, the death rate has been greatly reduced. Both anesthesia and operation on a poorly prepared thyrotoxic patient are the leading precipitating factors for this event. Furthermore, operation on an unprepared Graves' gland can be more difficult because severe bleeding may occur because the thyroid is often soft and very vascular. With proper preoperative preparation, however, operation on the thyroid gland in Graves' disease can be performed safely.

- Preparation of Graves' patient for operation
  - In *mild* cases of thyrotoxicosis with Graves' disease, iodine therapy alone has been used for preoperative preparation, although we do not recommend this approach routinely. Lugol's solution or a saturated solution of potassium iodide (SSKI), two or three drops twice daily, is given for 8 to 10 days preoperatively. This medication is taken in milk or orange juice to make it more palatable. Iodine therapy suppresses thyroid hormone release only in Graves' disease and should not be given to patients with toxic nodular goiter or toxic adenoma.
  - Most patients with Graves' disease are treated initially with antithyroid drugs, PTU or more commonly, methimazole (Tapazole) until they approach a euthyroid state. Then iodine is added to the regimen for 8 to 10 days before surgery. The iodine decreases the vascularity and increases the firmness of the gland. Sometimes, thyroxine is added to this regimen to prevent hypothyroidism and to decrease the size of the gland. Beta-adrenergic blockers such as propranolol (Inderal) are used commonly with the antithyroid drugs to decrease the pulse rate and eliminate the tremor. Other preoperative protocols using propranolol alone or with Lugol's solution are sometimes necessary, especially when allergic reactions to antithyroid medications have occurred. However, we do not use these routinely because they appear to be less safe.

OPERATION

- Following general anesthesia, the patient is placed in a supine position with the neck extended. A low collar incision is made, usually in a skin crease, and carried down through the subcutaneous tissue and platysma muscle. Currently, small incisions are the rule unless a large goiter is present.
- Superior and inferior subplatysmal flaps are developed, and the strap muscles are divided vertically in the midline and retracted laterally. Often, a large pyramidal lobe is present (**FIG 1**, **left**).

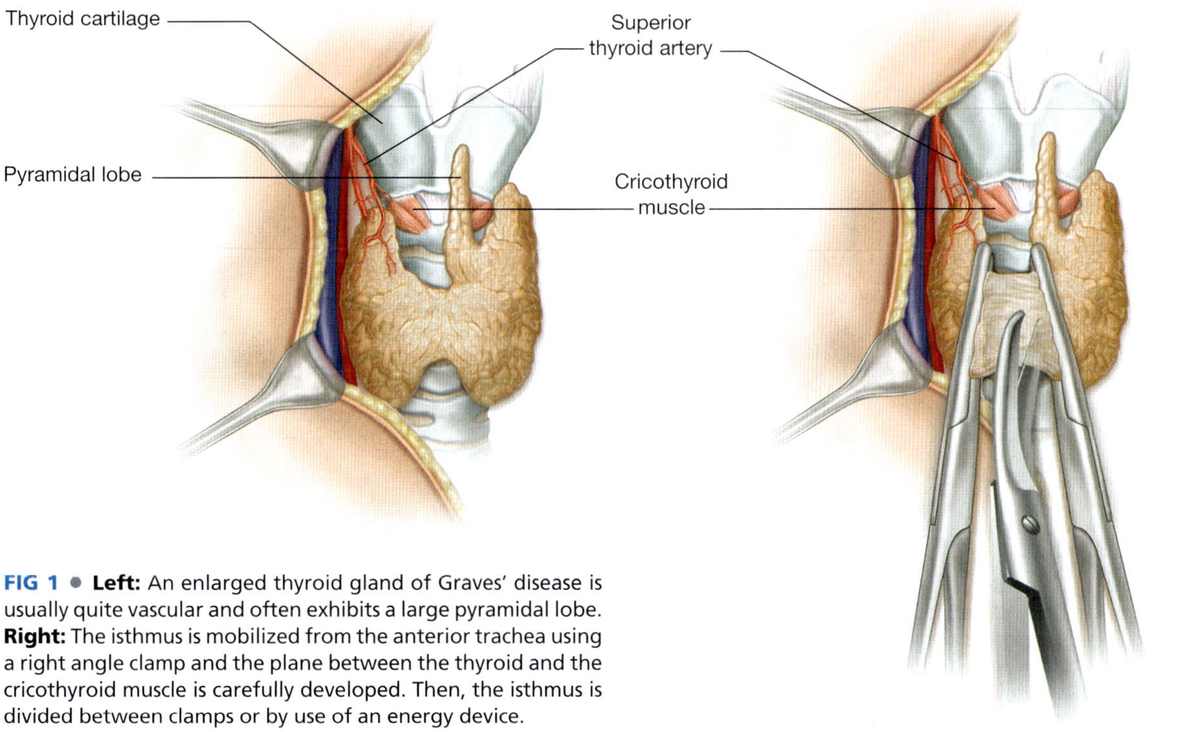

FIG 1 • **Left:** An enlarged thyroid gland of Graves' disease is usually quite vascular and often exhibits a large pyramidal lobe. **Right:** The isthmus is mobilized from the anterior trachea using a right angle clamp and the plane between the thyroid and the cricothyroid muscle is carefully developed. Then, the isthmus is divided between clamps or by use of an energy device.

- The thyroid isthmus is clamped and divided early in the course of operation for most patients with Graves' disease (**FIG 1**, **right**). Alternatively, an energy device can be used to transect the isthmus.
- The isthmus on each side is then sharply dissected from the front of the trachea in order to improve mobilization of the gland. The isthmus on each side is oversewn for hemostasis (**FIG 2**). The medial side of the thyroid lobe to be operated on first is then carefully dissected in a superficial plane toward the upper pole, developing a plane between the thyroid lobe and the cricothyroid muscle. Care is taken to preserve and not damage the external branch of the superior laryngeal nerve and the cricothyroid muscle.
- The thyroid lobe to be operated on first is mobilized by dividing the areolar tissue and any small vessels along its lateral surface.
- The upper pole vessels are then individually ligated along the front surface of the upper pole and not more cephalad in the neck. The right angle is kept "pointing out laterally" to prevent damage to the external branch of the superior laryngeal nerve (**FIG 2**). This nerve can often be visualized if the area is carefully evaluated.
- The thyroid lobe is then retracted medially again and the middle thyroid vein is identified, ligated, and divided (**FIG 3**). This vein is usually in a plane superficial to the inferior thyroid artery and to the recurrent laryngeal nerve, but all structures should be carefully evaluated before ligation.
- The inferior thyroid artery, a branch of the thyrocervical trunk which runs medially and enters the field deep to the carotid artery, as well as the recurrent laryngeal nerve are now carefully identified (**FIG 4**). Whenever

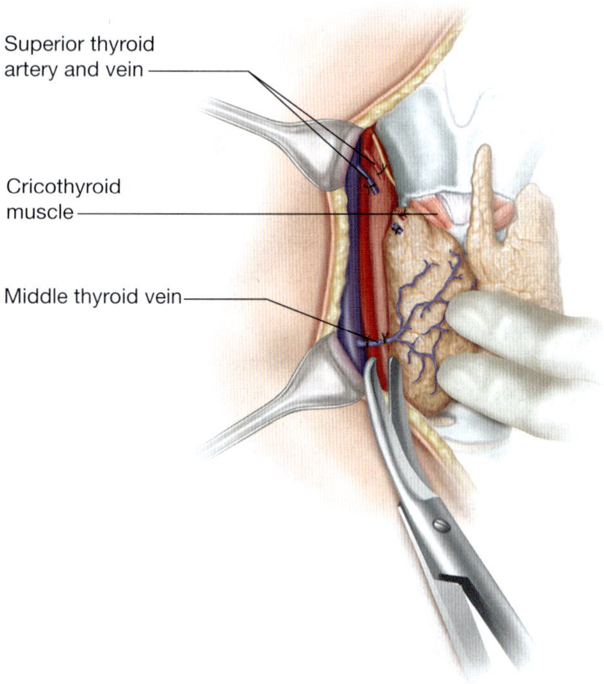

FIG 3 ● The thyroid lobe is retracted medially and care is taken to clearly identify the middle thyroid vein and to ligate and divide it. Be certain that the vein is separate from other structures before dividing it in order to avoid injury to the recurrent laryngeal nerve.

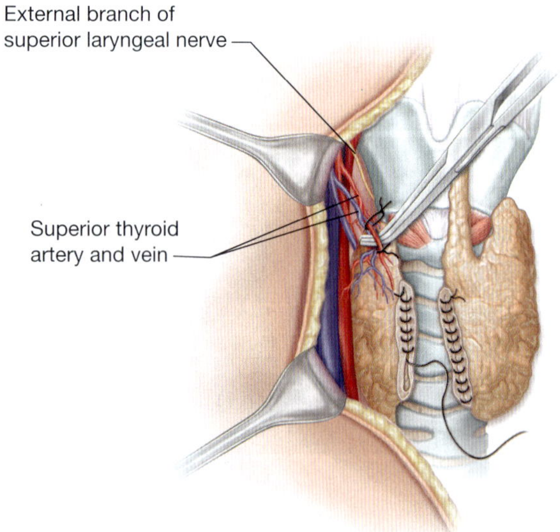

FIG 2 ● If the isthmus was clamped, it is oversewn by a running horizontal mattress suture behind the hemostat followed by a "baseball stitch" for hemostasis. The upper pole vessels are individually ligated on the anterior surface of the upper thyroid pole and divided. The points of the right angle should face away from the trachea and care is taken to identify the external branch of the superior laryngeal nerve when possible and not to injure it.

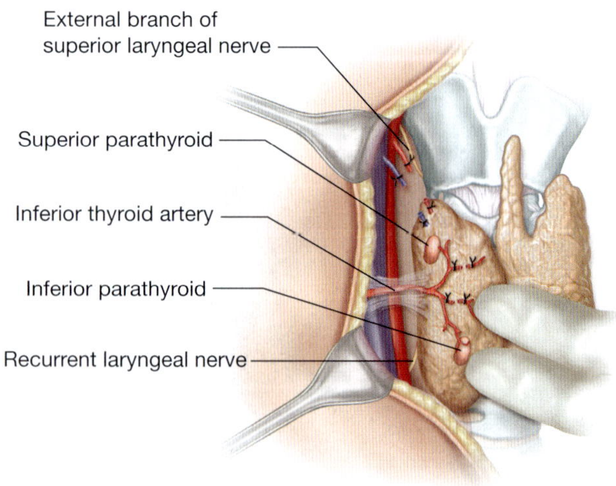

FIG 4 ● With further blunt dissection, the inferior thyroid artery, which runs transversely toward the thyroid lobe, is identified and the recurrent nerve is visualized. The inferior thyroid artery is not ligated as a single trunk but rather individual branches of it are ligated and divided on the surface of the lobe, and the lower parathyroid gland is moved off the thyroid lobe with its blood supply intact.

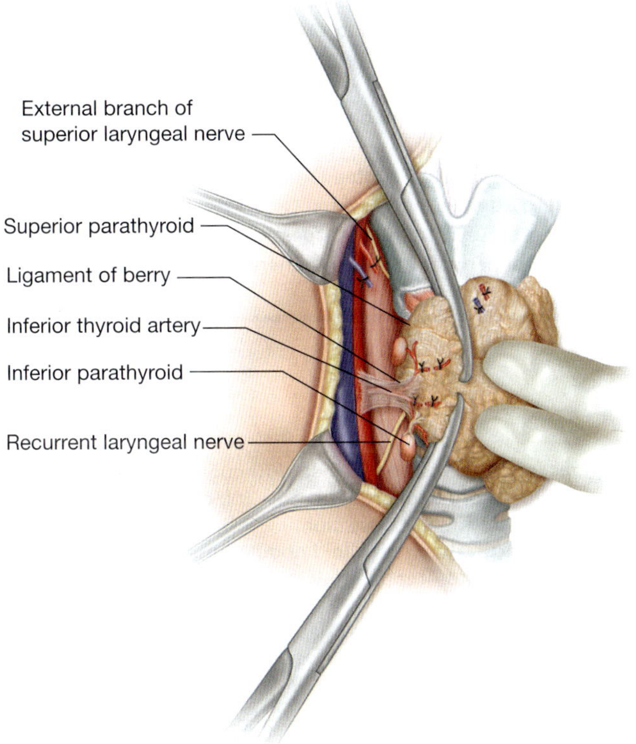

FIG 5 ● The recurrent laryngeal nerve should be visualized and followed up toward the ligament of Berry. The nerve should be treated gently and tissues "unroofed" from its anterior surface. Clamps are then applied (or an energy device used) only after the recurrent laryngeal nerve and parathyroids are seen to be safely preserved.

possible, the inferior thyroid artery is not ligated as a single trunk because this might devascularize the parathyroid glands. Rather, the small branches of the artery are individually ligated and divided along the surface of the thyroid lobe. The inferior parathyroid gland, which often is present high along the lower thyroid lobe, is mobilized with its blood supply and moved more posteriorly and laterally off the thyroid lobe.

- The carotid artery is now retracted laterally and the recurrent laryngeal nerve is more carefully identified, usually in the lower neck, and followed in an inferior to superior direction by "unroofing" the tissues from the front of the nerve (**FIG 5**). Remember that on the right side, the recurrent laryngeal nerve takes an oblique course from lateral to medial and from deep to superficial. On the left side, the nerve usually runs straight upward and is usually found in the lower neck much more medially than on the right side within or near the tracheoesophageal groove.
- If a subtotal lobectomy is to be done, before any clamps are placed on the thyroid lobe, the surgeon must be certain that the recurrent nerve has been identified and followed in a cephalad direction to near the ligament of Berry and that the nerve and parathyroid glands are clearly posterior and away from the sites to be clamped. Then hemostats are applied to the tissue and most of the lobe is resected (**FIG 5**). The remaining small thyroid remnant is oversewn for hemostasis. This resection can also be accomplished by using an energy device if one is far enough from the nerve so the heat does not damage it. Do not perform a subtotal thyroid lobectomy without visualizing the recurrent laryngeal nerve, for this is unsafe.
- At the end of the procedure for Graves' disease (**FIG 6**), a small, well-vascularized remnant of thyroid tissue can be left on each side, a procedure called bilateral subtotal lobectomies. In other instances, to achieve the same

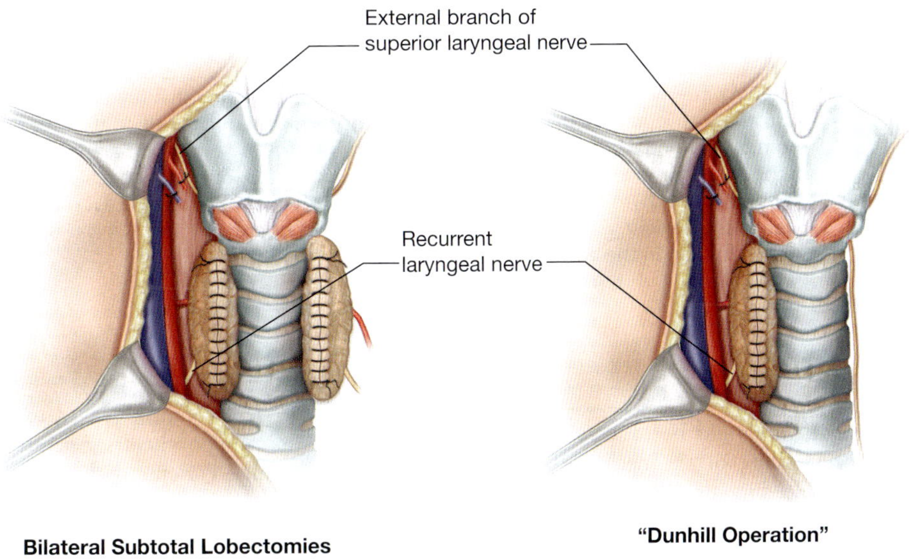

FIG 6 ● At the end of an operation for Graves' disease, each recurrent laryngeal nerve has been identified and preserved, and the parathyroid glands have been spared. Either small thyroid remnants are left bilaterally **(left)** or a total lobectomy and contralateral subtotal lobectomy **(right)** are performed, often called a "Dunhill operation."

result, a lobectomy can be performed on one side with a subtotal lobectomy on the other side, often called a Dunhill operation from the Australian surgeon who popularized this technique. Whichever operation is performed, it is important to leave small thyroid remnants especially in young patients in order to prevent a recurrence of disease. When severe ophthalmopathy is present, a total thyroidectomy may be most appropriate and many surgeons recommend total thyroidectomy instead of subtotal thyroidectomy more commonly for patients with graves' disease. However, always remember that Graves' disease is a benign disorder and our aim is to do an operation that does not cause a nerve injury or hypoparathyroidism.

- Many surgeons find a recurrent laryngeal nerve monitor to be helpful; although in current practice, its use is not mandatory.
- Finally, as stated, instead of suturing the thyroid, an energy device may be used. However, be careful when using these instruments, especially near the recurrent laryngeal nerve for the heat generated may damage it.

PEARLS AND PITFALLS

Preoperative considerations	▪ When operating on the thyroid, some surgeons raise the head of the bed. Although this may seem attractive because it decreases venous bleeding, it is more dangerous because it increases the chance of an air embolism if a major vein is opened during the dissection. ▪ The operation for Graves' disease is often more difficult than for colloid nodular disease because of an increase in vascularity and "stickiness" in some cases. Treatment with iodine preoperatively has been shown to decrease the blood flow to the thyroid. ▪ Although it may be best to check the vocal cords preoperatively in all patients, the surgeon must be sure that both vocal cords are moving well in any patient who has had a previous neck or chest operation or in others who are hoarse.
Recurrent laryngeal nerve	▪ Always visually identify the recurrent laryngeal nerve, carefully "unroof" it, and gently follow its course. Although temporary nerve injuries may occur when this practice is followed, rarely will the injury be permanent. ▪ Remember that nonrecurrent recurrent laryngeal nerves may occur especially on the right side of the neck. Each is associated with a vascular anomaly. ▪ Use of a recurrent laryngeal nerve monitor may be helpful especially in a reoperative thyroidectomy. However, this technique has not been shown to reduce nerve injuries and sometimes can be misleading to the casual user. ▪ If the nerve monitor demonstrates the loss of recurrent laryngeal nerve function on the first side of the neck, one should strongly consider halting the operation or limiting the contralateral resection in order to prevent the possibility of a bilateral nerve injury if one proceeds.
Parathyroid	▪ Carefully search for and try to save each parathyroid gland with a good blood supply. ▪ Do not ligate the inferior thyroid artery as a single trunk. Rather, ligate small branches on the surface of the thyroid lobe in order to preserve the delicate blood supply to the parathyroid glands. ▪ Autotransplant each parathyroid gland that looks devascularized, if it does not bleed well on biopsy or if it is accidently removed.
Postoperative care	▪ Observe patients carefully postoperatively. Delayed bleeding with a hematoma can occur. ▪ A postoperative neck hematoma is an emergency which requires rapid return to the operating room or opening of the wound at the bedside if respiratory symptoms are present. ▪ In the postoperative care of a patient with Graves' disease, one cannot reliably use the TSH value alone to assess thyroid function, for the TSH value may stay suppressed even for weeks postoperatively if the patient was still thyrotoxic at the time of operation. The FT4 is usually a better indicator of function in the early postoperative course.

POSTOPERATIVE CARE

- In the recovery room, the patient should be observed for difficulty breathing and for swelling of the neck, which might indicate postoperative bleeding or hematoma. Return the patient to the operating room as an emergency if an expanding hematoma is recognized. Some surgeons advise endoscopic evaluation of the vocal cords in each patient; however, this should definitely be done if respiratory impairment is present.
- A serum calcium and PTH value is helpful. Some obtain a PTH in the recovery room; however, the authors generally wait until the morning of the first operative day to routinely obtain these results. Patients with Graves' disease may be more prone to manifesting hypocalcemia than others, partly due to bone hunger.
- Severe symptomatic hypocalcemia may require intravenous calcium therapy followed by oral calcium and vitamin D therapy. However, most patients are treated with oral calcium, which is given liberally and do very well. Thyroid

Table 1: Ablative Treatment of Graves' Disease with Thyrotoxicosis

Method	Dose or Extent of Surgery	Onset of Response	Complications	Remarks
Surgery	Subtotal excision of gland	Immediate	Mortality <1% Permanent hypothyroidism 20%–30% or greater[a] Recurrent hyperthyroidism <15%[a] Vocal cord paralysis approximately 1% Hypoparathyroidism approximately 1%	Applicable in young patients, pregnant women, large goiter, or nodular gland
Radioiodine 5–10 mCi		Several weeks to months	Permanent hypothyroidism, at least 50%–70%, often with delayed onset; multiple treatments sometimes necessary in large goiters	Avoid in children or pregnant women

[a]*Depends on size of thyroid remnant which is left in neck. As more tissue is removed, the incidence of hypothyroidism is increased but recurrence rate is diminished.*

replacement is given to many patients soon after surgery unless they are still thyrotoxic with a tachycardia. Although TSH is usually the best indicator of thyroid function, the FT4 is often a better indication in Graves' patients postoperatively because their TSH value may be suppressed for a considerable period of time.

OUTCOMES

- Although radioiodine therapy is the usual treatment, thyroidectomy is a very successful treatment for the thyrotoxicosis of Graves' disease in selected patients (Table 1). A major benefit is the rapid return to a euthyroid state, which is much quicker than following radioiodine therapy. It can be used in very young patients and during pregnancy if necessary. In each of these instances, radioiodine therapy is contraindicated. It removes the goiter and any thyroid nodules which are present. Finally, in patients with severe ophthalmopathy, many studies have shown improvement of eye changes or stabilization in others following thyroidectomy, whereas following radioiodine, the eye changes in some patients become worse.
- Postoperative thyroid function is directly related to the size of the thyroid remnants which are left in the neck. The larger the size of the remnant thyroid, the greater the rate of recurrence of thyrotoxicosis. Most patients and endocrinologists want a cure for the thyrotoxicosis and thus small thyroid remnants are preferable. In young patients, the chance of recurrence is greater and very small remnants should be used. In patients with severe ophthalmopathy, total thyroidectomy should be performed and may be most beneficial. Finally, subtotal or near-total thyroidectomy results in a lower incidence of complications than total thyroidectomy in most surgeons' practice and thus remains the surgical procedure of choice, especially in young children.

COMPLICATIONS

- Thyroid storm
- Postoperative hemorrhage (with respiratory distress)
- Injury to the external branch of the superior laryngeal nerve
- Unilateral or bilateral recurrent laryngeal nerve injury
- Temporary or permanent hypoparathyroidism

SUGGESTED READINGS

1. Behar R, Arganini M, Wu TC, et al. Graves' disease and thyroid cancer. *Surgery*. 1986;105:1121–1126.
2. DeGroot LJ. Graves' disease and the manifestations of thyrotoxicosis. Thyroid Disease Manager Web site. http://www.thyroidmanager.org.
3. DeGroot LJ. Diagnosis and treatment of Graves' disease. Thyroid Disease Manager Web site. http://www.thyroidmanager.org.
4. Kaplan EL. The place of subtotal thyroidectomy in the treatment of Graves' disease. *Surgical Rounds*. 1984;7(1):22–31.
5. Kaplan EL, Angelos P. Surgery of the thyroid. In: DeGroot LJ, Jameson JL, eds. *Endocrinology*. 6th ed. Philadelphia, PA: Elsevier; 2009.
6. Kaplan EL, Angelos P, Grogan RH. Surgery of the thyroid gland. Thyroid Disease Manager Web site. http://www.thyroidmanager.org/thyroidbook.htm.
7. Kaplan EL, McCaffrey K. Subtotal thyroidectomy in the treatment of Graves' disease. In: Thompson NW, ed. *Endocrine Surgery Update*. Philadelphia, PA: Grune & Stratton; 1983:43–57.
8. Klementschitsch P, Shen KL, Kaplan EL. Reemergence of thyroidectomy as treatment for Graves' disease. *Surg Clin North Am*. 1979;59:35–42.
9. Sridama V, Reilly M, Kaplan EL, et al. Long-term follow-up study of compensated low dose 131-I therapy for Graves' disease. *New Engl J Med*. 1984;311:426–432.

Chapter 39 Minimally Invasive Video-Assisted Thyroidectomy

Paolo Miccoli Gabriele Materazzi

DEFINITION

- Minimally invasive video-assisted thyroidectomy (MIVAT) is an endoscopic procedure characterized by the use of external retraction, avoiding any gas inflation, in order to create an operative space in the neck.
- This approach to the thyroid has been used at our Department of Surgery for the last 15 years on more than 3,500 patients with results that can successfully rival those of standard open surgery.
- This is not an appropriate operation for any patient with thyroid disease; patients must be strictly selected. Only 10% to 30% of the cases[1] are appropriate for a MIVAT procedure.

PATIENT HISTORY AND PHYSICAL FINDINGS

- The inclusion criteria and the main contraindications are summarized in the following text. The most significant limit is represented by the size of both the nodule(s) and/or the gland as measured by means of an accurate ultrasonographic study obtained preoperatively. In countries where goiter is endemic, the gland volume can be relevantly independent from the nodule volume, and this aspect might be responsible for the necessity of converting the procedure.
- Ultrasonography can also be useful to exclude the presence of thyroiditis, which might make the dissection troublesome. In case ultrasonography only gives the suspicion of thyroiditis, autoantibodies should be measured in the serum. If thyroiditis is diagnosed preoperatively, this is a consideration to MIVAT.
- One of the most controversial aspects regarding the appropriateness of MIVAT is in the treatment of malignant thyroid disease. "Low-risk" papillary carcinoma constitutes an ideal indication for MIVAT,[2,3] but it is important to take into account the possibility of lymph node involvement in the neck. Great caution should be taken when there is the possibility of either metastatic lymph nodes or extracapsular invasion of the gland, both of which represent a contraindication to the minimally invasive endoscopic procedure.
- Indications
  - Multinodular goiter (thyroid volume less than 25 mL and nodules smaller than 3 cm)
  - Low-risk papillary carcinoma
  - Graves' disease
  - Microfollicular/Hürthle cell adenoma
  - *RET* gene mutation carriers (familial medullary thyroid carcinoma)
- Contraindications
  - Absolute
    - Previous neck surgery
    - Acute thyroiditis
    - Metastatic carcinoma (levels II to VI)
    - Locally advanced carcinoma
    - Sporadic medullary carcinoma
  - Relative
    - Previous neck irradiation
    - Short neck in an obese patient
    - Chronic thyroiditis

IMAGING AND OTHER DIAGNOSTIC STUDIES

- All patients should undergo (1) neck ultrasound in order to evaluate thyroid gland total volume (this should be less than 25 mL) and diameter of nodule/s (these should be less than 3 cm); (2) fine needle aspiration cytology of suspicious nodules; (3) blood tests in order to exclude thyrotoxicosis and acute thyroiditis before surgery; (4) basal serum calcitonin dosage is strongly suggested in order to exclude medullary carcinoma, which is a contraindication to MIVAT; (5) routine preoperative laryngoscopy is strongly recommended in all patients in order to identify asymptomatic vocal cord palsy.

TECHNIQUES

POSITIONING OF THE PATIENT AND DRAPING

- Patient is positioned in supine position without neck extension (**FIG 1**). Hyperextension must be avoided because it would reduce the operative space. Conventional neck preparation and draping is obtained. The skin is protected by means of a sterile film (Tegaderm®).

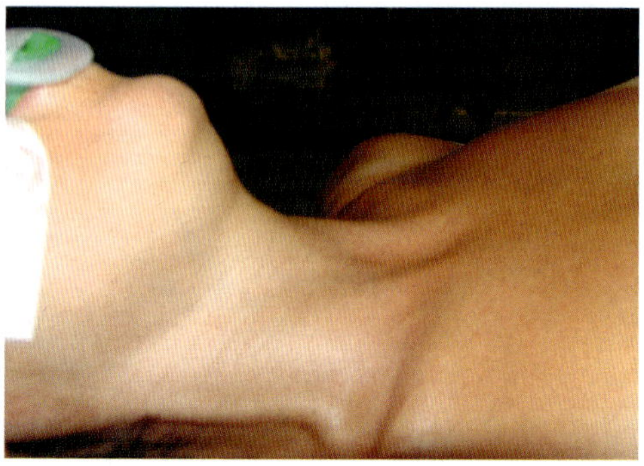

FIG 1 • Position of the patient on the operative table: Neck is not extended and skin is covered by sterile drapes.

POSITIONING OF THE SURGICAL TEAM

- Operation is performed by four surgeons: The first surgeon is on the right side of the table, the first assistant is on the left side of the table. The second assistant, who is holding the retractors, is at the head of the table. The third assistant, who is holding the endoscope, is on the left side of the table.The scrub nurse is behind the surgeon on the right side of the table (**FIG 2**).

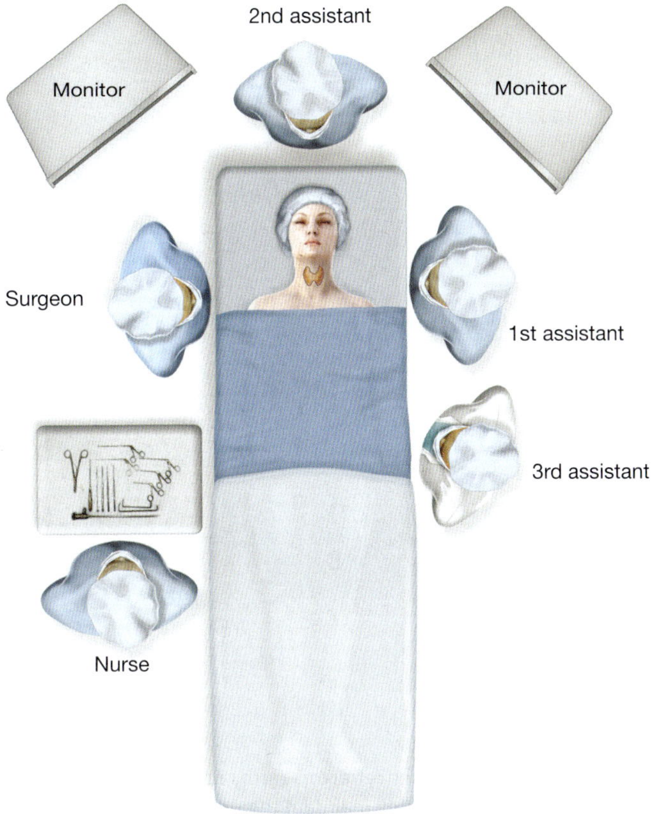

FIG 2 ● Operating room setup: Team

- The surgeon is on the right side of the table.
- The first assistant is on the left side of the table (opposite the surgeon).
- The second assistant is at the head of the table.
- The third assistant is on the left side of the table.
- The scrub nurse is behind the surgeon on the right side of the table.

INSTRUMENTATION

- Forward-oblique telescope 30 degrees, diameter 5 mm, length 30 cm; suction dissector with cutoff hole, with stylet, blunt, length 21 cm; ear forceps, very thin, serrated, working length 12.5 cm; conventional tissue retractor army navy type; small tissue retractor, double-ended, length 12 cm; clip applier for vascular clips; straight scissors, length 12.5 cm, Harmonic Scalpel CS14; electrocautery (monopolar) (**FIG 3**).

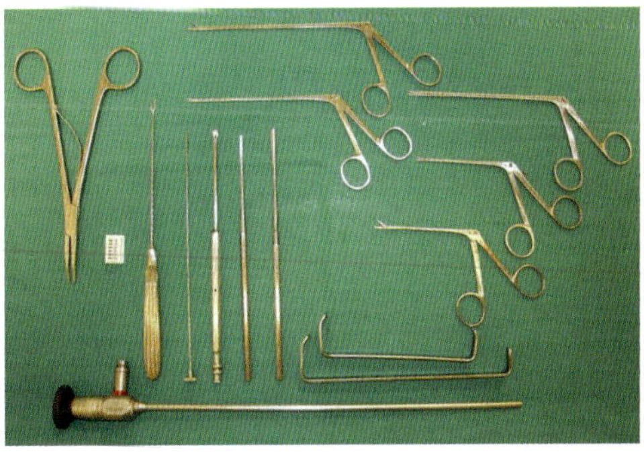

FIG 3 ● Instrumentation for MIVAT.

INCISION AND PREPARATION OF THE OPERATIVE SPACE

- A 1.5-cm horizontal skin incision is performed 2 cm above the sternal notch in the central cervical area (**FIG 4**). Subcutaneous fat and platysma are carefully dissected so as to avoid any minimum bleeding.
- Two small retractors are used to expose the midline, which has to be incised for 2 to 3 cm in an absolutely bloodless plane (**FIG 5**).
- The blunt dissection of the thyroid lobe from the strap muscles is performed through the skin incision by gentle retraction and using tiny spatulas. When the thyroid lobe is almost completely dissected from the strap muscles,

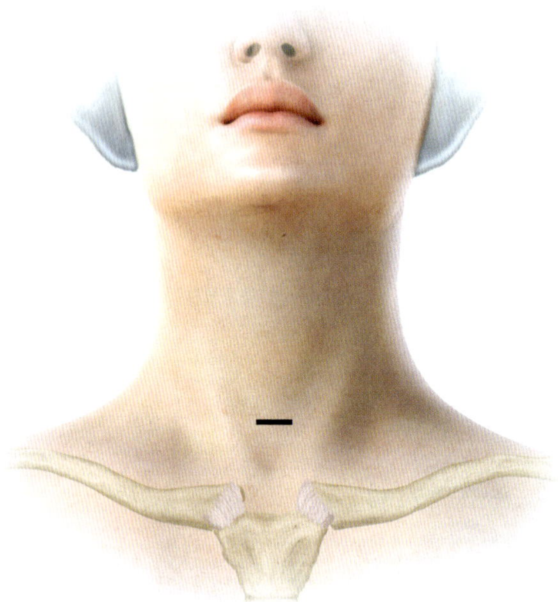

FIG 4 ● A 1.5-cm horizontal skin incision is performed 2 cm above the sternal notch in the central cervical area.

larger and deeper retractors (army navy type) can be inserted and they will maintain the operative space during all the endoscopic part of the procedure (FIG 6).

- Then, a 30-degree, 5-mm or 7-mm endoscope is introduced through the skin incision: From this moment on, the procedure is entirely endoscopic until the extraction of the lobe of the gland. Preparation of the thyrotracheal groove is completed under endoscopic vision by using small (2 mm in diameter) instruments such as spatulas, forceps, spatula-sucker, and scissors.

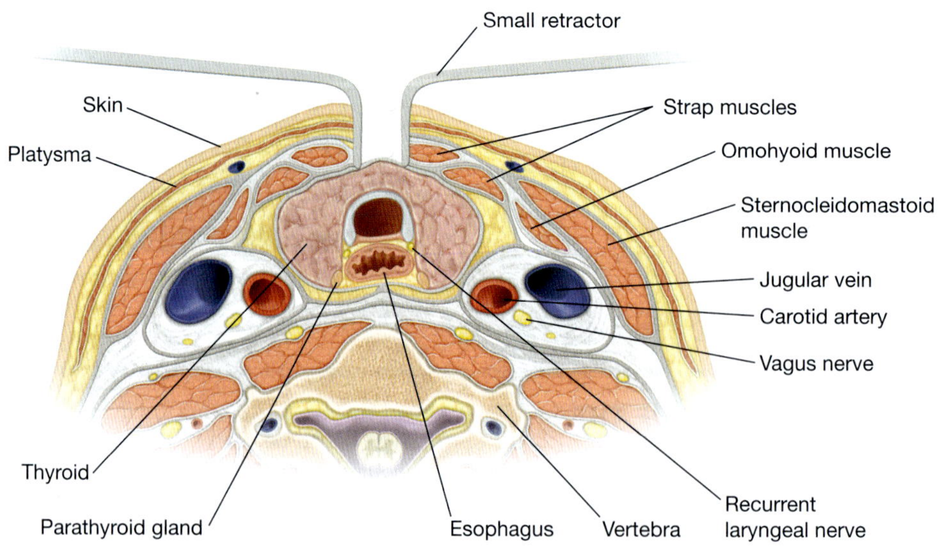

FIG 5 ● Two small retractors are used to expose the midline, which has to be incised for 2 to 3 cm on an absolutely bloodless plane.

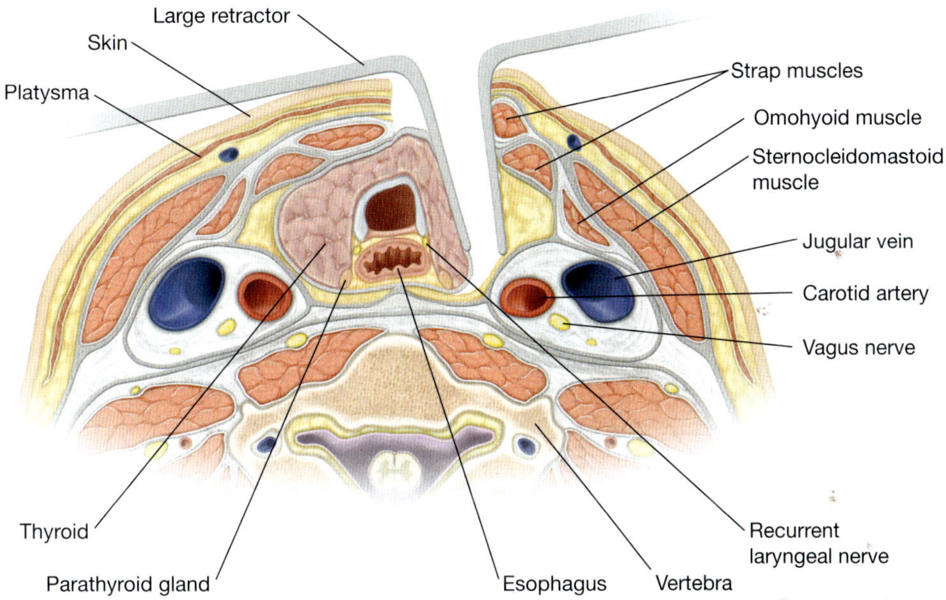

FIG 6 ● Access to the operative space during MIVAT: when the thyroid lobe is almost completely dissected from the strap muscles, larger and deeper retractors (army navy type) can be inserted and they will maintain the operative space during all the endoscopic part of the procedure.

SECTION OF THE MAIN THYROID VESSELS

- The first vessel to be ligated is the middle vein, when present, or the small veins between jugular vein and thyroid capsule. This step allows a better preparation of the thyrotracheal groove where the recurrent nerve will be later searched.
- During this step, the endoscope has to be held inside the camera with the 30-degree tip looking downward and in an orthogonal axis with the thyroid lobe and trachea.
- A further step is represented by the exposure of the upper pedicle, which must be carefully prepared, until an optimal visualization of the different branches is achieved. During this step, the endoscope should be rotated to 180 degrees with the 30-degree tip looking upward (**FIG 7**) and held in a parallel direction with the

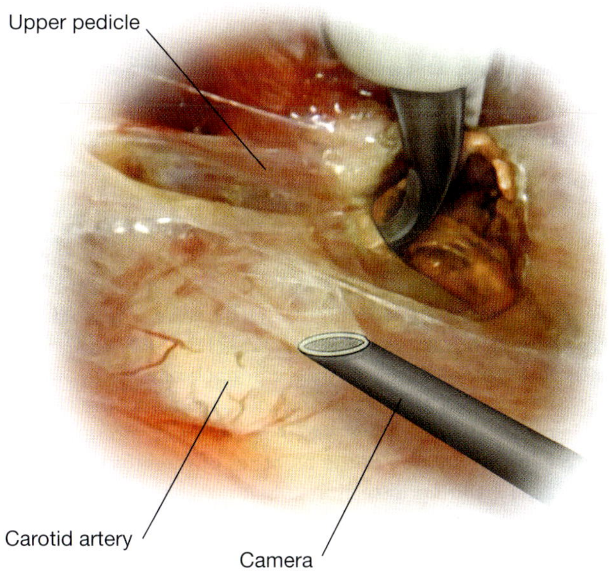

FIG 7 ● Upper pole section: During this step, the endoscope should be rotated to 180 degrees with the 30-degree tip looking upward and held in a parallel direction with the thyroid lobe and trachea in order to better visualize the upper portion of the operative space where the superior thyroid vein and artery are running.

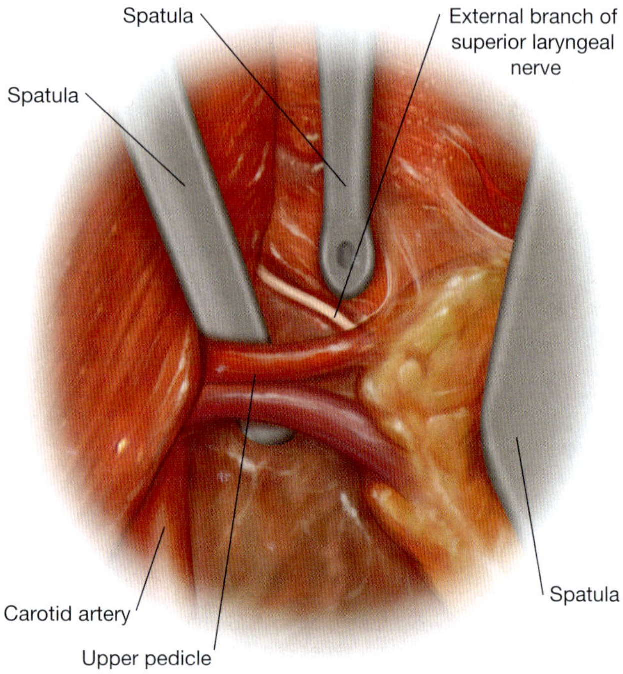

FIG 8 ● Identification of the external branch of the superior laryngeal nerve: The vessels (right side) are prepared by retracting downward and medially the thyroid lobe by means of the retractor and the spatula. A further spatula can be used to pull the vessels laterally. This will allow the external branch of the superior laryngeal nerve (SLN) to be easily identified during most procedures.

thyroid lobe and trachea in order to better visualize the upper portion of the operative space where the superior thyroid vein and artery are running.

- The upper pedicle is then prepared by retracting downward and medially the thyroid lobe by means of the retractor and the spatula. A further spatula can be used to pull the vessels laterally. This will allow the external branch of the superior laryngeal nerve to be easily identified during most procedures (**FIG 8**). Its injury can be avoided by keeping the inactive blade of Harmonic® in the posterior position so as to not transmit the heat to this delicate structure. At this point in time, section of the upper pedicle can be obtained by harmonic scalpel en bloc or selectively, depending on the diameter of the single vessels and/or the anatomic situation (**FIG 9**).

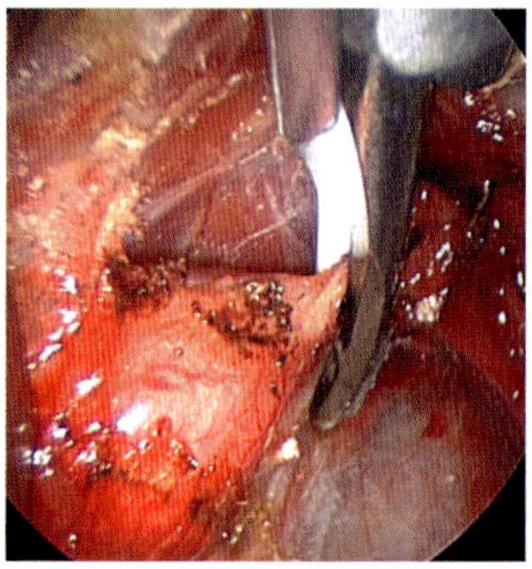

FIG 9 ● Section of the upper pedicle (left side) by harmonic scalpel. The inactive blade must be on the larynx in order to avoid any injury on laryngeal muscles and superior laryngeal nerve.

INFERIOR LARYNGEAL NERVE AND PARATHYROID GLANDS IDENTIFICATION AND DISSECTION

- After retracting medially and lifting up the thyroid lobe, the fascia can be opened by a gentle spatula retraction. During this step, the endoscope should be repositioned in an orthogonal axis with the thyroid lobe and trachea, looking downward with its 30-degree angle (**FIG 10**). The recurrent laryngeal nerve appears generally at this point in time, lying in the thyrotracheal groove, posterior to the Zuckerkandl tuberculum (posterior lobe), which is an important landmark in this step. This way, the recurrent nerve and the parathyroid glands are dissected and freed from the thyroid (**FIG 11A,B**).
- Dissection of the entire nerve from the mediastinum to its entrance into the larynx is not mandatory and might result in a time waste during the endoscopic phase. It is correct and very safe to identify the laryngeal nerve, to free it from the thyroid capsule as much as possible, but it is important to stress that the complete dissection of the nerve can be more easily obtained during the subsequent step, under direct vision, when the thyroid lobe has already been extracted.
- Both parathyroid glands are generally easily visualized during the endoscopic step; thanks to the camera magnification. Their vascular supply is preserved by selective division of the branches of the inferior thyroid artery. During dissection, when dealing with large vessels or small vessels close to the nerve, hemostasis can be achieved by 3-mm titanium vascular clips.

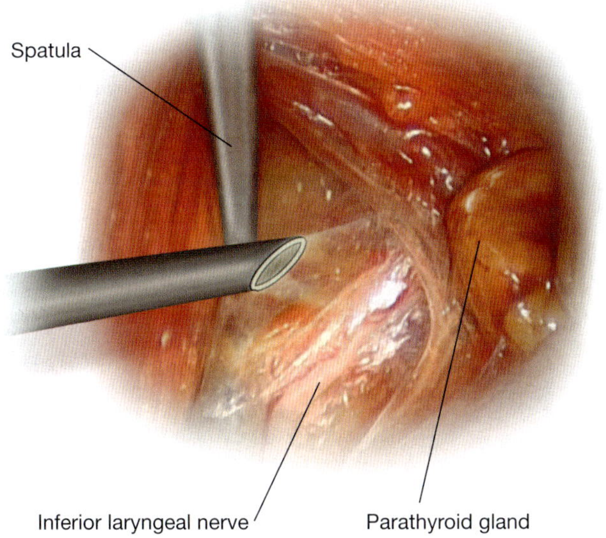

FIG 10 ● Inferior laryngeal nerve and parathyroids dissection: During this step, the endoscope should be repositioned in an orthogonal axis with the thyroid lobe and trachea, looking downward with its 30-degree angle.

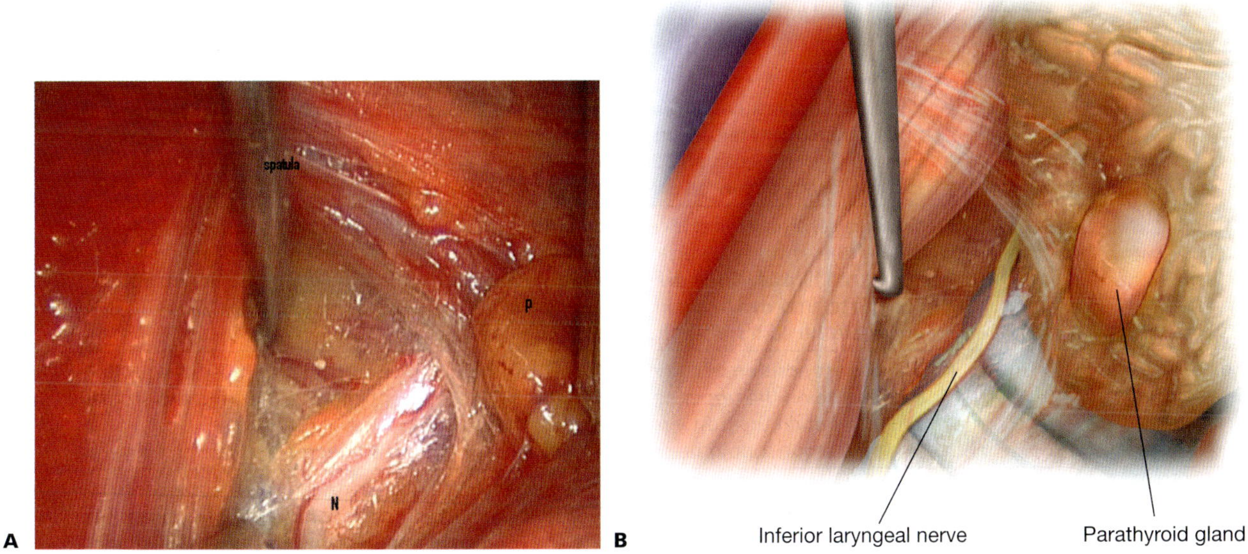

FIG 11 ● **A.** Endoscopic vision: dissection of the inferior laryngeal nerve. The recurrent laryngeal nerve *(n)* appears lying in the thyrotracheal groove. Parathyroid gland is also well visible *(p)*. **B.** Illustration of this step.

EXTRACTION OF THE LOBE AND RESECTION

- At this point in time, the lobe is completely freed. The endoscope and the retractors can be removed and the upper portion of the gland rotated and pulled out using conventional forceps. A gentle traction over the lobe allows the complete exteriorization of the gland (**FIG 12**). The operation is now conducted as an open surgery under direct vision. The lobe is freed from the trachea by ligating the small vessels and dissecting the Berry ligament. It is very important to check once again the laryngeal nerve at this point in time, so to avoid its injury before the final step. The isthmus is then dissected from the trachea and divided. After completely exposing the trachea, the lobe is finally removed.

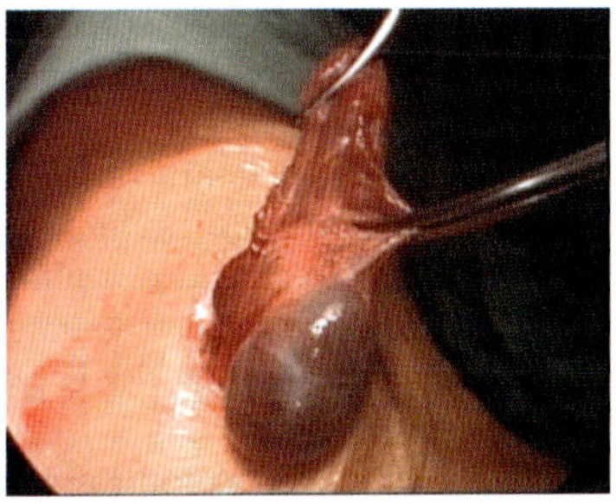

FIG 12 ● Thyroid lobe extraction. A gentle traction over the lobe allows the complete exteriorization of the gland.

CLOSURE

- Drainage is not necessary. The midline is then approached by a single stitch; platysma is closed by a subcuticular suture and a cyanoacrylate sealant is used for the skin (**FIGS 13** and **14**).

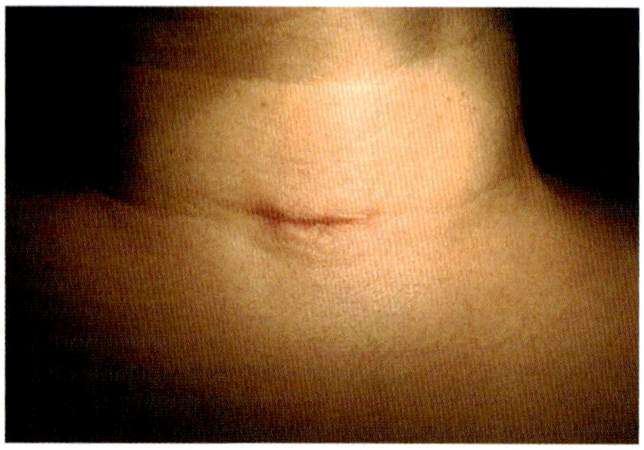

FIG 13 ● Skin is reapproximated and closed by means of glue.

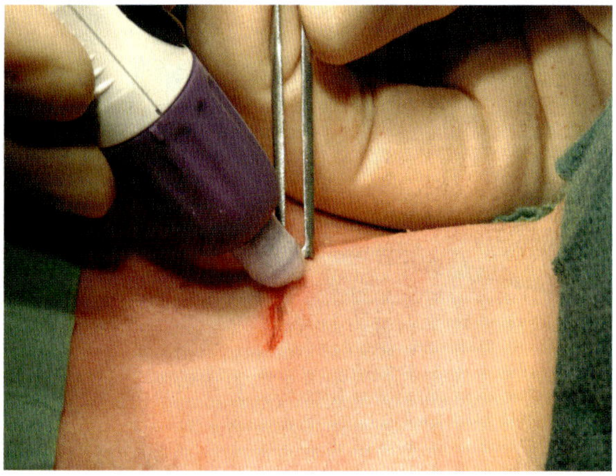

FIG 14 ● MIVAT: final result.

PEARLS AND PITFALLS

Indications	■ Perform preoperative ultrasound in order to evaluate thyroid volume (less than 25 mL) and nodule diameter (less than 3 cm). ■ Exclude thyrotoxicosis and acute thyroiditis ■ Exclude locally advanced or metastatic carcinoma
Incision	■ Create a central cervical incision two fingers above the sternal notch in order to easily allow for eventual conversion to cervicotomy. ■ Use a thin film of sterile drape on the electrocautery blade, leaving just the tip able to coagulate, in order to avoid damage to the skin or the superficial planes. ■ Avoid any bleeding from the anterior jugular veins.
Section of upper pedicle	■ The correct position of the retractors (both the first one on the strap muscles and the second one on the upper part of the thyroid lobe) is very important during this step, in order to obtain the best visualization of the vessels. ■ The endoscope should be rotated 180 degrees with the 30-degree tip looking upward.
Recurrent laryngeal nerve dissection	■ Avoid electrocautery (bipolar or monopolar) until both laryngeal nerves have been exposed. The Harmonic® device is used for almost all the vascular structures; but if the vessel is running particularly close to the inferior laryngeal nerve, then hemostasis is achieved by means of small vascular clips.
Closure	■ Close the midline with one single stitch, leaving some space in between the strap muscles, allowing quick blood evacuation in case of compressive hematoma.

POSTOPERATIVE CARE

- After surgery, patients undergoing MIVAT require strict observation during the first 5 to 10 hours on the ward. Dysphonia, airway obstruction, and neck swelling must be carefully checked. No drain is left, so careful surveillance for postoperative hematomas is required during the immediate postoperative period. Postoperative bleeding risk is very low and dramatically decreases after 5 hours.
- In case of postoperative hematoma, if compressive symptoms and airway obstruction are present, reintervention and immediate hematoma evacuation is required.
- Patients can start oral intake on the evening of the operative day and will be discharged the day after. On the first and second postoperative days, serum calcium must be checked in order to control hypoparathyroidism by substitutive therapy, as described in Table 1.
- Wound care is not really necessary after MIVAT because of the glue covering the skin, and postoperative pain will be controlled by means of both intravenous (IV) or oral analgesics.
- Voice impairments and subjective or objective dysphonia requires an immediate postoperative vocal cord check by an otolaryngologist. In the case of a normal postoperative course, a vocal cord check can be delayed until after 3 months.

Table 1: Management of Postoperative Hypocalcemia

Management of Hypocalcemia following Thyroidectomy on the First Postoperative Day	
Acute symptomatic	Calcium gluconate IV
Asymptomatic calcium ≤7.5 mg/dL[a]	Calcium (3 g) + vitamin D (0.5 μg) per os daily
Asymptomatic calcium 7.5–7.9 mg/dL	Calcium (1.5 g) per os daily

[a]*Normal range: 8 to 10 mg/dL.*

COMPLICATIONS

- Transient hypoparathyroidism and definitive hypoparathyroidism
- Transient monolateral inferior laryngeal nerve palsy and definitive monolateral inferior laryngeal nerve palsy
- Transient bilateral inferior laryngeal nerve palsy and definitive bilateral inferior laryngeal nerve palsy
- Hematoma (subcutaneous-conservative treatment; below strap muscles-reoperation)
  - Seroma
  - Wound infection

REFERENCES

1. Miccoli P, Materazzi G. Minimally invasive video assisted thyroidectomy (MIVAT). *Surg Clin North Am.* 2004;84:735–741.
2. Miccoli P, Elisei R, Materazzi G, et al. Minimally invasive video assisted thyroidectomy for papillary carcinoma: a prospective study about its completeness. *Surgery.* 2002;132:1070–1074.
3. Miccoli P, Pinchera A, Materazzi G, et al. Surgical treatment of low- and intermediate-risk papillary thyroid cancer with minimally invasive video-assisted thyroidectomy. *J Clin Endocrinol Metab.* 2009;94(5):1618–1622.

Chapter 40 Lymph Node Dissection in Thyroid Cancer

Gerard M. Doherty

DEFINITION

- Most thyroid cancer develops from the follicular cells of the thyroid gland (differentiated thyroid cancer includes papillary and follicular subtypes).
- Rare thyroid cancers develop from the C cells of the thyroid gland (medullary thyroid cancer).
- Thyroid cancer of any subtype can be associated with lymph node metastases in the neck.
- Clinical circumstances can indicate the need for cervical lymphadenectomy either as a therapeutic intervention for known metastases or as a prophylactic procedure for the diagnosis or therapy of occult metastases.
- The lymph node compartments of the neck are divided into "levels" to allow communication of the affected and dissected areas (**FIG 1**).
  - Level 6 is also known as the central neck and includes the lymph nodes medial to the carotid sheath on each side and bounded by the hyoid bone superiorly and the sternum inferiorly.
  - Levels 1 through 5 are also known as the lateral neck and include all of the node compartments lateral to the carotid sheath on each side.

PATIENT HISTORY AND PHYSICAL FINDINGS

- Thyroid cancer lymph node metastases can be palpable or, more often, nonpalpable but identifiable by imaging. Very small foci of thyroid cancer in lymph nodes may only be evident at microscopic pathology examination.

IMAGING AND OTHER DIAGNOSTIC STUDIES

- Patients with thyroid cancer should each have a staging ultrasound examination prior to operation.[1] This allows mapping of the lymph node status of each compartment in the neck (**FIG 2**).
- The level 6 lymph nodes are the most difficult to evaluate by ultrasound when the thyroid gland is still present, as these structures are in the same compartment.
- Patients with large tumors or gross adenopathy may be best studied by computed tomography (CT) scan with contrast or magnetic resonance scanning, as these modalities allow better examination of the areas low in the neck that may be obscured by gross disease on ultrasound (**FIG 3**).

SURGICAL MANAGEMENT

- Dissection of the level 6 lymph nodes is generally performed in conjunction with total thyroidectomy.
- The level 6 lymph nodes are removed by clearing the soft tissue that surrounds the thyroid gland. No additional incision or mobilization is necessary.
- Clearing these level 6 nodes involves additional manipulation of the soft tissue and vascular supply that surrounds the parathyroid glands. With these glands at additional risk of being damaged during operation, the performance of parathyroid autograft is particularly important to avoid permanent hypoparathyroidism[2] (**FIG 4**).

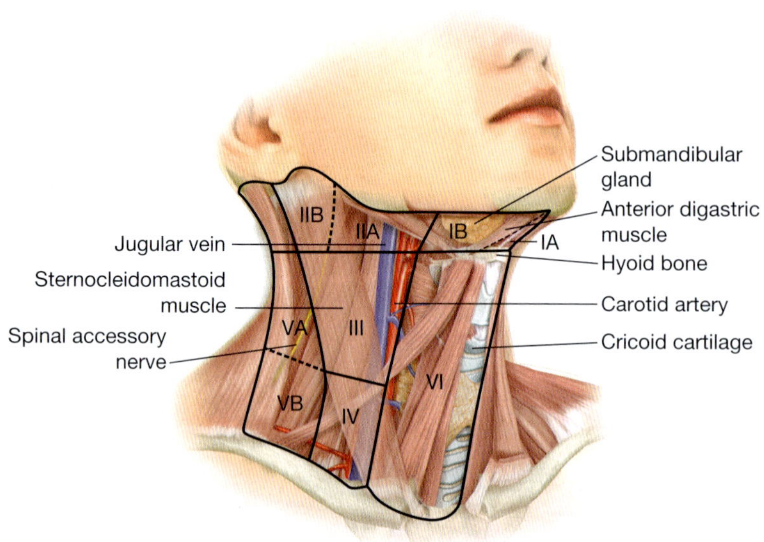

FIG 1 • Lymph node levels in the neck.

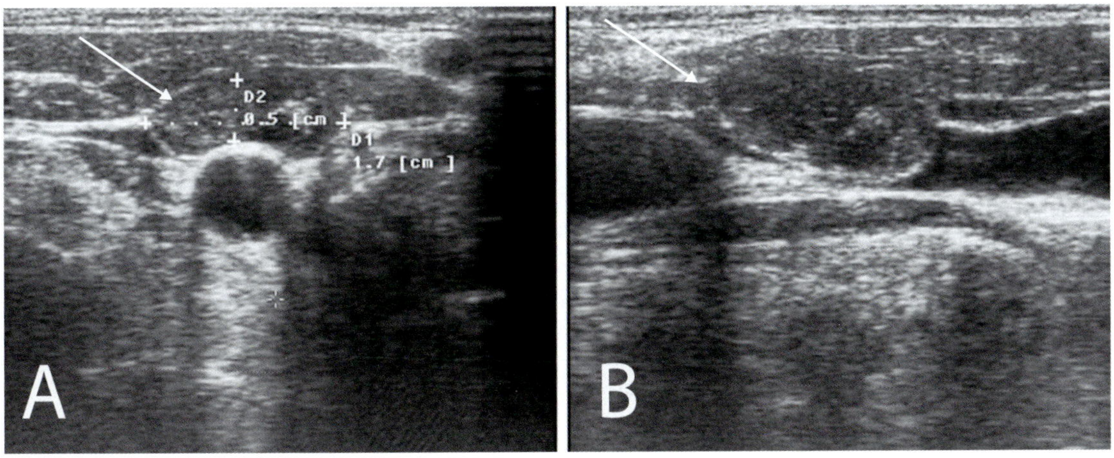

FIG 2 • Ultrasound demonstration of metastatic lymph nodes in thyroid cancer. **Panel A** shows a transverse view *(arrow)*, and **panel B** shows the longitudinal view *(arrow)*.

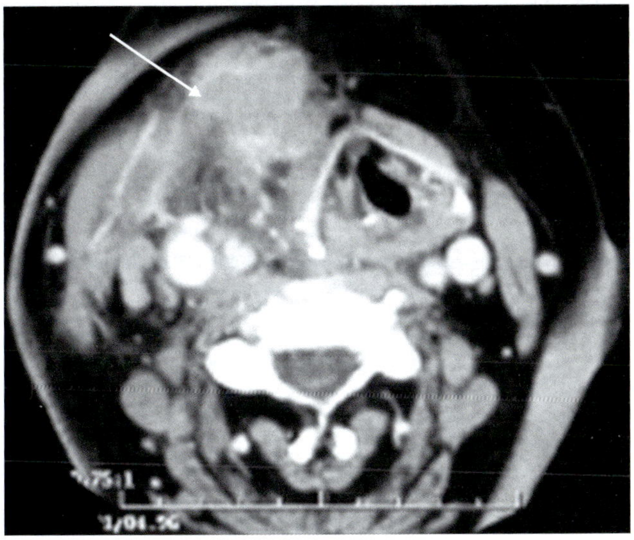

FIG 3 • CT scan of recurrent nodal disease in the lateral neck impinging upon the central compartment *(arrow)*. CT is useful in this instance as ultrasound cannot completely define the anatomy.

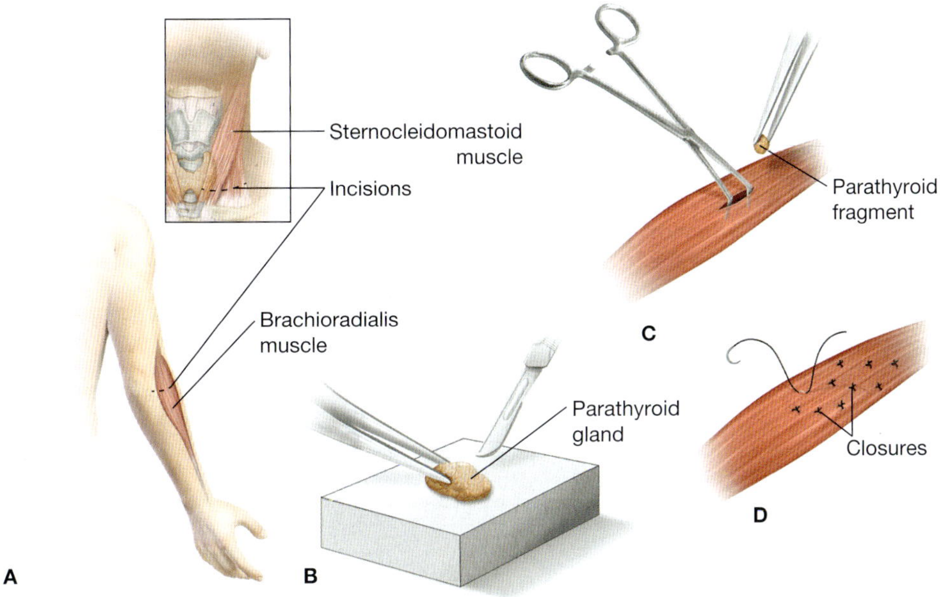

FIG 4 • Schematic of parathyroid autograft. If a parathyroid gland has been devascularized during dissection, then the best management is parathyroid autograft. **A.** Parathyroid glands can be grafted into any muscle; common choices include the neck muscles for normal glands and the brachioradialis muscle for abnormal glands. **B.** The gland should be minced into small pieces (1- to 2-mm in each dimension). **C,D.** The fragments are placed into individual muscle pockets. The pockets are secured with a stitch. The grafts typically require 10 to 12 weeks before measurable function.

Preoperative Planning

- Review of the preoperative ultrasound findings is critical to the proper inclusion of all suspicious lymph nodes.
- Especially in reoperations, ultrasound in the operating room after the induction of anesthesia and positioning can be helpful to localize small lymph nodes.
- A nerve stimulating and monitoring system can be helpful and is commonly used to identify and to test function of motor nerves during dissection. Testing of the vagus nerve is probably best accomplished by using a specialized nerve stimulator that includes electromyography (EMG) monitoring pads on the endotracheal tube to detect vocalis muscle contraction. Testing of motor nerves for which the enervated muscle is visible can be done with a simple nerve stimulator.

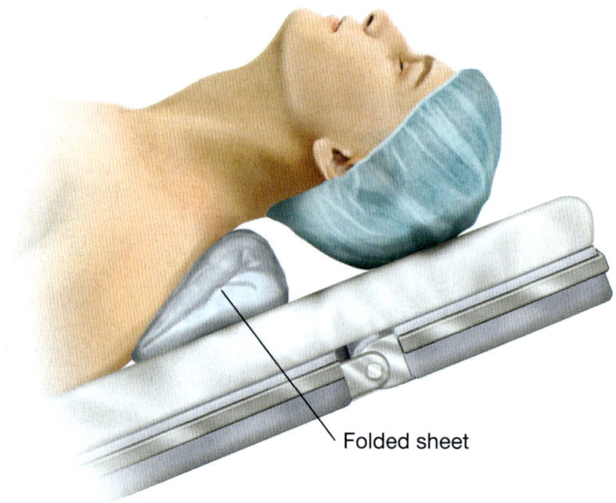

FIG 5 • Position of the neck should emphasize extension, but support. Overextension of the neck or lack of support for the head and neck can cause avoidable posterior neck stiffness postoperatively.

Positioning

- The patient should be supine and the head may be raised above the heart to decrease venous congestion in the neck (**FIG 5**).
- Airway management is of particular concern. Preoperative anesthesiology consultation should alleviate positioning concerns while ensuring proper airway safety during the procedure.
- A towel roll or thyroid air pillow can be placed beneath the shoulder blades to facilitate neck extension.
- Arms should be tucked.

TECHNIQUES

INCISION

- If a thyroidectomy is performed during the same anesthetic, the incision is extended laterally toward the posterior aspect of the neck; if not, then the dissection can generally be completed through a transverse incision at the level of the lower edge of the cricoid cartilage from the edge of the trachea to the anterior border of the trapezius muscle. The goal is to provide exposure of the anterolateral neck and posterior triangles.

RAISING SKIN AND PLATYSMA MUSCLE FLAPS

- Flaps are made superiorly, inferiorly, and posteriorly (**FIG 6**). The flaps should be in a plane superficial to the external jugular vein and should extend broadly over the compartments to be dissected. The facial vein can be divided and retracted superiorly. This has some benefit to retract and protect the marginal mandibular branch of the facial nerve. Erb's point can be identified as the area where the greater auricular nerve comes around the posterior edge of the sternocleidomastoid (SCM) muscle. This site is important to identify in order to protect the superficial sensory nerves that converge at that site.

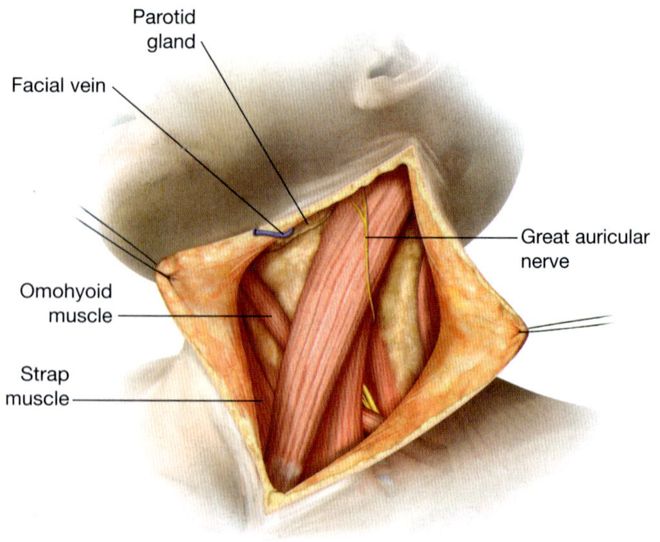

FIG 6 • The subplatysmal flaps should be generous to avoid struggling at the margins of dissection later in the case.

MOBILIZING THE STERNOCLEIDOMASTOID MUSCLE

- The fascia over the middle of the SCM muscle is incised longitudinally with careful preservation of the greater auricular nerve.
- The fascia is then stripped from the muscle over a broad area, unwrapping the muscle and following the fascial plane around the front edge of the muscle to its deep surface. The plane is continued deep to the muscle back to its posterior edge.
- The sensory nerves at Erb's point (greater auricular, lesser occipital, transverse cervical, and supraclavicular) are all preserved.
- The SCM muscle is encircled with a Penrose drain for traction to provide exposure (**FIG 7**).
- The omohyoid muscle is divided to improve exposure of the underlying nodal packet.

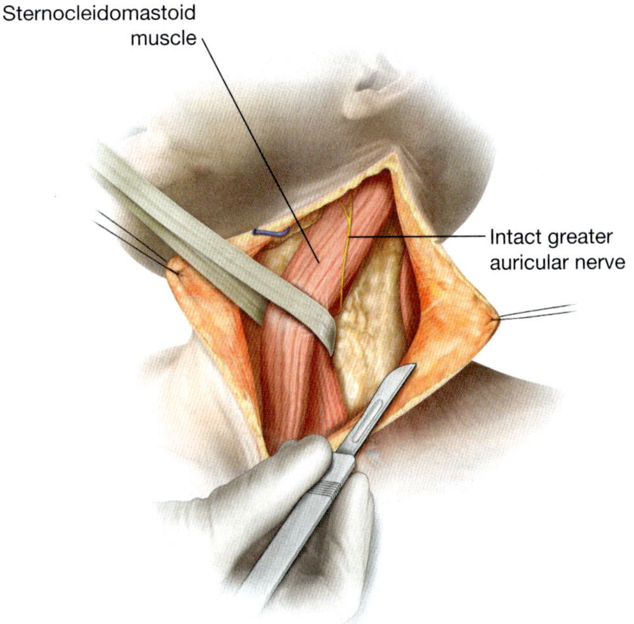

FIG 7 ● Once the SCM muscle has been mobilized, the fascia over the node packet can be incised laterally. This will allow separation of the fatty soft tissue from the anterior edge of the trapezius muscle. Great care is needed to identify the spinal accessory nerve without injury.

DISSECTION OF SOFT TISSUE SPECIMEN

- Dissection of the nodal packet can be initiated in a number of places (**FIG 8**). The posterior triangle is a common choice. The superficial fascia along the anterior edge of the trapezius muscle is carefully incised along the muscle edge to avoid inadvertent division of the spinal accessory motor nerve.
- The nodal packet attachments to the trapezius are taken down initially with blunt dissection, especially prior to identification of the spinal accessory nerve. Unless there is direct involvement of the nerve by tumor, the nerve should be preserved.
- The specimen is dissected from lateral to medial with attention to the underlying structures.
    - The supraclavicular sensory nerves fan out from Erb's point and divide the level 5 specimen into superficial and deep components. Removal of all nodes with preservation of the major branches of these nerves requires recognition of this and careful dissection.
- Once the dissection reaches the area deep to the SCM muscle, the jugular nodes (levels 2 to 4) are dissected either starting from the top (level 2) or the bottom (level 4) of the jugular chain, removing these nodes en bloc with the posterior triangle specimen.
- The jugular vein is generally preserved unless there is involvement of the vein by direct invasion or tumor thrombus. If the vein cannot be preserved, it is included in the specimen. There is no morbidity of including this in a unilateral dissection.
- The specimen is removed en bloc, marked, and prepared for pathologic examination.

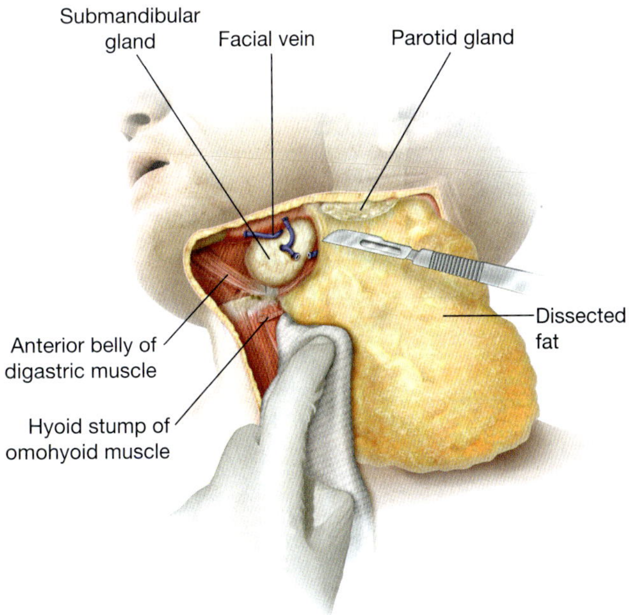

FIG 8 ● The dissection progresses with mobilization of the soft tissues away from the jugular vein (SCM not shown).

INSPECTION AND CLOSURE

- Once the specimen has been removed, the field is carefully inspected for residual soft tissue that can be removed (**FIG 9**). Nerves are tested for confirmation of function findings and hemostasis is ensured. Special inspection at the base of the jugular vein should ensure that there is no evidence of chyle leak.
  - A small drain is often placed to remove serum or chyle that could accumulate. If the operation has been straightforward and the disease burden low, then this may be omitted.
- The wound is closed in two layers, the platysma muscle layer with interrupted absorbable suture and the skin by whatever cosmetically advantageous method the surgeon chooses.

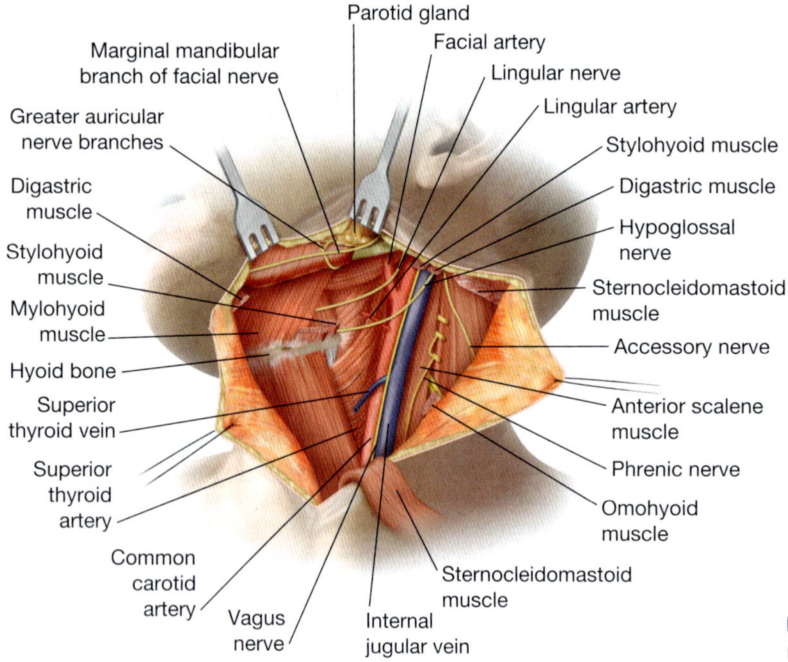

FIG 9 • Anatomy of the neck after the node-bearing soft tissues have been removed.

PEARLS AND PITFALLS

Indications	▪ Prophylactic lateral neck dissection is not generally indicated for thyroid cancer.
Raising of flaps	▪ The flaps plane must be accurately placed deep to platysma and superficial to external jugular vessels.
Mobilizing SCM muscle	▪ Avoid injury to the sensory nerves at Erb's point.
Dissecting specimen	▪ Identify the spinal accessory nerve early to avoid injury.
Ensuring hemostasis	▪ Small venous branches in the soft tissue deep to the clavicle, at the inferior margin of the dissection, can cause bothersome bleeding.
Avoiding chyle leak	▪ Pay careful attention to clear fluid welling up near the inferior-most visible portion of the jugular vein, on either side but especially the left.

POSTOPERATIVE CARE

- Drains should be inspected for lymphatic leak and patients instructed on drain care.
- Drains should be removed once output decreases to 30 mL or less per day.

OUTCOMES

- Functional outcomes are excellent if nerves are preserved.
- A minority of patients requires physical therapy to regain full range of shoulder motion.

COMPLICATIONS

- Nerve injury: spinal accessory nerve; vagus or recurrent laryngeal nerve injury (if central neck dissection is included in the procedure); brachial plexus
- Vascular injury: internal jugular vein; carotid artery causing neck hematoma, which can progress to airway compromise
- Thoracic duct injury leading to lymphatic leak, possibly requiring operative intervention for thoracic duct ligation
- Regional disease recurrence

REFERENCES

1. Cooper DS, Doherty GM, Haugen BR, et al. Revised American Thyroid Association management guidelines for patients with thyroid nodules and differentiated thyroid cancer. *Thyroid*. 2009;19:1167–1214.
2. Doherty GM. Complications of thyroid and parathyroid surgery. In: Mulholland MW, Doherty GM, eds. *Complications in Surgery*. 2nd ed. Philadelphia, PA: Lippincott Williams & Wilkins; 2011:550–566.

Chapter 41

Open Neck Exploration for Primary Hyperparathyroidism

Christopher R. McHenry

DEFINITION

- An open neck exploration for hyperparathyroidism (HPT) is defined as exposure of an abnormal parathyroid gland or glands using standard operative techniques through a single incision without endoscopic or videoscopic assistance. This includes bilateral neck exploration for patients with multiglandular disease and unilateral focused parathyroidectomy with intraoperative parathyroid hormone (PTH) monitoring for a single adenoma localized preoperatively.

DIFFERENTIAL DIAGNOSIS

- Primary HPT and malignancy account for 80% of all causes of hypercalcemia.
- Primary HPT accounts for 50% to 60% of all cases of hypercalcemia diagnosed in an ambulatory setting and approximately 30% of cases diagnosed in a hospital setting.
- There are many less common causes for hypercalcemia (Table 1).
- In patients with primary HPT, 85% to 90% will have a single adenoma, 5% to 10% hyperplasia, 3% to 4% double adenoma, and less than 1% carcinoma.

Table 1: Causes of Hypercalcemia

Hyperparathyroidism
Primary and tertiary
Malignancy
Osteolytic bone metastases
Tumor production of PTH-related polypeptide
Squamous cell carcinoma of the lung
Renal cell carcinoma
Bladder cancer
Hematologic malignancies
Leukemia
Lymphoma
Multiple myeloma
Granulomatous disease
Tuberculosis
Sarcoidosis
Fungal infection
Medications
Calcium
Vitamin A or D intoxication
Lithium
Thiazides
Milk-alkali syndrome
Miscellaneous
Hyperthyroidism
Paget's disease
Immobilization
Familial hypocalciuric hypercalcemia

PTH, parathyroid hormone.

PATIENT HISTORY AND PHYSICAL FINDINGS

- Primary HPT occurs in 1 out of every 500 women and 1 out of every 2,000 men. It most commonly occurs in women between the ages of 50 and 60 years.
- Most patients with primary HPT are diagnosed as a result of the incidental hypercalcemia detected on blood work that is obtained for an unrelated medical problem. Patients often have nonspecific symptoms such as fatigue, weakness, constipation, and depression.
- Patients with primary HPT may present with plethora of clinical manifestations (Table 2). Nephrolithiasis is the most common metabolic complication of primary HPT occurring in 15% to 20% of patients; however, only 2% to 5% of patients with kidney stones have primary HPT.
- Approximately 3% of patients may present with hyperparathyroid crisis manifested by severe hypercalcemia (serum calcium >14 mg/dL), nausea, vomiting, dehydration, and central nervous system dysfunction including coma.[1]
- Primary HPT is associated with a higher risk of cardiovascular disease and mortality that decreases after parathyroidectomy.[2]
- A prior history of head or neck radiation in childhood, radioiodine treatment, and long-term lithium therapy are associated with a greater prevalence of primary HPT.
- In 5% of patients, primary HPT is an inherited syndrome, underscoring the importance of obtaining a thorough family history. Familial HPT is inherited as an autosomal dominant

Table 2: Clinical Manifestation of Primary Hyperparathyroidism

Renal	**Psychiatric**
Nephrolithiasis	Depression
Nephrocalcinosis	Lethargy
Polyuria	Memory loss
Renal insufficiency	Confusion
	Hallucinations
	Coma
Skeletal	**Neuromuscular**
Generalized bone or joint pain	Fatigue
Osteopenia	Weakness
Osteoporosis	Malaise
Gout	
Pseudogout	
Pathologic bone fracture	
Osteitis fibrosa cystica	
Gastrointestinal	**Cardiovascular**
Constipation	Exacerbation of hypertension
Peptic ulcer disease	Cardiac calcification
Pancreatitis	Left ventricular hypertrophy
Nausea	Decreased QT interval
Vomiting	Conduction abnormalities
Abdominal pain	Heart block

Table 3: Familial Hyperparathyroidism

A. Familial isolated hyperparathyroidism

B. MEN I
Primary hyperparathyroidism
Gastroenteropancreatic tumors
Pituitary adenoma
Adrenocortical and thyroid tumors
Lipomas
Meningiomas
Facial angiofibromas
Bronchial, gastric, and thymic carcinoid tumors

C. MEN IIA
Medullary thyroid cancer
Pheochromocytoma
Primary hyperparathyroidism
Lichen planus amyloidosis
Hirschsprung disease

D. Hyperparathyroidism–jaw tumor syndrome
Ossifying fibromas of the mandible or maxilla
Renal cysts, hamartomas, and Wilms tumor
Uterine adenosarcoma, adenofibroma, leiomyoma, adenomyosis, and endometrial hyperplasia

syndrome with primary HPT occurring as an isolated entity or as part of multiple endocrine neoplasia (MEN) I, MEN IIA, or the hyperparathyroidism–jaw tumor syndrome (Table 3). Patients with hyperparathyroidism–jaw tumor syndrome have more severe hypercalcemia and a 10% to 15% incidence of parathyroid cancer.

- In most patients with primary HPT, the physical examination is normal. Less than 5% of patients with primary HPT will have a palpable parathyroid tumor. Patients with hyperparathyroid crisis are more likely to have a palpable neck mass.
- A palpable neck mass in patients with primary HPT should raise suspicion for parathyroid cancer or an associated thyroid nodule.
- Rare patients may have band keratopathy, a condition characterized by calcium phosphate deposition in the cornea, which can be identified by slit lamp examination.

IMAGING AND OTHER DIAGNOSTIC STUDIES

- A diagnosis of primary HPT is made by an elevated serum calcium level and an elevated or inappropriately normal intact serum PTH level.
- Up to 20% of patients have normocalcemic primary HPT with a serum calcium level in the normal range. Most patients with normocalcemic primary HPT are diagnosed as a result of evaluation for kidney stones, osteoporosis, or osteopenia. Vitamin D deficiency, excess phosphate intake, low calcium set point, and hypo- or hypermagnesemia may be contributory factors to normocalcemic HPT.
- Patients with primary HPT may have low or low normal serum phosphate and high serum chloride, alkaline phosphatase, and uric acid levels. Alkaline phosphatase is elevated in patients with bone disease.
- Patients may also have a mild metabolic acidosis, which occurs because of the inhibitory effect of PTH on phosphorus and bicarbonate reabsorption in the kidney.
- Prior to the introduction of sensitive immunoradiometric and chemiluminescence assays for measurement of intact PTH levels, a chloride to phosphorus ratio greater than 33:1 was used to make the diagnosis of primary HPT.
- Blood urea nitrogen, serum creatinine, and glomerular filtration rate should be measured and followed, because renal insufficiency is a known complication of primary HPT.
- Bone mineral density should be measured at the lumbar spine, hip, and distal radius using dual energy x-ray absorptiometry.
- A calcium:creatinine clearance ratio should be determined if familial hypocalciuric hypercalcemia (FHH) is suspected. FHH is a rare autosomal dominant disorder characterized by asymptomatic hypercalcemia, hypocalciuria, and variable PTH elevation that results from a higher renal setpoint for calcium secretion. Patients with FHH have one or more first-degree relatives with hypercalcemia, a calcium:creatinine clearance less than 0.01, and a 24-hour urine calcium less than 100 mg. Parathyroidectomy is not indicated.
- Once a diagnosis of primary HPT has been established, imaging should be performed to localize an abnormal parathyroid gland or glands. When an abnormal parathyroid gland can be localized preoperatively, a focused parathyroidectomy can be performed with intraoperative PTH measurement to confirm cure of the primary HPT. This minimizes dissection, shortens the operation, and reduces cost.
- Localization studies should only be performed once a diagnosis of HPT has been established and a decision to proceed with surgical therapy has been made. The role of localization studies is to help determine the site of the incision and where in the neck to begin the exploration.
- Office-based, high-resolution ultrasonography is the initial imaging study performed. A parathyroid adenoma appears as a homogeneous, hypoechoic, oval- or bean-shaped mass posterior to the thyroid gland (**FIG 1**). Occasionally, a parathyroid adenoma may be multilobulated. Ultrasound is also of value in identifying concomitant nodular thyroid disease.
- Technetium-99m-sestamibi with single-photon emission computed tomography (SPECT) is a combined functional and anatomic imaging study, which is obtained prior to operation. It is particularly beneficial for identifying ectopic parathyroid glands (**FIG 2**).
- Four-dimensional computed tomography and positron emission tomography/computed tomography (PET/CT) fusion imaging are other potentially valuable imaging studies to help localize abnormal parathyroid glands but are usually reserved for patients with persistent or recurrent HPT.

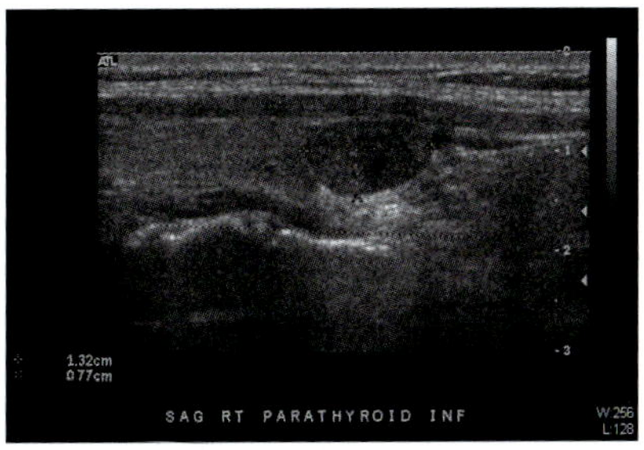

FIG 1 • High-resolution ultrasound image of 1.32 × 0.77 cm homogenous, hypoechoic mass inferior to the right lobe of the thyroid gland in a sagittal view. At operation, this was confirmed to be a right inferior parathyroid adenoma.

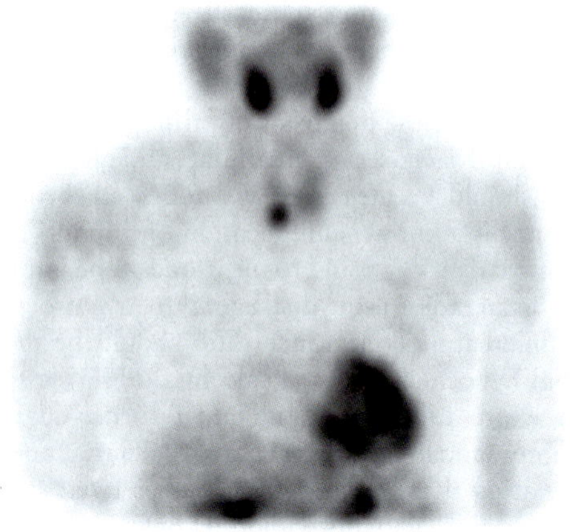

FIG 2 • Technetium-99m-sestamibi image demonstrating abnormal radiotracer accumulation inferior to the inferior pole of the right lobe of the thyroid gland.

- Intraoperative PTH monitoring is most valuable in patients with discordant lesions on ultrasound and technetium-99m-sestamibi. It has been suggested that intraoperative PTH monitoring is unnecessary in patients with concordant lesions detected on ultrasound and technetium-99m-sestamibi imaging.

SURGICAL MANAGEMENT

- All patients with primary HPT should be presented with option of surgical therapy, because parathyroidectomy is the only curative treatment. The classical symptoms of primary HPT (nephrolithiasis, osteoporosis, osteitis fibrosa cystica, and neuromuscular dysfunction) are well-established indications for surgery.
- In patients with asymptomatic primary HPT, indications for surgical therapy have been defined by the 2008 revised consensus guidelines sponsored by the National Institutes of Health[3] (Table 4). Parathyroidectomy is recommended in all patients younger than 50 years of age because at least 25% will develop one or more complications of HPT during their lifetime, which can be irreversible. Significant hypercalcemia, renal dysfunction, reduction in bone mineral density, and inability or unwillingness to participate in subsequent medical surveillance and follow-up are other indications for parathyroidectomy in patients with asymptomatic primary HPT.

Table 4: Indications for Surgical Therapy in Patients with Asymptomatic Primary Hyperparathyroidism as Established by the 2008 Revised National Institutes of Health Consensus Guidelines

Serum calcium >1 mg/dL above the upper limit of the normal range
Glomerular filtration rate <60 mL/min
Decreased bone density: T score of −2.5 or less at lumbar spine, femoral neck, hip, or distal radius
Age <50 years
When routine follow-up and medical surveillance is problematic or not possible

- Open neck exploration for primary HPT is performed as an outpatient procedure under general anesthesia or local anesthesia with sedation. Various intraoperative adjuncts may be used including ultrasound, PTH monitoring, and radio guidance.
- Intraoperative ultrasound may be used to help determine the best site for the incision.
- Intraoperative PTH monitoring may be used to help determine that all hyperfunctioning parathyroid tissue has been excised and to confirm cure of primary HPT.
- Administration of technetium-99m-sestamibi prior to operation and use of a gamma probe intraoperatively is used by some surgeons to help localize abnormal parathyroid tissue and confirm ex vivo that a sestamibi-avid parathyroid gland has been removed and that no sestamibi-avid glands remain in the neck. Some of the limitations of this technique include that hyperplastic parathyroid glands are most often not sestamibi-avid, and thyroid nodules may also retain sestamibi, producing false-positive results.
- For a single adenoma localized preoperatively, a unilateral focused parathyroidectomy with intraoperative PTH monitoring to confirm cure of primary HPT is performed.
- Bilateral neck exploration is indicated for patients with negative preoperative imaging or when bilateral disease is detected preoperatively and for patients with a higher likelihood of multiglandular disease such as patients with MEN I, MEN IIA, or lithium-associated HPT. It may also be necessary for patients with associated thyroid disease. Bilateral neck exploration may also be preferentially used in all patients with primary HPT.
- Patients with a double adenoma are treated with resection of the two enlarged glands.
- Patients with parathyroid hyperplasia are preferentially treated with subtotal parathyroidectomy, leaving a well-vascularized parathyroid remnant that approximates the weight and size of one normal parathyroid gland. A bilateral transcervical thymectomy is also performed because of a 5% to 15% incidence of supernumerary parathyroid glands, which are most commonly found in the thymus. Alternatively, a total parathyroidectomy and parathyroid autotransplantation into the brachioradialis muscle of the nondominant forearm may be performed (see Chapter 42).
- Patients with parathyroid cancer are treated with an en bloc resection of the tumor and the surrounding structures that are invaded. This usually involves resection of the lobe of the thyroid gland and the strap muscles.
- Patients with parathyroid cancer usually present with marked elevation in serum calcium and PTH levels and they may have a palpable neck mass. Parathyroid cancer typically has a gray-white appearance and diagnosis is confirmed by the presence of local invasion of surrounding structures (**FIG 3**).

Preoperative Planning

- Serum levels of 25-hydroxy-vitamin D and alkaline phosphatase are measured preoperatively. Patients with low 25-hydroxy-vitamin D and elevated alkaline phosphatase levels are at increased risk for symptomatic postoperative hypocalcemia.

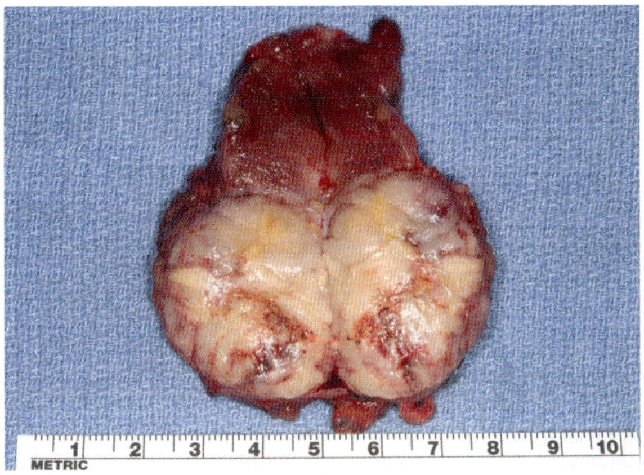

FIG 3 ● A parathyroid cancer with its typical gray-white appearance and the lobe of the thyroid gland, which was invaded by the cancer.

- A sequential compression device is preferably used for prophylaxis against deep vein thrombosis to minimize the risk of postoperative neck hematoma, which may occur with the use of subcutaneous heparin or Lovenox. Routine surgical antimicrobial prophylaxis is unnecessary.
- No special preoperative preparation is required except for patients who present with hyperparathyroid crisis. Hydration with a saline infusion, calciuresis, bisphosphonate therapy, and/or a calcimimetic agent are used to correct severe life-threatening hypercalcemia before proceeding with parathyroidectomy.[1]

POSITIONING

- The patient is positioned on the operating table with a roll placed lengthwise beneath the shoulders, the neck extended, and the head on a soft foam headrest. The patient's arms are tucked at the side (FIG 4).
- The bed is placed in slight reverse Trendelenburg to reduce venous pressure. The ventilatory tubing is directed off the back of the operating table to optimize the working space for the surgeon and assistants (FIG 4).
- The surgical field is widely prepped with ChloraPrep and allowed to dry for 3 minutes before sterile drapes are applied.

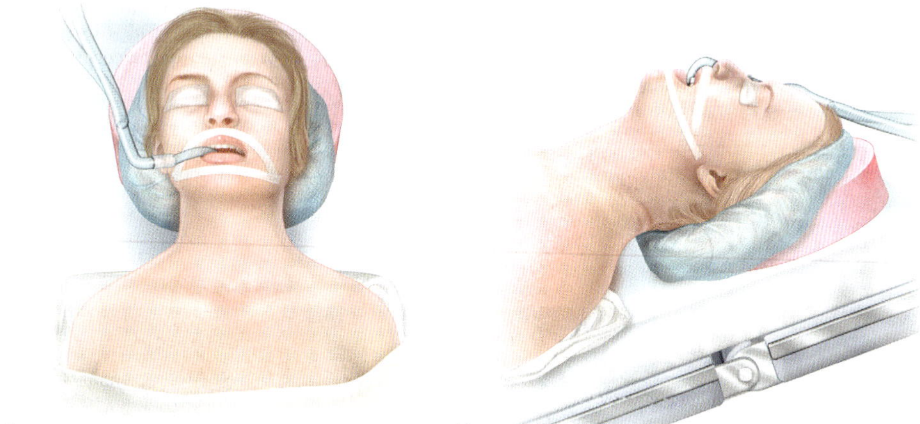

FIG 4 ● Anteroposterior and lateral views of patient who is positioned for parathyroid surgery. The patient's neck is extended with a soft roll placed beneath the shoulder blades and their head positioned on a soft foam pillow. The bed is placed in approximately 30 degrees of reverse Trendelenburg. The ventilator tubing is passed of the head of the bed.

INCISION

- The surface anatomy of the neck is identified before determining the site of the skin incision (FIG 5). For the best cosmetic result, it is often best to mark the site of the incision with the patient standing in the preoperative holding area. This will help to ensure that the incision is within a normal skin crease and is symmetrical. A curvilinear incision is made in the midline of the neck between the cricoid cartilage and the sternal notch.
- The site of the incision is based on preoperative localizing scans, the patient's natural skin creases, and other cosmetic considerations. Intraoperative ultrasound may sometimes be of help to decide the placement of the incision.

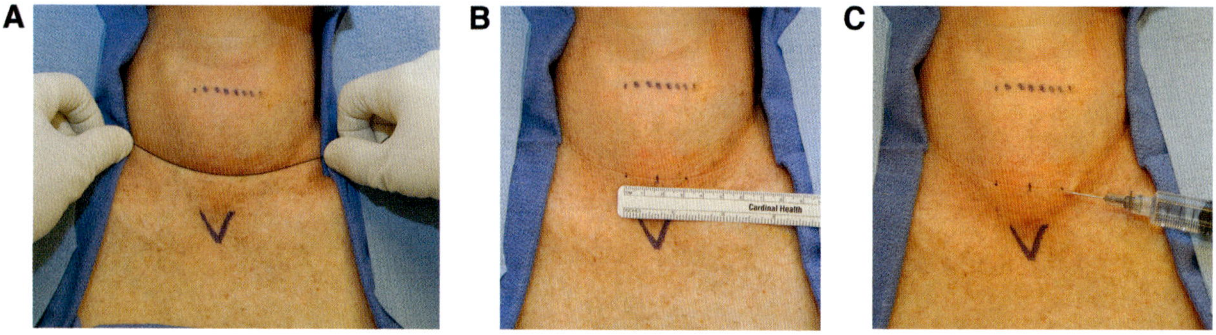

FIG 5 ● **A.** The sternal notch and cricoid cartilage are marked to help decide the most appropriate site for the incision. A 0 silk suture is used to mark the site of the incision. **B.** A 3-cm incision is marked in the midline. **C.** 0.5% Marcaine is used to anesthetize the site of the incision prior to making the incision to establish preoperative analgesia.

- A midline incision is cosmetically preferable and it allows easy access to both sides of the neck for exploration.
- Applying gentle pressure to the neck using a 0 silk suture marks the site of the incision. This is important to maintain symmetry and ensure a curvilinear incision (**FIG 5**).
- The midpoint of the incision is marked on the skin using the midpoint of the sternal notch as a landmark.
- A 2- to 4-cm incision in the midline of the neck is used for parathyroidectomy (**FIG 5**). Patients with a short, thick neck and/or morbid obesity may require a longer incision to improve exposure.
- 0.5% bupivacaine is used to anesthetize the site of the incision prior to making the incision to establish preemptive analgesia (**FIG 5**). This helps enhance patient comfort postoperatively.
- A no. 15 blade scalpel is used to incise the skin. The electrocautery is used to divide the subcutaneous tissue and the platysma muscle.

CREATION OF A WORKING SPACE

- Skin flaps are raised in a subplatysmal plane using skin hooks and small Richardson retractors to elevate the skin (**FIG 6**).
- The anterior jugular veins are identified and the plane of dissection is established immediately anterior to the veins (**FIG 6**).
- The superior skin flap is raised to the prominence of the thyroid cartilage and the inferior skin flap is raised to the sternal notch.
- The sternal heads of the sternocleidomastoid muscle are exposed laterally.

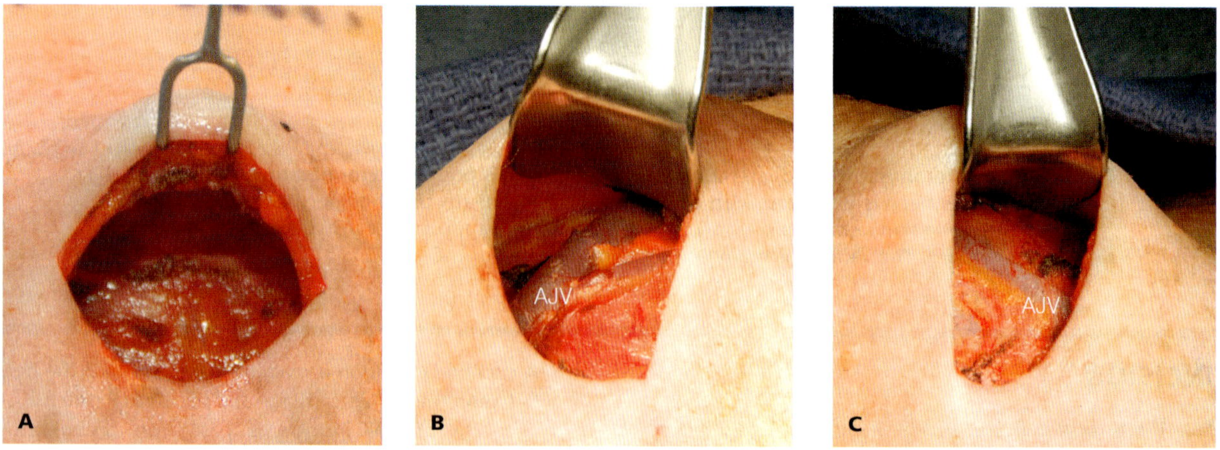

FIG 6 ● **(A)** Superior skin flaps raised in a subplatysmal plane using the anterior jugular veins (**B** and **C**) to create the plane of dissection.

EXPOSURE OF THE THYROID GLAND

- The sternohyoid muscles are separated in the midline along the median raphe with the electrocautery from the sternal notch inferiorly to the thyroid cartilage superiorly (**FIG 7**). The median raphe is an avascular plane consisting of the investing fascia of the thyroid gland.
- Separation of the sternohyoid muscles exposes the thyroid gland.
- The sternothyroid muscle is then dissected and elevated from the surface of the thyroid lobe (**FIG 8**). This is accomplished by blunt and sharp dissection of the intervening loose areolar tissue.

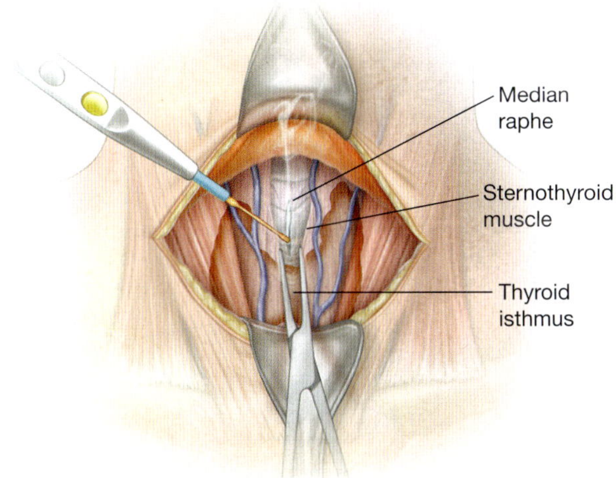

FIG 7 • The sternothyroid muscles are separated along the median raphe to expose the underlying thyroid gland.

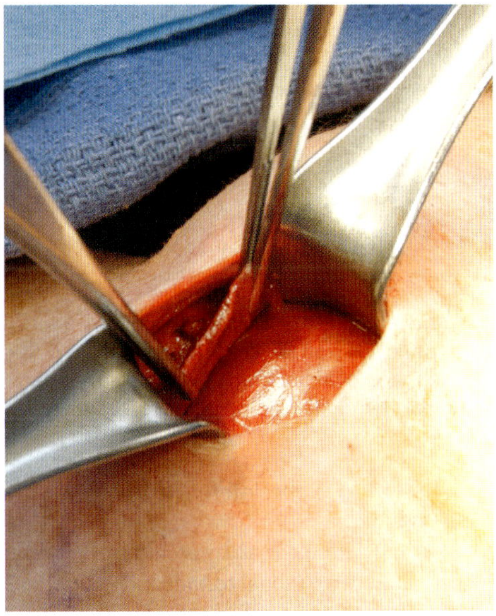

FIG 8 • The sternothyroid muscle is gently retracted with forceps and is freed from the underlying thyroid lobe.

MOBILIZATION OF THE THYROID LOBE AND EXPOSURE OF AN ABNORMAL PARATHYROID GLAND

- The sternothyroid and the sternohyoid muscles are retracted laterally.
- The lobe of the thyroid gland is elevated anteriorly and medially. An Allis clamp applied to the thyroid lobe facilitates retraction and optimizes exposure in a small working space.
- The middle thyroid vein is identified. It may be divided if necessary for improved exposure.
- It is important to maintain a bloodless field. Blood staining of the tissues can make it more difficult to identify normal and abnormal parathyroid tissue.
- The initial search for an abnormal parathyroid gland is based on preoperative localization studies. Exploration of the normal anatomic location for a superior or inferior parathyroid gland is completed first.
- Abnormal parathyroid glands are larger, more firm, and darker in color than normal parathyroid glands (**FIG 9**).
- In adults, a normal parathyroid gland is yellow-tan in color and oval-, spherical- or bean-shaped. It is usually 5 mm in maximum dimension and, on average, weighs 35 to 50 mg (**FIG 10**). In general, there is no need to biopsy a normal-appearing parathyroid gland.
- The normal location for a superior parathyroid gland is posterior and superior to the recurrent laryngeal nerve. It is approximately 1 cm cephalad to the junction of the inferior thyroid artery and the recurrent laryngeal nerve where the recurrent laryngeal nerve enters the

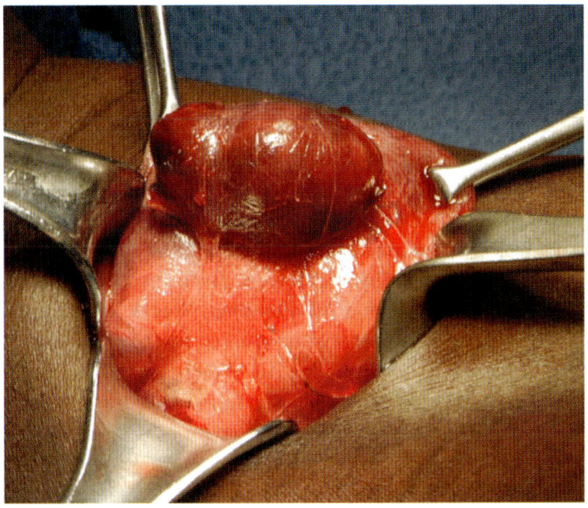

FIG 9 • Anteromedial rotation of the lobe of the thyroid gland to expose a large abnormal parathyroid gland that is firm and dark in color.

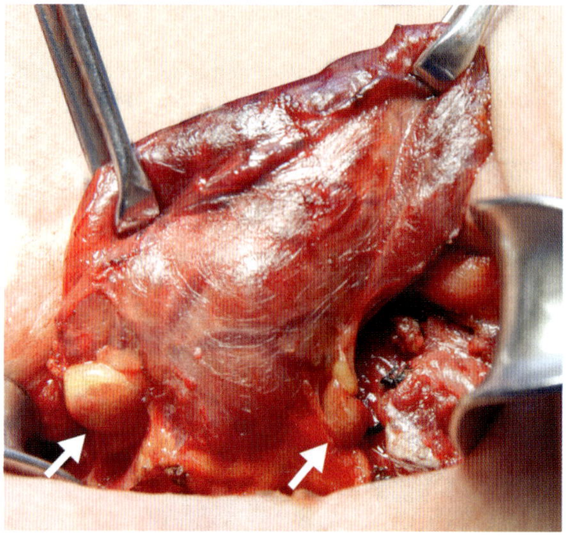

FIG 10 ● Two normal parathyroid glands are seen in their normal anatomic position *(arrows)*. Both have a typical yellow-tan color and are oval in shape. The superior parathyroid gland is surrounded by the adipose tissue.

larynx posterior to the inferior pharyngeal constrictor muscle (**FIG 11**).

- The normal location for an inferior parathyroid gland is approximately 1 cm caudal to the junction of the inferior thyroid artery and the recurrent laryngeal nerve on the posterior lateral aspect of the inferior pole of the thyroid lobe. It is usually anterior to the recurrent laryngeal nerve (**FIG 11**).
- Approximately 16% of patients with primary HPT will have ectopic parathyroid glands.[4] The inferior parathyroid gland is more likely to be in an ectopic location related to its more extensive embryologic migration.
- When a parathyroid gland is not found in its normal anatomic location, a search for an ectopic gland should be completed.
- The most common location for an ectopic inferior parathyroid gland is in the thymus. Other ectopic locations are the thyrothymic ligament, the anterior superior mediastinum, intrathyroidal, the carotid sheath, and undescended in a submandibular location (see Chapter 42 and Chapter 45).
- The most common location for an ectopic superior parathyroid gland is the tracheoesophageal groove. Other ectopic locations are retroesophageal, retropharyngeal, posterior mediastinal, and intrathyroidal.
- A transcervical thymectomy is performed to resect an intrathymic parathyroid adenoma. This is accomplished by exposing the cervical tongue of the thymus beneath the sternothyroid muscle. The thymus is anterior to the inferior thyroid veins and is often immediately adjacent to the inferior pole of the thyroid lobe. The recurrent laryngeal nerve is routinely exposed and dissected into the chest to avoid injury. The connective tissue anterior to the thymus is divided. The thymic veins, which drain into the innominate veins, are divided with an electrothermal bipolar vessel-sealing system. Gentle traction is applied

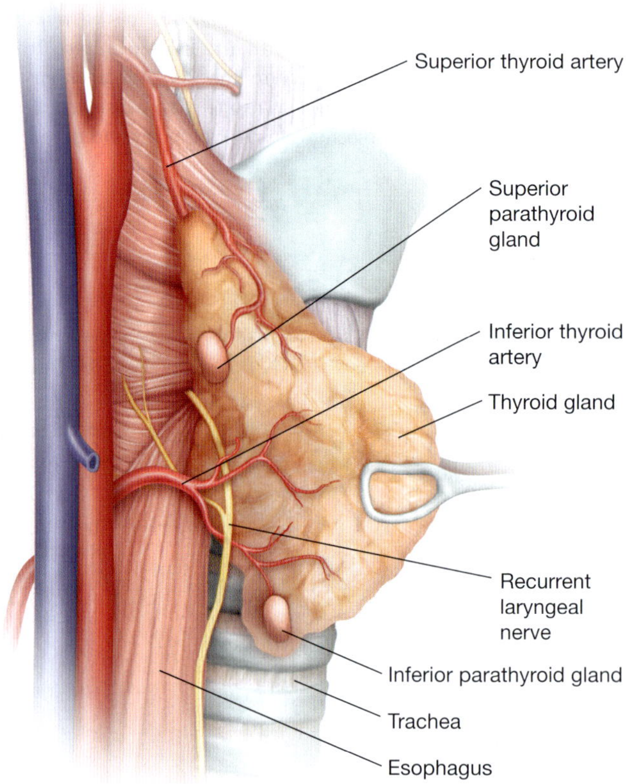

FIG 11 ● Anteromedial rotation of the lobe of the thyroid gland to expose the normal superior and inferior parathyroid glands seen with the right lobe of the thyroid gland retracted anteriorly and medially.

to the cervical tongue of the thymus with a right-angle clamp, progressively elevating more and more of the retrosternal thymic tissue into the operative field.

- An intrathyroidal parathyroid adenoma (**FIG 12**), found in approximately 1% of patients with primary HPT, can usually be enucleated and does not require resection of the lobe of the thyroid gland.

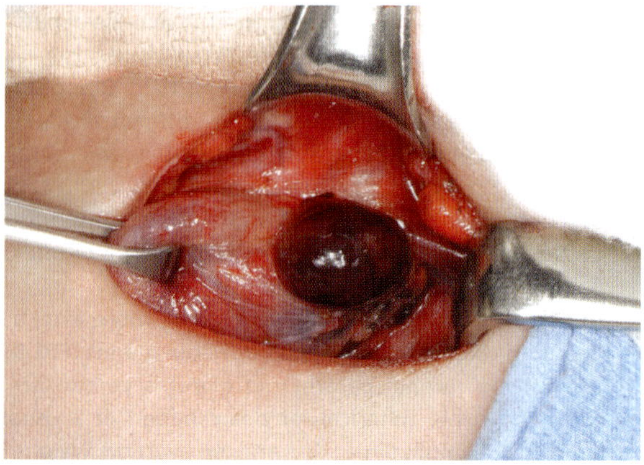

FIG 12 ● Enucleation of an intrathyroidal parathyroid adenoma.

- Division of the superior pole vessels may be helpful when a superior parathyroid gland is not found in its normal anatomic location and it is necessary to search ectopic sites.
- For patients who undergo bilateral neck exploration for multiglandular disease, parathyroid gland location is most often symmetrical.

RESECTION OF AN ABNORMAL PARATHYROID GLAND

- Initially, the enlarged parathyroid gland is dissected anteriorly, laterally, and posteriorly. The medial dissection is left until the end (**FIG 13**).
- An enlarged parathyroid gland is gently mobilized by separating it from the surrounding areolar tissue using blunt dissection with a fine curved hemostat until all that remains is the vascular pedicle.
- Care should be taken to avoid violation of the capsule of the abnormal parathyroid gland, which can lead to parathyroid cell deposition into the soft tissue or parathyromatosis, which is a cause for recurrent HPT.
- The surgeon should always be aware of the recurrent laryngeal nerve, but it is not necessary to routinely expose it nor is nerve monitoring necessary during parathyroidectomy. This is left up to surgeon discretion.
- Care should be taken to stay close to the enlarged parathyroid gland when it is being dissected to avoid injury to the recurrent laryngeal nerve.
- Exposure of the recurrent laryngeal nerve is more often necessary when searching for and removing an enlarged superior parathyroid gland. The superior parathyroid gland is usually posterior to the recurrent laryngeal nerve and the nerve may need to be dissected to resect the gland.
- After mobilization of a parathyroid adenoma has been completed and prior to ligating the vascular pedicle, 3 mL of blood is obtained from the internal jugular vein, a peripheral vein or an arterial line for intraoperative PTH monitoring (**FIG 14**). The vascular pedicle is then ligated and divided and the enlarged parathyroid gland is weighed and submitted to pathology for paraffin evaluation. An additional 3 mL of blood is obtained 5 and 10 minutes after resection of an abnormal parathyroid gland for intraoperative PTH measurement.
- A more than 50% decline in PTH compared to the pre-excision or preoperative PTH value is predictive of cure, although a more than 50% decline compared to the preoperative value is preferred before deciding that no additional exploration is necessary. Because of some variability in the half-life of intact PTH, which is normally between 3 and 5 minutes, it may be necessary to obtain an additional intact PTH level before making a decision to proceed with additional exploration. Intact PTH levels that fail to decline by more than 50% suggest that there is persistent hyperfunctioning parathyroid tissue.
- Frozen section exam of an excised parathyroid adenoma is unnecessary if intraoperative PTH monitoring is used. Frozen section exam may be of value to distinguish normal or hyperplastic parathyroid tissue from nodal or thyroid tissue. It may also be useful in patients who undergo thyroidectomy for a nodule with an inconclusive fine needle aspiration biopsy or an incidentally discovered thyroid nodule that has not been previously biopsied.

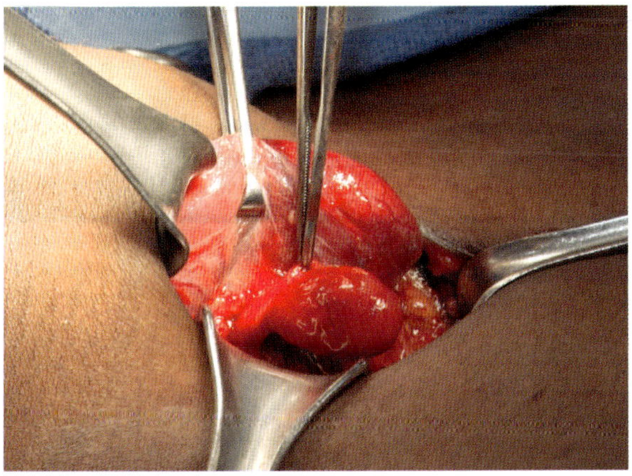

FIG 13 • A large, superior parathyroid adenoma that has been completely mobilized and all that remains is the medial vascular pedicle.

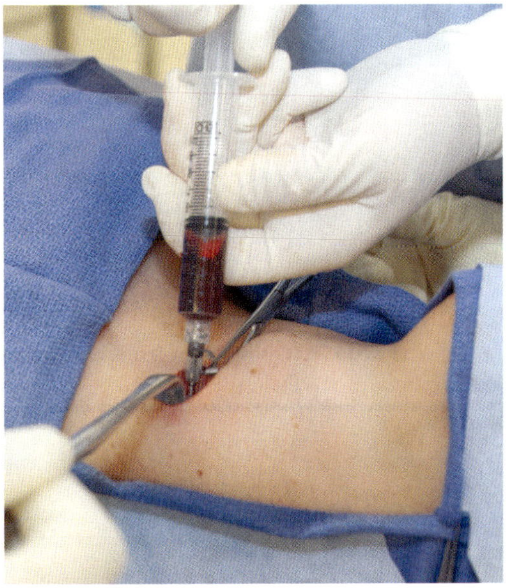

FIG 14 • Blood is obtained from the internal jugular vein for intraoperative PTH monitoring. The thyroid lobe is retracted with an Allis clamp. The strap muscles are retracted laterally and the common carotid artery is identified. The internal jugular vein is anterior and lateral to the common carotid artery.

SURGICAL SITE CLOSURE

- The surgical site is closed while awaiting the results of the intraoperative PTH measurements, which have a minimum 20-minute turnaround time. The wound is examined for hemostasis. Venipuncture sites in the internal jugular vein close with some brief, gentle pressure.
- The sternohyoid muscles are reapproximated in the midline with a running absorbable suture, leaving a 3-cm opening at the inferior aspect of the incision (**FIG 15**). This is done to prevent blood from collecting in an enclosed space if bleeding should occur postoperatively. It allows the blood to drain into the subcutaneous space, delaying the onset of respiratory compromise, which occurs from impairment of the venous return from the larynx and laryngeal edema.
- The subcutaneous tissue is reapproximated with absorbable suture. The skin is closed with absorbable suture placed in a subcuticular fashion and Mastisol and Steri-Strips or Dermabond is applied (**FIG 16**).

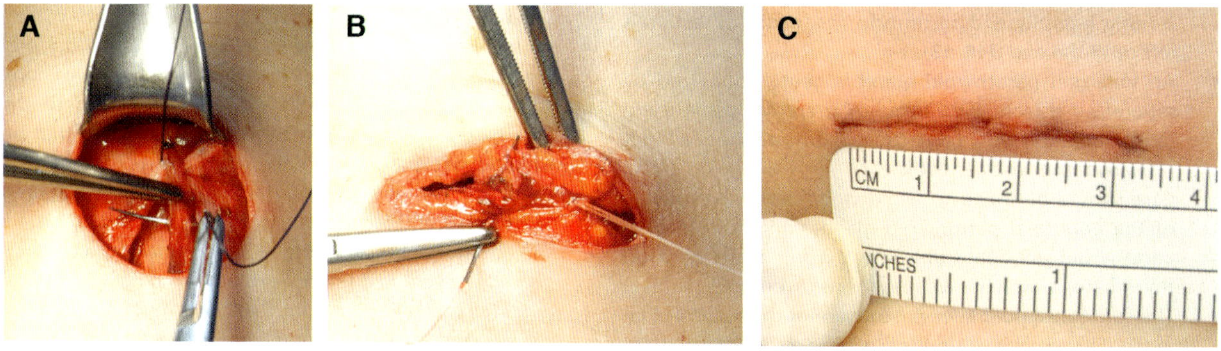

FIG 15 ● **A.** The sternohyoid muscles are reapproximated in the midline with a running absorbable suture. **B.** The subcutaneous tissue is reapproximated in the midline with interrupted absorbable suture. **C.** The skin is closed with an absorbable suture placed in a subcuticular fashion.

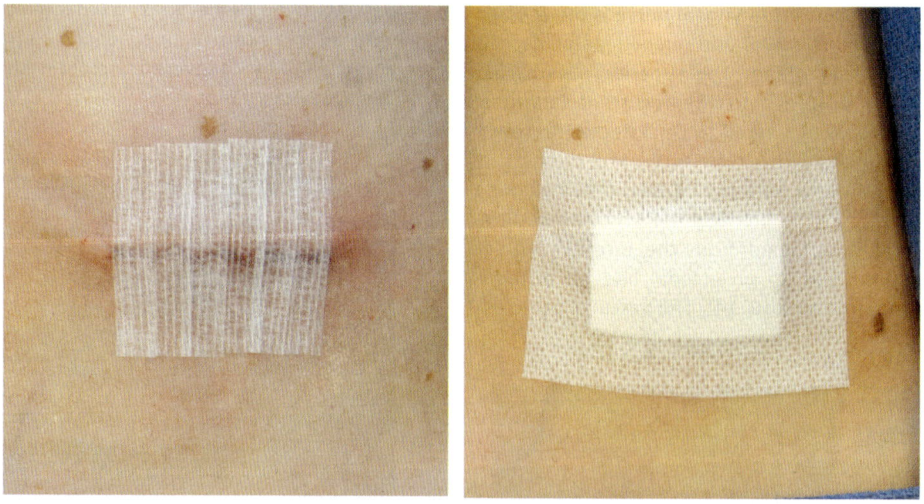

FIG 16 ● Mastisol, Steri-Strips, and a dressing are applied. Alternatively, Dermabond may be used.

PEARLS AND PITFALLS

Incision	■ For the best cosmetic result, mark the site of the incision with the patient standing in the preoperative holding area. This will help to ensure that the incision is within a normal skin crease and is symmetrical.
Raising skin flaps	■ Use the anterior jugular veins to help develop the skin flaps. For the most part, the plane just anterior to the veins is avascular.
Mobilization of the thyroid lobe	■ Use an Allis clamp to apply traction and elevate the thyroid lobe anteromedially. This will allow you to optimize exposure and use a smaller incision.
Parathyroid dissection	■ An enlarged parathyroid gland is surrounded by areolar tissue anteriorly, laterally, and posteriorly. The vascular pedicle is medial in location. The gland is mobilized primarily by blunt dissection, staying close to the gland to avoid the recurrent laryngeal nerve. The vascular pedicle is ligated last. The capsule of the parathyroid gland should not be violated. This can lead to parathyroid cell implantation in the soft tissues (parathyromatosis) and recurrent HPT.
Ectopic parathyroid glands	■ A gland that is described as inferior on a localizing scan may actually be a superior gland that has descended posteriorly from its normal anatomic location. The most common location for a supernumerary or an ectopic inferior parathyroid gland is in the thymus and is resected by performing a transcervical thymectomy. The most common location for an ectopic superior parathyroid gland is in the tracheoesophageal groove. An intrathyroidal parathyroid adenoma can usually be enucleated and normally does not require thyroid lobectomy.
Multiglandular disease	■ Parathyroid glands are most often symmetrical in location.

POSTOPERATIVE CARE

- Patients are discharged home after routine recovery in the postambulatory care unit. They are instructed to keep their dressing on for 48 hours and keep the Steri-Strips on until they return for their first follow-up visit in 2 weeks.
- Patients are instructed about the potential for neck hematoma and symptoms of hypocalcemia. They are told to come directly to the emergency department if they experience neck swelling that is out of the ordinary or they have difficulty breathing. They are asked to call if they develop symptoms of hypocalcemia and are told to begin oral calcium 500 to 1,000 mg three times daily.
- A serum calcium level is obtained at their first follow-up visit and in 6 months to confirm curative parathyroidectomy. Patients are followed yearly thereafter with a serum calcium level to assess for recurrent disease.

OUTCOMES

- The cure rate for primary HPT with parathyroidectomy performed by an experienced surgeon is 95% to 99%.
- Parathyroidectomy for primary HPT results in improvement in health quality-of-life measures including energy level, muscle strength, fine motor skills, and neurocognitive deficits.[5–7]
- Parathyroidectomy for primary HPT results in improvement of bone density.[8]
- After parathyroidectomy, there is complete resolution of the skeletal abnormalities associated with osteitis fibrosa cystica and the reduced concentrating ability of the renal tubules. In 90% of patients, kidney stone formation resolves.
- Parathyroidectomy may halt progressive and irreversible renal insufficiency and hypertension, although hypertension is unlikely to remit.
- The increased cardiovascular mortality associated with primary HPT is reversed with parathyroidectomy.[2]
- Recurrent HPT, defined as hypercalcemia with an elevated or inappropriately normal serum PTH level that develops 6 months following curative parathyroidectomy, occurs in 1% to 3% of patients.
- Approximately 25% of patients have postparathyroidectomy secondary HPT manifested by a normal serum calcium level with an elevated serum PTH level following curative parathyroidectomy. The pathogenesis is not completely understood. Low vitamin D levels, impaired kidney function, and bone remineralization has been suggested as contributory factors. This entity is important to recognize because it can be confused with recurrent disease, but it is rarely of clinical significance.

COMPLICATIONS

- The potential complications from parathyroidectomy include bleeding with neck hematoma that can lead to acute respiratory compromise, hypocalcemia, permanent hypoparathyroidism, recurrent laryngeal nerve injury, transient thyrotoxicosis, and persistent HPT.
- Recurrent laryngeal nerve injury and significant bleeding and neck hematoma are rare following parathyroidectomy, occurring in less than 1% of patients. They occur less often than in patients who undergo thyroidectomy because there is less tissue dissection—most of which is blunt—and no major vessels are ligated and divided.
- Symptomatic hypocalcemia is uncommon after resection of a single adenoma. Patients with elevated preoperative alkaline phosphatase levels are at higher risk for symptomatic hypocalcemia from "bone hunger" following parathyroidectomy. Patients who undergo subtotal or total parathyroidectomy are at higher risk for developing symptomatic postparathyroidectomy hypocalcemia and permanent hypoparathyroidism.
- Permanent hypoparathyroidism may occur in patients following subtotal parathyroidectomy when the remnant fails and total parathyroidectomy when the autotransplant fails.

- Persistent HPT may occur as a result of an ectopic adenoma, a supernumerary parathyroid gland, unrecognized multiglandular disease in patients with false-positive intraoperative PTH results (>50% decline), and an adenoma in a normal anatomic position unrecognized as a result of surgeon inexperience.
- Transient thyrotoxicosis may occur in one-third of patients following parathyroidectomy. It is thought to be the result of thyroid gland manipulation and it is self-limited. Beta-blocker therapy may be used for patients who are symptomatic.
- Recurrent HPT occurs in 1% to 3% of patients and should raise concern for MEN I or MEN IIA.

REFERENCES

1. Phitayakorn R, McHenry CR. Hyperparathyroid crisis: the use of bisphosphonates as a bridge to parathyroidectomy: a case series and review of the literature. *J Amer Coll Surg*. 2008;206: 1106–1115.
2. Nilsson IL, Yin L, Lundgren E, et al. Clinical presentation of primary hyperparathyroidism in Europe: nationwide cohort analysis on mortality from nonmalignant causes. *J Bone Miner Res*. 2002;17(suppl 2):N68–N74.
3. Bilezikian JP, Khan AA, Potts JT Jr. Guidelines for the management of asymptomatic primary hyperparathyroidism: summary statement from the third international workshop. *J Clin Endocrinol Metab*. 2009;94(2):335–339.
4. Phitayakorn R, McHenry CR. Incidence and location of ectopic abnormal parathyroid tissue. *Am J Surg*. 2006;191:418–423.
5. Pasieka JL, Parsons LL. Prospective surgical outcome study of relief of symptoms following surgery in patients with primary hyperparathyroidism. *World J Surg*. 1998;22:513–519.
6. Roman SA, Sosa JA, Mayes L, et al. Parathyroidectomy improves neurocognitive deficits in patients with primary hyperparathyroidism. *Surgery*. 2005;138:1121–1128; discussion 1128–1129.
7. Edwards ME, Rotramel A, Beyer T, et al. Improvement in the health-related quality-of-life symptoms of hyperparathyroidism is durable on long-term follow up. *Surgery*. 2006;140:655–663.
8. Rubin MR, Bilezikian JP, McMahon DJ, et al. The natural history of primary hyperparathyroidism with or without parathyroid surgery after 15 years. *J Clin Endocrinol Metab*. 2008;93(9):3462–3470.

Chapter 42 Subtotal Parathyroidectomy or Total with Autologous Graft

Brian D. Saunders

DEFINITION

- Parathyroidectomy is a functional surgical procedure performed to remove all or nearly all of a patient's hyperactive parathyroid tissue. Primary hyperparathyroidism is the most common pathologic entity requiring parathyroidectomy. Although roughly 85% to 90% of primary hyperparathyroidism involves a single overactive parathyroid gland, there are somatic, as well as inherited, conditions that result in multiglandular parathyroid pathology.[1] Further, secondary and occasionally tertiary hyperparathyroidism may require surgical resection of more than one parathyroid gland. Subtotal parathyroidectomy is the removal of all but a small portion of one parathyroid gland from the neck. This usually equates to removing three and a half parathyroid glands. The remnant portion of parathyroid tissue is left on its native blood supply and in its normal anatomic position. An alternative to a subtotal resection of parathyroid tissue is a total or complete removal of parathyroid tissue (e.g., all four glands) and the immediate transplantation of autologous parathyroid tissue into a heterotopic position.

DIFFERENTIAL DIAGNOSIS

- The necessity for a multiglandular resection of parathyroid tissue may be recognized preoperatively or intraoperatively. There are a number of etiologies for hyperparathyroidism that are always multiglandular in nature and, as such, would warrant preoperative planning for either a subtotal parathyroidectomy or a total parathyroidectomy with parathyroid autotransplantation. These include multiple endocrine neoplasia (MEN) type I– and type IIa–related primary hyperparathyroidism and secondary hyperparathyroidism related to renal failure. Other pathophysiologic conditions leading to hyperparathyroidism may involve the overactivity of more than one gland. Intraoperative recognition of multiple enlarged glands, or recognition through intraoperative parathormone monitoring data, may lead the surgeon to subtotally resect the parathyroids or perform a total parathyroidectomy with immediate transplant. These include sporadic primary hyperparathyroidism due to multiglandular hyperplasia, lithium-related primary hyperparathyroidism, tertiary hyperparathyroidism, and CDC73-related causes of hyperparathyroidism.[2] This latter category is a familial hyperparathyroidism caused by germline mutations in the CDC73 gene (also known as HRPT2 or parafibromin) and includes familial, isolated hyperparathyroidism and hyperparathyroidism–jaw tumor syndrome.[3]

PATIENT HISTORY AND PHYSICAL FINDINGS

- Hyperparathyroidism is a biochemical diagnosis. The evaluation of a patient for hyperparathyroidism may begin with an incidental note of an elevated calcium level on a laboratory report or with interrogating a patient's calcium level based on the patient's presenting signs or symptoms. Patients with recurrent nephrolithiasis (especially calcium-based kidney stones) or osteoporotic (e.g., fragility or nontraumatic) bone fractures should be evaluated for hypercalcemia and hyperparathyroidism. Other, less specific, symptoms that may warrant a biochemical investigation for hyperparathyroidism include fatigue; musculoskeletal aches and pains; neurocognitive decline; mood lability; abdominal pain; and recurrent, otherwise unexplained, pancreatitis.
- A detailed family history should be sought to evaluate the possibility of an inherited cause of hyperparathyroidism. The patient should be queried about family members with pituitary tumors, other cases of parathyroid disease, medullary thyroid cancer, pheochromocytomas, enteropancreatic neuroendocrine tumors (especially gastrin-producing tumors), and ossifying fibromas of the mandible.
- Patients with suspected inherited causes of hyperparathyroidism should be counseled to seek genetic counseling and testing as this may impact operative planning, future disease surveillance, and the health of relatives.
- Renal-related secondary hyperparathyroidism is a constant and expected biochemical finding in all patients with chronic kidney dysfunction. The degree of hyperparathormonemia is routinely followed by treating nephrologists, especially in patients who have progressed to some form of renal replacement therapy (peritoneal or hemodialysis). National management guidelines exist for the target parathyroid hormone (PTH) level for each stage of chronic kidney disease.[4]
- Physical examination findings for patients with hyperparathyroidism are uncommon. Certainly, the neck of each patient proposed for a parathyroidectomy should be thoroughly examined. The identification of a palpable mass would warrant further imaging investigation. It is distinctly unusual to palpate a parathyroid adenoma. A palpable mass with severe hyperparathyroidism should raise the specter of the unusual entity of parathyroid carcinoma. Often, though, a palpable central neck mass in a patient with hyperparathyroidism is an incidentally discovered thyroid nodule.
- For patients planned to undergo a total parathyroidectomy with immediate autologous parathyroid transplantation, a detailed inspection of the forearms should be undertaken. It is important to note the handedness of the patient, as the parathyroid autograft is usually placed in the nondominant forearm. In patients with preexisting or impending renal failure, note should be made of arteriovenous fistula position. Great care should be taken to avoid injuring a functional fistula or disturbing the bed of a soon-to-be constructed fistula.

IMAGING AND OTHER DIAGNOSTIC STUDIES

- Hyperparathyroidism (whether primary, secondary, or tertiary) is a biochemical diagnosis. This must be made to the satisfaction of the surgeon prior to contemplating any procedure. The surgeon should consider imaging studies only after a diagnosis has been secured and the need for an operation has been established.
- Known multiglandular parathyroid disease processes that will require preoperative planning for a subtotal parathyroidectomy or a total parathyroidectomy with autologous graft do not require parathyroid imaging as both sides of the neck will need to be explored and all four of the parathyroid glands identified.
- High-resolution ultrasonography of the neck (whether performed by the surgeon or a radiologist) is an excellent modality to attempt to localize enlarged parathyroid glands. Parathyroid adenomas appear as hypoechoic, ovoid masses that are separable from the thyroid gland. Upper parathyroid adenomas that lie in the tracheoesophageal groove will often be mobile with graded compression of the ultrasound probe (**FIG 1A,B**). Parathyroid adenomas adjacent to the thyroid can usually be well seen, although ectopic parathyroid adenomas (e.g., posterior to the clavicular heads) may be difficult to visualize due to limitations of the ultrasound waves in travelling through bone. Ultrasonography will also aid in the identification of concurrent thyroid pathology, which may then be dealt with at the time of the parathyroid operation.
- Nuclear medicine parathyroid scans using technetium sestamibi as a tracer can accurately identify overactive parathyroid glands about 85% of the time.[5] When performed with a concurrent single-photon emission computed tomography (SPECT)/computed tomography (CT) scan, this overlay of functional and structural imaging provides an excellent anatomic map of disease localization invaluable to the operating surgeon (**FIG 2A,B**). One caveat is that small parathyroid adenomas in close association with the thyroid gland may be difficult to visualize with this imaging technique.

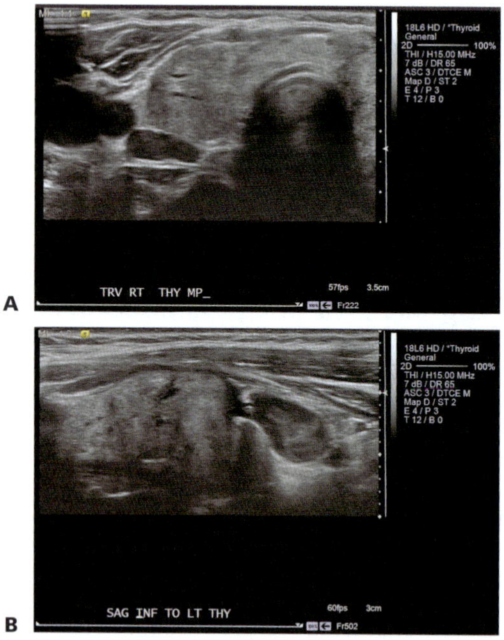

FIG 1 • High-resolution cervical ultrasound demonstrating clear parathyroid adenomata. **A.** Right thyroid lobe with a hypoechoic right upper parathyroid adenoma in the tracheoesophageal groove. **B.** Sagittal ultrasound view of the left thyroid lobe with a hypoechoic left inferior parathyroid adenoma.

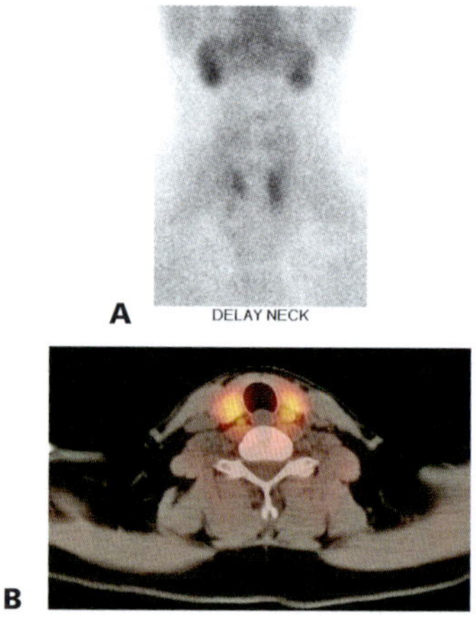

FIG 2 • Nuclear medicine parathyroid scan. **A.** 2-hour delayed planar view showing bilateral parathyroid adenomata. **B.** Fused sestamibi-SPECT/CT scan showing bilateral sestamibi-avid parathyroid lesions posterior to each lobe of the thyroid gland.

- Neck CT scan or magnetic resonance imaging (MRI) is occasionally used to image parathyroid glands. Newer CT scan imaging protocols are becoming more widespread, such as 4D CT scans. This takes advantage of the timing of the intravenous (IV) contrast bolus, the vascularity of the parathyroid tumors, and the delayed washout of hyperactive parathyroid lesions.
- More invasive modalities of parathyroid localization include selective venous sampling for PTH measurement. This technique requires experienced interventional radiologists and is best reserved for the reoperative setting.
- Imaging prior to reoperative parathyroid surgery is essential to minimize exploration in a scarred operative field and to minimize iatrogenic morbidity. It is ideal to have two concordant imaging studies prior to all reoperative parathyroid surgery (see Chapter 45).

SURGICAL MANAGEMENT

Preoperative Planning

- Prior to any parathyroid operation, all diagnostic biochemical data should be reviewed to confirm to the surgeon's satisfaction that a diagnosis of surgically correctable hyperparathyroidism is present in the patient.
- If an autologous parathyroid transplant is planned, confirmation with the patient as to which upper extremity will be the recipient site should be sought.
- The wound classification for parathyroid surgery is clean. It is rare for parenteral antibiotics to be indicated prior to parathyroid surgery. Individual patient characteristics (e.g., cardiac valvular lesions, implanted prosthetic hardware), however, should always be considered.
- Local or general anesthesia may be used.

Positioning

- The patient is positioned supine on the operating room (OR) table with the arms tucked either at the sides or lying on the abdomen. A sheet, fastened with towel clips, is used to secure the arms next to the patient and to allow for removal of the arm boards from the OR table (**FIG 3**).
- If a parathyroid transplant is planned to the patient's forearm, this arm can be extended from the patient and reprepped and draped at the time of that portion of the procedure (after the parathyroid tissue has been removed from the neck).
- A towel roll or other small bump is placed behind the patient's shoulder to aid in extension of the neck.
- The bed is positioned with the head up, the feet down, and in some slight Trendelenburg. This is known as the semi-Fowler's position or the beach chair position.
- Some surgeons will rotate the OR table 90 degrees to have the head of the patient away from the anesthesia providers and thus more accessible to the surgical team.

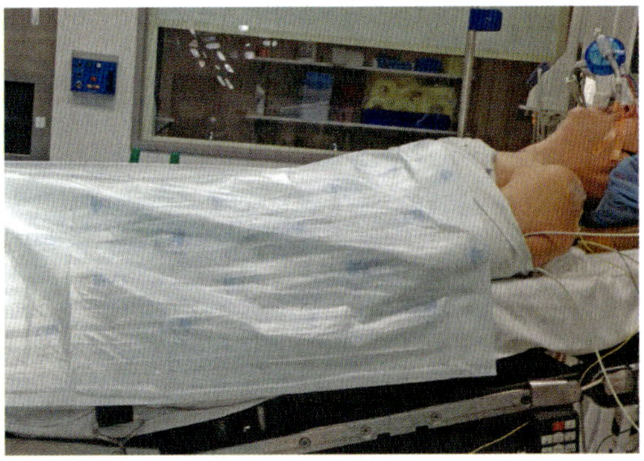

FIG 3 • The patient is positioned on the OR table with the arms tucked, a roll behind the shoulders, and the head elevated.

PLACEMENT OF INCISION

- A transverse incision is made in the line of a skin crease roughly 1 cm caudal to the cricoid cartilage or two fingerbreadths cephalad to the suprasternal notch. The incision may be between 3 and 5 cm in length and is centered on the midline of the neck (**FIG 4**). Some surgeons will infiltrate the region of the incision with a local anesthetic combined with epinephrine. Placement of the incision within a natural skin line or crease of the neck is more important for postoperative cosmesis than the length of the incision (**FIG 5**).

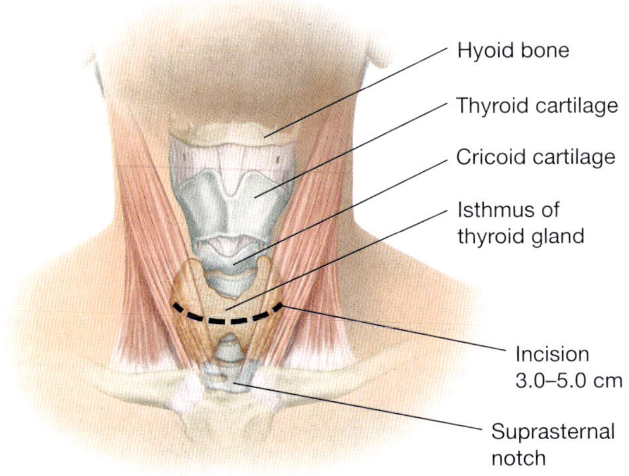

FIG 4 • Surface anatomy and relationships for parathyroid incision placement.

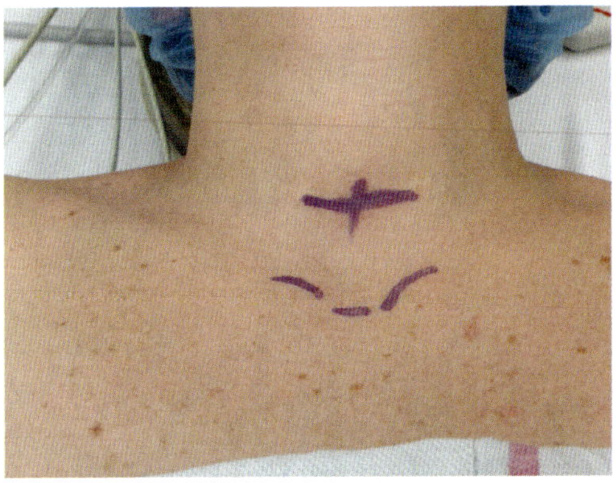

FIG 5 • Diagram of planned parathyroidectomy incision, with clavicular heads and sternal notch marked for reference.

CREATION OF FLAPS

- Dissection is deepened through the subcutaneous tissues and through the platysma muscle with electrocautery. Subplatysmal flaps are created superiorly, inferiorly, and laterally with a combination of electrocautery and blunt dissection (**FIG 6**).
- Care must be taken to avoid injury to the paired anterior jugular veins. Should a rent be made in one of these veins, it is best to ligate the vein rather than attempt to cauterize the vein.
- The superior flap should extend to the level of the thyroid cartilage and the inferior flap down to the sternal notch.

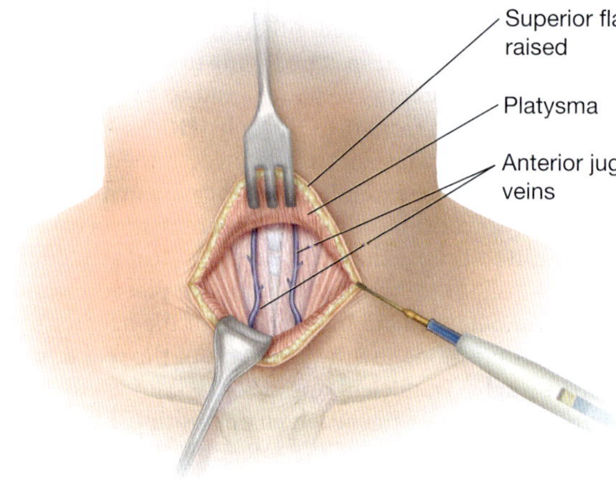

FIG 6 • Myocutaneous flaps are raised superiorly, inferiorly, and laterally to facilitate skin retraction and to expose the various sites to be explored.

ENTRY INTO THE DEEP CENTRAL NECK SPACE

- The avascular, midline raphe between the sternohyoid and sternothyroid muscles on each side is entered with electrocautery. This midline is best identified by digital palpation of the midline of the underlying trachea. These strap muscles should be separated to expose the underlying thyroid isthmus (**FIG 7**).
- The layers of the strap muscles are separated into two by dividing the connective tissue in the layer between the sternohyoid and the sternothyroid muscles. The lateral extent of this dissection is the lateral borders of these muscles and the carotid sheath. This exposes the internal jugular vein, a site from which to draw a baseline blood sample for intraoperative PTH monitoring[6] (**FIG 8**).
- An alternate site for PTH sampling is a peripheral venipuncture (often in the lower extremity) performed by the anesthesiologist. If an arterial catheter is present for anesthetic monitoring, it is acceptable to use an arterial blood sample for PTH monitoring.

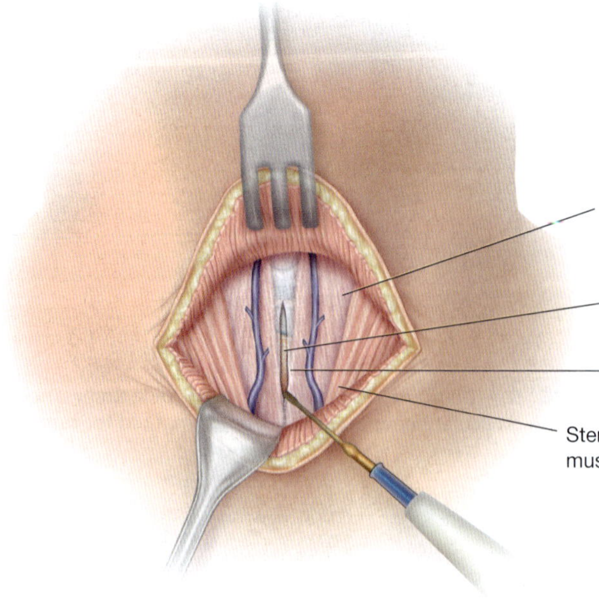

FIG 7 • The strap muscles (sternohyoid and sternothyroid) are separated in the midline with electrocautery to expose the underlying thyroid isthmus.

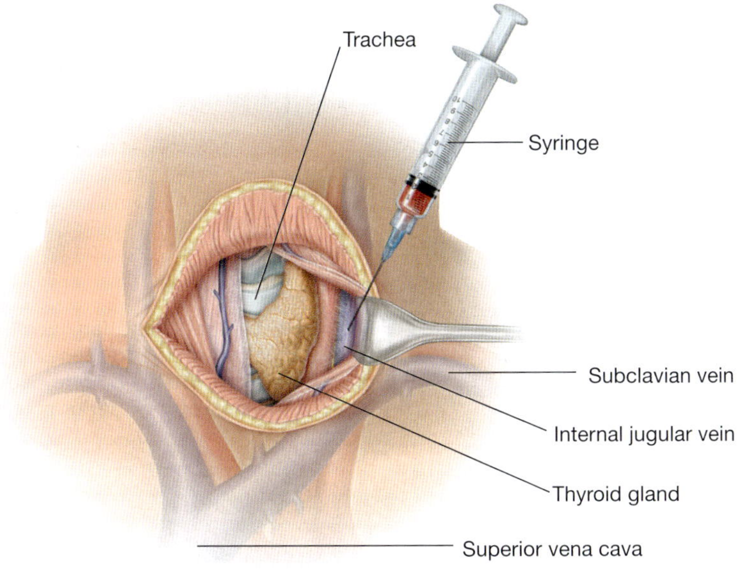

FIG 8 ● Blood is drawn from the internal jugular vein to test for PTH levels.

- The space between the sternothyroid muscle and the thyroid lobe is developed with a combination of blunt dissection and electrocautery. The operation must necessarily begin on one side of the neck, but an identical procedure will be done on the contralateral side of the neck to identify all four parathyroid glands. This space lateral to the thyroid lobe and medial to the carotid artery is developed back to the level of the prevertebral fascia. The crossing middle thyroid vein may need to be divided. This may be accomplished with metallic clips, suture, or through any of the available powered surgical devices (**FIG 9**). Caution must be taken to avoid searching for parathyroid tissue too soon, as it is possible for the tumor to be more posterior than one has opened, or remaining with either the thyroid or the carotid sheath.
- The recurrent laryngeal nerve may be identified at this point, coursing superiorly in the tracheoesophageal groove (**FIG 10**).

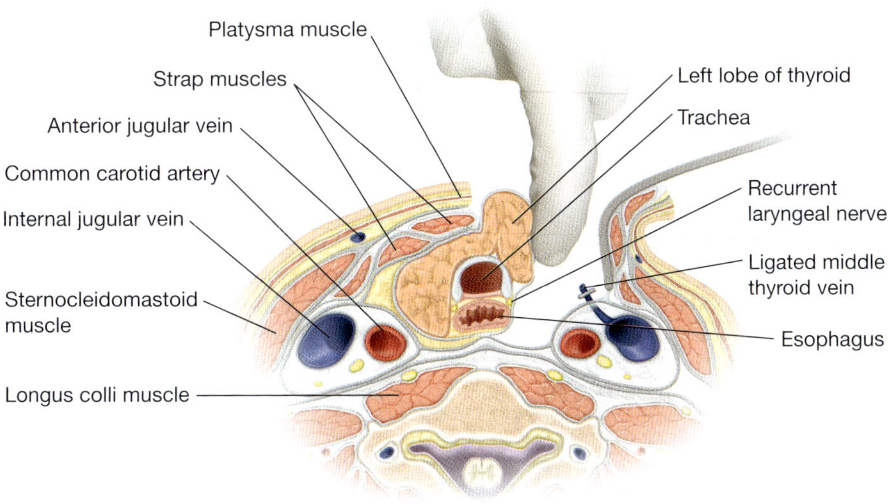

FIG 9 ● Initial dissection for a parathyroidectomy includes separating the strap muscles off the underlying thyroid lobe. The plane just medial to the carotid sheath is followed posteriorly to the level of the spine. The only transversely crossing structure is the middle thyroid vein, which can be ligated. All soft tissue, along with the thyroid lobe, is kept under the surgeon's finger.

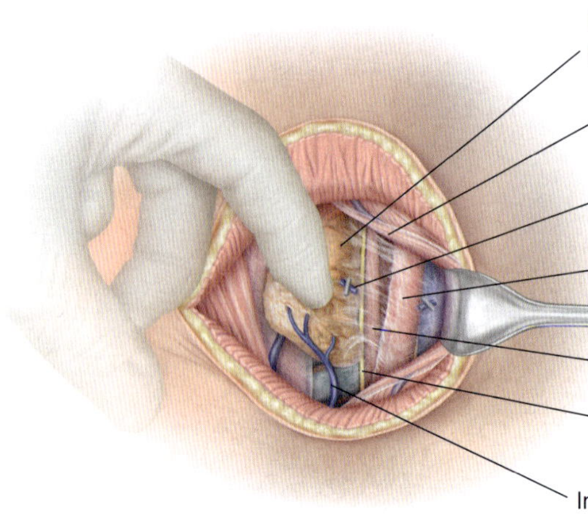

FIG 10 • The recurrent laryngeal nerve courses superiorly in the tracheoesophageal groove and can often be identified most easily at the level of the inferior pole of the thyroid gland.

IDENTIFICATION OF SUPERIOR PARATHYROID GLANDS

- The superior parathyroid glands lie posterior to the upper pole of the thyroid lobe. To explore this space, the thyroid lobe is rolled anteromedially using one's finger or a Kittner dissector. The superior parathyroid glands are posterior to the recurrent laryngeal nerve as it passes underneath the tubercle of Zuckerkandl and just posterolateral to the ligament of Berry (**FIG 11**). Their position is more constant than that of the inferior parathyroid glands. There is often symmetry between sides of the neck, and if one cannot locate a superior parathyroid gland on one side, it is often advisable to locate it on the contralateral side.

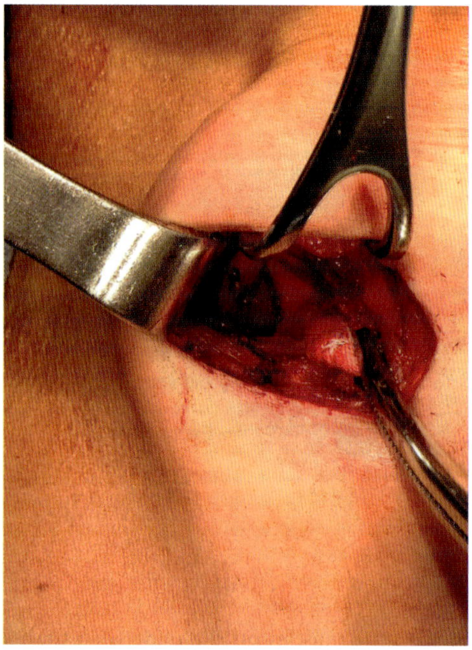

FIG 11 • Right superior parathyroid adenoma lying posterior to the right thyroid lobe (rolled anteriorly with Kittner dissector). The right strap musculature is seen retracted laterally.

- Due to limited space for enlargement, superior parathyroid adenomas often grow caudad and ultimately lie in a pseudoectopic position in the tracheoesophageal groove, low in the neck. The blood supply, however, remains in the eutopic position near the upper pole of the thyroid lobe. Caution must be taken elevating these low-lying superior parathyroid adenomas out of the tracheoesophageal groove as they often lie with the recurrent laryngeal nerve draped over them.
- Ectopic positions for the superior parathyroid glands include low in the tracheoesophageal groove, retroesophageal, retrotracheal, within the carotid sheath, and within the thyroid gland.
- Exploration of the carotid sheath begins with retraction of the sternothyroid muscle laterally to expose the carotid artery. Gentle blunt dissection anterior to the carotid artery allows separation of the carotid artery from the internal jugular vein just lateral to it. Posterior in the carotid sheath is the vagus nerve. Exposure of the carotid sheath for about 5 to 6 cm in a cephalocaudal direction allows one to search for a soft, brown nodule consistent with a parathyroid adenoma (**FIG 12**). Care must be taken not to mistake nodules posterior to the carotid sheath for parathyroid adenomas as these may in fact be ganglia of the sympathetic chain.
- Once identified, the parathyroid tumor should be dissected back to its single vascular pedicle. Great care should be taken to avoid entry into the parathyroid capsule and the potential for spilling and seeding parathyroid tumor cells in the central neck space (known as parathyromatosis).
- Any uncertainty in the visual identification of parathyroid tissue should prompt a biopsy sent for frozen section analysis. A small fragment of tumor can be taken with a pair of scissors. Gentle pressure can control any slight ooze from the biopsied gland.
- Once the superior gland has been identified, it should remain in place until the inferior gland has been identified.
- This same procedure will be used to identify the superior parathyroid glands on each side of the neck.

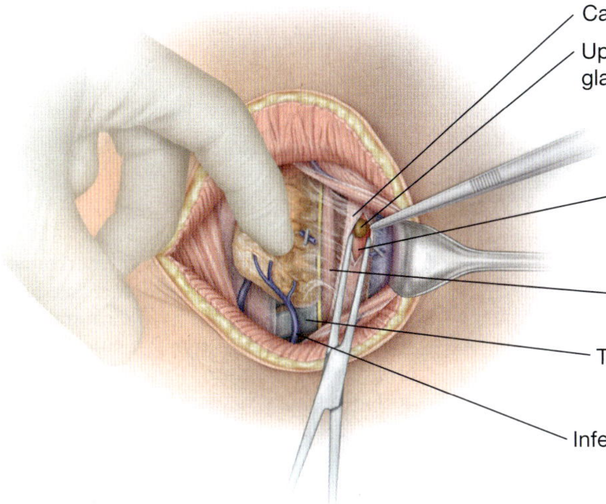

FIG 12 ● Exploration of the carotid sheath for a missing or ectopic superior parathyroid gland. The soft tissue covering the carotid artery is opened, and this space can be explored from the retropharyngeal region into the posterior superior mediastinum.

IDENTIFICATION OF INFERIOR PARATHYROID GLANDS

- The inferior parathyroid glands have a slightly more variable location than the superior parathyroid glands related to the greater distance of migration during embryologic development. The typical location for these glands is just caudal and slightly posterior to the inferior tip of the lower pole of the thyroid lobe. The inferior parathyroid glands often lie in a plane equal to the trachea. They are uniformly anterior to the recurrent laryngeal nerve (**FIG 13**).

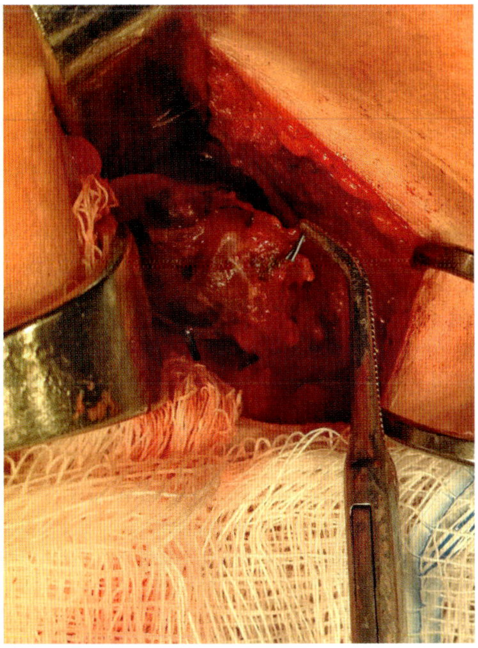

FIG 13 ● Left inferior parathyroid adenoma retracted away from the inferior pole of the thyroid gland.

- As the inferior parathyroid gland enlarges, it may descend with gravity into the fatty tissue caudal to the thyroid lobe and into the anterior superior mediastinum. Gentle dissection in this region can allow for identification of a parathyroid adenoma without causing bleeding.
- The inferior parathyroid glands may lie in the connective tissue ligament that attaches the lower pole of the thyroid to the cervical horn of the thymus (the so-called thyrothymic ligament).
- Ectopic positions for the inferior parathyroid glands include the thyrothymic ligament, the cervical portions of the thymus, the intrathoracic thymus, undescended within the neck, and with the thyroid gland itself. Each of these spaces needs to be examined for a missing parathyroid gland. There is often symmetry of location of the inferior parathyroid glands, and inability to find one inferior parathyroid gland should prompt attempts at identification of the contralateral inferior parathyroid gland as a guide.
- A transcervical thymectomy may be done to identify missing or ectopically located inferior parathyroid glands. This procedure is begun by dissecting the fatty tissue in the anterior superior mediastinum just posterior to the clavicular head and just lateral to the trachea. A search is undertaken for the canary yellow color of the remnant thymus. Gentle traction in a cephalad direction will allow one to extract the thymus from the mediastinum. An encasing membrane will often need to be opened to fully allow the thymus to be removed. The cervical thymic remnant will thin out to a small attachment often containing a blood vessel that should be clipped or suture ligated (**FIG 14**).
- Once the inferior parathyroid adenoma is identified, it should be dissected back to its vascular pedicle. Any question as to its identity should prompt a small sample to be taken with scissors for frozen section biopsy.
- An identical procedure will be followed to identify the inferior parathyroid tumor on the contralateral side.

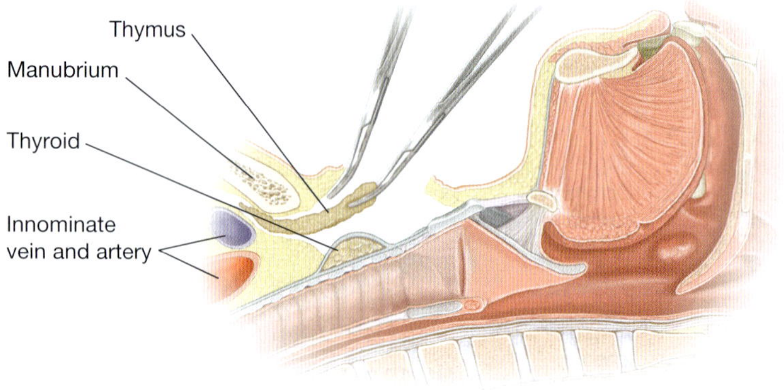

FIG 14 ● A transcervical thymectomy can be accomplished to identify ectopic inferior parathyroid glands that lie caudal to the sternal notch. The thymic tissue is grasped and gently pulled up from the mediastinum and into the cervical incision.

FROZEN SECTION PATHOLOGIC ANALYSIS

- It is often advisable to confirm the identity of the four parathyroid glands identified with frozen section.
- Frozen section is used to confirm identification as parathyroid tissue more so than to quantify cellularity of the parathyroid gland. It is nearly impossible to reliably determine parathyroid hyperplasia from a parathyroid adenoma on frozen section (**FIG 15A,B**).

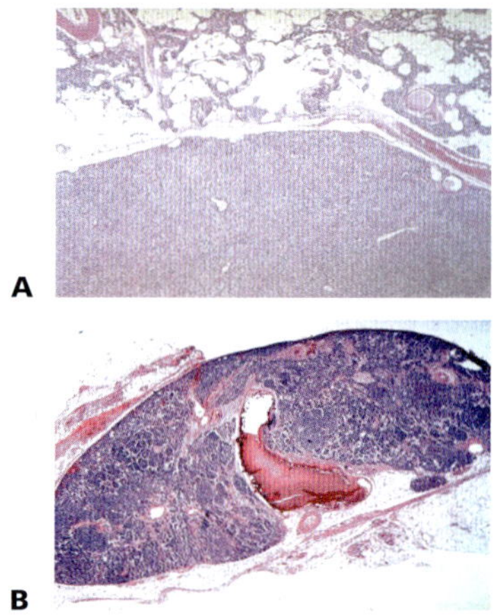

FIG 15 ● Low-power photomicrographs of **(A)** a parathyroid adenoma and **(B)** a hyperplastic parathyroid gland. The adenoma has a characteristic compressed rim of normal parathyroid tissue, with admixed adipocytes and parathyroid chief cells.

SUBTOTAL RESECTION OF PARATHYROIDS

- If a subtotal resection of the parathyroid glands is to be done, one plans to resect three and a half of the four glands. This is best done by dividing one of the glands first and continually checking on its viability as the resection of the second through fourth glands ensues to avoid an inadvertent total parathyroidectomy.
- In general, the remnant of parathyroid gland to remain on its native blood supply in the neck should be a portion of the most normal-appearing gland of the four identified.
- If possible, a remnant inferior gland should be left, as this remnant will sit more anterior, and anterior to the recurrent laryngeal nerve, making it easier to reoperate upon if necessary.
- A sufficient parathyroid remnant is about 30 to 50 mg of tissue or the size of a normal parathyroid gland.
- The parathyroid remnant is created by placing a metallic clip or clips across the gland and sharply dividing the distal segment of the gland away from the remnant (**FIG 16**).
- The remnant may also be tagged with a Prolene suture to aid in future identification if a reoperation becomes necessary. Great care should be taken when placing this marking stitch to avoid injury to the end arteriole feeding the parathyroid gland.
- The second through fourth glands are removed by dividing the vascular pedicle of the gland. The vascular pedicle can be clipped or tied as per surgeon preference.

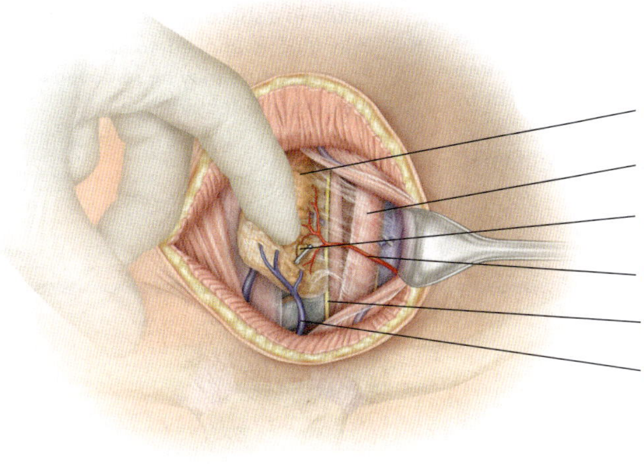

FIG 16 ● A remnant of a left lower parathyroid gland is left on its native blood supply. A metallic surgical clip is placed to divide the gland and to mark in the case that a future reoperative parathyroid surgery becomes necessary. Great care must be taken to ensure that the clip is not placed across the blood supply to the parathyroid remnant.

TOTAL PARATHYROIDECTOMY

- A total parathyroidectomy involves the removal of all parathyroid tissue (usually four glands) from the neck.
- Each gland is fully dissected back to its vascular pedicle, which is clipped or ligated and then divided.
- The parathyroid tissue to be transplanted is identified and kept moist. Great care should be taken to avoid this tissue from mistakenly being handed off the sterile field (**FIG 17**).

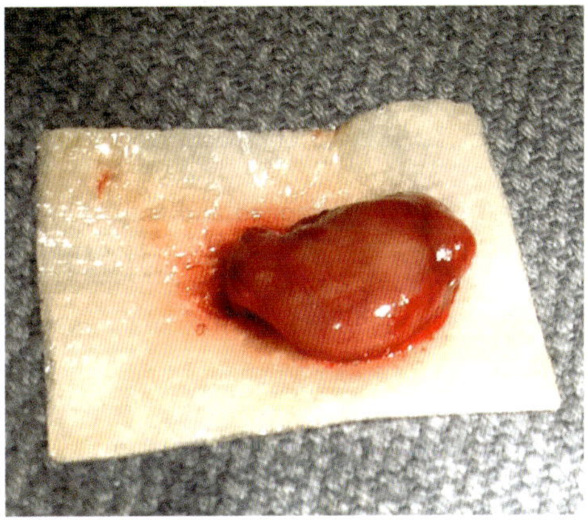

FIG 17 ● Ex vivo right superior parathyroid adenoma.

INTRAOPERATIVE PARATHYROID HORMONE MONITORING

- If intraoperative PTH monitoring is being used, a postresection PTH value should be drawn and sent at 5, 10, or 15 minutes postresection of all parathyroid tissue. Timing is per the surgeon's protocol. Longer time points (15 minutes) are usually used if the PTH specimen is being drawn from a central vein (internal jugular). Shorter time points may be used if the specimen is from a peripheral venipuncture or a radial arterial line.[6]
- Resolution of hyperparathyroidism and long-term eucalcemia is well predicted by postresection PTH values that are at least 50% of the baseline value and into the normal range (<40 pg/mL).[7]

HEMOSTASIS

- Careful attention to hemostasis is of paramount importance throughout the entire parathyroidectomy to ease in parathyroid identification.
- Postoperative neck hematomas are a rare but potentially disastrous complication following parathyroidectomy.
- Prior to wound closure, a Valsalva maneuver is requested to decrease venous return and to identify any slight bleeding in the operative bed.
- Topical hemostatic agents may be placed in the tracheoesophageal groove and inferior to the thyroid lobes.
- Routine placement of closed suction drains is not required.

WOUND CLOSURE

- The two layers of strap musculature are closed in the midline in either one layer or two separate layers. Three to four interrupted, absorbable stitches are sufficient to reapproximate these muscles.
- The platysma muscle layer is reapproximated with interrupted, buried, absorbable sutures.
- The skin edges are brought together with a 3-0 Prolene suture in a subcuticular stitch.
- Skin glue is applied to the wound, and once dry, the Prolene suture may be removed immediately. No further dressings are required.

IMMEDIATE PARATHYROID AUTOTRANSPLANTATION

- If a total parathyroidectomy has been performed, one must reimplant autologous parathyroid tissue to avoid permanent hypoparathyroidism.
- Roughly 30 to 50 mg of parathyroid tissue should be transplanted.
- The upper extremity in which the parathyroid graft is to be placed is extended out from the patient and supported on an arm board (**FIG 18**).
- The transplant site is into the brachioradialis muscle on the dorsal aspect of the forearm (usually the nondominant forearm). Again, thought must be given to the location of a current or future hemodialysis access in those patients on chronic renal replacement therapy.
- The dorsal forearm is prepped and draped in the usual fashion.
- A 3- to 4-cm longitudinal incision is made, and dissection is deepened through the subcutaneous tissue to the fascia overlying the brachioradialis muscle (**FIG 19A,B**).

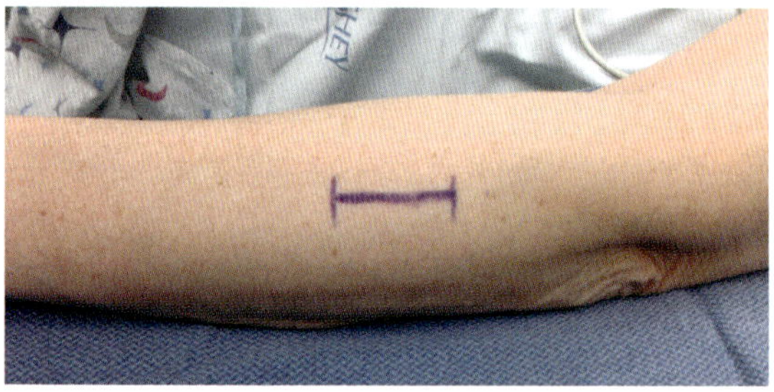

FIG 18 • The heterotopic transplant site is marked prior to surgical prepping and draping. The transplant site is the brachioradialis muscle of the nondominant forearm.

- The fragment of parathyroid tissue to be transplanted is then cut into 1-mm^3 fragments, totaling about 15 fragments (**FIG 20**).
- A small muscle pocket is made in the brachioradialis muscle with the tip of a dissecting instrument, and a single

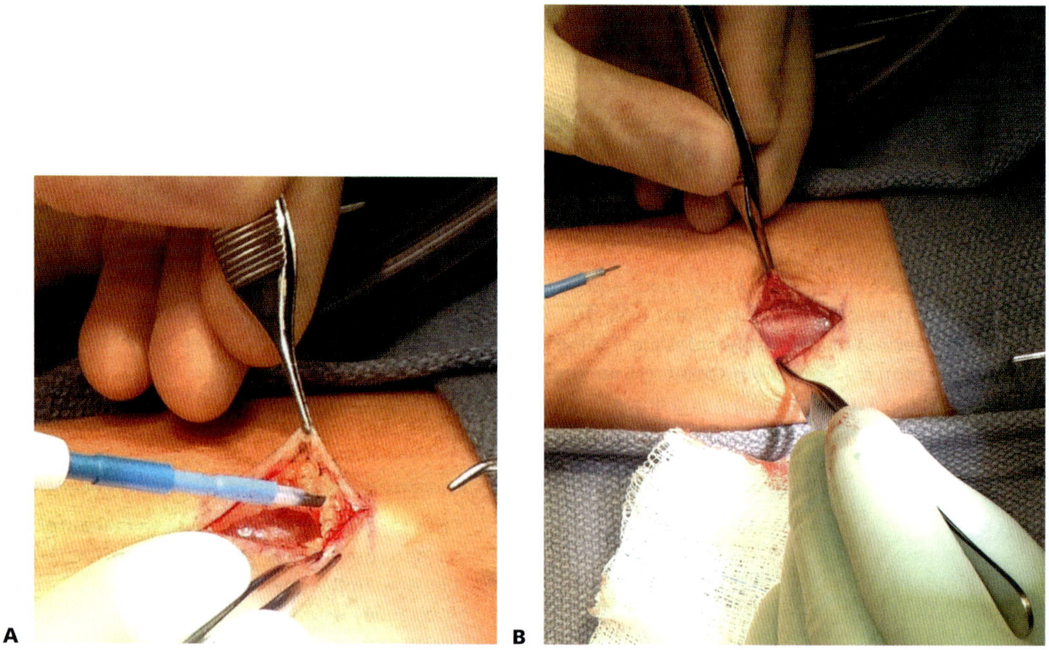

FIG 19 • Preparing the recipient site for parathyroid tissue. **A.** Dissection through subcutaneous tissue to the level of the brachioradialis muscle. **B.** Exposed brachioradialis muscle.

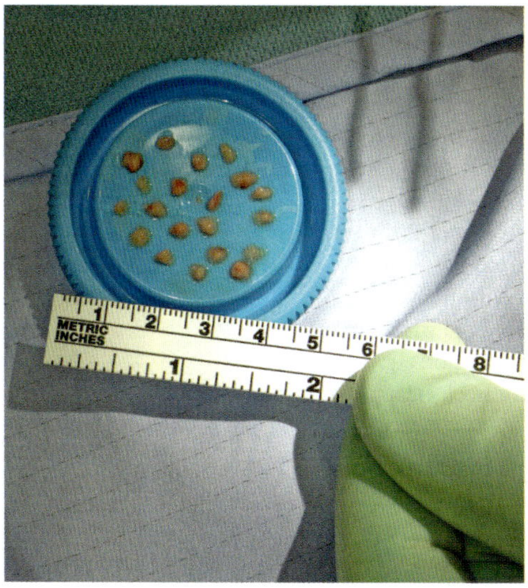

FIG 20 ● Minced parathyroid to be transplanted. Numerous 1-mm^3 fragments of parathyroid tissue await placement into individual muscle pockets.

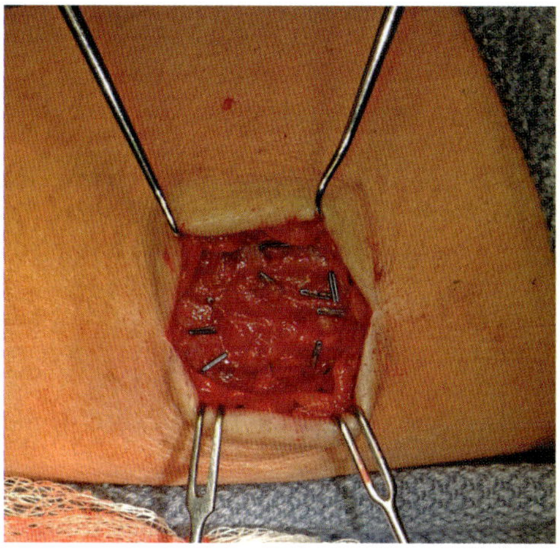

FIG 21 ● Parathyroid autotransplantation completed, with muscle pockets loosely approximated with metallic clips.

fragment of parathyroid tissue is placed into this pocket. The edges of the pocket are loosely approximated with an absorbable suture or a metallic clip.

- This procedure is repeated until each fragment of parathyroid tissue has been placed into a separate muscle pocket (**FIG 21**).
- Great care needs to be taken to avoid any bleeding in these muscle pockets as the initial nutrient supply of the parathyroid graft requires contact with the vascularized muscle.
- The wound is then closed in layers, using interrupted, absorbable sutures to close the deep dermal layers and tissue adhesive to reapproximate the skin edges (**FIG 22**).

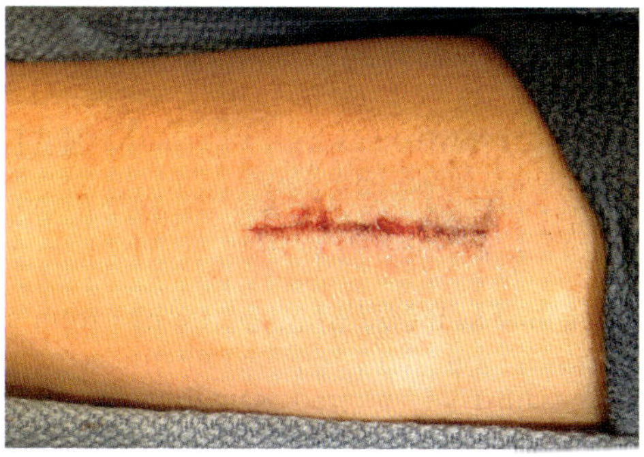

FIG 22 ● The transplant incision is closed with skin glue.

PEARLS AND PITFALLS

Indications	■ Hyperparathyroidism is a biochemical diagnosis, and this needs to be secured prior to cervical imaging or planning an operation.
Identification of parathyroids	■ Dissection in the central neck space should free the carotid sheath medially and include all the tissue down to the prevertebral fascia.
Excision of parathyroid adenomas	■ Parathyroid glands have a singular blood supply and should be dissected back to this vessel prior to ligation and division to avoid injury to critical adjacent structures such as the recurrent laryngeal nerve.
Hemostasis	■ A bloodless field greatly aids in the identification of parathyroid glands from their surrounding tissue. ■ A hematoma at the site of a parathyroid transplant greatly jeopardizes the viability of the autologous graft.
Placement of autologous graft	■ The parathyroid autotransplant may be placed in either the dorsal forearm or the presternal area.
Postoperative hypocalcemia	■ Anticipate and aggressively treat the hypocalcemia that accompanies either a subtotal parathyroidectomy or certainly a total parathyroidectomy with autologous graft.

POSTOPERATIVE CARE

- Patients undergoing subtotal parathyroidectomy or total parathyroidectomy with autologous graft should be admitted for at least 1 day to monitor postoperative calcium and PTH levels.
- Patients having undergone a forearm parathyroid transplant should have a limb alert placed, and blood pressures, IV sites, and venipunctures should be avoided in the transplant arm.
- Acetaminophen or ibuprofen is often sufficient for the pain related to the procedure. Occasionally, opioid agents are needed for a short time postoperatively.
- Endocrinology consultation can be sought as needed by the surgical team.
- Oral calcium and possibly vitamin D (in the form of calcitriol) should be started immediately and titrated if hypocalcemia occurs.
- Patients having undergone a total parathyroidectomy will have an obligate period of hypoparathyroidism until their autograft begins to function.
- Parenteral calcium should be restricted to severely low serum calcium levels and/or patients with symptomatic hypocalcemia.
- Symptoms of hypocalcemia include perioral and digital numbness or tingling, muscle aches/spasms, carpopedal spasms, facial nerve hyperactivity (Chvostek's sign), respiratory muscle insufficiency, and tetany.

OUTCOMES

- The long-term outcome as measured by eucalcemia from a subtotal parathyroidectomy and a total parathyroidectomy with immediate parathyroid autotransplantation are very similar. Both have a small rate of recurrent hyperparathyroidism (as a result of the natural history of the parathyroid disease). This recurrence may occur 10 to 20 years after the index operation.[8]
- Immediate transplantation of autologous parathyroid tissue has successful engraftment approximately 95% of the time. Most parathyroid grafts will gain function in about 8 weeks.[9]

COMPLICATIONS

- Compressive cervical hematoma
- Laryngeal nerve injuries (external branch of the superior laryngeal nerve or recurrent laryngeal nerve)
- Sympathetic chain/stellate ganglion injury
- Prolonged or permanent hypoparathyroidism
- Inability to extirpate all hyperactive tissue with resultant persistent hyperparathyroidism
- Tracheal injury
- Esophageal injury
- Lymph or chylous leak
- Wound infection
- Unsightly neck or arm scarring

REFERENCES

1. Wermers RA, Khosala S, Atkinson EJ, et al. Incidence of primary hyperparathyroidism in Rochester, Minnesota, 1993-2001: an update on the changing epidemiology of the disease. *J Bone Miner Res.* 2006;21:171–177.
2. Saunders BD, Saunders EFH, Gauger PG. Lithium therapy and hyperparathyroidism: an evidence-based assessment. *World J Surg.* 2009;33(11):2314–2323.
3. Pichardo-Lowden AR, Manni A, Saunders BD, et al. Familial hyperparathyroidism due to a germline mutation of the CDC73 gene: implications for management and age-appropriate testing of relatives at risk. *Endocr Pract.* 2011;17(4):602–609.
4. National Kidney Foundation. K/DOQI clinical practice guidelines for bone metabolism and disease in chronic kidney disease. *Am J Kidney Dis.* 2003;42(4)(suppl 3):S1–S201.
5. Sharma J, Mazzaglia P, Milas M, et al. Radionuclide imaging for hyperparathyroidism (HPT): which is the best technetium-99m sestamibi modality? *Surgery.* 2006;140:856–863.
6. Woodrum DT, Saunders BD, England BG, et al. The influence of sample site on intraoperative PTH monitoring during parathyroidectomy. *Surgery.* 2004;136(6):1169–1175.
7. Heller KS, Blumberg SN. Relation of final intraoperative parathyroid hormone level and outcome following parathyroidectomy. *Arch Otolaryngol Head Neck Surg.* 2009;135(11):1103–1107.
8. Richards ML, Wormuth J, Bingener J, et al. Parathyroidectomy in secondary hyperparathyroidism: is there an optimal operative management? *Surgery.* 2006;139:174–180.
9. Feldman AL, Sharaf RN, Skarulis MC, et al. Results of heterotopic parathyroid autotransplantation: a 13-year experience. *Surgery.* 1996;126(6);1042–1048.

Chapter **43**

Minimally Invasive Parathyroidectomy

Peter Angelos Raymon H. Grogan

DEFINITION

- Although there is no uniformly agreed upon definition of a "minimally invasive parathyroidectomy" (MIP), most surgeons accept that this term refers to an operation to remove the parathyroid gland that is a focused or unilateral exploration done through a small incision.[1] Some surgeons stress that MIP should also refer to an operation done without general anesthesia in an outpatient setting. However, we believe that because the choice of anesthesia and determination of whether a patient is discharged on the day of surgery is dependent on the patient (and not always the operation), we do not limit MIP to outpatient procedures without general anesthetic. We believe that MIP is the treatment of choice for primary hyperparathyroidism (HPT) when the location of the abnormal parathyroid gland has been well localized preoperatively.[2,3]
- MIP is effective and recommended for the treatment of sporadic primary HPT but not in cases of familial HPT (e.g., multiple endocrine neoplasia type 1 or 2), secondary HPT, or tertiary HPT. In all of the latter categories, the high likelihood of multigland disease necessitates the exploration of all four glands.
- Although MIP is effective in both primary operations as well as in reoperative cases, we will focus on primary operations in the following description. The decision making for reoperative parathyroidectomy is complicated by the scarring that will be present in the neck and the potential difficulty with performing a four gland exploration. For this reason, preoperative localization becomes much more important in reoperative cases and is beyond the scope of this chapter.

DIAGNOSIS AND INDICATIONS FOR SURGERY

- The diagnosis of HPT is made by the finding of an elevated calcium level with an elevated intact parathyroid hormone (iPTH) level. It is possible to have normocalcemic HPT if the calcium level is at the upper range of normal but the iPTH is elevated. Alternatively, patients sometimes have elevated calcium levels with the iPTH level being inappropriately in the high normal range. It is important when making the diagnosis of HPT to assess both calcium and iPTH levels so that the relative values of these tests can be compared. In a patient with normally functioning parathyroid glands, a high calcium should be associated with a low iPTH level.
- In order to confirm the diagnosis of HPT and rule out familial benign hypocalciuric hypercalcemia (FBHH), a 24-hour urine calcium should be obtained. In FBHH, the urinary calcium is expected to be very low. A normal or elevated 24-hour urine calcium level effectively rules out FBHH. An elevated 24-hour urine calcium increases the risk of kidney stones.
- The indications for surgery in HPT are well described in several National Institutes of Health (NIH) consensus conferences over the last few decades.[4] Most surgeons and endocrinologists currently agree that patients with HPT who are symptomatic or have marked elevations in serum calcium should have surgery. A history of kidney stones and the presence of osteoporosis are widely accepted as indications for surgery. It is common for patients with HPT to have additional symptoms that may be associated with the disease, including low energy, bone pain, decreased proximal extremity muscle strength, decreased ability to concentrate, and reductions in short-term memory. Although all of these symptoms may be caused by conditions other than HPT, they are very common in patients with HPT and may influence the decision to recommend surgery.
- The diagnosis of HPT in a young patient (<50 years old) also is a relative indication for parathyroidectomy because such patients will have more years to develop osteoporosis and other problems associated with HPT. In addition, for women of childbearing age, HPT also appears to increase the risks of spontaneous abortion.
- There is currently no approved medical treatment for primary HPT. For this reason, the choice for patients and physicians is between parathyroidectomy and continued observation.

IMAGING AND OTHER DIAGNOSTIC STUDIES

- Once the decision is made to proceed to surgical treatment, localization studies to attempt to identify the location of the abnormal parathyroid gland are indicated. We recommend the routine use of technetium-99m (Tc-99m) sestamibi scan and ultrasound evaluation of the thyroid gland.[5]
- Sestamibi scanning has high rates of sensitivity and specificity and is effective in localizing not only parathyroid adenomas in the neck but also in ectopic locations such as undescended glands in the neck or intrathoracic glands. Unfortunately, in cases of multigland disease, sestamibi scanning is least likely to identify the location of abnormal glands. Sestamibi is taken up by both thyroid and parathyroid cells. It is more rapidly cleared from thyroid cells than from abnormal parathyroid cells. For this reason, a comparison of early and delayed scans often reveals the presence of a persistent focus of increased activity in the abnormal parathyroid gland. With the use of fused sestamibi–computed tomography (CT) scanning or three-dimensional single photon emission computed tomography (SPECT) reconstructions, it is often possible to determine

whether the focus of uptake is anterior in the neck (at or near the level of the thyroid lobe) or more posterior. Because the superior parathyroid gland is located posterior to the recurrent laryngeal, posterior parathyroid glands on scans are most likely superior glands, whereas anterior glands are more likely to be inferior glands.

- Ultrasonography is an effective noninvasive means of identifying abnormal parathyroid glands. The study can be performed in the radiology department or by surgeons in the clinic or operating room. Ultrasonography is effective in identifying enlarged parathyroid glands that are close to the thyroid gland. Abnormal parathyroid glands usually appear as hypoechoic lesions either posterior or inferior to the thyroid gland. Parathyroid glands that are located posterior to the esophagus and those in the mediastinum are less likely to be visualized on ultrasound.
- Ultrasound is very effective at identifying thyroid nodules, which may be a source of increased uptake on sestamibi scans. We believe that thyroid nodules greater than 1 cm or with suspicious characteristics should be evaluated with fine needle aspiration cytology prior to planned parathyroidectomy. This strategy limits the chances of missing a nonpalpable thyroid malignancy and thus reduces the likelihood for reoperative neck surgery.
- In cases of primary HPT when patients have negative preoperative localization studies, we recommend proceeding with surgery and planning on a four-gland exploration (see Chapter 41). Some surgeons would obtain a four-dimensional CT scan of neck and chest prior to exploring the patient. However, we believe that additional evidence is required before this approach should be routinely adopted.

SURGICAL MANAGEMENT

- MIP can be performed either with local anesthesia and sedation or with general anesthesia, depending on surgeon and patient preference. We have found that because inferior parathyroid adenomas are located more anteriorly in the neck, these glands are more amenable to resection without using general anesthesia. Large posteriorly located superior parathyroid adenomas often are more challenging to remove without general anesthetic because of the need to rotate the thyroid lobe medially to gain access to the space posterior to the esophagus. Although it is possible to access these glands even when the patient is not asleep, surgeons should be cognizant of the challenge and choose the appropriate patient for such an approach.
- Identification of the optimal skin crease for a cosmetic incision is best done with the patient sitting up while awake. Although extending the neck in the operating room may change the location of skin creases, marking them prior to entering the operating room increases the likelihood of a good cosmetic result.
- After the patient has been either intubated or appropriately sedated, the use of superficial cervical plexus block may be used to facilitate local anesthesia if the patient has not received a general anesthetic or to improve postoperative pain control if a general anesthetic is used.
- The superficial cervical plexus block is a safe, effective technique to provide cutaneous anesthesia to the C2, C3, and C4 dermatomes. We perform a two-point (transverse and inferior), bilateral superficial blockade to allow complete local anesthesia of the midline Kocher incision, which, if done correctly, will last for several hours after the procedure. Anecdotally, this should also allow for reduced general anesthesia intraoperatively, particularly for superficial lower parathyroidectomies. We use 10 mL of 0.25% bupivacaine without epinephrine for each side of the neck.
- After induction of general anesthesia, the patient's neck is extended with a beanbag or shoulder roll. The midpoint of the posterior border of the sternocleidomastoid muscle is identified, and a 22-gauge needle is inserted subcutaneously (no more than 1 cm) at this anatomic landmark (**FIG 1**). Check to be sure the needle is not inserted into a vein by pulling back on the plunger of the syringe. First, 5 mL of anesthetic are injected straight toward the midline of the neck (transverse injection) just posterior to the muscle. The needle is then repositioned without removing it from the skin so that it is now pointing at the sternal notch. The remaining 5 mL of anesthetic is then injected inferiorly along the posterior border of the muscle (inferior injection). The other side of the neck is then injected in a similar manner.
- If done correctly, there is minimal risk associated with this technique. The main risk of this procedure occurs if the injection is done too deep. If injected too deep into the neck, branches of the brachial plexus can be anesthetized, and the patient may have a temporary paralysis of the ipsilateral upper extremity. A deep injection can also anesthetize the phrenic nerve and lead to temporary diaphragmatic paralysis. For this reason, if the injection is being done without general anesthetic while the patient is awake, it is important that bilateral blockade is not performed simultaneously on both sides of the neck. Finally, if the injection infiltrates superiorly, the greater auricular branch of the plexus will be blocked, and the patient will have numbness of the skin overlying the parotid and the earlobe. This is a common side effect that the patient should be told to be aware of in the immediate postoperative period.

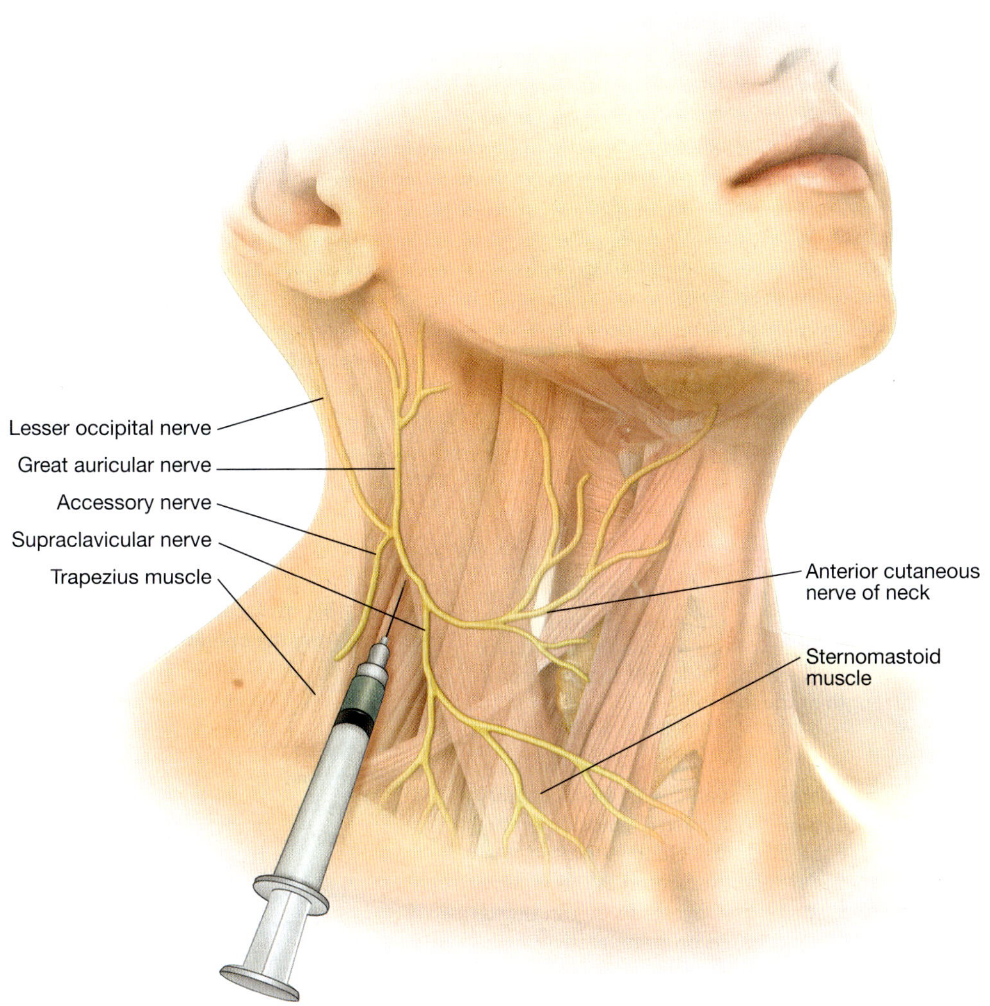

FIG 1 • A 22-gauge needle is inserted no more than 1 cm subcutaneously at the midpoint of the posterior border of the sternocleidomastoid muscle. After assuring the needle is not in a vein, 5 mL of anesthetic is injected toward the midline of the neck (transverse injection). The needle is repositioned without removing it toward the sternal notch. The remaining 5 mL of anesthetic is then injected inferiorly along the posterior border of the muscle (inferior injection).

- Optimal positioning for parathyroidectomy is with the patient's neck gently extended but well supported. Prior to prepping the skin, we routinely perform an intraoperative ultrasound of the neck to ensure the choice of the optimal location for the skin incision (**FIG 2**). In addition, intraoperative ultrasound often allows the surgeon to confirm the location of the adenoma and focuses the subsequent surgical exploration.
- After prepping the skin, it is critical that if the patient has not received a general anesthetic, care must be taken when placing drapes to ensure that the operative field is fully separated from the space below the drapes. Patients who are receiving sedation and local anesthesia usually are also given supplemental oxygen by the anesthesiologist during the operation. This is commonly done with nasal cannula and results in relatively high oxygen concentrations below the drapes. If that oxygen comes in contact with a spark from electrocautery used during the performance of the parathyroidectomy, the risk of fire is increased. For this reason, when draping the patient, an occlusive dressing or adherent drapes are important to separate the operative field from the space below the drapes (**FIG 3**).
- A small (2 to 3 cm) incision in the midline is made in a skin crease. Although some surgeons prefer an incision shifted toward the side of the parathyroid adenoma, we prefer using a midline incision so that if it becomes necessary to explore both sides, the same incision can often be used. If it is necessary to lengthen the incision, this is usually only a minimal increase in incision size.

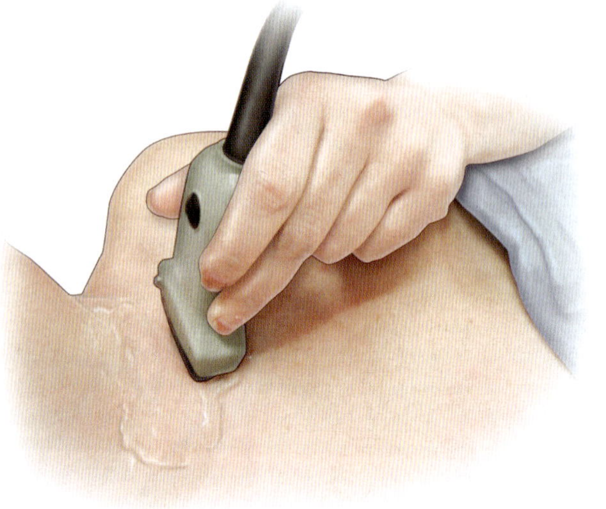

FIG 2 ● Ultrasound of the neck is performed prior to prepping the patient's neck. The ultrasound is particularly useful in determining the optimal location for the small neck incision. Note that the mark on the neck is of the skin crease but not the actual length of the incision.

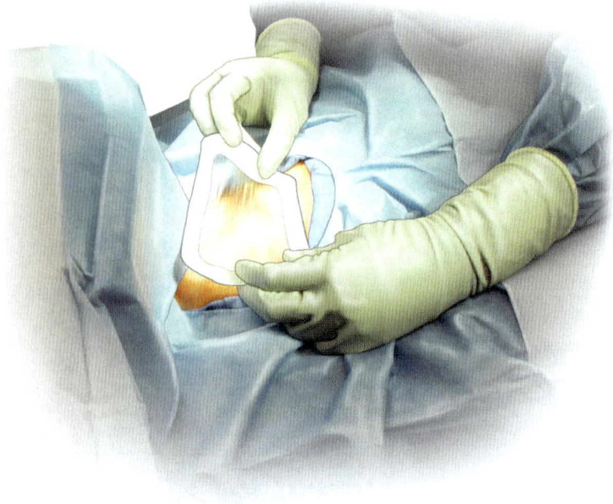

FIG 3 ● Occlusive barrier dressing being placed. This is very important if the patient is not intubated and supplemental oxygen is used. The barrier dressing separates the space under the drapes from the operative field and reduces the risk of fire.

- Small subplatysmal flaps are created with electrocautery to allow the skin incision to be moved up or down depending on where the abnormal gland is located. The midline strap muscles are then separated in the midline so that the thyroid lobe on the involved side can be rotated medially (**FIG 4**). If, based on preoperative imaging, the abnormal parathyroid appears to be the inferior parathyroid, then the dissection is focused on the area near the inferior pole of the thyroid or in the thyrothymic tract where inferior parathyroid glands are most commonly located. If the abnormal parathyroid gland appears to be a superior gland, then dissection is focused on the more posterior tissue. The entire thyroid lobe is mobilized medially such that the space posterior to the esophagus can be adequately explored.
- Once an abnormal parathyroid gland is identified, the vascular pedicle should be carefully identified, ligated, and divided (**FIG 5**). Once adequate hemostasis is achieved, the incision is closed.

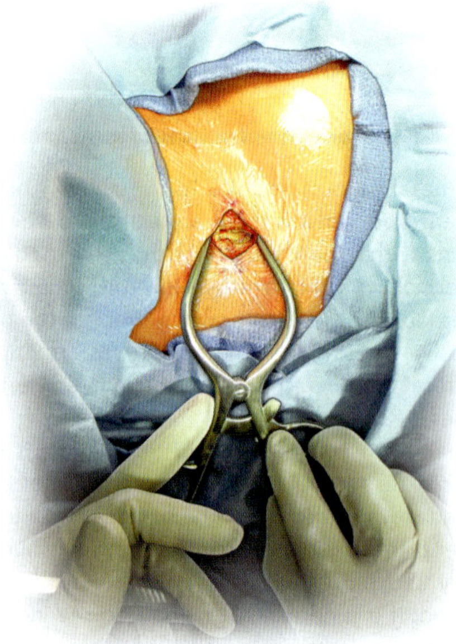

FIG 4 ● Small skin incision after the subplatysmal flaps have been created and the midline strap muscles have been separated to expose the thyroid gland below.

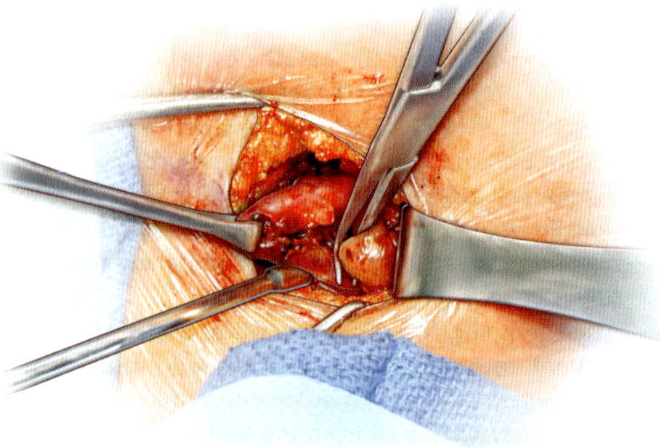

FIG 5 ● Parathyroid adenoma is identified in proximity to the thyroid gland. The parathyroid adenoma is separated from the surrounding tissue, taking care not to enter the capsule of the gland. The vascular pedicle is identified, ligated, and divided.

INTRAOPERATIVE DECISION MAKING WITH INTRAOPERATIVE PARATHYROID HORMONE

- We believe that intraoperative PTH assay is an important component of any MIP. iPTH has such a short half-life that if the abnormal parathyroid gland is removed and the other glands are normal, the PTH levels will drop by more than 50% in 5 to 10 minutes for the vast majority of patients. In most circumstances, a second peripheral intravenous catheter is placed prior to positioning the patient. Blood samples are then drawn through this intravenous catheter, taking care to ensure adequate blood is drawn to avoid a dilute sample from the intravenous fluid. We routinely draw four samples. The first is drawn after the skin preparation prior to making an incision ("preincision"). The second is drawn after finding the parathyroid adenoma prior to dividing its blood supply ("preexcision"). Postexcision levels are then drawn at 5 and 10 minutes after removing the parathyroid adenoma.
- Although many papers have been written on identifying the optimal criteria for intraoperative drop in PTH, we believe that a drop of 50% from the first baseline level at 5 or 10 minutes postexcision, as long as the value is within normal range, is strongly predictive of a successful operation.[6] If the preincision PTH level is very high and the preexcision level is even higher, it is sometimes necessary to draw levels beyond 10 minutes postexcision in order to see an adequate drop in PTH levels. We believe that with positive preoperative localization studies and a dramatic drop in PTH after excising the adenoma, the likelihood of a second abnormal parathyroid gland is exceedingly low and a four-gland exploration is not indicated.

CLOSURE

- As long as the skin incision is located in a skin crease or at least in line with skin creases, the likelihood of a cosmetically appealing scar is very high. We routinely close the skin with an absorbable suture in the platysma and subdermal level to take tension off the skin edges. The skin is closed with a 5-0 monofilament subcuticular suture with no knots. If an absorbable suture is used, Steri-Strips are applied and the suture is then cut flush with the skin. If a nonabsorbable suture is used, skin glue is placed over the incision prior to pulling the subcuticular stitch out in the operating room. Most patients have excellent cosmetic results.

POSTOPERATIVE CARE

- Assuming no other medical issues, many patients can be discharged after a successful MIP. Because a focused exploration has been undertaken, only one side of the neck has been dissected. Patients are generally given extra oral calcium for several days to prevent transient symptomatic hypocalcemia while the remaining parathyroid glands recover from having been suppressed. The extra calcium can be rapidly weaned. Patients are allowed to shower the day after surgery and the only restriction in activity is to avoid driving a car until there is no neck pain in turning and the patient is off pain medication.

OUTCOMES

- The outcomes after MIP have been shown to be excellent in several large series.[7,8] Patients recover rapidly and many have improvements in energy level with decreased bone pain in the weeks to months after surgery. The long-term risks of recurrent HPT are not different in many large series when comparing MIP with four-gland exploration.

COMPLICATIONS

- The primary risk of MIP is the small possibility of recurrent laryngeal nerve injury resulting in hoarseness. The risk of permanent hoarseness is in the 1% to 2% range in most large series of parathyroidectomies. Use of MIP in comparison to four-gland exploration does not seem to affect risk of recurrent laryngeal nerve injury. By contrast, the risk of permanent hypoparathyroidism, which is approximately 1% with a four-gland exploration, is eliminated with an MIP approach.
- Other potential complications of MIP include bleeding and infection. Both of these risks are extremely low with a parathyroidectomy and are not increased by use of MIP.

REFERENCES

1. Grant CS, Thompson G, Farley D, et al. Primary hyperparathyroidism surgical management since the introduction of minimally invasive parathyroidectomy: Mayo Clinic experience. *Arch Surg*. 2005;140(5):472–478; discussion 478–479.
2. Udelsman R, Lin Z, Donovan P. The superiority of minimally invasive parathyroidectomy based on 1650 consecutive patients with primary hyperparathyroidism. *Ann Surg*. 2011;253(3): 585–591.
3. Kuntsman JW, Udelsman R. Superiority of minimally invasive parathyroidectomy. *Adv Surg*. 2012;46:171–180.
4. Bilezikian JP, Khan AA, Potts JT Jr. Guidelines for the management of asymptomatic primary hyperparathyroidism: summary statement from the third international workshop. *J Clin Endocrinol Metab*. 2009;94(2):335.
5. Siperstein A, Berber E, Mackey R, et al. Prospective evaluation of sestamibi scan, ultrasonography, and rapid PTH to predict the success of limited exploration for sporadic primary hyperparathyroidism. *Surgery*. 2004;136(4):872–880.
6. Chiu B, Sturgeon C, Angelos, P. Which intraoperative parathyroid hormone assay criterion best predicts operative success? A study of 352 consecutive patients. *Arch Surg*. 2006;141:483–487.
7. McGill JF, Sturgeon C, Kaplan S, et al. How does the operative strategy for primary hyperparathyroidism impact the findings and cure rate? A comparison of 800 parathyroidectomies. *J Am Coll Surg*. 2008;207:246–249.
8. Zanocco K, Angelos P, Sturgeon C. Cost-effectiveness analysis of parathyroidectomy for asymptomatic primary hyperparathyroidism. *Surgery*. 2006;140:874–881; discussion 881–882.

Chapter 44 Endoscopic Parathyroidectomy by Lateral Approach

Jean-François Henry

DEFINITION

- A minimally invasive parathyroidectomy (MIP) may be defined as an operation requiring a small and discrete incision for a very direct access to the parathyroid glands, resulting in a focused dissection. MIP may be divided in two groups: open MIP performed under direct vision via a small cervical incision[1] and various endoscopic MIP performed partially or totally with the help of an endoscope. Today, three different types of endoscopic parathyroidectomies can be considered to be an option for surgeons: (1) Video-assisted parathyroidectomy,[2] which is a mini-open procedure performed partially with the help of the endoscope. (2) Endoscopic techniques using an extracervical approach. These techniques have the advantage of leaving no scar in the neck area but cannot reasonably be described as minimally invasive as they require more dissection than conventional open surgery. (3) Pure endoscopic techniques using a cervical access. These operations are performed totally with the help of the endoscope and include constant gas insufflations. Two pure endoscopic techniques have been described: the endoscopic parathyroidectomy by midline approach[3] and the endoscopic parathyroidectomy by lateral approach (EPLA).[4] EPLA develops the plane between the carotid sheath laterally and the strap muscles medially. This "back-door route" does not require complete dissection of the thyroid lobe from the strap muscles. It allows direct access to the posterior aspect of the thyroid lobe and it does not require anterior and medial retraction of the thyroid lobe during the entire procedure.

DIFFERENTIAL DIAGNOSIS

- Today, the diagnosis of primary hyperparathyroidism (PHPT) can be made with near certainty by documenting an increased serum intact parathormone (iPTH) level in a patient with increased ionized or total calcium. It is therefore necessary to eliminate all other causes of hypercalcemia and iPTH elevation. As for iPTH elevation, renal dysfunction and vitamin D deficiency are well known. Among causes of hypercalcemia, thought should be given to the syndrome of benign familial hypocalciuric hypercalcemia (BFHH), where the hypercalcemia is associated with normal or slightly raised levels of iPTH coexisting with hypocalciuria.

PATIENT HISTORY AND PHYSICAL FINDINGS

- The patient must be carefully selected. Not all patients presenting with HPT are candidates for an EPLA, as EPLA does not allow for a bilateral exploration.[5] Patients who are suspected to have multiglandular disease (MGD), including patients with secondary hyperparathyroidism (HPT) or patients with familial primary HPT, are not eligible for this procedure. Suspicion of parathyroid carcinoma is also an absolute contraindication. A history of neck irradiation, the presence of a large goiter and previous surgery in the thyroid vicinity are relative contraindications. EPLA can be performed in patients who have previously undergone a contralateral neck operation (Table 1).
- When considering EPLA, the adenoma must be solitary and clearly localized by preoperative imaging studies. Whether preoperative localizations techniques can rule out MGD with sufficient accuracy is questionable. Therefore, as with other minimally invasive techniques, the risk of missing MGD justifies the use of a quick intraoperative parathormone assay (QPTH).[6] The less definitive the localizations studies, the more imperative the need for QPTH.
- When patients are selected on the basis of the abovementioned criteria, no more than 50% of patients are eligible for this procedure (**FIG 1**).
- EPLA is technically more challenging than standard cervical exploration and its performance should be confined to tertiary centers. The surgeon must be experienced in conventional parathyroid surgery. Mentoring by a surgeon who has experience with endoscopic neck procedures is also recommended.

IMAGING AND OTHER DIAGNOSTIC STUDIES

- Only noninvasive tests should be considered. When these tests are negative, EPLA is not indicated and the traditional open cervicotomy is preferable. The topographic diagnosis should ideally be established by convergence of the results of two different investigations, one providing good anatomic information and the other providing functional information.
- High-resolution ultrasonography (US) and technetium-99m (Tc-99m) sestamibi scan are used most commonly in combination.[7] US can only assess the cervical region but gives good anatomic information, including useful information about the thyroid gland. The patient should be examined in the supine position with the neck in hyperextension. A pillow can be placed under the shoulders if the patient has a short neck. A high-frequency linear transducer

Table 1: Absolute and Relative Contraindications for Endoscopic Parathyroidectomy by Lateral Approach

Absolute contraindications
Suspicion of parathyroid carcinoma
Large goiter
Secondary or tertiary HPT
Familial HPT
Suspicion of MGD
No localization
Relative contraindications
Previous surgery
History of neck irradiation
Large tumor (>3 cm)
Inferior adenoma located anteriorly

HPT, hyperparathyroidism; MGD, multiglandular disease.

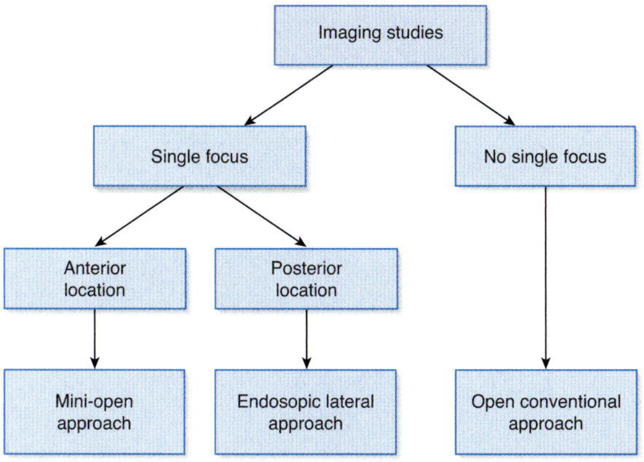

FIG 1 • Algorithm for the surgical management of patients eligible for an endoscopic parathyroidectomy by lateral approach.

(7.5 to 10 MHz) is used to obtain optimal depth penetration of 3 to 4 cm. A bilateral and comparative scan should be performed in transverse section, then in longitudinal section. In transverse section, the examination concentrates on an area defined by the longus colli muscles posteriorly, the thyroid gland anteriorly, the trachea medially, and the carotid artery laterally. The scan is then performed in cranial and caudal directions. An additional scan can be performed with the head of the patient turned away to the side and during deglutition to optimize the lateroesophageal images. The anterosuperior mediastinum is examined by inclining the transducer deeply in a retrosternal direction. The examiner should note the precise location with respect to surrounding structures, particularly to the thyroid gland, and the depth from the skin. Finally, a color flow Doppler or a power flow Doppler will be performed to test the vascularization of the area and define the artery branches involved.

- Two protocols for sestamibi scanning can be used: the single isotope dual phase protocol and the substraction protocol. The dual protocol requires early (15 minutes postinjection) and delayed images (at 1 and 2 to 3 hours, depending on thyroid washout). In cases of multinodular thyroid disease, additional further delayed images are sometimes needed. When a subtraction protocol is used, Tc-99m sestamibi is used in conjunction with another radionuclide specific to the thyroid. Tc-99m pertechnetate and ^{123}I are the most widely used radioisotopes for thyroid scintigraphy. The main advantage of using ^{123}I is that thyroid and parathyroid images can be acquired simultaneously in a dual energy window setup. The disadvantage is the cost of the protocol related to ^{123}I. Parathyroid scintigraphy should include views of the neck and the mediastinum. Single-photon emission computed tomography (SPECT) can be helpful for more precise localization of adenomas, as it provides simultaneous three-dimensional (3-D) information on both neck and superior mediastinum.
- Instead of US and Tc-99m sestamibi scan, four-dimensional computed tomography (4D-CT)[8] or the use of computed axial tomography-methoxyisobutyl isonitrile (MIBI) image fusion,[9] when available, may be preferable.
- Consideration for EPLA depends on the results of preoperative imaging. EPLA should be strongly considered when the parathyroid adenoma is in close proximity to the recurrent laryngeal nerve, as the nerve is at risk during MIP. Therefore, EPLA is the procedure of choice in all cases where the parathyroid adenomas are deeply located in the neck.
- Three locations of parathyroid adenomas with regard to the recurrent laryngeal nerve can be described (**FIG 2**).[4] Location 1 is posterior to the two superior thirds of the thyroid lobe (**FIGS 3** and **4**). These adenomas are superior glands. Location 2 is at the level of or below the inferior pole of the thyroid lobe but in a plane posterior to it (**FIGS 5** and **6**). These adenomas may be either a superior gland that has migrated posteriorly and in a downward direction or an inferior gland that has fallen posteriorly. These glands can also migrate into the superior and posterior mediastinum. Location 3 is at the level of or below the inferior pole of the thyroid lobe but in a superficial plane (**FIGS 7** and **8**). These adenomas are always inferior glands and can be found in close contact with the tip of the inferior pole of the thyroid lobe but also along the thyrothymic ligament or into the superior pole of the thymus.

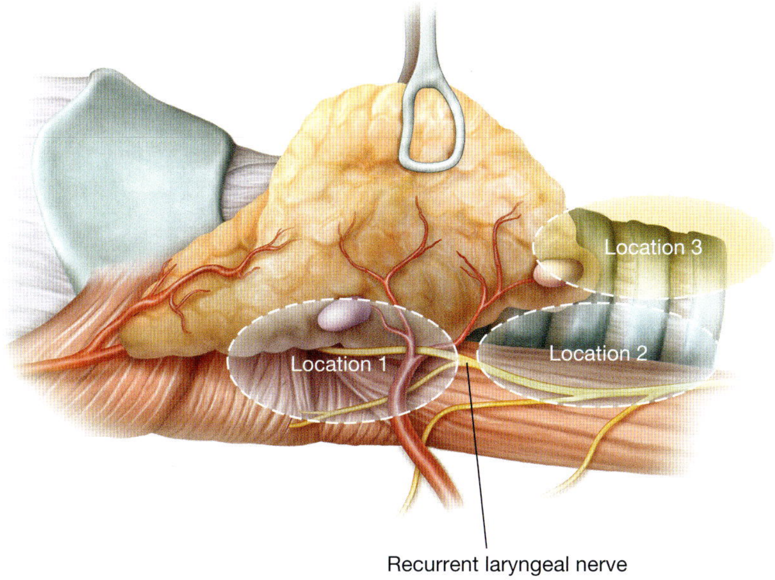

FIG 2 • The three different locations of parathyroid adenomas with regard to the recurrent laryngeal nerve. Location 1, posterior to the two superior thirds of the thyroid lobe; location 2, at the level of or below the inferior pole of the thyroid lobe but in a plane posterior to it; location 3, at the level of or below the inferior pole of the thyroid lobe but in a superficial plane.

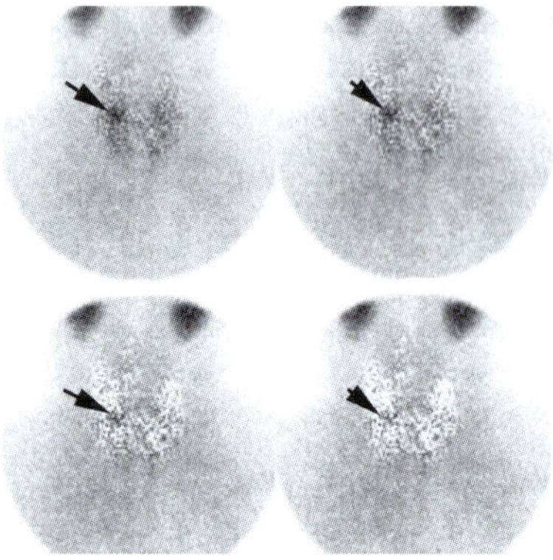

FIG 3 • Parathyroid Tc-99m sestamibi scintigraphy; subtraction protocol. The subtraction image demonstrates a right parathyroid adenoma at the level of the middle third of the right thyroid lobe *(arrow)*.

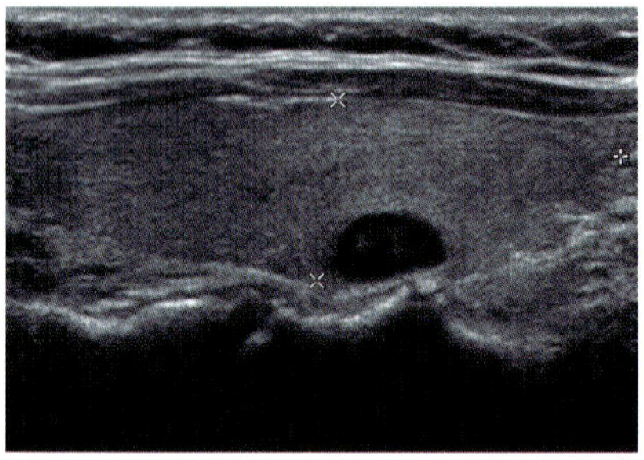

FIG 4 • Ultrasound (same patient in **FIG 3**). Right parathyroid adenoma posterior to the middle third of the thyroid lobe: right superior parathyroid adenoma in location 1. EPLA is indicated.

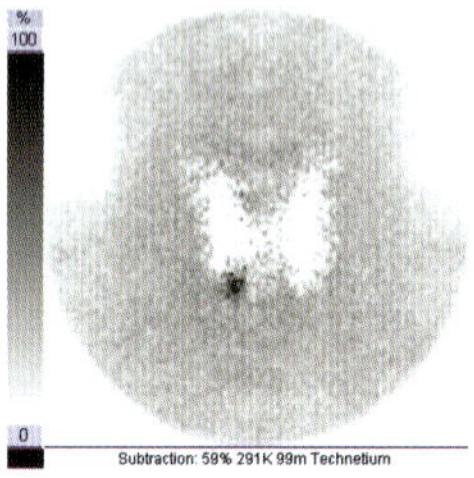

FIG 5 • Parathyroid Tc-99m sestamibi scintigraphy; subtraction protocol. The subtraction image demonstrates a right parathyroid adenoma at the level of the inferior third of the right thyroid lobe.

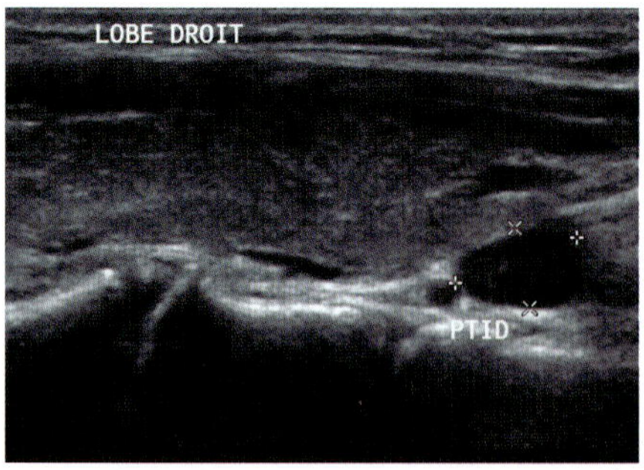

FIG 6 • Ultrasound (same patient in **FIG 5**). Right parathyroid adenoma posterior to the inferior third of the thyroid lobe: right, more probably inferior, parathyroid adenoma in location 2. EPLA is indicated.

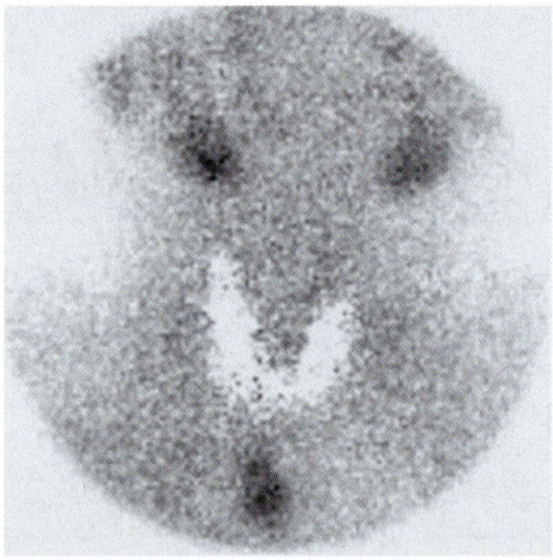

FIG 7 • Parathyroid Tc-99m sestamibi scintigraphy; subtraction protocol. The subtraction image demonstrates a right parathyroid adenoma below the inferior pole of the thyroid lobe.

- Adenomas in locations 1 and 2 are deeply located and are in the vicinity of the recurrent laryngeal nerve. The nerve is at risk and its clear identification during the procedure is recommended. The lateral view, provided by EPLA, permits its easy identification and allows a secure dissection. On the other hand, adenomas in location 3 are at distance from the nerve, which runs more deeply. Its identification is not essential. An anterior mini-open approach without the help of the endoscope is indicated.
- In conclusion, the need to know preoperatively when the nerve is at risk reinforces the role of preoperative imaging studies. Depending on whether the patient has a deep-seated adenoma or a superficial-seated adenoma, the surgeon can choose between EPLA and an anterior mini-open approach.
- The main interest of using an endoscope is not that one can perform a parathyroidectomy through a small incision but that one can perform a safe parathyroidectomy through a small incision.

SURGICAL MANAGEMENT

Preoperative Planning

- Prior to surgery, the patient undergoes a vocal cord check.
- The procedure is performed under general anesthesia with endotracheal intubation. Trocars are poorly tolerated by

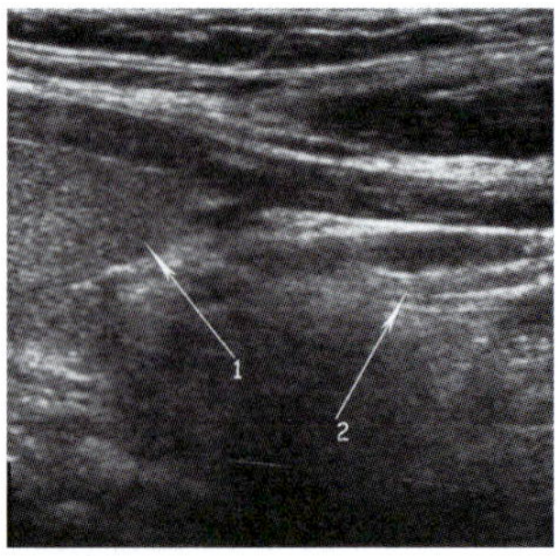

FIG 8 • Ultrasound (same patient in **FIG 7**). The adenoma *(2)* is in the superficial plane, below the inferior pole of the thyroid lobe *(1)*, along the thyrothymic tract: right inferior parathyroid adenoma in location 3. There is no need for the endoscope. A mini-open procedure is indicated.

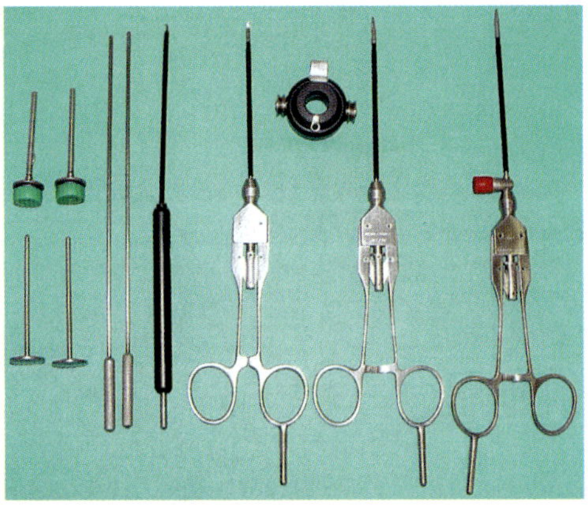

FIG 9 ● Instruments of 3-mm trocars (Medtronic Xomed, MicroFrance, Saint Aubin Le Monial, France).

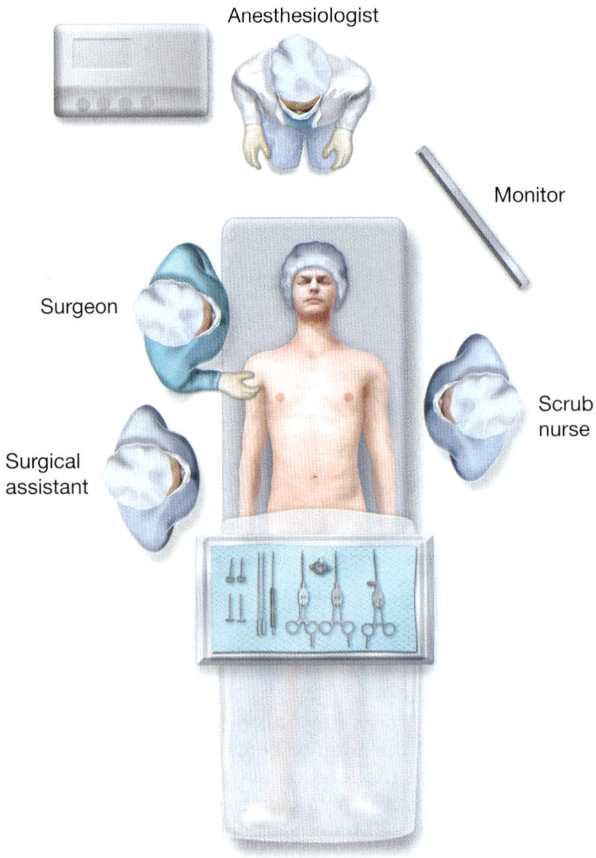

FIG 10 ● Operating room organization.

patients under local or regional anesthesia. In addition, swallowing and spontaneous breathing present impediments when dissecting in a small operative space.

- The surgical instruments required include a 10-mm trocar, which will accommodate a 0-degree fiberoptic endoscope, and two 3-mm trocars, which will receive a series of purpose-made instruments (Medtronic Xomed, MicroFrance) including blunt-tipped dissectors, graspers, scissors, a diathermy hook, and an aspiration canula. These instruments measure 25 cm in length (**FIG 9**).
- In patients presenting with small parathyroid adenomas less than 2 cm in diameter, a 5-mm trocar and a 5-mm 0-degree endoscope can be used.
- QPTH assays are performed before and at the time of incision, directly before parathyroid excision and, subsequently, 5 and 15 minutes after parathyroid excision. Parathyroidectomy is considered successful when QPTH value falls by greater than 50% with respect to the highest preexcision level and into normal range (10 to 65 pg/mL).[5]
- The surgical team consists of the operator, first assistant, and a scrub nurse. The surgeon and first assistant stand on the side of the diseased gland, with the scrub nurse facing them. The monitor is placed next to the scrub nurse and directly in front of the surgeon (**FIG 10**).

Positioning

- The patient is positioned in the supine position. The head is placed in a neutral position without hyperextension to avoid tensing the sternocleidomastoid muscle (SCM) and the strap muscles. Complete relaxation and suppleness of these muscles are essential to prevent narrowing down the operative space given that this is maintained with low-pressure gas insufflation. The patient is prepped and draped as for standard parathyroid surgery.

THE BACK-DOOR APPROACH

- An initial 12- to 15-mm transverse skin incision (optic trocar incision) is made on the anterior border of the SCM, at the level of the thyroid isthmus (**FIG 11**). It will permit the creation of a space through which the 10-mm trocar will be introduced. This incision is placed such that in the event of conversion, it can be extended medially to result in a symmetric collar incision.
- After division of the platysma, the anterior border of the SCM is identified and the investing layer of cervical fascia is incised. This allows access to the plane of dissection between the SCM laterally and the strap muscles medially, just inferior to the omohyoid muscle (**FIG 12**).
- The fascia connecting the posterior aspect of the thyroid lobe medially to the carotid sheath laterally is gently divided with scissors (**FIG 13**). A middle thyroid vein may be encountered. It is ligated without any difficulty through the incision.
- A small moist gauze is then inserted through the incision and packed deeply in an upward and downward direction into the initially created space (**FIG 14**). This blind maneuver enlarges the cavity and permits a surprisingly quick, efficient, and bloodless exposure of the operative field.

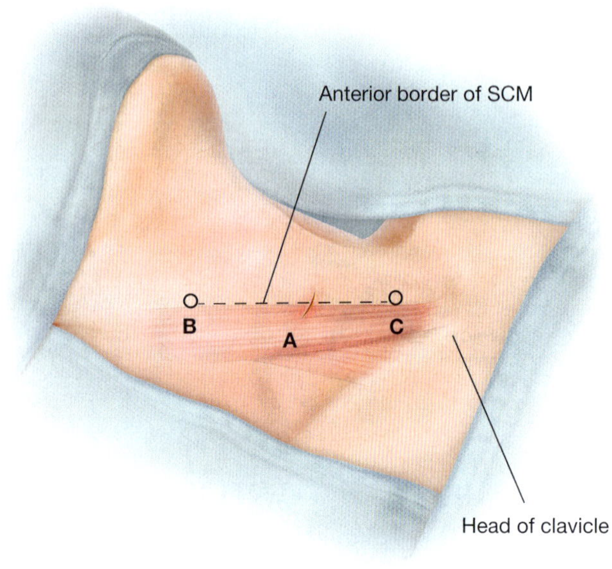

FIG 11 • Trocar sites. All three trocars are positioned on the line of the anterior border of the SCM. Main trocar *(A)* is placed at the level of the thyroid isthmus. Trocars *B* and *C* should be 3 to 4 cm apart and will be used for the 2-mm instruments. SCM, sternocleidomastoid muscle.

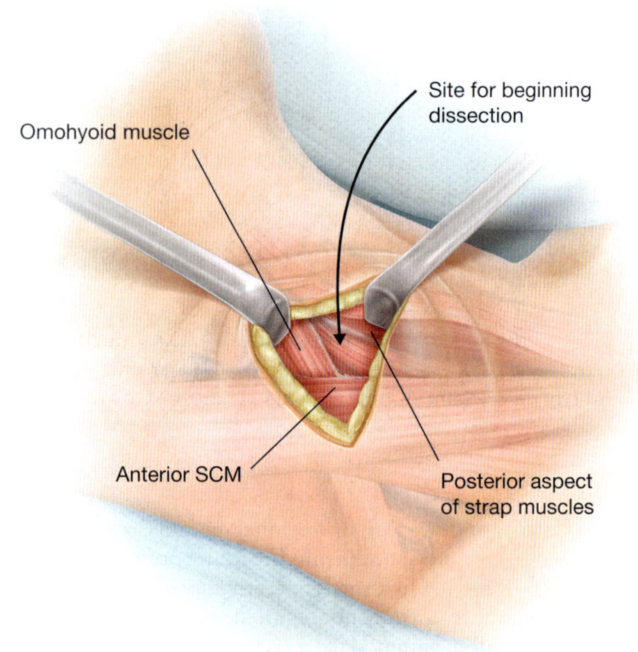

FIG 12 • The access to the plane of dissection between the SCM laterally and the strap muscles medially is just inferior to the omohyoid muscle. SCM, sternocleidomastoid muscle.

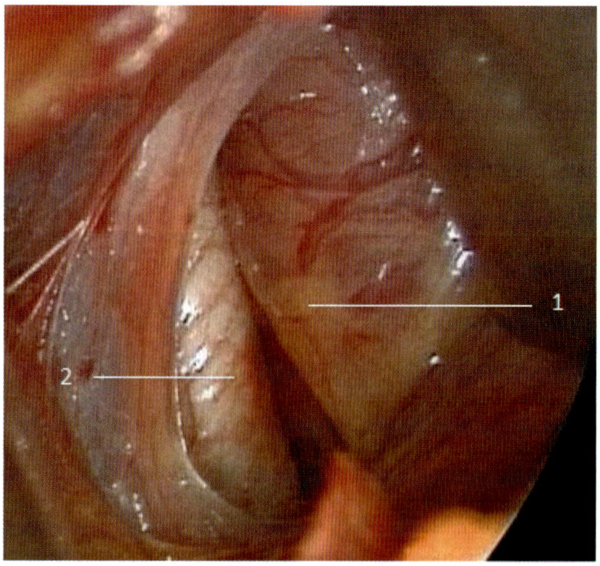

FIG 13 • The back-door approach uses the plane between the posterior aspect of the thyroid lobe medially *(1)* to the carotid sheath laterally *(2)*.

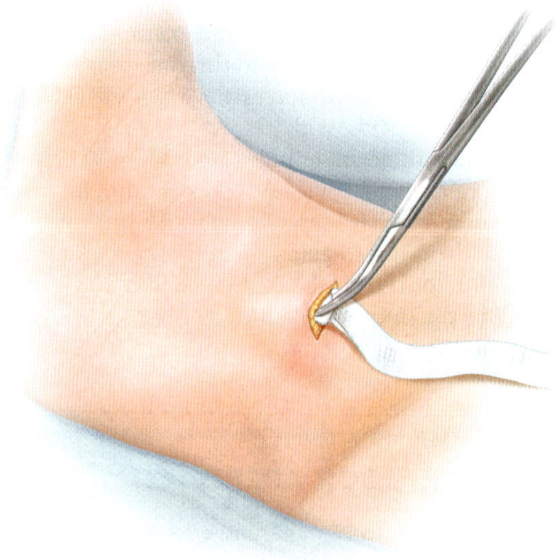

FIG 14 • Creating space for endoscopic exploration. A small moist gauze roll is inserted through the incision and packed deeply into the initially created space.

INSTALLATION OF THE TWO 3-MM WORKING TROCARS

- The two 3-mm trocars are placed on the line situated along the anterior border of the SCM, in their respective positions, above (5 to 6 cm) and below (3 to 4 cm) the main optic trocar incision. Safe trocar placement is achieved by tunnelling a 2.5-mm drain introducer needle inserted from within the main incision through to the skin. The direction this guide takes must follow the anterior border of the SCM. During this maneuver, one must constantly be aware of the internal jugular vein situated posteriorly, the external jugular vein situated cranially, and the anterior jugular vein situated caudally. The 3-mm trocar is placed over the tip of the introducer needle, which has pierced the skin from inside out and railroaded into the operative space (**FIG 15**). Each appropriately positioned 3-mm trocar is then loosely fixed to the skin with a nonabsorbable monofilament stitch to prevent involuntary removal.

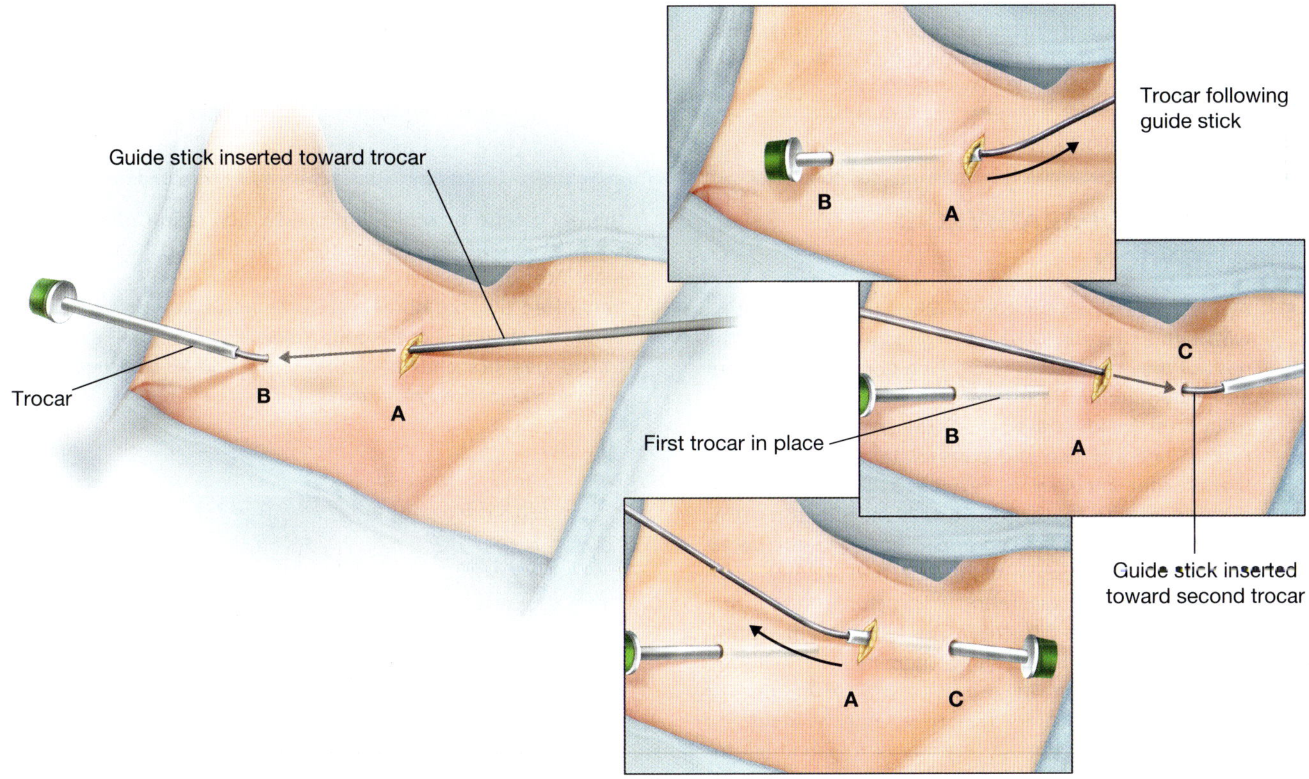

FIG 15 • Installation of the 3-mm trocars. The transparietal path of both trocars is made through the incision *(A)*, from the inside to the outside, using a guide stick. The pathway of the guide stick must follow the anterior border of the SCM. Then, the 3-mm trocar is placed over the tip of the guide stick and railroaded into the operative space.

INSTALLATION OF THE 10-MM OPTIC TROCAR

- A purse-string stitch is placed around the main wound. It incorporates not only the skin but also the anterior border of the SCM laterally and the posterior border of the sternothyroid muscle medially. At this stage, the gauze roll is removed, the 10-mm trocar inserted and held in position with the purse-string suture.
- The purse string is subsequently threaded through an eyelet mounted on a specifically designed device encircling the trocar and secured to this (**FIG 16**). This arrangement guarantees air tightness, allows the amplification of the operative space, and prevents the trocar from slipping out of the wound.
- The three trocars are now positioned. The assistant takes care of the endoscope and the surgeon works through the other two trocars (**FIG 17**).

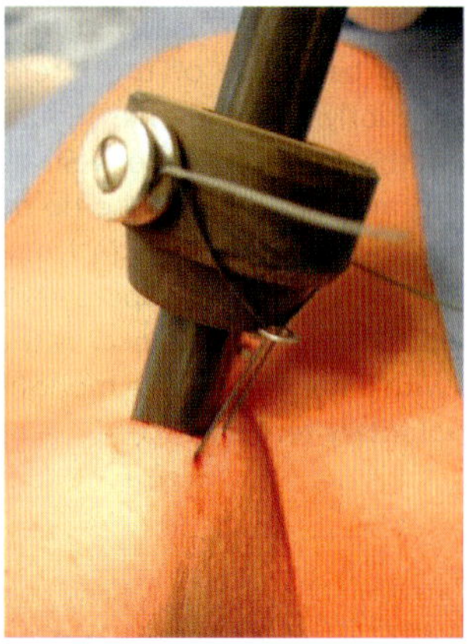

FIG 16 ● Installation of the main trocar. A purse-string stitch is placed around the main wound and is tied on a specifically designed device encircling the main trocar.

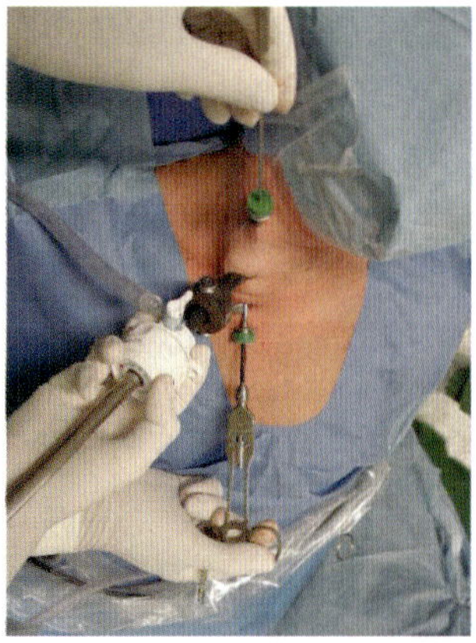

FIG 17 ● The three trocars are positioned. Insufflation (8 mmHg) is installed. The assistant holds the camera and the operator works through the other two 3-mm trocars. Endoscopic exploration can start.

ENDOSCOPIC PARATHYROID EXPLORATION

- A pneumocervicotomy is established using insufflation with carbon dioxide (CO_2) at low pressure (8 mmHg). The gas not only maintains the working operative space but also may tamponade off minor bleeders. First, the carotid must be identified. Then, the space between the carotid laterally and the posterolateral aspect of the thyroid lobe medially is developed. The dissection is performed with the help of two blunt-tipped metallic dissectors. Ligatures or clip applications are not necessary. The combination of blunt dissection and gas insufflation allows easy separation of structures, minimizing the need for sharp dissection. This facilitates identification of the key structures and landmarks that will permit a safe dissection. The inferior thyroid artery and, of course, the recurrent laryngeal nerve must be identified first. The inferior thyroid artery is a useful landmark for locating the recurrent laryngeal nerve. The easiest site to identify the nerve is at the level of the lower pole of the thyroid gland, just caudally to the trunk of the artery. On the left side, the nerve ascends at the depth of the tracheoesophageal groove. On the right side, the nerve courses more obliquely. The magnification allowed by the endoscope provides improved visualization of the vasa nervorum running along the nerve and help its identification.
- Very often one can observe that the nerve branches far below its laryngeal entry point (**FIG 18**). Also, small extralaryngeal branches extending to the adjacent trachea and esophagus are easily seen.

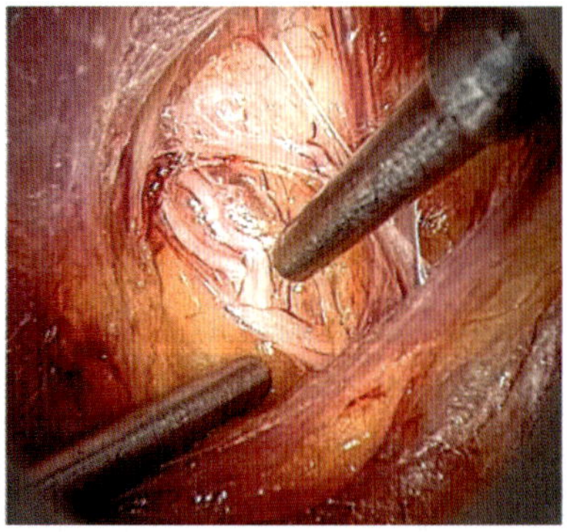

FIG 18 ● Endoscopic exploration on the right side: identification of the right recurrent laryngeal nerve. In this case, the nerve branches far below its laryngeal entry point.

IDENTIFICATION OF THE PARATHYROID ADENOMA

- Based on the results of the preoperative imaging studies, the surgeon may suspect an adenoma in location 1 or 2.
- All glands in location 1 are superior parathyroid adenomas. The search for them requires the dissection of the upper two-thirds of posterior aspect of the thyroid lobe (**FIG 19**). Small superior adenomas usually remain located in their orthotopic site, floating in a loose, fatty setting immediately adjacent to the inferior thyroid artery. Large superior adenomas tend to migrate posteriorly and downward. Therefore, if they are not found in immediate contact with the thyroid capsule, they should be sought beside or behind the esophagus.
- Glands in location 2 may be also superior parathyroid adenomas. Their migration may drag them down very low, well below the inferior thyroid artery, behind whose

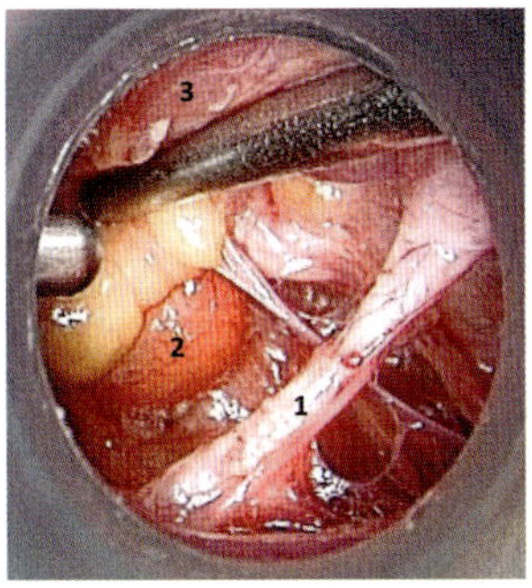

FIG 19 ● Endoscopic exploration on the right side: inferior thyroid artery *(1)*, superior parathyroid adenoma *(2)* posterior to the middle third of the thyroid lobe *(3)*. The adenoma is located in location 1.

trunk they cross during their descent. Endoscopic exploration behind the inferior thyroid artery, along the esophagus, and down into the posterior mediastinum can be easily accomplished by this back-door approach. These adenomas are revealed by their vascular pedicle, which is easily dissected at the level of the inferior thyroid artery. They emerge with simple traction on it and their elongated shape is amenable to expeditious extraction.

- The search of inferior parathyroid adenomas in location 2 requires the exploration of the lower third of the posterior aspect of the thyroid lobe. Sometimes, they are identified immediately after introducing the endoscope. They tend to descend posteriorly and in a downward direction to acquire a paratracheal or a paraesophageal position. It is in these cases that they become intimate with the recurrent laryngeal nerve. Their posterior surface may adhere to the nerve. In these cases, the lateral view allows a secure dissection of the nerve.
- Although searching for the ipsilateral gland is not mandatory, it can often be identified when it is in location 1 or 2 (**FIG 20**).

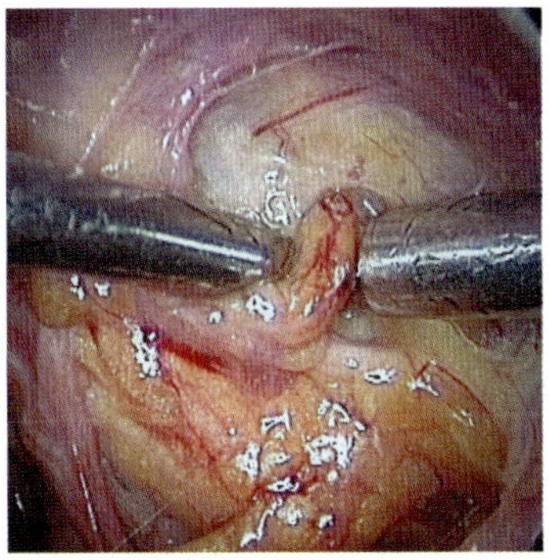

FIG 20 ● Identification of the ipsilateral inferior parathyroid gland. The gland is normal.

DISSECTION OF THE PARATHYROID ADENOMA

- The adenoma must never be grasped to avoid parathyroid fracture and potential risk of parathyromatosis. The adenoma is progressively freed from adjacent structures by blunt dissection with the help of two blunt-tipped metallic dissectors (**FIG 21**). One dissector retracts the adenoma, providing tension, while the other instrument is used to dissect the gland away from surrounding structures and loose areolar tissue until complete mobilization is achieved. When the pedicle is isolated (**FIG 22**), the terminal vascular branches are grasped, skeletonized, and electrocoagulated with the 3-mm diathermy hook (**FIG 23**).

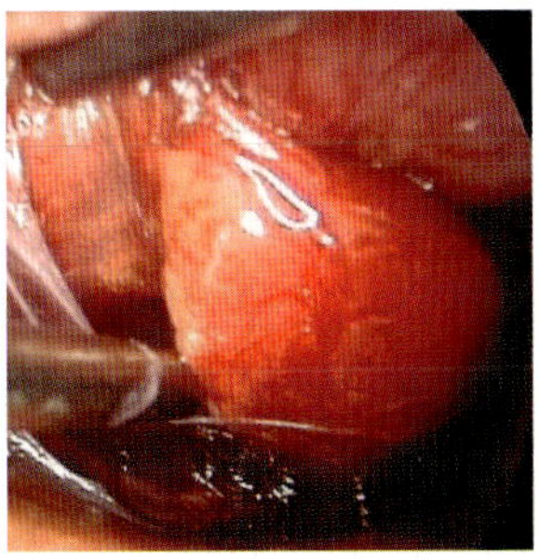

FIG 21 ● Endoscopic dissection of the superior parathyroid adenoma with the help of two blunt-tipped dissectors. The gland should not be grasped to avoid capsular disruption.

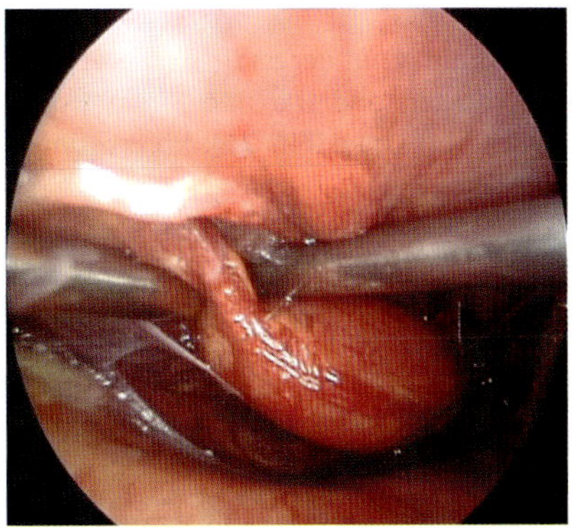

FIG 22 ● Dissection of the vascular pedicle of the superior parathyroid adenoma.

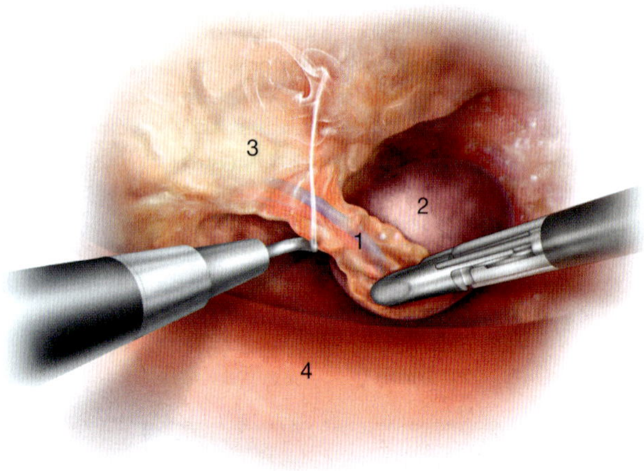

FIG 23 • Electrocoagulation of the terminal vascular branches *(1)* of the superior parathyroid adenoma *(2)* with the 3-mm diathermy hook. *3*, thyroid lobe; *4*, carotid artery.

EXTRACTION OF THE PARATHYROID ADENOMA

- Most parathyroid adenomas can be extracted through the 10-mm trocar. In performing this step, after removing the 10-mm endoscope, a grasper and a 5-mm lens are simultaneously introduced into the 10-mm trocar. The pedicle of the adenoma is grasped and the adenoma is drawn into the trocar (**FIG 24**), the trocar containing the specimen is then removed.
- Larger adenomas that cannot be drawn into the 10-mm trocar are extracted directly through the trocar site under direct vision. There is no need to place them in a sterile plastic bag during this maneuver. After checking hemostasis, the two 3-mm trocars are removed.

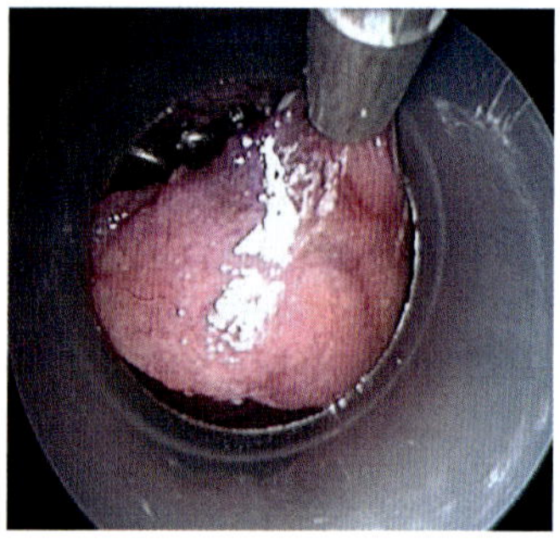

FIG 24 • Extraction of the parathyroid adenoma. The pedicle of the adenoma is grasped and the adenoma is drawn into the trocar.

CLOSURE

- A surgical drain is not necessary. The platysma is sutured. The skin incision and the two 3-mm trocars sites are closed with fibrin glue (**FIG 25**). No dressing is required.

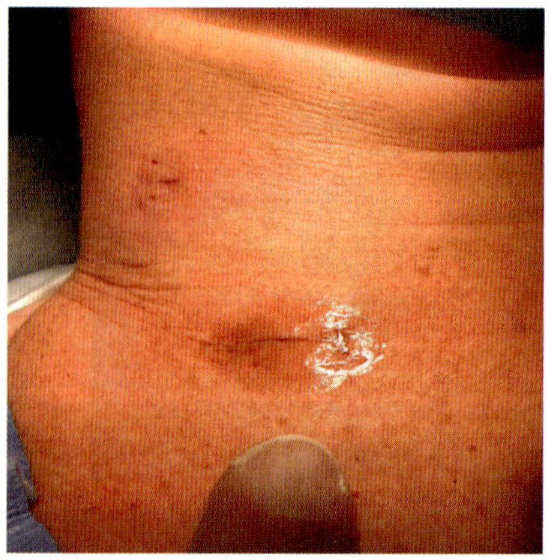

FIG 25 • Fibrin glue is used to close the skin.

PEARLS AND PITFALLS

Indications	■ Only patients with sporadic primary HPT, in whom a single adenoma has been clearly localized by preoperative imaging studies, are potential candidates for EPLA. ■ Based on the results of preoperative imaging studies, EPLA should be reserved for patients presenting with parathyroid adenomas deeply located in the neck.
QPTH assay	■ The availability of the QPTH assay is of utmost importance. This test is especially useful when localization studies are less certain.
Installation of trocars	■ Place all three trocars on the line of the anterior border of the SCM and fix them to the skin to prevent involuntary removal. ■ Optic trocar incision should be created such that in the event of conversion, it can be extended medially to result in a traditional cervicotomy. ■ The transparietal path of the working trocars should be made through the optic trocar incision, from the inside to the outside.
Working space	■ Place the head in a neutral position to avoid tensing the SCM and the strap muscles. ■ In order to enlarge the working area, before introducing the optic trocar, stuff a small moist gauze, upward and downward, deeply into the initially created space, and then remove it.
Endoscopic exploration	■ Bear in mind that because the working space is very small, the endoscope is very close to the anatomic structures, which will therefore appear highly magnified. There is a definite risk of removing a normal gland that appears enlarged under endoscopic vision.
Endoscopic dissection	■ Never grasp the adenoma to avoid parathyroid fracture. The dissection can be performed entirely with the two blunt-tipped palpators.

POSTOPERATIVE CARE

- The patient may remain in the operating room or, in case of long processing for the QPTH assay, may be transferred to the postanesthesia care unit after extubation. In this latter case, if the results of QPTH are not consistent with successful removal of parathyroid adenoma, the patient must be returned to the operating room. In both cases, conversion to bilateral neck exploration is performed if the QPTH value does not fall by greater than 50% and into normal range (10 to 65 pg/mL).
- Patients have determination of serum parathyroid hormone (PTH) 4 hours after excision of the adenoma, then on day 1 and day 8 after surgery. Calcemia and phosphoremia are also systematically evaluated on day 1 and day 8.
- The serum PTH level reaches its nadir 4 hours after excision of the adenoma and, in most patients, the serum calcium reaches its lowest level within 48 to 72 hours after surgery. Because the parathyroid exploration is unilateral, postoperative hypoparathyroidism is not observed. However, postoperative hypocalcemia can be observed in patients with severe skeletal depletion of calcium, resulting in "bone hunger." If symptoms appear, calcium and vitamin D derivatives should be administrated.
- Usually, patients are discharged the day after surgery.
- Postoperative vocal cord evaluation must be performed systematically.

OUTCOMES

- After EPLA, more than 95% of patients are normocalcemic. However, it should be kept in mind that these excellent results are obtained in a group of carefully selected patients.[4]
- EPLA does not appear to be clearly superior to other MIP technique in terms of recurrent disease or postoperative complications.[10]
- As with other techniques of single-gland excision through a limited neck exploration, EPLA does not lead to an increased incidence of persistent/recurrent HPT[10]; it is associated with a better postoperative course in terms of pain and it produces better cosmetic results compared to bilateral neck exploration[11] (**FIG 26**). Prevalence and severity of postoperative hypocalcemia are lowered.[12]

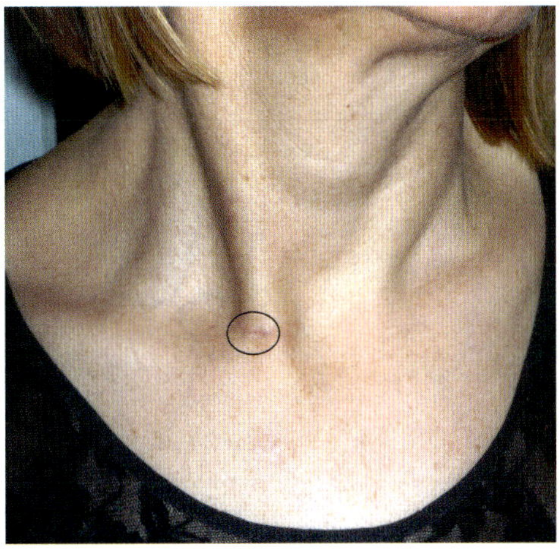

FIG 26 • Cervical scar 1 month after surgery.

COMPLICATIONS

- Hematoma
- Inferior laryngeal nerve injury
- Parathyroid adenoma not found: conversion
- Capsular rupture of adenoma
- False-positive result of preoperative imaging studies
- False-negative result of QPTH assay

REFERENCES

1. Udelsman R, Donovan PI, Sokoll LJ. One hundred consecutive minimally invasive parathyroid explorations. *Ann Surg*. 2000;232:331–339.
2. Miccoli P, Bendinelli C, Vignali E, et al. Endoscopic parathyroidectomy: report of an initial experience. *Surgery*. 1998;124:1077–1080.
3. Gagner M, Rubino F. Endoscopic parathyroidectomy. In: Schwartz AE, Pertsemlidis D, Gagner M, eds. *Endocrine Surgery*. New York, NY: Marcel Dekker; 2004:289–296.
4. Henry JF, Sebag F, Cherenko M, et al. Endoscopic parathyroidectomy: why and when? *World J Surg*. 2008;32:2509–2515.
5. Mihai R, Barczynski M, Iacobone M, et al. Surgical strategy for sporadic primary hyperparathyroidism: an evidence-based approach to surgical strategy, patient selection, surgical access, and reoperations. *Langenbecks Arch Surg*. 2009;394:785–798.
6. Harrison BJ, Triponez F. Intraoperative adjuncts in surgery for primary hyperparathyroidism. *Langenbecks Arch Surg*. 2009;394:799–809.
7. Mihai R, Simon D, Hellman P. Imaging for primary hyperparathyroidism: an evidence-based analysis. *Langenbecks Arch Surg*. 2009;394:765–784.
8. Rodgers SE, Hunter GJ, Hamberg LM. Improved preoperative planning for directed parathyroidectomy with 4-dimensional computed tomography. *Surgery*. 2006;140:932–941.
9. Profanter C, Prommegger R, Gabriel M, et al. Computer axial tomography-MIBI image fusion for preoperative localization in primary hyperparathyroidism. *Am J Surg*. 2004;187:383–387.
10. Bergenfelz OA, Hellman P, Harrison B, et al. Positional statement of the European Society of Endocrine Surgery on modern techniques in pHPT surgery. *Langenbecks Arch Surg*. 2009;394:761–764.
11. Henry JF, Raffaeli M, Iacobone M, et al. Video-assisted parathyroidectomy via the lateral approach vs conventional surgery in the treatment of sporadic primary hyperparathyroidism. *Surg Endosc*. 2001;15:1116–1119.
12. Westerdalh J, Bergenfelz A. Unilateral versus bilateral neck exploration for primary hyperparathyroidism: five-year follow-up of a randomized controlled trial. *Ann Surg*. 2007;246:976–980.

Chapter 45

Reoperative Parathyroidectomy

Barnard J. A. Palmer   William B. Inabnet, III

DEFINITIONS

- Reoperative parathyroid surgery occurs in multiple clinical settings but is most frequently performed as the result of failed exploration, recurrent, or persistent hyperparathyroidism.
- Persistent hyperparathyroidism is defined as hypercalcemia that remains or recurs within 6 months of an initial parathyroid operation.
- Recurrent hyperparathyroidism is the reappearance of hypercalcemia after a period of 6 months of postoperative normocalcemia following successful surgery.

PATIENT HISTORY AND PHYSICAL FINDINGS

- A detailed history of the patient's disease should be performed, focusing on the management to date.
- Biochemical confirmation of persistent or recurrent hyperparathyroidism is the initial step in management. A 24-hour collection for calcium is recommended.[1,2]
- The benefits of reoperation must be weighed against the risks of continued hyperparathyroidism and the surgical complications for each individual patient. Nonsurgical management can be considered if the sequela of continued parathyroid disease is relatively low risk or the risk of operation is high.
- Surgical history is an essential component of reoperative parathyroid surgery. The surgeon must understand reasons for initial operative failure.[3]
- Operative and pathology reports should be carefully reviewed, focusing on the extent of exploration, glands identified and removed, whether confirmed by biopsy, if marked, and if reimplanted.

IMAGING AND OTHER DIAGNOSTIC STUDIES

- Extensive preoperative planning is key to successful reoperative surgery.
- Previous operative reports, imaging, and pathology results should be obtained and reviewed to understand the cause of failure.[2]
- Localization studies are an essential portion of preoperative planning and should be performed in all reoperative parathyroid patients. Ultrasound, sestamibi, computed tomography (CT) (parathyroid protocol, 4-D) (**FIG 1**), single-photon emission computed tomography–computed tomography (SPECT/CT), and fluorodeoxyglucose-positron emission tomography (FDG-PET) can be used for localization and to rule out multigland disease. Preoperative location of abnormal glands can significantly alter the operative approach particularly if aberrant glands lie in the mediastinum.
- Fine needle aspiration (FNA) with measurement of parathyroid hormone (PTH) can confirm parathyroid tissue in questionable lesions or parathyroid adenomatosis identified by ultrasound.
- Invasive localization studies such as selective venous sampling (**FIG 2**) or arteriography should be reserved for when noninvasive studies fail to localize pathology.

SURGICAL MANAGEMENT

Preoperative Planning

- The imaging must be thoroughly reviewed to plan the operative approach.
- Prior operative notes are reviewed and operative steps clearly determined prior to reexploration.
- Positively localized lesions lend themselves to focused reexplorations, whereas more extensive exploration is required for multigland or nonlocalized diseases.
- Preoperative flexible laryngoscopy is recommended prior to reoperative surgery to document vocal cord function and guide the extent of surgery.
- Frozen section and intraoperative PTH assays are useful adjuncts to confirm parathyroid identification and biochemical cure.

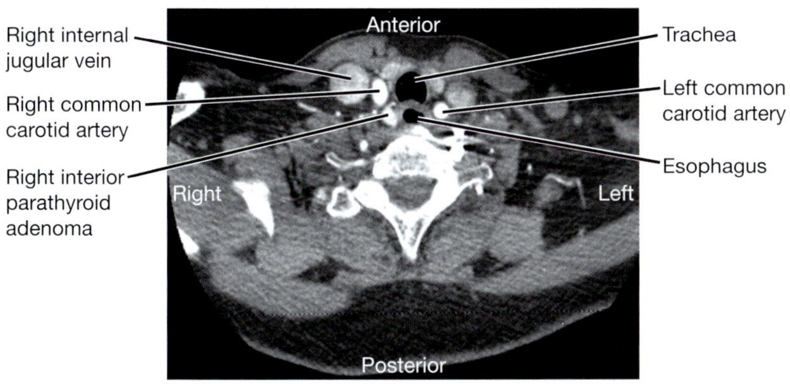

FIG 1 • Parathyroid CT demonstrates a contrast-enhancing lesion posterior to the right common carotid artery, posterolateral to the trachea, and lateral to the esophagus, representing a right inferior parathyroid adenoma.

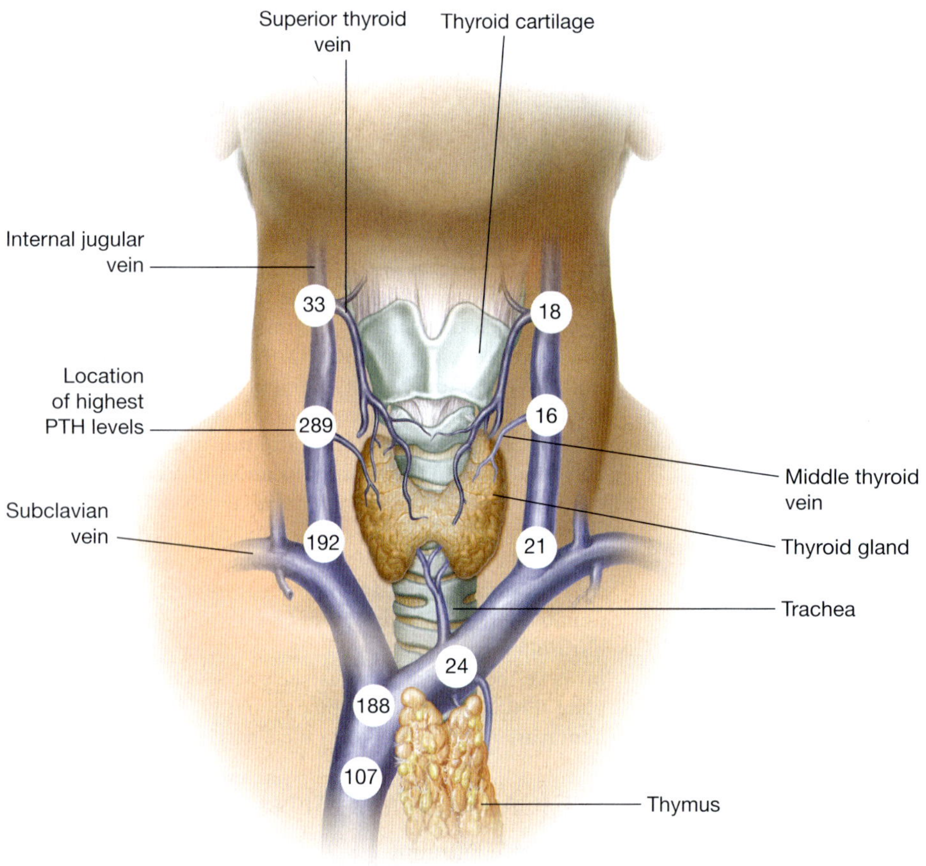

FIG 2 • Selective venous sampling schematic lists PTH levels at different anatomic locations and is consistent with a right midlobe parathyroid adenoma.

Positioning

- The patient is positioned either supine or in the semi-Fowler position. Both arms are tucked and neck extension is achieved with a shoulder roll (**FIG 3**).
- Surgical prep must be wide enough to allow access superiorly to angle of mandible and inferiorly to xiphoid in the instance that sternotomy is necessary.
- General endotracheal anesthesia permits the use of intraoperative nerve monitoring.

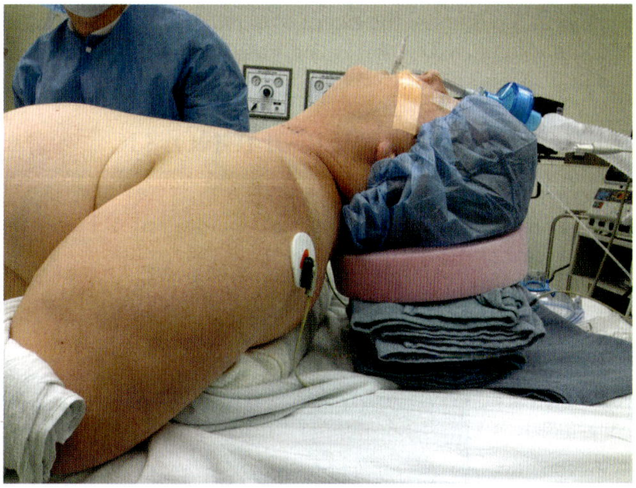

FIG 3 • The patient is placed supine with both arms tucked. A shoulder roll provides additional neck extension, which elevates the trachea anteriorly and superior mediastinal structures cephalad.

CERVICAL REEXPLORATION

Incision and Flap Elevation

- Skin incisions are placed as indicated by the preoperative localizing studies, preferably in a natural cervical skin crease or the old incision (unless the scar is too low or high). Width of incision is dependent on depth of neck but is large enough to allow access superiorly to the level of the hyoid bone and inferiorly to the anterior mediastinum (**FIG 4**).
- Incisions may be placed over the site of pathology for a directed approach if preoperatively localized.
- Skin and platysma are divided and subplatysmal flaps superficial to the anterior jugular veins are elevated superiorly to the thyroid notch, inferiorly to the sternal notch, and laterally to anterior borders of the sternocleidomastoid muscles (SCM).

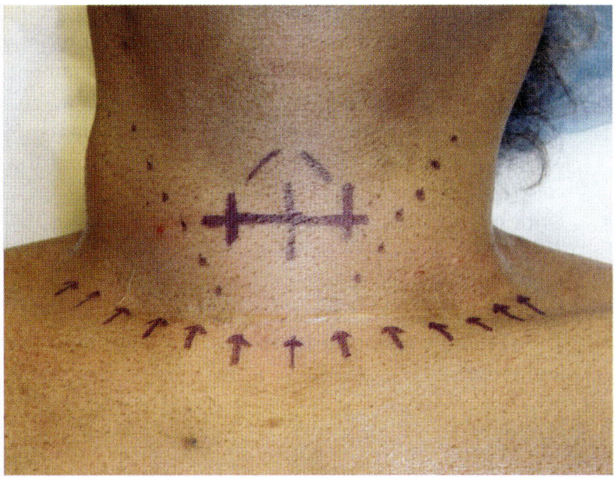

FIG 4 ● Skin incisions are placed in a natural skin crease and is adjusted according to preoperative localization and planned approach. Classic, large, inferior incisions have been substituted by more superior smaller incisions or incisions directly over parathyroid lesions. Lateral incisions can be made for a posterolateral approach with entry between the anterior border of the sternocleidomastoid and lateral border of the strap muscles. *Upward arrows* on the pictures show a classic incision versus a small superior incision as indicated by the *solid transverse line markings*.

Cervical Approach[3]

- Surgical approach to the reoperative neck is done via focused exploration or by classic midline, posterolateral, or thyrothymic ligament approaches.
- Focused explorations for preoperatively localized ectopic glands not accessible via prior cervicotomy should be adjusted to location and surgeon experience with incisions placed according to imaging.
- Revision cervicotomy is indicated when multigland disease is suspected or when abnormal glands are not localized preoperatively. The previous incision is used and the cervical scar revised prior to opening the midline raphe by vertical separation of strap muscles (see Chapters 45 and 48).
- The back door or ***posterolateral*** approach should be considered when there is extensive scar tissue or when seeking a posteriorly localized gland. The lateral portion of a prior wound is used and entry to the neck is achieved between the lateral border of the straps and anterior portion of the SCM (**FIG 5**).

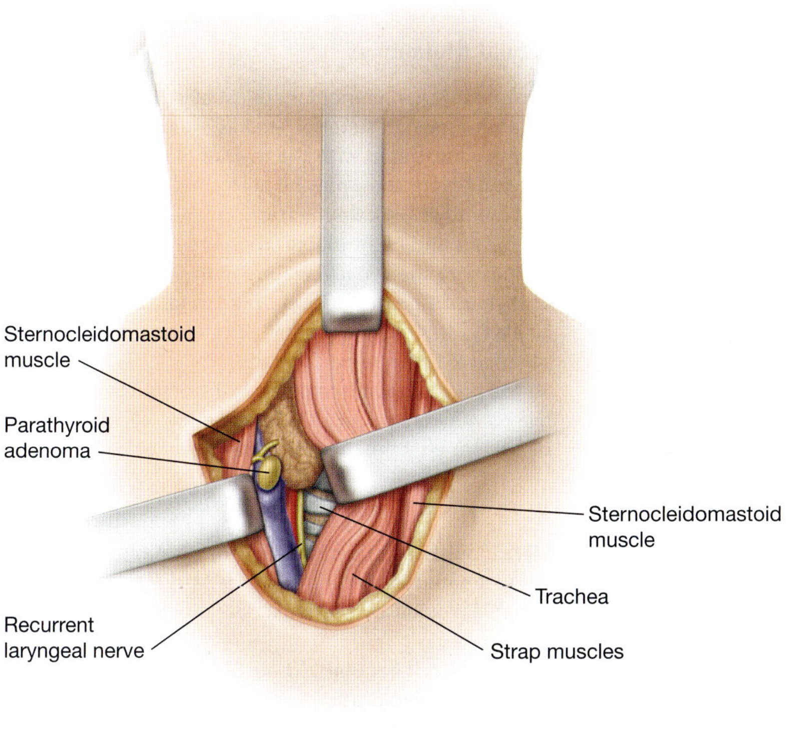

FIG 5 ● The posterolateral approach to the neck is similar to the classic approach except that subsequent access is achieved along the medial border of the SCM and lateral to the sternohyoid-sternothyroid, minimizing dissection through midline scar. The omohyoid muscle is divided as necessary.

- The front door or ***thyrothymic*** ligament approach should be considered when adenomas are localized anteriorly along the inferior thyroid pole or thyrothymic ligament. Infrahyoid muscles may be divided as inferiorly as possible to allow direct access to the thyrothymic ligaments, avoiding dissection between the strap muscles and thyroid capsule.
- Once deep to the strap muscles, retraction of the thyroid involves elevation of the strap muscles off the gland and medial thyroid rotation. A Kittner, thyroid clamp, or figure-of-eight suture assists thyroid retraction.
- The recurrent laryngeal nerve (RLN) is then identified and preserved.

Exploration

- Steps are systematically planned and based on preoperative imaging.
- If an abnormal gland is localized preoperatively, commence with focused exploration.
- Start by exploring the normal locations of the missing glands. The superior glands are generally at the mid to upper one-third of the thyroid in the expected position 85% of the time, at the inferior border of the thyroid cartilage posterior to the RLN and the superior portion of the inferior thyroid artery.
- The inferior glands are classically located near the posterior aspect of the thyroid pole, anterior to the RLN from the inferior thyroid artery to the inferior thyroid pole or along thyrothymic ligament (see Chapter 41, **FIG 11**).
- If unable to locate in normal positions, search expected aberrant positions.
- Ectopic superior glands are generally displaced posteriorly or inferiorly, becoming more posterior as they travel inferiorly.
- Search circumferentially around the superior thyroid pedicle and visceral sheath of the thyroid capsule with thyroid palpation.
- Follow the tracheoesophageal groove inferiorly down to the posterior mediastinum (**FIG 6**).
- Inferior glands have a greater range of position but nearly 25% are along the thyrothymic ligament or upper pole of the thymus. They are rarely posterior and become more anterior the lower they are.
- Search and digitally explore the posterior and inferior thyroid gland.
- Inspect the thyrothymic ligament, incise the thymic sheath, and pull the thymic lobe cephalad to inspect the thymus (see **FIG 8**).
- Explore the carotid sheath up to the angle of the mandible (**FIG 7**).

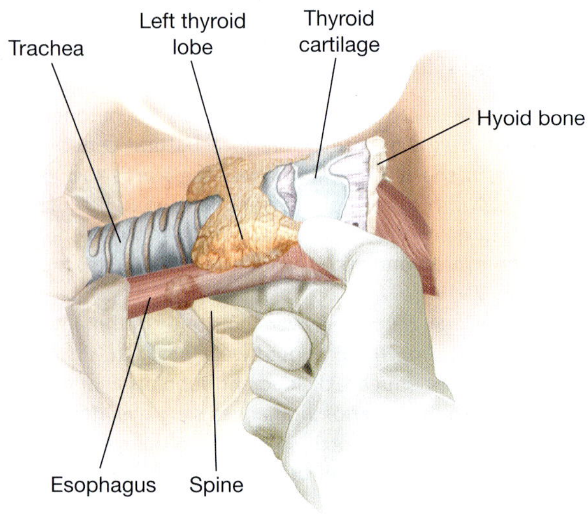

FIG 6 ● The lateral wall of the esophagus and the tracheoesophageal groove are exposed from the hypopharynx superiorly down to the mediastinum. Missing glands may be found in the prevertebral space and the search for parathyroids in this region is augmented by digital palpation.

Gland Identification and Excision

- Normal parathyroids are approximately 3 × 2 × 4 mm and tan in appearance.
- Abnormal glands have a characteristic rubbery feel and reddish brown appearance.
- They are freed from the surrounding tissue and the vascular pedicle is clamped and divided.
- Parathyroid confirmation can be achieved through histologic examination. Biopsy of the antihilar tip of the gland using sharp dissection is performed with great care to not disturb the fragile blood supply.
- Intraoperative PTH monitoring improves the cure rate and guides the extent of exploration.
- A drop in PTH by 50% of baseline and within normal limits at 10 minutes is indicative of cure. If operating for multigland disease (as opposed to a missed adenoma), the PTH level at 10 minutes should also be within normal limits.
- Exploration continues if levels do not fall precipitously and the process is repeated until an appropriate drop is achieved.

Additional Maneuvers

- Because inferior adenomas are usually displaced into the anterior aspect of superior mediastinum, they may be intimately associated with the thymus gland.
- Cervical thymectomy may be performed in the case of absent glands (**FIG 8**). Gentle traction cephalad with sequential grasps and blunt mobilization are used to deliver the thymus into the cervical wound with the aim of removal of thymus tissue to the level of the innominate vein.
- Similarly, thyroid lobectomy on the side of a missing parathyroid may be performed.
- Staged procedures are common with nonlocalized reoperative parathyroid surgery. Closure and relocalization should be performed if the offending gland cannot be found.

Closure

- Meticulous hemostasis is achieved; strap muscles are reapproximated in midline (or to SCM if lateral approach done), followed by platysma reapproximation and skin closure.
- Drains are not regularly used unless there is extensive dissection or exploration.

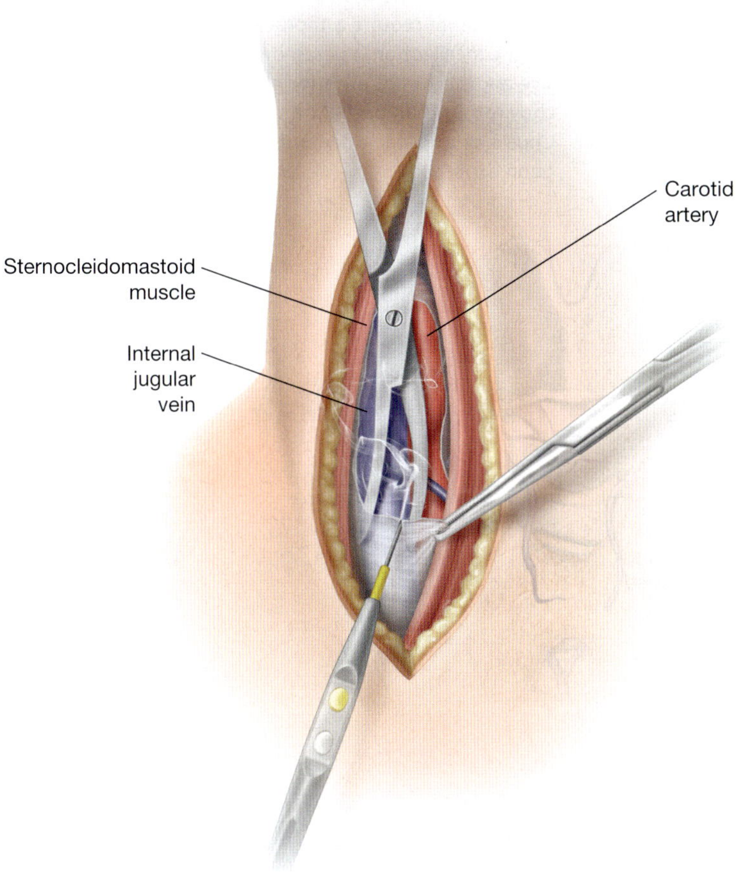

FIG 7 • If the search fails to disclose an adenoma, the carotid sheath is opened.

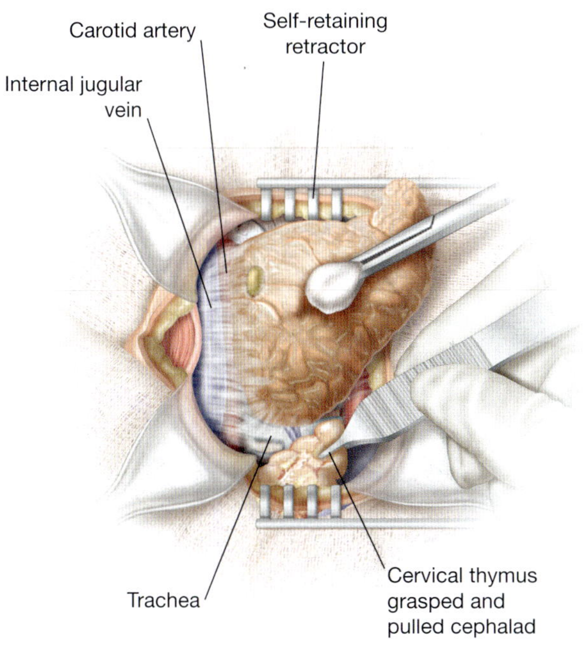

FIG 8 • Because it is not infrequent that parathyroid glands are found partially embedded in the thymus, cervical thymectomy may be performed in the case of a missing gland. The superior aspect of the thymus is grasped and pulled by continuous traction from the chest. It can be grabbed sequentially and lifted cephalad until the often single posterior vessel is seen and divided. If a gland remains missing, it is the practice of some surgeons to perform a thyroid lobectomy on the affected side. The mediastinum should not be split unless there is definite evidence of a mediastinal tumor by preoperative imaging.

MEDIASTINAL EXPLORATION[1,3]

Approach

- Mediastinal exploration should not be performed without localization evidence of a hyperfunctioning gland in the mediastinum. Preferably, two different localizing studies should identify gland location prior to surgery.
- Most adenomas in the posterior mediastinum or anterior mediastinum above the aortic arch can be approached and excised through neck.
- Those deep in the anterior mediastinum or in the middle mediastinum require a thoracic approach (**FIG 9**).
- Precise localization is paramount and may allow less invasive approaches of anterior mediastinotomy or thoracoscopy rather than partial or median sternotomy (**FIG 10**).
- Choice of approach depends on gland location and surgeon expertise.

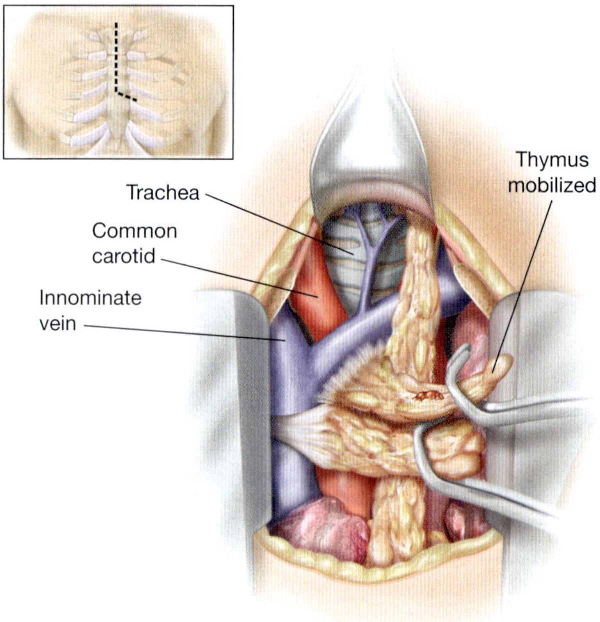

FIG 9 • Median sternotomy or partial sternotomy to 3 cm below the predicted level of the adenoma provides access to the mediastinum (inset shows where the incision would be on the chest). The area of exploration is bound by the innominate vein superiorly and the pericardium inferiorly. Adenomas commonly lie in the thymic remnant in the anterior mediastinum.

A

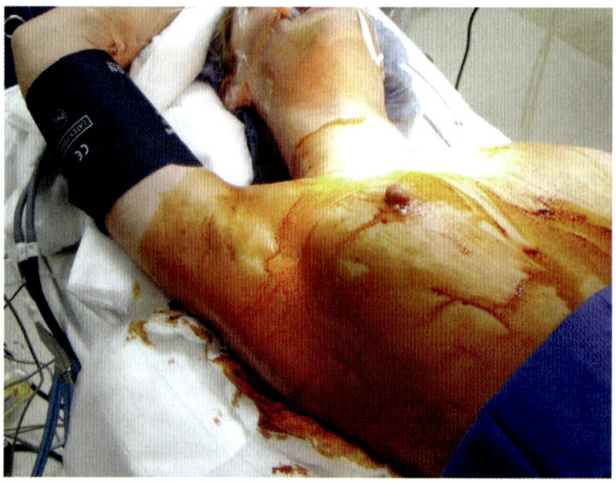

B

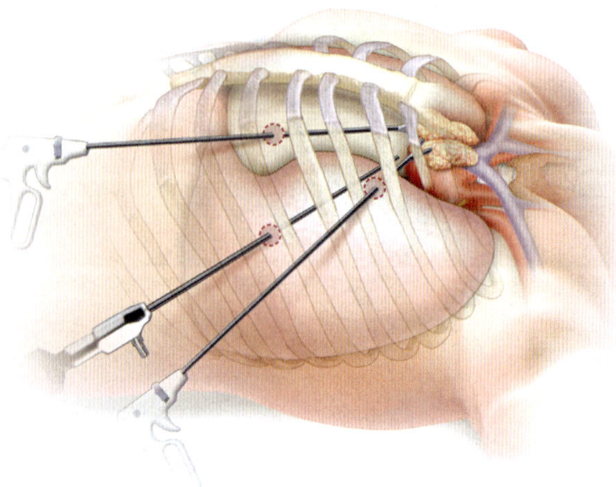

FIG 10 • Thoracic approaches should not be performed without positive localization studies. **A.** The image indicates positioning for a thoracoscopic approach. The patient is supine, with the ipsilateral arm elevated above the head to allow transthoracic access between ribs. **B.** Position placement for thoracoscopic trocars.

PARATHYROID REIMPLANTATION

Procedure

- For multigland disease or when the vasculature of remaining parathyroid tissue is compromised, parathyroid reimplantation may be performed to preserve function. Grafts have a high success rate but may take several weeks to function.
- Approximately 50 mg of the most normal-appearing parathyroid tissue is minced into 1-mm pieces and placed into muscular pockets in the forearm. Alternatively, it may be placed in the subcutaneous tissue overlying the forearm or anterior chest wall (**FIG 11**).

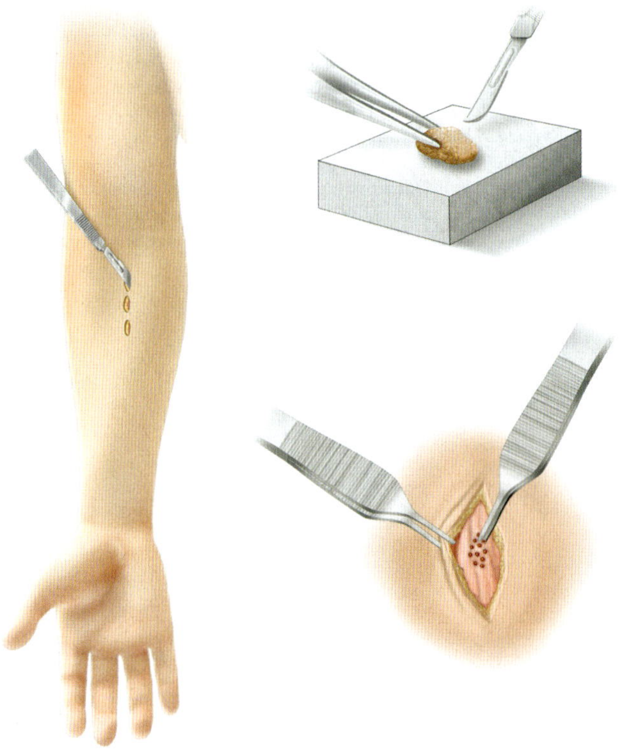

FIG 11 ● Parathyroid tissue to reimplant is minced into 1-mm pieces and placed into intramuscular pockets in the forearm as seen in the figure. Alternatively, they can be placed subcutaneously in the forearm or on the anterior chest wall.

PEARLS AND PITFALLS

Indications	■ Complete history and physical with symptoms and severity of hypercalcemia should be obtained. Biochemical diagnosis of recurrent or persistent hyperparathyroidism must be confirmed.
Preoperative planning	■ Review of initial operative notes and pathology is required. ■ Preoperative localization provides a map for reoperative surgery.
Placement of incision	■ Incisions are created, keeping in mind the localization of pathology and the operative plan. ■ Cosmesis is improved when placed in a natural skin crease.
Cervical approach	■ Entry into the neck may be via focused, posterolateral, thyrothymic ligament, or revision midline cervicotomy approach.
Exploration	■ Eutopic locations for superior and inferior glands should first be searched. ■ Exploration in expected ectopic sites along the tracheoesophageal groove, carotid sheath, thyrothymic ligament, cervical thymus, and intrathyroid should follow.
Mediastinal lesions	■ Accurate preoperative localization allows the least invasive procedure for lesions in the mediastinum, which may be approached via cervical or thoracoscopic approach.
Additional maneuvers	■ Cervical thymectomy or ipsilateral thyroid lobectomy can be performed when an offending gland cannot be located. ■ Parathyroid reimplantation provides a useful adjunct to patients with multigland disease.
Closure	■ Layered closure without drain

POSTOPERATIVE CARE

- Patients should be monitored for respiratory compromise in the immediate postoperative period.
- Patients with reimplantation, extensive dissection, gland or vascular manipulation, or multiple gland removal are at increased risk of postoperative hypoparathyroidism.
- Postoperative hypocalcemia can be mitigated with calcium and vitamin D prophylaxis versus expectant monitoring of serum calcium and PTH. Calcium supplements are generally continued for 3 to 6 months to avoid reactive secondary hyperparathyroidism from a chronic hypocalcemic state.

OUTCOMES

- Success rates between 82% and 98% are expected of reoperative parathyroid surgery, with rates as low as 37% to 73% in multigland disease.
- RLN injury ranges from 0% to 2.7%, whereas permanent hypocalcemia rates vary from 1% to 18%.

COMPLICATIONS

- Neck seroma
- Hematoma
- Infection
- Voice change
- RLN injury
- Hypocalcemia, hypoparathyroidism
- Failure of cure, recurrence

REFERENCES

1. Hubbard JGH, Inabnet WB, Lo C-Y. *Endocrine Surgery: Principles and Practice*. London, United Kingdom: Springer-Verlag; 2009.
2. Inabnet WB, Lee JA. Parathyroid disease, syndromes and pathophysiology. In: Lennard TWJ, ed. *Endocrine Surgery: A Companion to Specialist Surgical Practice*. 4th ed. Philadelphia, PA: Saunders Elsevier; 2009:1–20.
3. Henry JF, Sebag F. Operative strategy for the management of parathyroid disease. In: Lennard TWJ, ed. *Endocrine Surgery: A Companion to Specialist Surgical Practice*. 4th ed. Philadelphia, PA: Saunders Elsevier; 2009:20–38.

Chapter 46 Adrenalectomy: Open Anterior

Barbra S. Miller

DEFINITION

- Adrenal masses may be functional or nonfunctional and benign or malignant. Most are incidentally discovered when imaging is obtained for other reasons. Laparoscopic adrenalectomy is the gold standard for appropriately sized benign (most often functional) adrenal masses and for some metastatic tumors to the adrenal gland (see Chapters 49 and 50). If adrenocortical carcinoma is a concern, adrenalectomy by an open approach should be performed.[1] Several genetic syndromes are associated with adrenal abnormalities and appropriate testing should be obtained if indicated.

DIFFERENTIAL DIAGNOSIS

- Adenoma
- Metastatic cancer
- Pheochromocytoma
- Ganglioneuroma
- Primary adrenocortical carcinoma
- Cyst
- Adjacent paraganglioma
- Soft tissue tumor

PATIENT HISTORY AND PHYSICAL FINDINGS

- All adrenal abnormalities should be evaluated in a systematic fashion, including a thorough history and physical examination investigating the possibility of a hormone-secreting mass. This includes the possibility of a pheochromocytoma, Cushing's syndrome, primary hyperaldosteronism, and hypertestosteronemia. Specifically, the patient should be questioned regarding poorly controlled hypertension, diabetes, edema, diaphoresis, tachycardia, palpitations, sudden severe headaches, flushing, and easy bruising. The physical exam should look for evidence of central obesity, edema, peripheral wasting, core muscle weakness, a buffalo hump, striae, thin skin, and facial plethora. Because the adrenal gland is situated in the retroperitoneum, unless it is extremely large, palpation of the mass is usually unable to be achieved.

IMAGING AND OTHER DIAGNOSTIC STUDIES

- All adrenal masses should undergo appropriate biochemical testing. Even in the absence of signs or symptoms, patients should have at a minimum the following: potassium, aldosterone, renin, plasma fractionated metanephrines (followed by 24-hour urine metanephrines and normetanephrines, catecholamines, and vanillylmandelic acid [VMA] if plasma values are abnormal), 24-hour urine-free cortisol, and adrenocorticotropic hormone (ACTH). Some physicians may also perform a low-dose dexamethasone suppression test and obtain dehydroepiandrosterone-sulfate (DHEA-S) and free testosterone, among other laboratory tests.
- Imaging studies should include an adrenal protocol computed tomography (CT) scan (to assess imaging characteristics and calculate washout percentage of contrast from the tumor) or magnetic resonance imaging (MRI) (to assess for loss of signal intensity between in and out of phase images) and a positron emission tomography (PET) scan if malignancy is questioned (**FIG 1**).
- Additional imaging studies may be required depending on the functionality of the tumor (metaiodobenzylguanidine [MIBG] for pheochromocytoma in select cases, adrenal vein sampling for hyperaldosteronism, etc.).
- Fine needle aspiration or core biopsy is not recommended if adrenocortical carcinoma is suspected but may be useful if metastasis to the adrenal gland is in the differential and the adrenal tumor is the most accessible site of metastasis for biopsy in the setting of multiple sites of metastatic disease. If biopsy is performed, it is imperative to first biochemically rule out a pheochromocytoma.

SURGICAL MANAGEMENT

- Adrenal tumors, if benign appearing by imaging criteria, nonfunctional, and therefore not requiring resection, should be reevaluated with at least one additional CT scan or MRI 6 to 12 months after the initial imaging study to ensure stability in size and internal imaging characteristics. Some advocate for a longer period of follow-up imaging for 2 years with reevaluation of biochemistry for 4 more years.[2]
- Functional tumors leading to hormone excess, indeterminate masses, and those suspected of being adrenocortical carcinoma or isolated metastatic disease from another primary tumor without evidence of widespread metastatic disease should be removed.

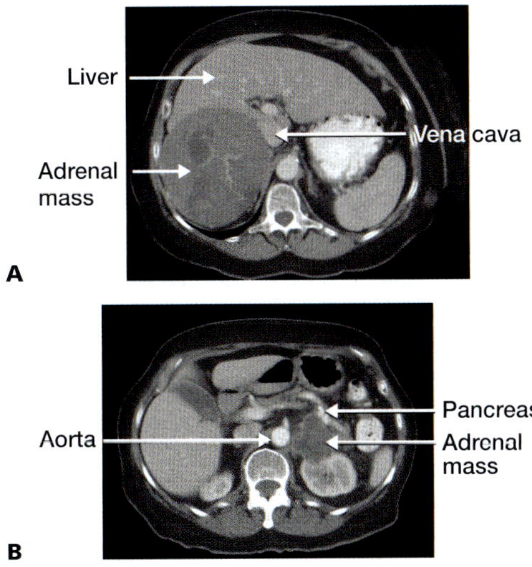

FIG 1 • **A.** CT scan showing large heterogeneous right adrenal mass concerning for adrenocortical carcinoma. **B.** CT scan showing a large left adrenal mass.

Preoperative Planning

- The surgeon must evaluate available imaging studies for tumor involvement of adjacent organs, vessels, and lymphadenopathy. Invasion of major vessels (vena cava) or adjacent organs may require additional teams or different approaches to the tumor. As CT tends to overestimate invasion of adjacent vessels, MRI with magnetic resonance venogram can be especially helpful to assess for vena cava invasion or intracaval tumor thrombus.
- The risks, benefits, and alternatives to surgery are discussed with the patient, including potential need for steroid supplementation in the postoperative setting. Patients with pheochromocytomas should be adequately alpha blocked and volume replete. Beta blockade may also be necessary. In patients with hyperaldosteronism, a potassium level should be checked the morning of surgery and treated if necessary.
- Routine prophylactic antibiotics and deep vein thrombosis (DVT) prophylaxis is administered prior to surgery, and sequential compression devices are applied.
- A general endotracheal anesthetic is administered and an epidural is often placed for postoperative pain management.
- Common to all approaches, skin preparation with clipping rather than shaving is preferred, and the surgical area is prepped and draped in a sterile fashion.

Positioning

- The patient is placed supine on the table with arms out to the side, and all pressure points are padded appropriately (**FIG 2**).

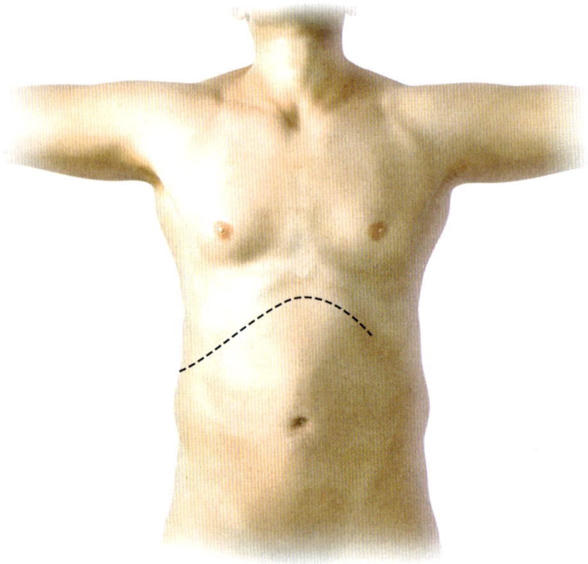

FIG 2 • The patient is placed supine on the table with arms out. Pressure points are padded. An incision is marked 2 cm inferior to the costal margin and carried from the lateral abdominal wall across the midline to facilitate exposure.

TECHNIQUES

RIGHT ADRENALECTOMY

Exposure

- A wide right subcostal incision is made and carried across the midline to the midleft abdomen. The subcutaneous fat, fascia, abdominal wall musculature, and posterior fascia are incised with cautery. The peritoneum is entered sharply with scissors and the incision opened to its full length. The ligamentum teres is divided between sutures and the peritoneal cavity is inspected in a systematic manner, assessing for evidence of metastatic disease or other abnormalities. The falciform ligament, triangular, and coronary ligaments of the left and right lobes of the liver are divided to allow for full mobility of the liver during retraction (**FIGS 3** and **4**).
- Ultrasound of the liver is also performed to assess for metastatic disease not identified on preoperative imaging, and the vena cava may also be evaluated sonographically for evidence of intracaval tumor thrombus or direct tumor invasion.
- The hepatic flexure of the colon may need to be mobilized, and if a Kocher maneuver is needed, it should be done at this time. The right lobe of the liver is retracted medially to expose the retroperitoneum and allow access to the area of the tumor and vena cava. A retractor system is placed. The Omni retractor provides excellent retraction as well as the critically important ability to retract the costal margin and ribs as superiorly and anteriorly as possible. A large saline-soaked towel is placed against the bowel with retractors to not only provide exposure but also to exclude the rest of the peritoneal cavity and minimize potential seeding of the peritoneal cavity by a malignant tumor (**FIG 5**).

Dissection

- The posterior peritoneal lining over the retroperitoneum is incised over the superior half of the right kidney and carried from medial to lateral out to the side of the abdominal wall. Medial dissection should proceed carefully to the vena cava, making sure not to divide branches of the renal artery supplying the upper portion of the kidney or venous branches draining to the renal vein. Small branches supplying and draining the adrenal gland should be carefully ligated and divided. Any lymph nodes posterior to the renal hilum should be included in the dissection (**FIGS 6** and **7**).
- The fat overlying and just superior to the kidney is mobilized from inferior to superior, making this tissue the inferior margin, using cautery, silk sutures, and other hemostatic devices as needed, making sure not to create a nonexistent plane between the inferior aspect of the tumor and the superior aspect of the kidney. The peritoneal lining should remain intact over the anterior

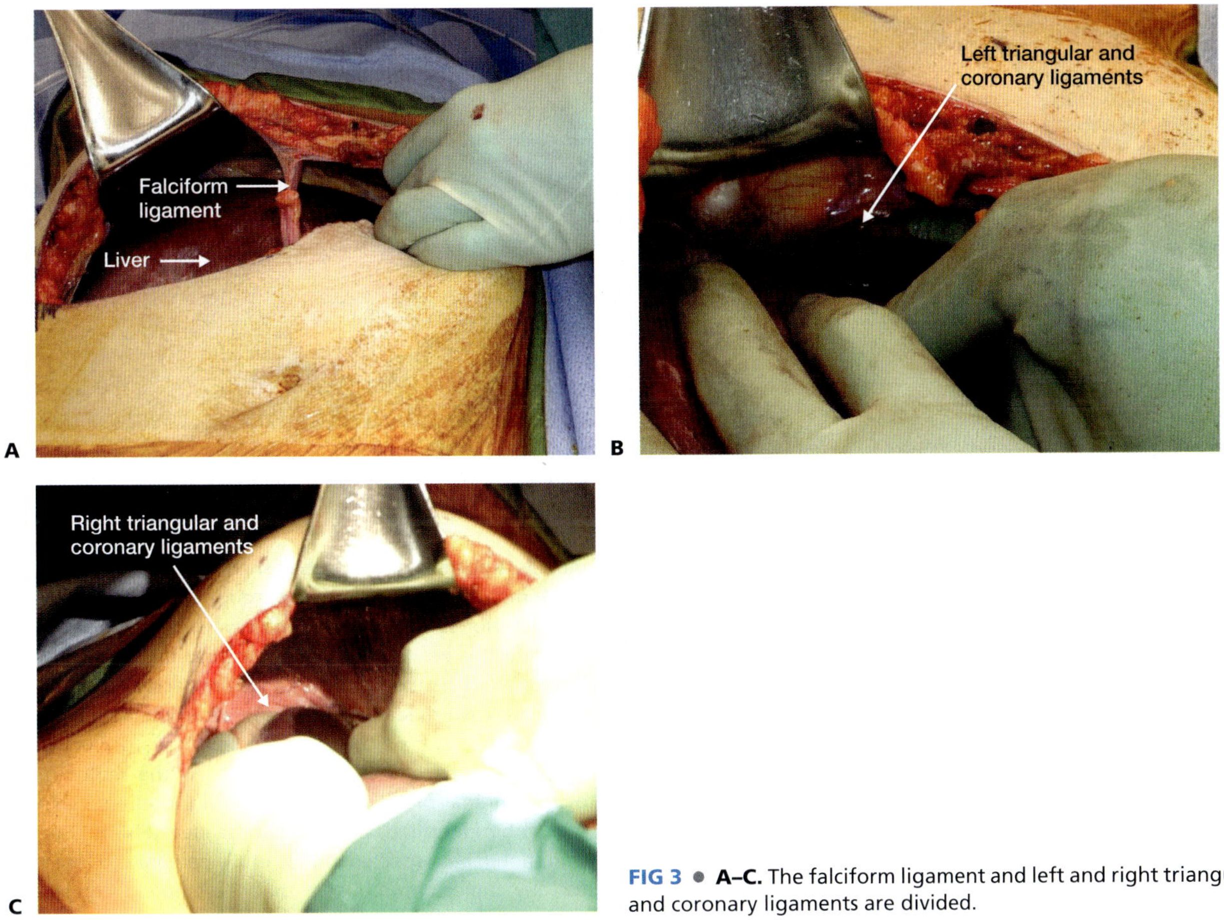

FIG 3 • **A–C.** The falciform ligament and left and right triangular and coronary ligaments are divided.

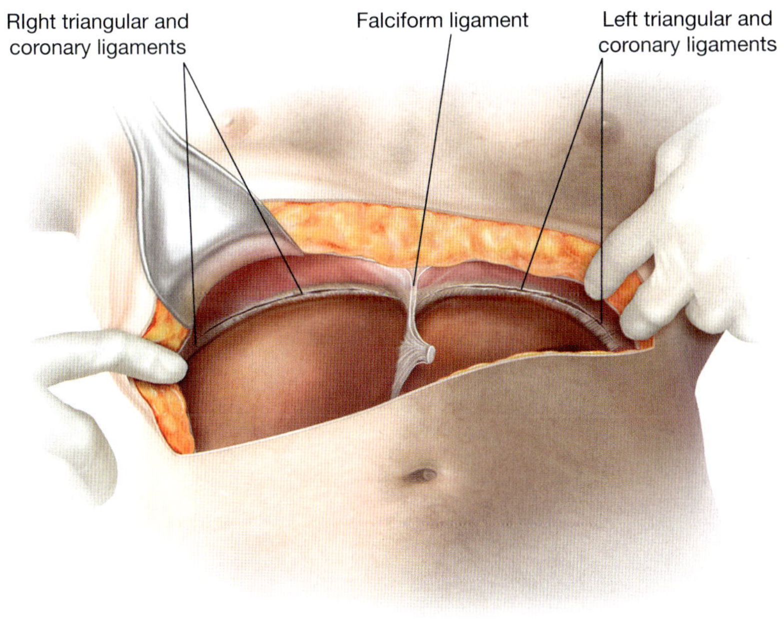

FIG 4 • With the ligamentum teres, falciform ligament, and triangular and coronary ligaments divided, this allows adequate retraction of the liver and access to the tumor and vena cava.

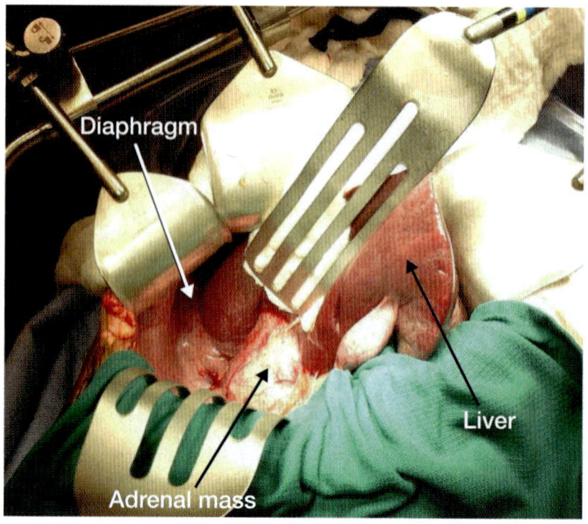

FIG 5 ● A retractor system is placed to retract the ribs superiorly and anteriorly and to retract the liver medially. A moist towel is placed inferiorly to retract the bowel and exclude the rest of the peritoneal cavity.

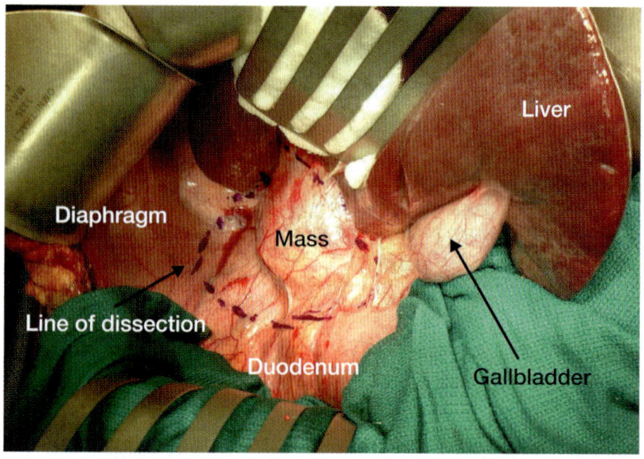

FIG 7 ● The intended line of dissection to include the tumor and all retroperitoneal soft tissue is marked.

aspect of the tumor to serve as the anterior margin if not already invaded by the tumor (**FIG 8**).

- The dissection continues superiorly along the diaphragm, making sure to ligate and divide any feeding vessels, most commonly branches from the inferior phrenic vessels.
- Posterior dissection should proceed from lateral to medial, making sure to remove all fat posterior to the tumor in an en bloc fashion. If the tumor invades the muscle, a portion of the muscle should be included with the tumor to ensure negative margins.
- The anterior surface of the vena cava should be identified and the peritoneal lining overlying this should be incised along its length. Using a vein retractor to retract the vena cava medially, soft tissue attachments medial to the gland and posterior to the vena cava, including lymphatics, are ligated and divided. As the midpoint of the adrenal gland is reached, the right adrenal vein should be identified, ligated, and divided (**FIG 9**). The vein should be inspected and carefully palpated to assess for any tumor thrombus so that the tumor thrombus

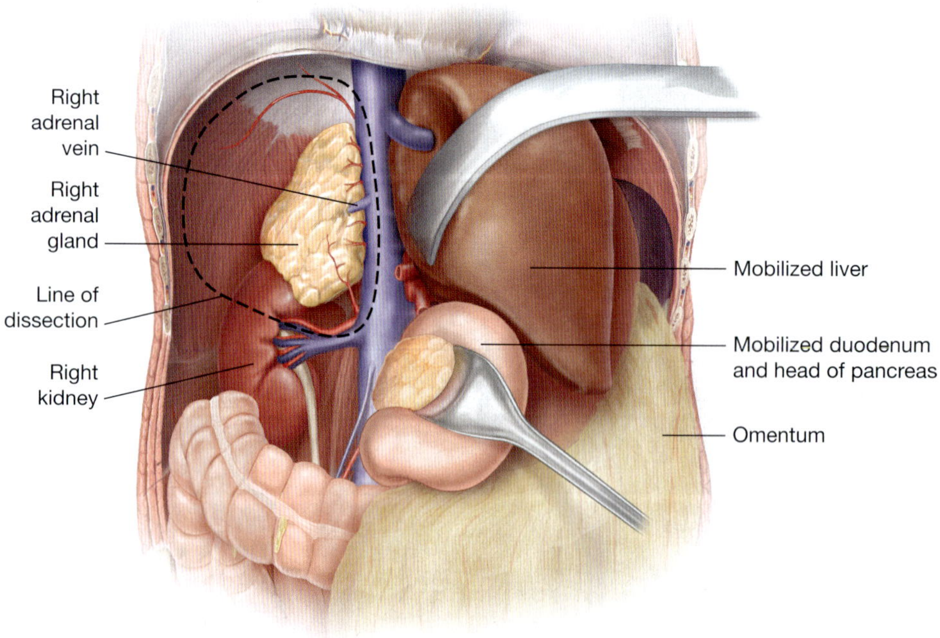

FIG 6 ● With the liver retracted medially, the adrenal vein and inferior vena cava are exposed. The *dotted line* demonstrates the intended line of dissection.

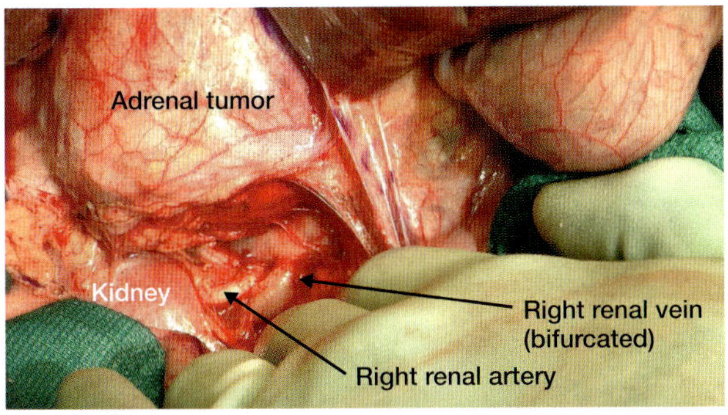

FIG 8 ● The inferior portion of the dissection is shown. A branch of the right renal artery is seen between two branches of the right renal vein.

can be included with the specimen in an en bloc fashion. Advanced techniques for managing large tumor thrombi within the vena cava are beyond the scope of this chapter. If removing a pheochromocytoma, the anesthesiologist should be warned well in advance prior to ligating the adrenal vein in anticipation of ensuing hypotension. The dissection is continued superiorly until all medial attachments have been released (**FIG 10**).

- The adrenal gland and the periadrenal soft tissue are removed, marked with orienting sutures for the pathologist, and sent to the pathology lab (**FIG 11**).

Closure

- A small amount of water should be used for irrigation and final hemostasis is achieved. The area encompassed by the dissection should be marked with large clips to assist with postoperative external beam radiation therapy if needed.
- A drain may be placed if desired but is not required in many cases.
- The retractor system is removed, the organs replaced in their normal anatomic positions, and the abdominal wall musculature is closed in two separate layers. The subcutaneous tissue may be reapproximated with interrupted absorbable sutures if needed and the skin closed with staples or suture. A sterile dressing is applied.

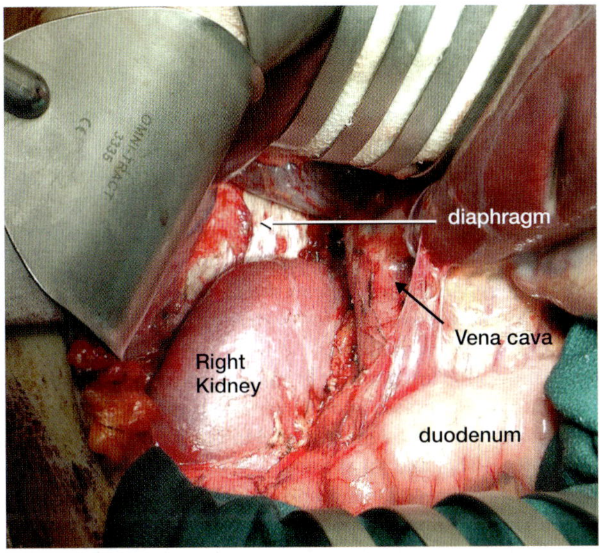

FIG 10 ● The adrenal tumor and all retroperitoneal soft tissue has been removed en bloc. The right kidney has migrated superiorly against the diaphragm to fill the space.

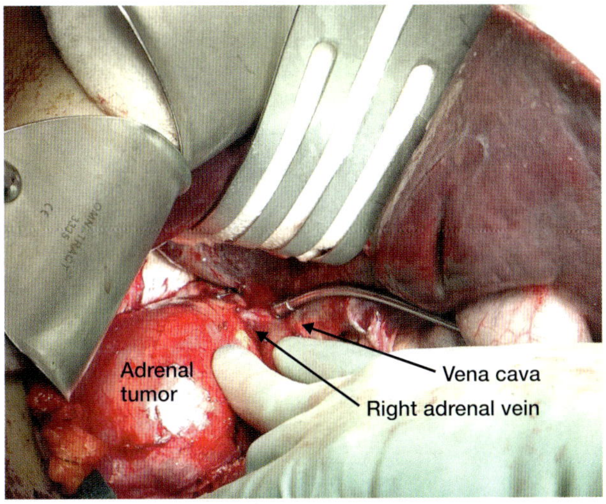

FIG 9 ● The right adrenal vein has been dissected free of its attachments. More superiorly along the vena cava, a second vein from the adrenal to the inferior vena cava has been clipped and divided.

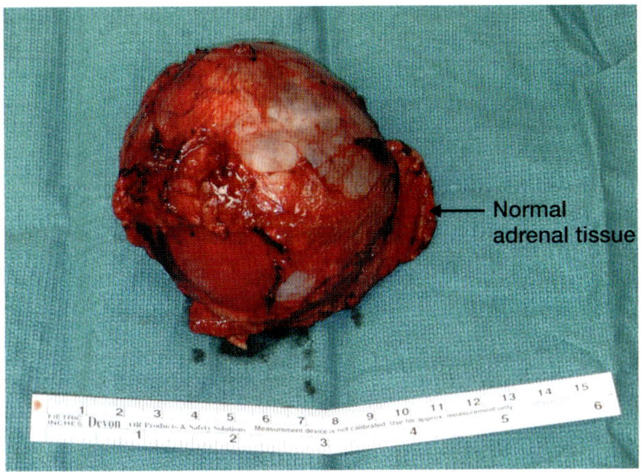

FIG 11 ● A small portion of normal adrenal tissue remains and is seen at the right side of the gland in this image. Surrounding soft tissue and the overlying anterior peritoneal lining remain on the anterior surface of the gland.

LEFT ADRENALECTOMY

Exposure

- A wide left subcostal incision is made and carried across the midline to the midright abdomen (**FIG 12**). The subcutaneous fat, fascia, abdominal wall musculature, and posterior fascia are incised with cautery. The peritoneum is entered sharply with scissors and the incision opened to its full length. The ligamentum teres is divided between sutures and the peritoneal cavity is inspected in a systematic manner, assessing for evidence of metastatic disease or other abnormalities.
- Ultrasound of the liver is also performed to assess for metastatic disease and the vena cava may also be evaluated for evidence of intracaval tumor thrombus from the left adrenal and renal veins.
- The falciform ligament and left triangular and coronary ligaments of the left lobe of the liver are divided to allow for mobility of the liver during retraction (**FIG 13**).
- The descending colon is mobilized along the line of Toldt and the colon reflected medially. The mobilization is continued superiorly to divide the splenic attachments to the abdominal side wall and the diaphragm. The spleen, stomach, pancreas, splenic flexure, and colon should be reflected medially, allowing exposure of the left retroperitoneum (**FIG 14**). A retractor system is placed. A large saline-soaked towel with retractors is placed against the bowel, pancreas, spleen to not only provide exposure but also to exclude the rest of the peritoneal cavity to minimize potential seeding of the peritoneal cavity by a malignant tumor. The left side of the aorta should be clearly appreciable if the exposure is adequate.

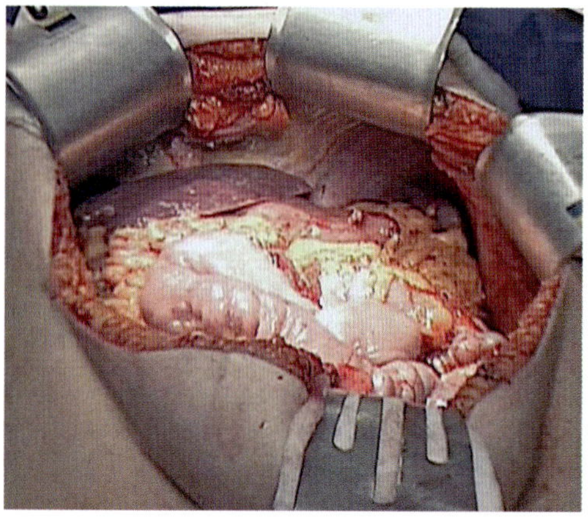

FIG 13 • The falciform ligament and left triangular and coronary ligaments are divided, allowing exposure of the left upper abdomen and mobility of the liver.

Dissection

- Because the peritoneal covering on the left has been reflected with the spleen and pancreas, the surgeon should make every effort to manipulate the tumor surface as little as possible (no-touch technique). The soft tissue overlying the superior half of the left kidney is incised and carried from medial to lateral out to the side of the abdominal wall. Inferior dissection should proceed carefully to the aorta medially along the left renal vein, making sure not to divide branches of the posteriorly situated renal artery supplying the upper portion of the kidney or venous branches draining to the renal vein. Small branches supplying and draining the adrenal gland should be carefully ligated and divided. Any lymph nodes posterior to the renal hilum should be included in the dissection.
- The left adrenal vein will be identified at the medial aspect of the left renal vein as it courses anterior to the aorta (**FIG 15**). It generally enters the adrenal gland in the 7 o'clock position. It should be ligated and divided. The adrenal vein and renal vein should be inspected and carefully palpated to assess for any tumor thrombus so that the tumor thrombus can be included with the

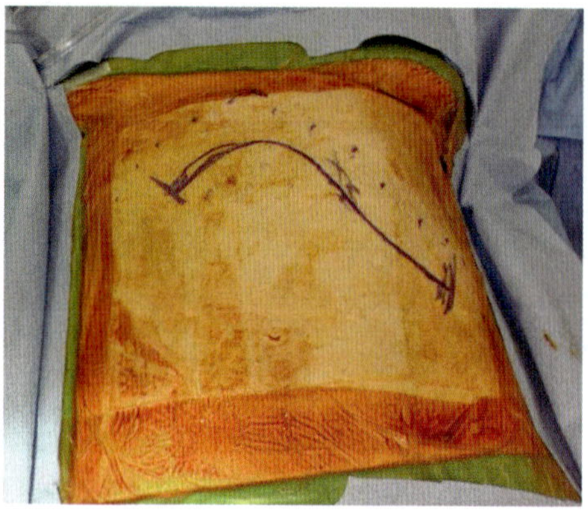

FIG 12 • The patient is placed supine on the table with arms out. Pressure points are padded. A wide left subcostal incision is marked 2 cm inferior to the costal margin and carried across the midline to the right abdomen to facilitate exposure.

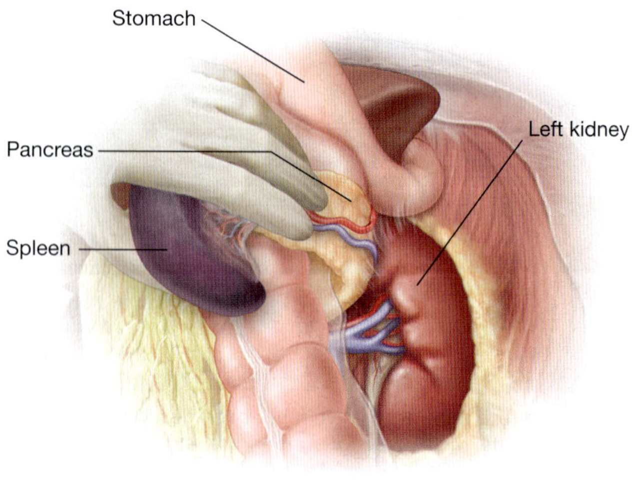

FIG 14 • The spleen, stomach, and pancreas are mobilized medially.

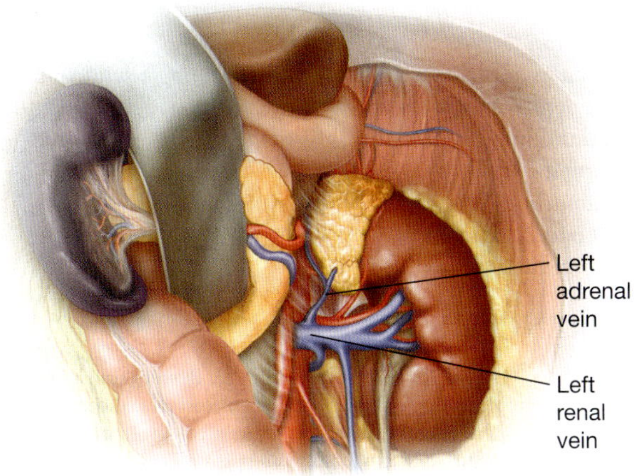

FIG 15 ● With retractors in place, the left retroperitoneum is exposed and excluded from the rest of the peritoneal cavity. The left side of the aorta, renal vein, and adrenal vein are visualized, with the left adrenal vein identified at the medial aspect of the left renal vein. The adrenal vein can be ligated and divided at its junction with the renal vein.

specimen in an en bloc fashion. Advanced techniques for managing large tumor thrombi within the renal vein and vena cava are not discussed in this chapter.

- The fat overlying and just superior to the kidney is mobilized from inferior to superior, making this tissue the inferior margin, using cautery, silk sutures, and other hemostatic devices as needed, making sure not to create a nonexistent plane between the inferior aspect of the tumor and the superior aspect of the kidney.
- Lateral dissection should continue along the abdominal side wall. The dissection continues superiorly along the diaphragm, making sure to ligate and divide any feeding vessels, most commonly branches from the inferior phrenic vessels.
- Posterior dissection should proceed from lateral to medial, making sure to remove all fat and any involved muscle posterior to the tumor in an en bloc fashion.
- The left lateral surface of the aorta should be identified, and the soft tissue attachments including small vessels and lymphatics are ligated and divided. If removing a pheochromocytoma, the anesthesiologist should be warned well in advance prior to ligating the adrenal vein in anticipation of ensuing hypotension. The dissection is continued superiorly until all medial attachments have been released. Any lymph nodes along the aorta or identified near the superior mesenteric artery or celiac axis should be included with the specimen.
- The adrenal gland and the periadrenal soft tissue are removed, marked with orienting suture for the pathologist, and sent to the pathology lab.

Closure

- A small amount of water should be used for irrigation and final hemostasis is achieved. The area encompassed by the dissection should be marked with large clips to assist with postoperative external beam radiation therapy if needed. A drain may be placed.
- The retractor system is removed, the organs replaced in their normal anatomic position, and the abdominal wall musculature is closed in two separate layers. The subcutaneous tissue may be reapproximated with interrupted absorbable sutures if needed and the skin closed with staples or suture. A sterile dressing is applied.

PEARLS AND PITFALLS

Bleeding—arterial and venous	■ May result from disruption of the vena cava, renal vein or artery, and aorta. Kitners, sponge sticks, and vascular clamps are helpful. Obtain proximal and distal control prior to potentially dangerous maneuvers.
Liver mobilization	■ Mobilize right and left lobes to obtain best exposure for right adrenalectomy. Mobilize left lobe to obtain best exposure for left adrenalectomy.
Tumor capsule penetration	■ Avoid this as penetration leads to peritoneal spread, which will result in recurrence and often shortened survival compared to alternate sites of recurrence. En bloc resection is critical to prevent creating a plane through microscopically positive tumor margins.

POSTOPERATIVE CARE

- Most patients will not need intensive care unit (ICU) care, although pheochromocytoma patients often need closer monitoring for the first 24 hours, depending on intraoperative stability and volume status.
- Hydrocortisone should be given administered to patients with overt Cushing's syndrome. A cosyntropin stimulation test can be performed the morning after surgery in subclinical or mild Cushing's cases if there is a question about the requirement for steroid supplementation.
- Electrolytes should be checked the morning after surgery. Patients undergoing surgery for primary hyperaldosteronism may experience rebound hyperkalemia.
- After bilateral adrenalectomy, high-dose intravenous (IV) hydrocortisone should be weaned to replacement

dose oral hydrocortisone and fludrocortisone 0.1 mg daily.

- Antihypertensive medications are withheld in the immediate postoperative setting and reinstituted as needed.
- Routine postoperative care is pursued and patients are discharged 3 to 7 days after surgery.
- Follow-up is typically 1 to 2 weeks after surgery with endocrine testing as needed.

OUTCOMES

- Although laparoscopic surgery has become the gold standard for benign adrenal disease due to decreased bleeding, infection, pain, and hospital stay, open adrenalectomy is still performed if conversion from laparoscopic adrenalectomy is required for various reasons, for very large adrenal tumors, and when adrenocortical carcinoma is in the differential diagnosis, as some studies have found a significantly higher incidence of incomplete positive margin resections, a higher incidence of and shorter time to tumor bed and peritoneal cavity recurrence, and decreased survival compared to laparoscopic surgery.[3–5] A greater number of oncologic principles of resection can be respected with open surgery for adrenal cancer compared to a laparoscopic approach.

COMPLICATIONS

- Bleeding
- Infection
- Adrenal insufficiency in those with Cushing's syndrome
- Postoperative hypotension in those with pheochromocytoma
- Rebound hyperkalemia in those with Conn's syndrome
- Lymphatic leak
- Pneumothorax
- Neurogenic pain
- Abdominal wall laxity

REFERENCES

1. Miller BS, Gauger PG, Hammer GD, et al. Resection of adrenocortical carcinoma is less complete and local recurrence occurs sooner and more often after laparoscopic adrenalectomy than after open adrenalectomy. *Surgery*. 2012;152(6):1150–1157.
2. Young WF. The incidentally discovered adrenal mass. *N Engl J Med*. 2007;356:601–610.
3. Gonzalez RJ, Shapiro S, Sarlis N, et al. Laparoscopic resection of adrenal cortical carcinoma: a cautionary note. *Surgery*. 2005;138:1078–1085.
4. Leboulleux S, Deanderis D, Al Ghuzian A, et al. Adrenocortical carcinoma: is the surgical approach a risk factor of peritoneal carcinomatosis? *Eur J Endocrinol*. 2010;162:1147–1153.
5. Porpiglia F, Miller BS, Manfredi M, et al. A debate on laparoscopic versus open adrenalectomy for adrenocortical carcinoma. *Horm Cancer*. 2011;2(6):372–377.

Chapter 47 Adrenalectomy: Open Thoracoabdominal

Barbra S. Miller

DEFINITION

- Adrenal masses may be benign or malignant. If adrenocortical carcinoma is a concern, adrenalectomy by an open approach should be performed. Adrenal masses may be functional or nonfunctional with regard to excess hormone secretion. Several genetic syndromes are associated with adrenal abnormalities and should be evaluated if indicated.

DIFFERENTIAL DIAGNOSIS

- Primary adrenal adenoma
- Primary adrenocortical carcinoma
- Cyst
- Metastatic cancer
- Pheochromocytoma
- Ganglioneuroma
- Adjacent paraganglioma
- Soft tissue tumor

PATIENT HISTORY AND PHYSICAL FINDINGS

- All adrenal abnormalities should be evaluated in a systematic fashion, including a thorough history and physical examination investigating the possibility of a hormone-secreting mass. This includes the possibility of a pheochromocytoma, Cushing's syndrome, primary hyperaldosteronism, and hypertestosteronemia. Specifically, the patient should be questioned regarding poorly controlled hypertension, diabetes, edema, diaphoresis, tachycardia, palpitations, sudden severe headaches, flushing, and easy bruising. The physical exam should look for evidence of central obesity, edema, peripheral wasting, core muscle weakness, a buffalo hump, striae, thin skin, and facial plethora. Because the adrenal gland is situated in the retroperitoneum, unless it is extremely large, palpation of the mass is usually unable to be achieved.

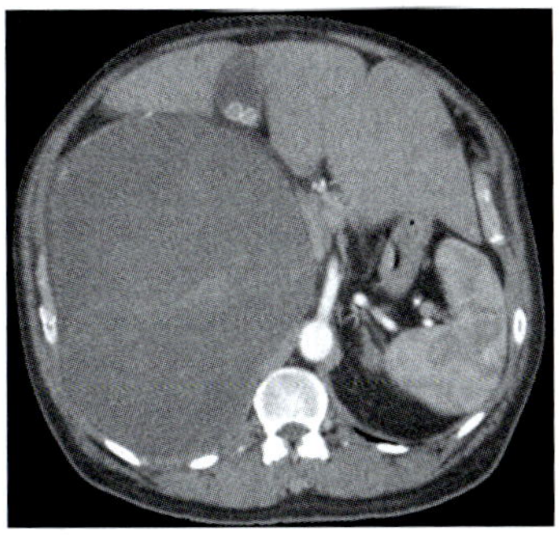

FIG 1 • CT image (axial cut) showing large heterogeneous right adrenal mass concerning for adrenocortical carcinoma.

IMAGING AND OTHER DIAGNOSTIC STUDIES

- All adrenal masses should undergo appropriate biochemical testing. Even in the absence of signs or symptoms, patients should have at a minimum the following: potassium, aldosterone, renin, plasma fractionated metanephrines (followed by 24-hour urine metanephrines and normetanephrines, catecholamines, and vanillylmandelic acid [VMA] if plasma values are abnormal), 24-hour urine-free cortisol, and adrenocorticotropic hormone (ACTH). Some physicians may also perform a low-dose dexamethasone suppression test, dehydroepiandrosterone-sulfate (DHEA-S), and free testosterone, among other laboratory tests.
- Imaging studies (**FIGS 1** and **2**) should include an adrenal protocol computed tomography (CT) scan (noncontrast, contrast, 15-minute–delayed scan to calculate washout percentage of contrast from the tumor) or magnetic resonance imaging (MRI) (to assess for loss of signal intensity between in and out of phase images) and a positron emission tomography (PET) scan if malignancy is questioned.
- Additional imaging studies may be required depending on the functionality of the tumor (metaiodobenzylguanidine [MIBG] for pheochromocytoma in select cases, adrenal vein sampling for hyperaldosteronism, etc.).
- Fine needle aspiration or core biopsy is not recommended if adrenocortical carcinoma is possible but may be useful if metastasis to the adrenal gland is in the differential and the adrenal tumor is the most accessible site of metastasis in the setting of multiple sites of metastatic disease. If biopsy is performed, it is imperative to first biochemically rule out pheochromocytoma as a diagnosis.

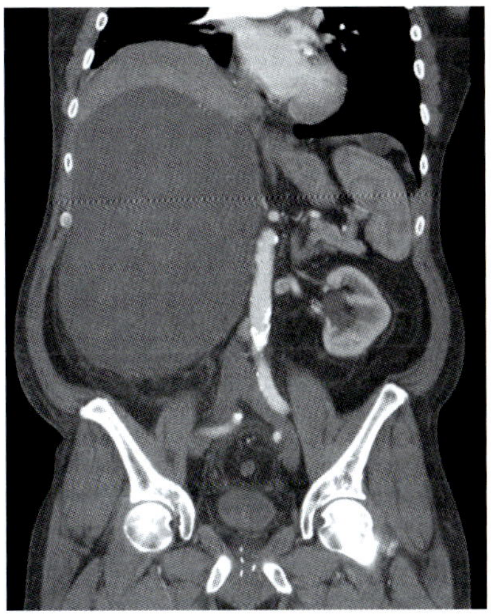

FIG 2 • CT image (coronal cut) showing large heterogeneous right adrenal mass concerning for adrenocortical carcinoma.

SURGICAL MANAGEMENT

- Adrenal tumors, if benign appearing by imaging criteria and hormonally nonfunctional, should be reevaluated with at least one additional CT scan or MRI 6 to 12 months after the initial imaging study to ensure stability in size and internal imaging characteristics. Some advocate for a longer period of follow-up imaging for 2 years with reevaluation of biochemistry for 4 more years.[1]
- Functional tumors leading to hormone excess, indeterminate masses, and those suspected of being adrenocortical carcinoma or isolated metastatic disease from another primary tumor without evidence of widespread metastatic disease should be removed.
- Adrenalectomy may be performed by anterior, posterior, or thoracoabdominal approach. The thoracoabdominal approach is particularly useful for providing excellent exposure and access to large adrenal tumors.[2–5] Although excellent exposure can be achieved by an anterior approach in most cases, the thoracoabdominal approach is most beneficial in patients who have undergone prior abdominal surgery, thereby avoiding the time and potential morbidity associated with extensive lysis of adhesions.

Preoperative Planning

- The surgeon must evaluate available imaging studies for possible involvement of adjacent organs and vessels and lymphadenopathy. Invasion of major vessels (vena cava) or adjacent organs may require additional teams or different approaches to the tumor. As CT tends to overestimate invasion of adjacent vessels, MRI with magnetic resonance venogram can be especially helpful to assess for vena cava invasion or intracaval tumor thrombus.
- The risks, benefits, and alternatives to surgery are discussed with the patient including potential need for steroid supplementation in the postoperative setting. Patients with pheochromocytomas should be adequately alpha blocked and volume replete. Beta blockade may also be necessary. A potassium level should be checked the morning of surgery and treated as necessary in patients with hyperaldosteronism.
- Routine prophylactic antibiotics and deep vein thrombosis (DVT) prophylaxis are administered prior to surgery, and sequential compression devices are applied.
- A general endotracheal anesthetic is administered. A dual lumen endotracheal tube may be placed for improved exposure but in general is not required.
- An epidural is often placed for postoperative pain management.
- Common to all approaches, skin preparation with clipping rather than shaving is prepared, and the surgical area is prepped and draped in a sterile fashion.

Positioning

- For a right adrenalectomy, the patient is placed in semi–left lateral decubitus position on a beanbag with an axillary roll beneath the left axilla. The right arm is held in place parallel over the left arm with a thoracic arm holder (**FIG 3**). For a left adrenalectomy, the opposite setup is performed. The pelvis remains flat. This allows access to the chest and abdomen. The bed is flexed to increase the space between the ribs and the pelvis.
- All pressure points are padded appropriately.
- The patient is prepped and draped.

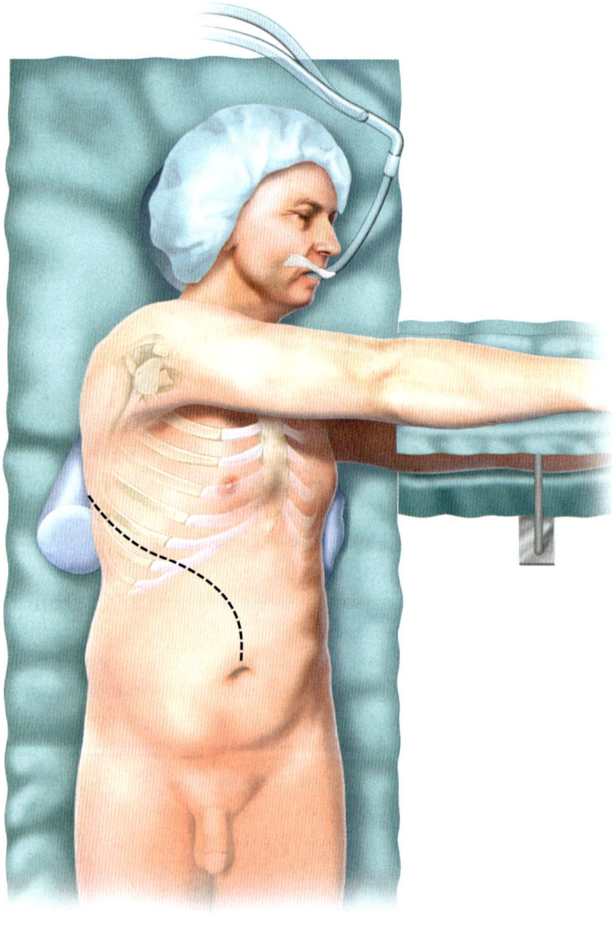

FIG 3 • The patient is placed in semi–left lateral decubitus position on a beanbag with an axillary roll beneath the left axilla. The chest is nearly fully lateral, and the pelvis remains flat (corkscrew twist). The right arm is held in place parallel over the left arm with a thoracic arm holder.

RIGHT ADRENALECTOMY

Exposure

- An incision is made 2 cm inferior to the tip of the right scapula and extended to a point midway between the xiphoid process and the umbilicus (**FIG 4**). If necessary, the incision can then be carried inferiorly along the midline of the abdomen. The subcutaneous tissue and muscle are divided, sparing the latissimus dorsi and incising the serratus anterior. The chest is entered at the 8th intercostal space, the pulmonary ligament divided, and the lung retracted superiorly. The diaphragm is incised 2 to 4 cm from its attachments, sparing the phrenic nerve. Several marking stitches should be placed intermittently on either side of the divided diaphragm to aid with reapproximation at the end of the case (**FIG 5**). The costochondral cartilage is divided. A portion may be excised. The abdominal incision is extended and the peritoneal cavity is entered. A self-retaining retractor system can be placed.
- The diaphragmatic attachments to the right lobe of the liver are released with electrocautery as is the falciform ligament. The ligamentum teres is ligated and divided with silk ligatures. If the adrenal tumor is adherent to the diaphragm, that portion of the diaphragm should be removed en bloc with the tumor and can be reconstructed with mesh or other material. Inspection of the peritoneal cavity is performed as much as possible in a systematic

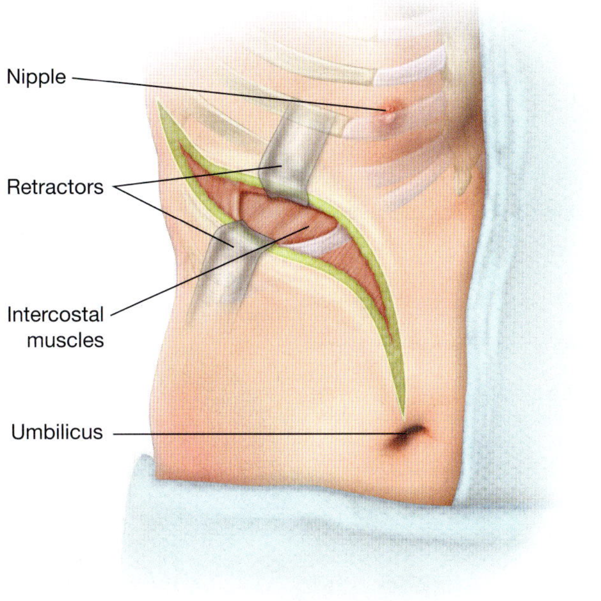

FIG 4 • An incision is made 2 cm inferior to the tip of the right scapula and extended to a point midway between the xiphoid process and the umbilicus. The incision can then be carried inferiorly along the midline of the abdomen. The subcutaneous tissue and muscle are divided, sparing the latissimus dorsi and incising the serratus anterior. The chest is entered at the 8th intercostal space.

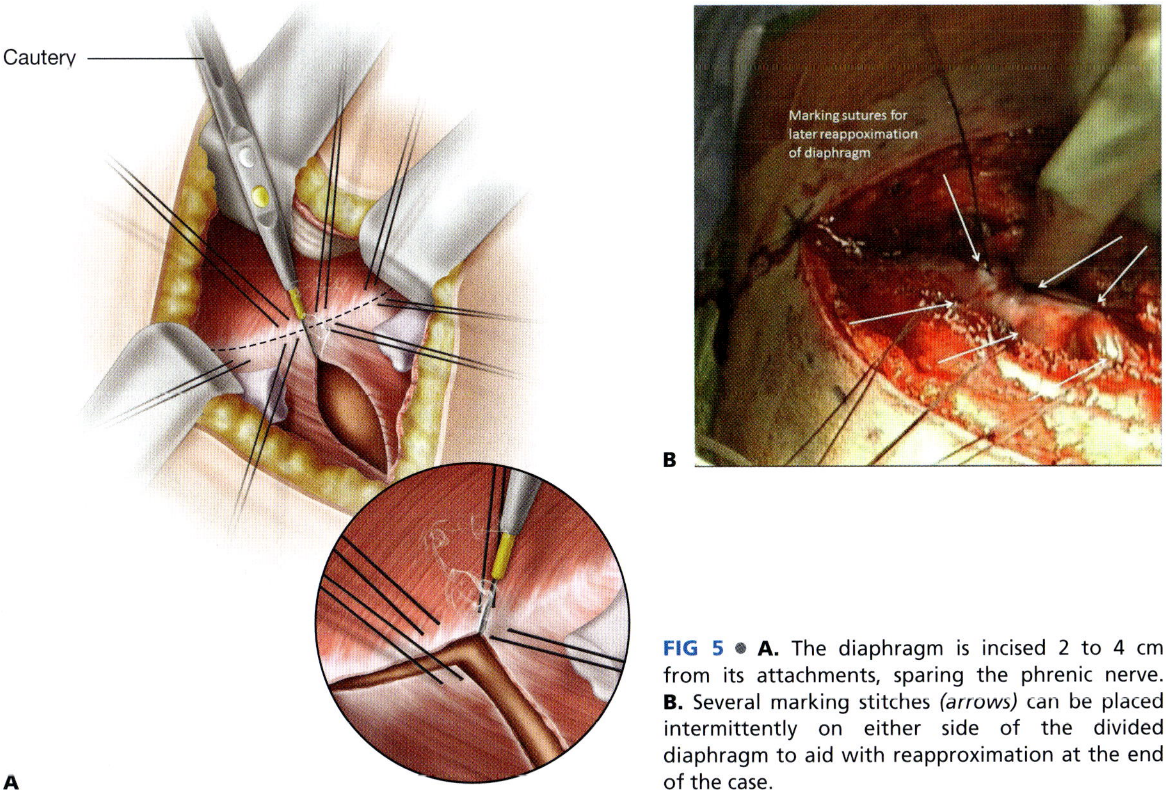

FIG 5 • **A.** The diaphragm is incised 2 to 4 cm from its attachments, sparing the phrenic nerve. **B.** Several marking stitches *(arrows)* can be placed intermittently on either side of the divided diaphragm to aid with reapproximation at the end of the case.

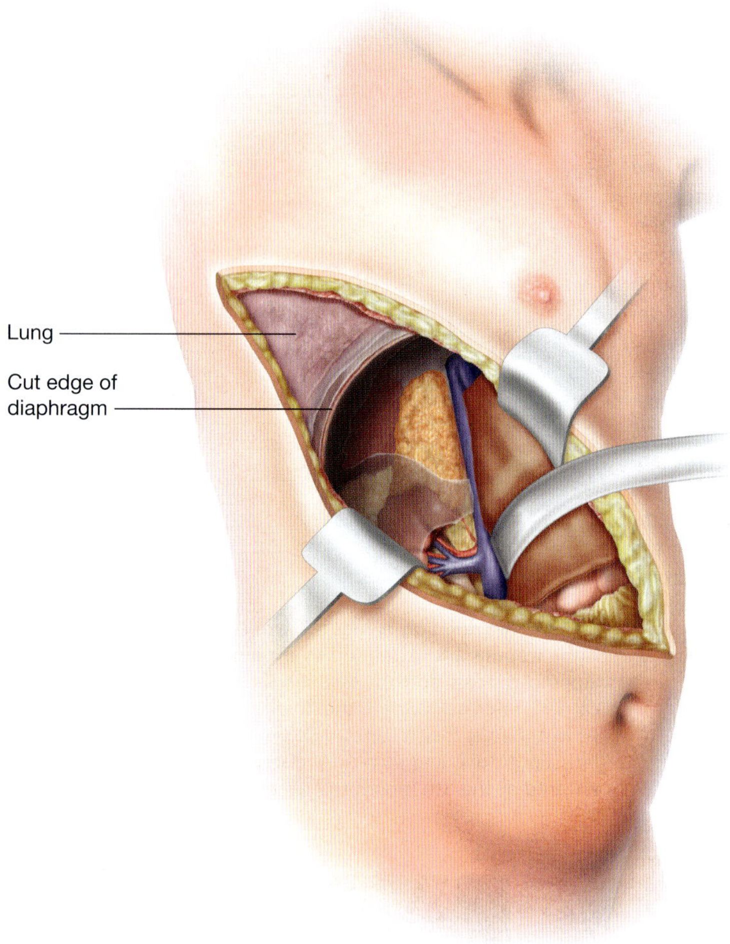

FIG 6 • The diaphragmatic attachments to the right lobe of the liver are released with electrocautery as is the falciform ligament. Both lobes of the liver are mobilized. A portion of the diaphragm should be removed en bloc with any adherent tumor.

fashion and an ultrasound of the liver is performed. The right lobe of the liver is retracted toward the left side, allowing access to the retrohepatic inferior vena cava (**FIG 6**).

Dissection

- The posterior peritoneal lining over the retroperitoneum in incised over the superior half of the right kidney and carried from medial to lateral out to the side of the abdominal wall (**FIG 7**). Medial dissection should proceed carefully to the vena cava, making sure not to divide branches of the renal artery supplying the upper portion of the kidney or venous branches draining to the renal vein. Small branches supplying and draining the adrenal gland should be carefully ligated and divided. Any lymph nodes posterior to the renal hilum should be included in the dissection.
- The fat overlying and just superior to the kidney is mobilized from inferior to superior, making this tissue the

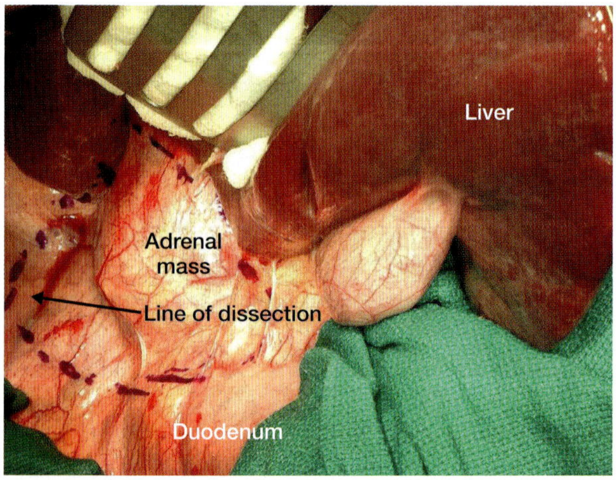

FIG 7 • The posterior lining over the retroperitoneal fat and kidney is incised over the superior half of the right kidney and carried from medial to lateral out to the side of the abdominal wall.

inferior margin, using cautery, silk sutures, and other hemostatic devices as needed, making sure not to create a nonexistent plane between the inferior aspect of the tumor and the superior aspect of the kidney. The peritoneal lining should remain intact over the anterior aspect of the tumor to serve as the anterior margin if not already invaded by the tumor. The dissection continues superiorly along the diaphragm, making sure to ligate and divide any feeding vessels, most commonly branches from the inferior phrenic vessels. Posterior dissection should proceed from lateral to medial, making sure to remove all fat posterior to the tumor in an en bloc fashion. If the tumor invades the muscle, a portion of the muscle should be included with the tumor to ensure negative margins.

- The anterior surface of the vena cava should be identified and the peritoneal lining overlying this should be incised along its length. Using a vein retractor to retract the vena cava medially, soft tissue attachments, including small vessels and lymphatics, are ligated and divided. As the midpoint of the adrenal gland is reached, the right adrenal vein should be identified, ligated, and divided. The vein should be inspected and carefully palpated to assess for any tumor thrombus so that the tumor thrombus can be included with the specimen in an en bloc fashion. Advanced techniques for managing large tumor thrombi within the vena cava are not discussed in this chapter. If removing a pheochromocytoma, the anesthesiologist should be warned well in advance prior to ligating the adrenal vein in anticipation of ensuing hypotension. The dissection is continued superiorly until all medial attachments have been released. Retraction of the vena cava allows access to posterior tissue, which should be removed as well. The adrenal gland and the periadrenal soft tissue are removed, marked with orienting suture for the pathologist, and sent to the pathology lab.

Closure

- A small amount of water should be used for irrigation and final hemostasis is achieved. The area encompassed by the dissection should be marked with large clips to assist with postoperative external beam radiation therapy if needed. A drain may be placed in the adrenal bed, and a chest tube is placed.
- Closure is begun, and the bed is taken out of the flexed position. A chest tube is placed. The diaphragm is repaired with no. 1 polydioxanone (PDS) suture in a running locking or interrupted fashion.
- At the junction of the diaphragm and abdominal fascia, a no. 2 Vicryl figure-of-eight suture is used to reapproximate the tissue en masse. If a portion of the costochondral cartilage has not been excised, it may be reapproximated using a microdrill and a no. 2 Vicryl suture. The ribs are also reapproximated with no. 2 Vicryl sutures, with or without the microdrill (**FIGS 8** and **9**).

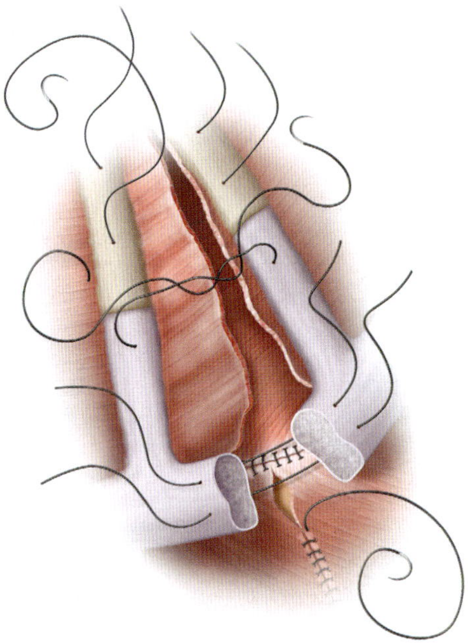

FIG 8 ● A portion of the costal margin can be excised to minimize postoperative rubbing of the ends and costochondritis. If a portion of the costochondral cartilage has not been excised, it may be reapproximated using a microdrill and a no. 2 Vicryl suture. The ribs are reapproximated with no. 2 Vicryl sutures, with or without the microdrill.

A rib approximator device helps decrease the tension required to tie the sutures. The abdominal midline is reapproximated with running no. 1 PDS suture. The chest wall musculature is closed in two separate layers using no. 1 Vicryl suture. The skin is closed with staples and a sterile dressing is applied (**FIG 10**).

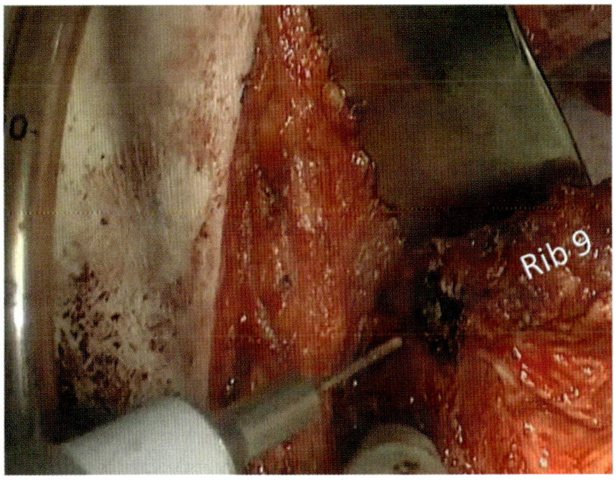

FIG 9 ● The microdrill is used to help reapproximate the ribs.

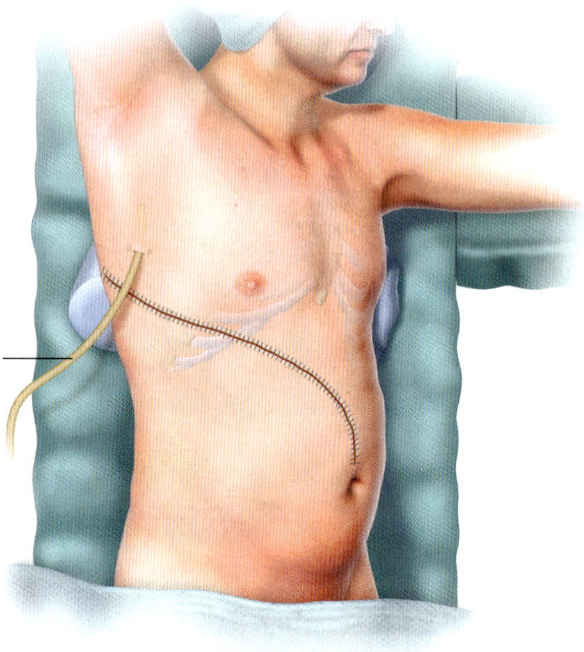

FIG 10 • During closure, a chest tube is inserted. The abdominal midline is reapproximated in a single layer. The chest wall musculature is closed in several layers. The skin is closed with staples and a sterile dressing is applied.

LEFT ADRENALECTOMY

Exposure

- An incision is made 2 cm inferior to the tip of the right scapula and extended to a point midway between the xiphoid process and the umbilicus (**FIGS 11** and **12**). If necessary, the incision can then be carried inferiorly along the midline of the abdomen. The subcutaneous tissue and muscle are divided, sparing the latissimus dorsi and incising the serratus anterior. The chest is entered at the 8th intercostal space, the pulmonary ligament divided, and the lung retracted superiorly. The diaphragm is incised 2 to 4 cm from its attachments, sparing the phrenic nerve. Several marking stitches should be placed intermittently on either side of the divided diaphragm to aid with reapproximation at the end of the case. The costochondral cartilage is divided. A portion may be excised. The abdominal incision is extended and the peritoneal cavity is entered. A self-retaining retractor system is placed.
- The diaphragmatic attachments to the spleen are released with electrocautery and reflected toward the right side along with the stomach and pancreas. If the adrenal tumor is adherent to the diaphragm, that portion of the diaphragm should be removed en bloc with the tumor and can be reconstructed with mesh or other material. The splenocolic attachments will require release and the omentum is released from the colon. The ligamentum teres is ligated and divided with silk ligatures.
- Inspection of the peritoneal cavity is performed as much as possible in a systematic fashion, and an ultrasound of the liver is performed.
- The left lobe of the liver is retracted toward the right side, allowing for better mobilization of the stomach, spleen, and pancreas.
- A large saline-soaked towel with retractors is placed against the bowel, pancreas, and spleen to not only provide exposure but also to exclude the rest of the

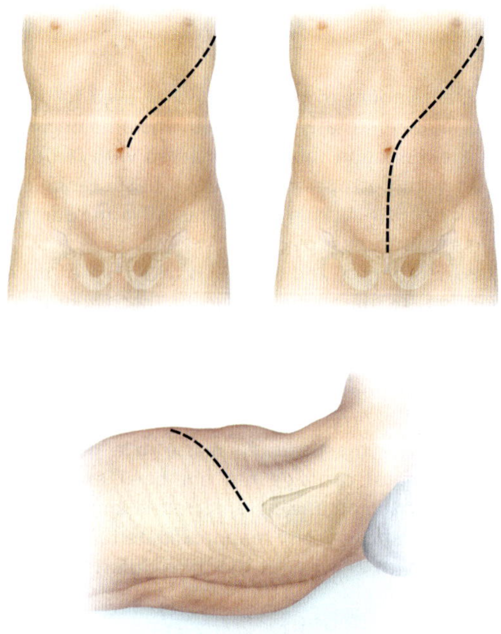

FIG 11 • Options for left thoracoabdominal incision for adrenalectomy.

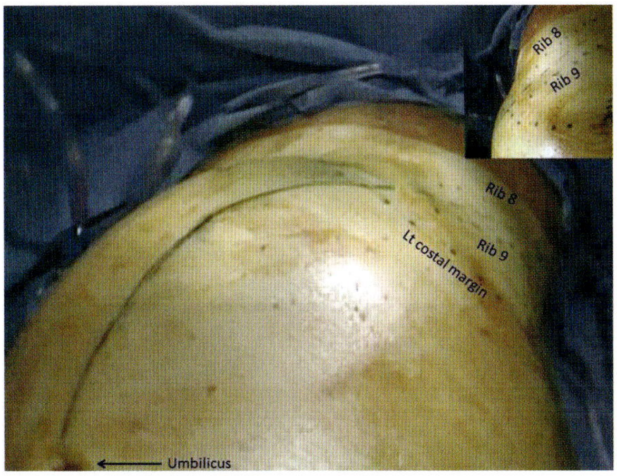

FIG 12 • An incision is made 2 cm inferior to the tip of the right scapula and extended to a point midway between the xiphoid process and the umbilicus.

peritoneal cavity to minimize potential seeding of the peritoneal cavity. The left side of the aorta should be appreciable if the exposure is adequate (**FIG 13**).

Dissection

- Because the peritoneal covering on the left has been reflected with the spleen and pancreas, the surgeon should make every effort to manipulate the tumor surface as little as possible (no-touch technique). The soft tissue overlying the superior half of the left kidney is incised and carried from medial to lateral out to the side of the abdominal wall. Inferior dissection should proceed carefully to the aorta medially along the left renal vein, making sure not to divide branches of the posteriorly situated renal artery supplying the upper portion of the kidney or venous branches draining to the renal vein. Small branches supplying and draining the adrenal gland should be carefully ligated and divided. Any lymph nodes posterior to the renal hilum should be included with the dissection. The left adrenal vein will be identified at the medial aspect of the left renal vein as it courses anterior to the aorta. It generally enters the adrenal gland in the 7 o'clock position. It should be ligated and divided. The adrenal vein and renal vein should be inspected and carefully palpated to assess for any tumor thrombus so that the tumor thrombus can be included with the specimen in an en bloc fashion. Advanced techniques for managing large tumor thrombi within the renal vein and vena cava are not discussed in this chapter. The fat overlying and just superior to the kidney is mobilized from inferior to superior, making this tissue the inferior margin, using cautery, silk sutures, and other hemostatic devices as needed, making sure not to create a nonexistent plane between the inferior aspect of the tumor and the superior aspect of the kidney. Lateral dissection should continue along the abdominal side wall. The dissection continues superiorly along the diaphragm, making sure to ligate and divide any feeding vessels, most commonly branches from the inferior phrenic vessels. Posterior dissection should proceed from lateral to medial, making sure to remove all fat posterior to the tumor in an en bloc fashion. If the tumor invades the muscle, a portion of the muscle should be included with the tumor to ensure negative margins. The left lateral surface of the aorta should be identified, and the soft tissue attachments including small vessels and lymphatics are ligated and divided. If removing a pheochromocytoma, the anesthesiologist should be warned well in advance prior to ligating the adrenal vein in anticipation of ensuing hypotension. The dissection is continued superiorly until all medial attachments have been released. Any lymph nodes along the aorta or identified near the superior mesenteric artery or celiac axis should be included with the specimen. The adrenal gland and the periadrenal soft tissue is removed, marked with orienting suture for the pathologist, and sent to the pathology lab.

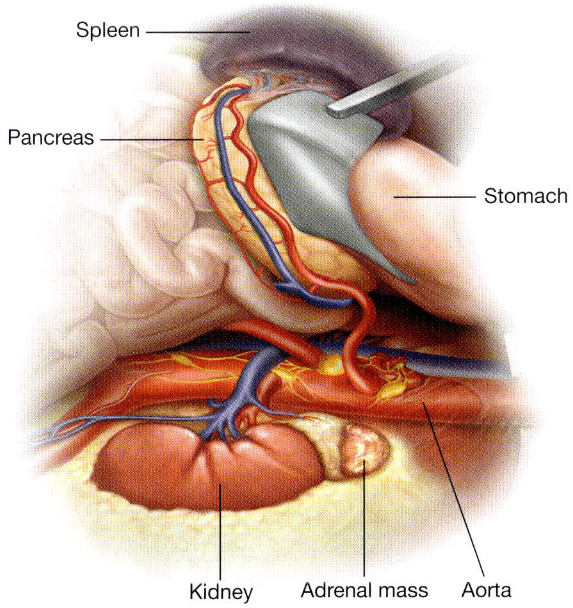

FIG 13 • With the stomach, pancreas, and spleen retracted medially, the aorta, adrenal mass, and kidney are exposed and excluded from the rest of the peritoneal cavity.

Closure

- A small amount of water should be used for irrigation and final hemostasis achieved. The area encompassed by the dissection should be marked with large clips to assist with postoperative external beam radiation therapy if needed. A drain may be placed in the adrenal bed, and a chest tube is placed. Closure is begun, and the bed is taken out of the flexed position. The diaphragm is repaired with no. 1 PDS suture in a running locking or interrupted fashion. At the junction of the diaphragm and abdominal fascia, a no. 2 Vicryl figure-of-eight suture is used to reapproximate the tissue en masse. If a portion of the costochondral cartilage has not been excised, it may be reapproximated using a microdrill and a no. 2 Vicryl suture. The ribs are also reapproximated with no. 2 Vicryl sutures, with or without the microdrill. A rib approximator device helps decrease the tension required to tie the sutures. The abdominal midline is reapproximated with running no. 1 PDS suture. The chest wall musculature is closed in two separate layers using no. 1 Vicryl suture. The skin is closed with staples and a sterile dressing is applied.

PEARLS AND PITFALLS

Atelectasis	▪ Ensure excellent respiratory care and pulmonary toilet due to increased pain limiting respiratory effort.
Bleeding	▪ Access to the suprahepatic inferior vena cava is improved during left adrenalectomy with this approach, allowing for easier vascular control.
Pain	▪ Thoracoabdominal incisions are associated with greater pain than other incisions. Local anesthetic blocks may be helpful.
Neurovascular bundle of rib	▪ Avoid transection of the bundle and damage to the nerve by incising along the superior border of the rib.
Phrenic nerve palsy	▪ Take care to stay away from the phrenic nerve when incising the diaphragm.

POSTOPERATIVE CARE

- Most patients will need intensive care unit (ICU) care for 24 to 48 hours, either for pulmonary care or for resuscitation. The chest tube may be managed in standard fashion and removed when appropriate.
- Hydrocortisone should be administered to patients with overt Cushing's syndrome. A cosyntropin stimulation test can be performed the morning after surgery in subclinical or mild Cushing's cases if there is a question about the requirement for steroid supplementation. After bilateral adrenalectomy, high-dose intravenous (IV) hydrocortisone should be weaned to replacement dose oral hydrocortisone and fludrocortisone 0.1 mg daily. Electrolytes should be checked the morning after surgery. Patients undergoing surgery for primary hyperaldosteronism may experience rebound hyperkalemia. Antihypertensive medications are withheld in the immediate postoperative setting and reinstituted as needed. Routine postoperative care is pursued and patients are discharged approximately 5 to 7 days after surgery. Follow-up is typically 1 to 2 weeks after surgery with endocrine testing as needed.

OUTCOMES

- Excellent outcomes can be expected with low morbidity if aggressive respiratory care and pain control is initiated early in the postoperative period.

COMPLICATIONS

- Prolonged atelectasis: 21%
- Prolonged ileus: 9%
- Phrenic nerve injury and diaphragmatic paralysis
- Chronic pain

REFERENCES

1. Young WF. The incidentally discovered adrenal mass. *N Engl J Med*. 2007;356:601–610.
2. Gusani NJ, Avella D, Staveley-O'Carroll KF, et al. Thoracoabdominal incision: a forgotten tool. *Oper Tech Gen Surg*. 2008;10(2):107–110.
3. Karakousis CP, Pourshahmir M. Thoracoabdominal incisions and resection of upper retroperitoneal sarcomas. *J Surg Oncol*. 1999;72: 150–155.
4. Lumsden AB, Colborn GL, Sreeram S, et al. The surgical anatomy and technique of the thoracoabdominal incision. *Surg Clin North Am*. 1993;73(4):633–644.
5. Yang M, Zhao X. Retrospective study of the efficacy and complication of thoracoabdominal incision for nephrectomy: a comparison with flank approach. *Front Med China*. 2009;3(2):191–196.

Chapter 48 Adrenalectomy: Open Posterior

Barbra S. Miller

DEFINITION

- Adrenal masses may be benign or malignant and functional or nonfunctional with regard to excess hormone secretion. An open posterior approach should be considered if:
  - An anterior, lateral, or posterior retroperitoneoscopic approach is not feasible in a patient with a benign or metastatic adrenal tumor.
  - An open anterior approach is not feasible in patients who have undergone previous extensive upper abdominal surgery and are presumed to have dense adhesions limiting access.
  - Conversion from a retroperitoneoscopic posterior approach to an open approach is required.
  - Both adrenals need to be removed and repositioning of the patient during the case is to be avoided.

DIFFERENTIAL DIAGNOSIS

- Primary adrenal adenoma
- Primary adrenocortical carcinoma
- Cyst
- Metastatic cancer
- Pheochromocytoma
- Ganglioneuroma
- Adjacent paraganglioma
- Soft tissue tumor

PATIENT HISTORY AND PHYSICAL FINDINGS

- All adrenal abnormalities should be evaluated in a systematic fashion, including a thorough history and physical examination investigating the possibility of a hormone-secreting mass. This includes the possibility of a pheochromocytoma, Cushing's syndrome, primary hyperaldosteronism, and hypertestosteronemia. Specifically, the patient should be questioned regarding poorly controlled hypertension, diabetes, edema, diaphoresis, tachycardia, palpitations, sudden severe headaches, flushing, and easy bruising. The physical exam should look for evidence of central obesity, edema, peripheral wasting, core muscle weakness, a buffalo hump, striae, thin skin, and facial plethora. Because the adrenal gland is situated in the retroperitoneum, unless it is extremely large, palpation of the mass is usually unable to be achieved.

IMAGING AND OTHER DIAGNOSTIC STUDIES

- All adrenal masses should undergo appropriate biochemical testing. Even in the absence of signs or symptoms, patients should have at a minimum: potassium, aldosterone, renin, plasma fractionated metanephrines (followed by 24-hour urine metanephrines and normetanephrines, catecholamines, and vanillylmandelic acid (VMA) if plasma values are abnormal), 24-hour urine-free cortisol, and adrenocorticotropic hormone (ACTH). Some physicians may also perform a low-dose dexamethasone suppression test and obtain dehydroepiandrosterone Sulfate (DHEA-S) and free testosterone, among other laboratory tests.
- Imaging studies should include an adrenal protocol computed tomography (CT) scan (to assess imaging characteristics and calculate washout percentage of contrast from the tumor) or magnetic resonance imaging (MRI) (to assess decrease in signal between in and out of phase images) and 18F-Fluorodeoxyglucose (18FDG) positron emission tomography (PET) CT if malignancy is questioned (**FIG 1**).
- Additional imaging studies may be required depending on the functionality of the tumor (metaiodobenzylguanidine [MIBG] for some pheochromocytoma patients, adrenal vein sampling for hyperaldosteronism, etc.).
- Fine needle aspiration or core biopsy is not recommended if adrenocortical carcinoma is questioned. FNA may be useful if metastasis to the adrenal gland is in the differential and the adrenal tumor is the most accessible site of metastasis in the setting of multiple sites of metastatic disease. If biopsy is performed, it is imperative to first biochemically rule out pheochromocytoma.

SURGICAL MANAGEMENT

- Adrenal tumors, if benign appearing by imaging criteria, nonfunctional, and therefore not requiring resection, should be reevaluated with at least one additional CT scan or MRI 6 to 12 months after the initial imaging study to ensure stability in size and internal imaging characteristics. Some advocate for a longer period of follow-up imaging for 2 years with reevaluation of biochemistry for 4 years.[1]
- Functional tumors leading to hormone excess, indeterminate masses, and those suspected of being adrenocortical carcinoma or isolated metastatic disease from another primary tumor without evidence of widespread metastatic disease should be removed.

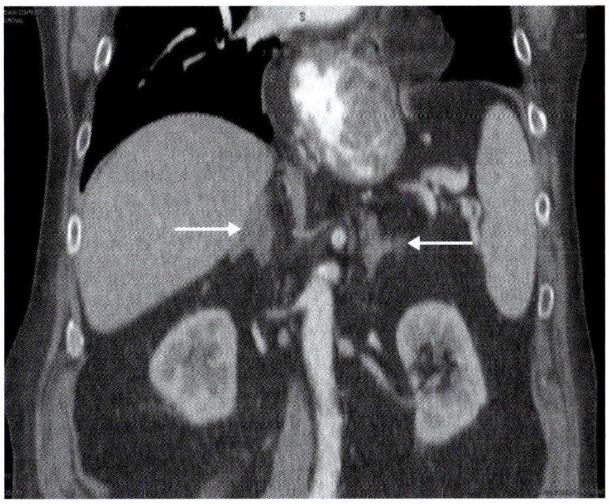

FIG 1 • Bilateral hyperplastic adrenal glands *(arrows)* with benign imaging characteristics are shown in an obese patient with Cushing's disease requiring bilateral adrenalectomy.

Preoperative Planning

- The surgeon must evaluate available imaging studies for possible adrenocortical carcinoma or tumor involvement of adjacent organs, vessels, and lymphadenopathy. An open posterior approach is not optimal for removing adrenocortical carcinomas or large tumors, as the working space is limited by the rib cage and does not allow for multivisceral resections. These types of tumors should be approached by an open anterior or thoracoabdominal approach.
- The surgeon should evaluate the position of the adrenal gland with respect to the overlying rib that will need to be resected as well as any visible vasculature supplying or draining the adrenal gland.
- The risks, benefits, and alternatives to surgery are discussed with the patient including potential need for steroid supplementation in the postoperative setting. Patients with pheochromocytomas should be adequately alpha blocked and volume replete. Beta blockade may also be necessary. A potassium level should be checked the morning of surgery and treated as necessary in patients with Conn's syndrome (hyperaldosteronism).
- Routine prophylactic antibiotics and deep vein thrombosis (DVT) prophylaxis are administered prior to surgery, and sequential compression devices are applied.
- A general endotracheal anesthetic is administered.
- Common to all approaches, skin preparation with clipping rather than shaving is prepared, and the surgical area is prepped and draped in a sterile fashion.

Positioning

- Patients are intubated and a Foley catheter is placed prior to placing the patient in a modified prone position. Several methods for positioning may be used, including use of the Wilson frame, the Cloward surgical saddle, gel rolls, and flexion of the table (**FIG 2**). All of these have the common goal of creating a gentle flexion of the spine. Space is also created for the abdominal contents to shift away from the retroperitoneum.
- All pressure points are padded appropriately.

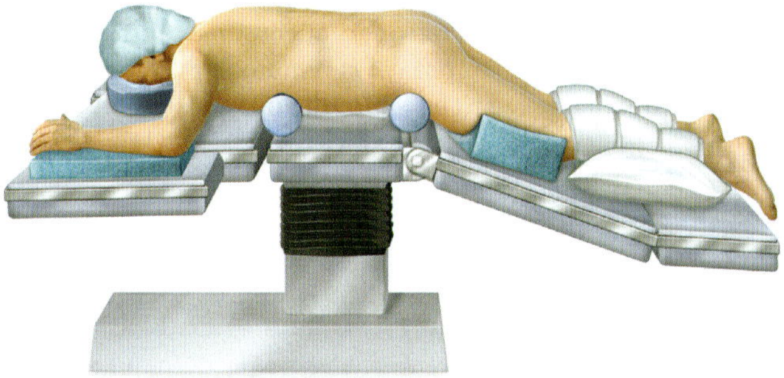

FIG 2 • The patient is placed in a modified prone position. Pressure points are padded.

TECHNIQUES

LEFT ADRENALECTOMY

Exposure

- A curvilinear incision is made from a paramedian position (4 to 5 cm from the spine) over the left 10th rib and carried inferolaterally toward the iliac crest. Alternatively, a straighter incision over the 11th or 12th rib, depending on the position of the gland on CT scan, with a more vertical upward incision medially may be made (**FIGS 3** and **4**).
- The subcutaneous tissue and musculature (latissimus dorsi and lumbodorsal fascia) are divided. The sacrospinalis is retracted medially with a handheld retractor. The 12th rib (and occasionally the 11th rib) is cleared of its attachments in a subperiosteal fashion using cautery and a Doyen or periosteal elevator, making sure to preserve the neurovascular bundle (**FIGS 5** and **6**). The rib is transected as far medially as possible with bone cutters and removed in its entirety. Bone wax may be used to assist with hemostasis.
- Entrance into the diaphragm and pleura should be avoided and the diaphragm is reflected superiorly. The retroperitoneal fat will be evident (**FIG 7**).

Dissection

- Using retractors to separate the tissue and rib(s), Gerota's fascia is incised after identifying the upper pole of the kidney. The surgeon's hand places downward (inferior and toward the peritoneal cavity) pressure on the kidney to facilitate exposure of the adrenal gland (**FIG 8**).
- The inferior, lateral, superior, and medial attachments may be divided in similar fashion to the standard open anterior approach, but the peritoneum overlying the anterior surface of the gland as described in the anterior open approach is not included with the specimen. The inferior attachments should be left until last, as they assist in retraction and exposure of the gland.
- The left adrenal vein should be ligated and divided when encountered during the course of dissection of the inferior attachments and will be found medially near the junction of the superior aspect of the left renal vein with the lateral aspect of the aorta in a 5 o'clock position due to the prone position. The left adrenal vein will be slightly posterior while in the prone position beneath some of the fatty attachments between the adrenal gland and left renal vein.
- The adrenal gland with the periadrenal soft tissue is removed en bloc, marked with orienting sutures for the pathologist, and sent to the pathology lab.

Closure

- A small amount of water should be used for irrigation and final hemostasis is achieved. A drain may be placed if desired but is not required in most cases.
- The musculature and subcutaneous tissue are closed in layers and the skin closed with staples or suture. A sterile dressing is applied.

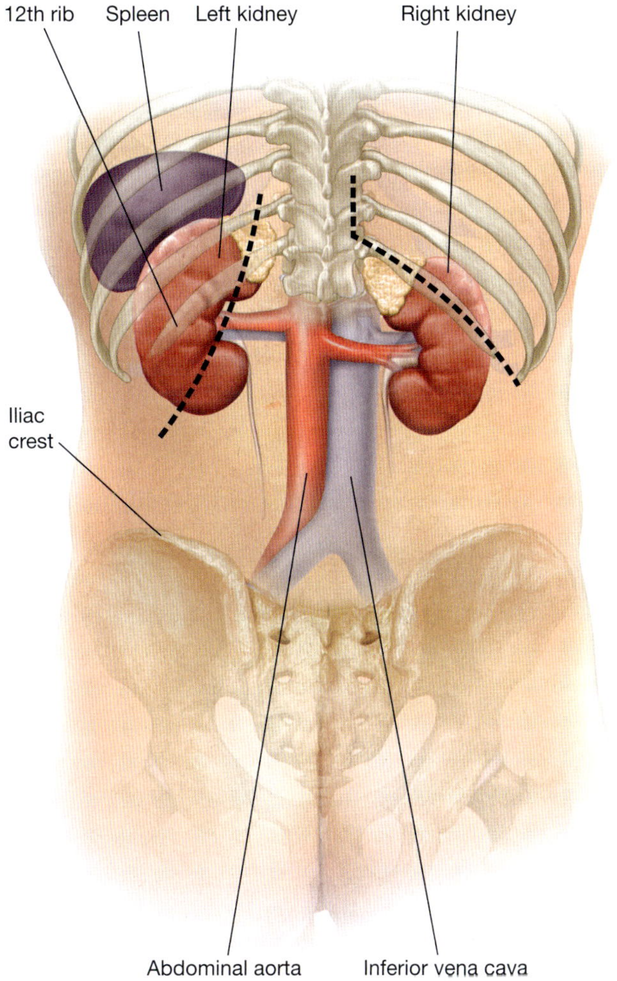

FIG 3 ● The incision can be made in a linear or curvilinear fashion to facilitate access to the 11th and 12th ribs.

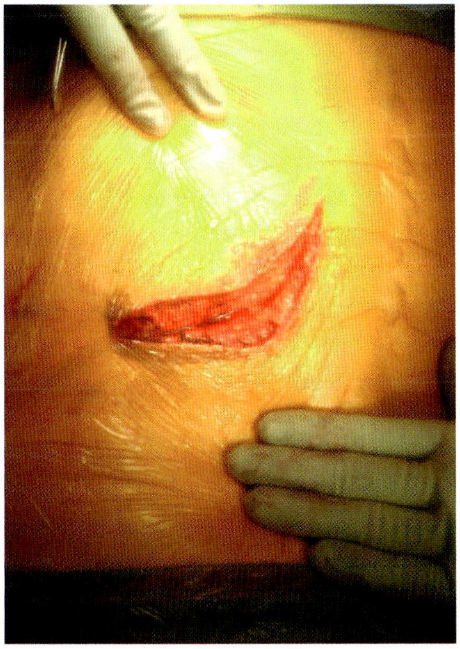

FIG 4 ● Intraoperative image of curvilinear incision carried from 10th rib medially across the 11th rib and inferior to the 12th rib laterally.

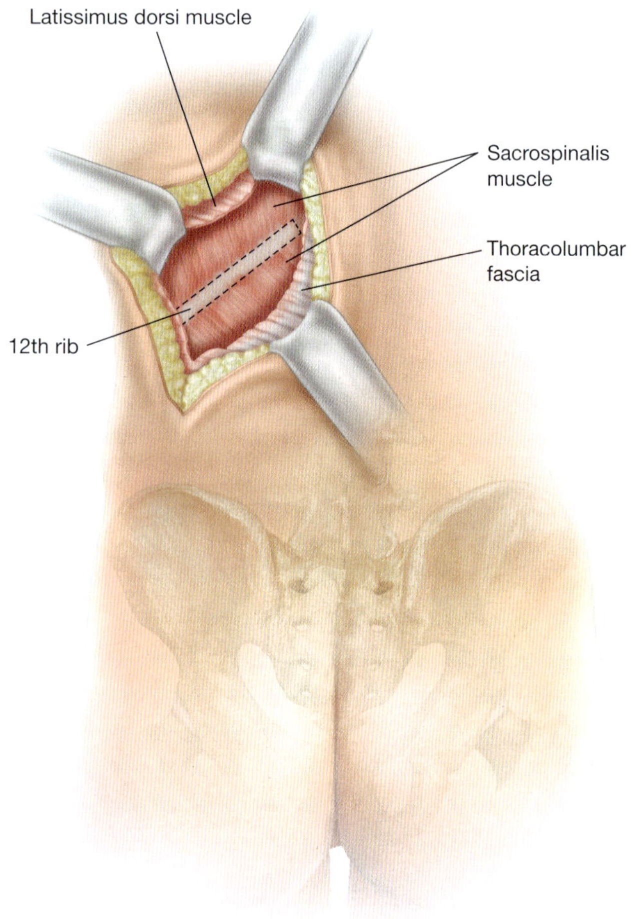

FIG 5 • Schematic of exposure of the 12th rib that is cleared of its attachments in a subperiosteal fashion using cautery and a Doyen or periosteal elevator, making sure to preserve the neurovascular bundle.

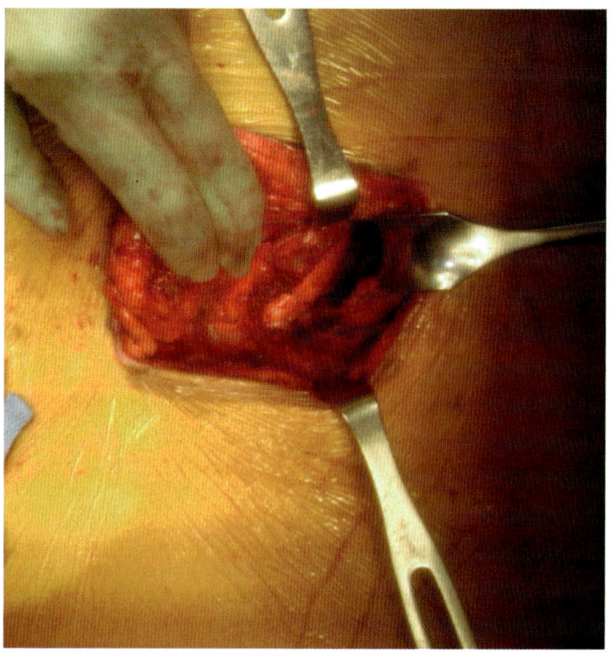

FIG 6 • Intraoperative photo showing exposure of the 12th rib.

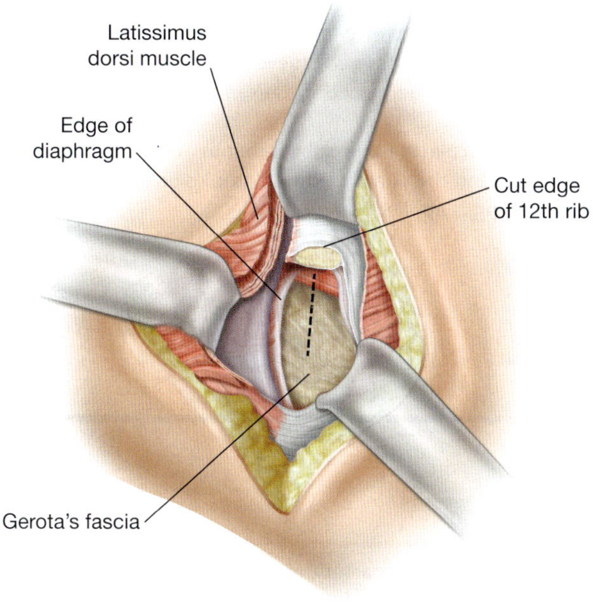

FIG 7 ● After removal of the 12th rib, Gerota's fascia and the retroperitoneal fat is evident.

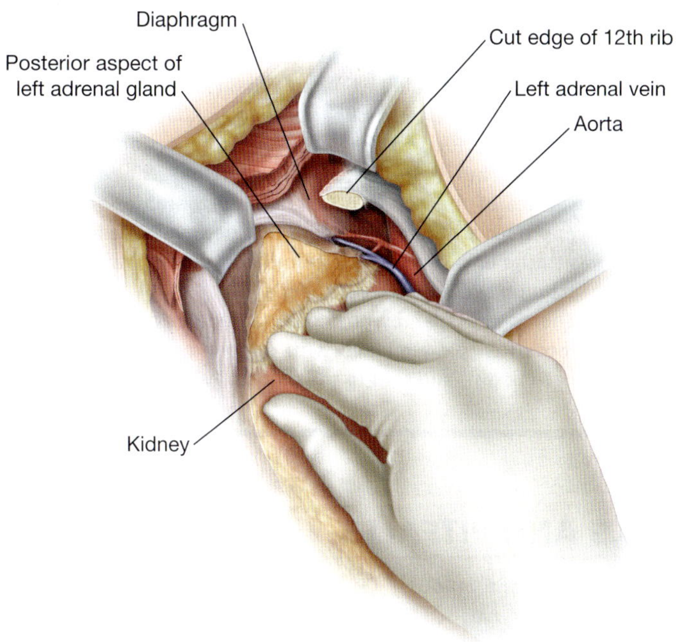

FIG 8 ● The left adrenal gland is best exposed using retractors and downward retraction using the hand on the upper pole of the kidney. The left adrenal vein is located in a 5 o'clock position.

RIGHT ADRENALECTOMY

Exposure

- A curvilinear incision is made from a paramedian position (4 to 5 cm from the spine) over the right 10th rib and carried inferolaterally toward the iliac crest. Alternatively, a straighter incision over the 11th or 12th rib, depending on the position of the gland on CT scan, with a more vertical upward incision medially may be made.
- The subcutaneous tissue and musculature (latissimus dorsi and lumbodorsal fascia) are divided. The sacrospinalis is retracted medially with a handheld retractor. The 12th rib (and occasionally the 11th rib) is cleared of its attachments in a subperiosteal fashion using cautery and a Doyen or periosteal elevator, making sure to preserve the neurovascular bundle. The rib is transected as far medially as possible with bone cutters and removed in its entirety. Bone wax may be used to assist with hemostasis.
- Entrance into the diaphragm and pleura should be avoided and is reflected superiorly. The retroperitoneal fat will be evident.

Dissection

- Using retractors to separate the tissue and rib(s), Gerota's fascia is incised after identifying the area of the upper pole of the kidney. The surgeon's hand places downward (inferior and toward the peritoneal cavity) pressure on the kidney to facilitate exposure of the adrenal gland (**FIG 9**).

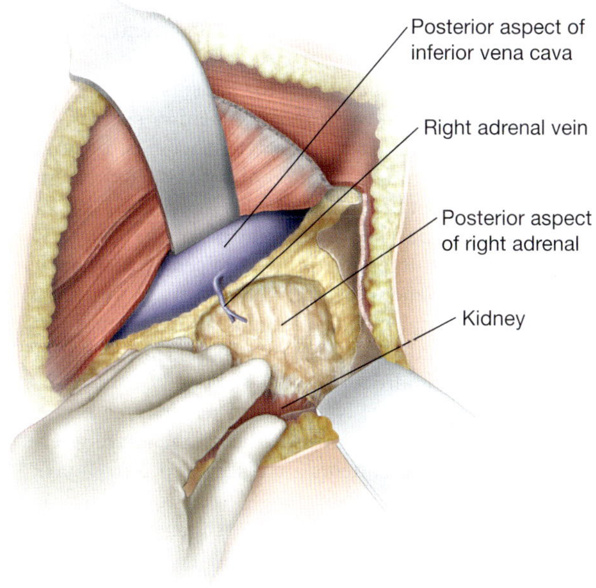

FIG 9 ● The right adrenal gland is best exposed using retractors and downward retraction using the hand on the upper pole of the kidney. The right adrenal vein is located in a 9 o'clock position.

- The right adrenal vein will be found along the medial aspect of the gland in a more anterior position off of the inferior vena cava (IVC) due to the prone position of the patient and should be ligated and divided.
- The inferior, lateral, superior, and medial attachments may be divided in similar fashion to the standard approach, but the peritoneum overlying the anterior surface of the gland as described in the anterior open approach is not included with the specimen. The inferior attachments should be left until last, as they assist in retraction and exposure of the gland.
- The adrenal gland with the periadrenal soft tissue is removed en bloc, marked with orienting sutures for the pathologist, and sent to the pathology lab.

Closure

- A small amount of water should be used for irrigation and final hemostasis is achieved.
- A drain may be placed if desired but is not required in many cases.
- The musculature and subcutaneous tissue are closed in layers and the skin closed with staples or suture. A sterile dressing is applied.

PEARLS AND PITFALLS

Bleeding—arterial and venous	■ May result from disruption of the vena cava, renal vein or artery, and aorta. A laparoscopic knot pusher, Allis clamp, and/or Kitner may be helpful given limited access due to the overlying ribs.
Diaphragmatic penetration	■ May occur upon entry to the retroperitoneum. May be closed in standard fashion.
Neurovascular bundle injury	■ Chronic pain may result if care is not taken to spare the bundle when removing the rib or upon closure of the wound.

POSTOPERATIVE CARE

- Most patients will not need intensive care unit (ICU) care, although pheochromocytoma patients often need closer monitoring for the first 24 hours, depending on intraoperative stability and volume status.
- Hydrocortisone should be given to patients with overt Cushing's syndrome. A cosyntropin stimulation test can be performed the morning after surgery in subclinical or mild Cushing's cases if there is a question about the requirement for steroid supplementation.
- Electrolytes should be checked the morning after surgery. Patients undergoing surgery for primary hyperaldosteronism may experience rebound hyperkalemia.
- After bilateral adrenalectomy, high-dose intravenous (IV) hydrocortisone should be weaned to replacement dose oral hydrocortisone and fludrocortisone 0.1 mg daily.
- Routine postoperative care is pursued. Diets may be begun early, as ileus is not usually an issue due to the entirely retroperitoneal dissection. Patients are discharged 2 to 3 days after surgery.
- Follow-up is typically 1 to 2 weeks after surgery with endocrine testing as indicated.

OUTCOMES

- Outcomes in general are quite good; however, hospital stay is longer, pain is greater, and morbidity can be higher compared to other approaches.[2]
- Neurologic changes due to injury of the neurovascular bundle coursing along the inferior aspect of the rib can be problematic.

COMPLICATIONS

- Bleeding
- Infection
- Adrenal insufficiency in those with Cushing's syndrome
- Postoperative hypotension in those with pheochromocytoma
- Rebound hyperkalemia in those with Conn's syndrome
- Lymphatic leak
- Pneumothorax
- Neurogenic pain
- Laxity of flank musculature

REFERENCES

1. Young WF. The incidentally discovered adrenal mass. *N Engl J Med*. 2007;356:601–610.
2. Thompson GB, Grant CS, van Heerden JA, et al. Laparoscopic versus open posterior adrenalectomy: a case-control study of 100 patients. *Surgery*. 1997;122(6):1132–1136.

Chapter 49 Laparoscopic Retroperitoneal Adrenalectomy

Michael G. Johnston James A. Lee

INDICATIONS

- Adrenalectomy is indicated for a variety of different clinical scenarios, including patients with (1) a functional tumor; (2) a solid adrenal mass larger than 3 to 4 cm, due to increasing risk of adrenocortical carcinoma; (3) growth of 0.5 cm or greater in 6 months based on serial cross-sectional imaging, again due to a risk of adrenocortical carcinoma; and (4) isolated metastasis from a remote primary malignancy.
- Laparoscopic adrenalectomy is now considered standard practice due to its shorter duration of postoperative pain, shorter hospitalization, and faster return to work compared to an open procedure.
- Contraindications to the transabdominal laparoscopic approach include severe cardiopulmonary disease and coagulopathy. Relative contraindications include prior intraabdominal surgery and very large tumor size.
- The laparoscopic retroperitoneal approach is based on the historical open posterior approach. This approach is gaining popularity as it offers advantages over a laparoscopic transabdominal approach. These advantages include faster operating times, potentially less postoperative pain, a lower risk of complications (especially of incisional hernia), and improved intraoperative hemostasis as the surgeon has the ability to increase the insufflation pressure to 30 mmHg (a maneuver not feasible in a laparoscopic transabdominal approach given the negative impact on central venous return and renal perfusion).
- The laparoscopic retroperitoneal approach does have some potential drawbacks. There is a slightly longer learning curve associated with the nontraditional "back-door" anatomic view. This approach may also be more difficult in patients with large tumors or who are morbidly obese.
- The posterior approach is the ideal approach for bilateral procedures because it eliminates the need for patient repositioning. It is also preferable for patients who have had previous transabdominal operations.
- Absolute contraindications to the laparoscopic retroperitoneal approach include the need to explore the rest of the abdomen and coagulopathy.
- Relative contraindications include an adrenal mass greater than 8 cm due to the smaller working space, patient body mass index greater than 45 due to the patient's pannus and visceral fat compressing the retroperitoneal working space. Severe cardiopulmonary disease is also a relative contraindication but may be less of an issue than for the transabdominal laparoscopic approach, as the diaphragm is not compressed to the same extent. Theoretically, increased ocular pressures are also a relative contraindication, as an extended time in a prone position would put the optic nerve at risk. This is usually only a problem for very long operations, however, and the vast majority of laparoscopic retroperitoneal adrenalectomies should not threaten the optic nerve.

PREOPERATIVE PLANNING

- As with any endocrine disease, the workup of adrenal disease typically follows a logical progression, from making a biochemical diagnosis to localizing the lesion to determining the indications for an operation. In deciding if an operation is indicated, the two principal questions to be answered are (1) "Is the mass functional?" and (2) "What is the risk for cancer (either primary or metastatic disease)?" Most functional tumors and most malignant lesions should be considered for resection, taking into account the patient's overall health, prognosis, and preferences.
  - Aldosteronoma. Ideally, the potassium level should be normalized preoperatively. Potassium supplements and/or aldosterone antagonists may be employed to achieve this goal. Maintain or optimize the antihypertensive regimen preoperatively.
  - Pheochromocytoma. Give the patient an α-blocker such as phenoxybenzamine. Start at 10 mg twice daily and increase the frequency and dose as tolerated until the patient becomes slightly symptomatic (including mild orthostasis and stuffy nose). A selective α-blocker is a good alternative in an older male patient due to less reflex tachycardia and potential prostatism benefits. In addition, some patients may be candidates for calcium channel therapy instead. As α-blockade proceeds, it is critical to replete the intravascular space with liberal fluid and some additional salt intake preoperatively. β-Blockade may be started a few days prior to the operation if the patient becomes tachycardic. Do *not* start β-blockade prior to adequate α-blockade or the resulting unopposed α-mediated vasoconstriction may cause stroke, myocardial infarction, and even death. Close communication with the anesthesia team is critical throughout the operation as manipulation of the tumor may cause wide swings in hemodynamics. Ensure that the anesthesia team is equipped with short-acting vasoactive agents to control or support intraoperative blood pressure as needed.
  - Cortisol-producing tumor. Give stress-dose steroids prior to induction. The patient will require a careful steroid taper postoperatively and endocrinology consultation is recommended. Although no level I data is available, perioperative antibiotics should be considered due to the relative immunosuppressed state in a patient with cortisol excess.
  - Adrenocortical carcinoma. Primary adrenal cancers may manifest any or all of the biochemical irregularities found in the aforementioned tumors and should be addressed as appropriate. It is important to assess the vasculature for evidence of venous invasion and tumor thrombus, ideally with a magnetic resonance venogram or formal venogram. The

laparoscopic retroperitoneal approach should not be used in cases of very large or locally invasive adrenal tumors.

ANATOMY

- The retroperitoneal space is bounded by the peritoneum laterally, the paraspinous muscle medially, the rib cage posteriorly (i.e., away from table), the kidney/adrenal gland/peritoneum anteriorly (i.e., toward the table), and the diaphragm superiorly.
- The superior pole of the kidney and the paraspinous muscle serve as the major landmarks.

PATIENT POSITIONING

- A modification of the "Walz position"
- Intubate, obtain intravenous/arterial access as indicated, and place a urinary catheter while patient is still on stretcher. Administer stress-dose steroids and perioperative antibiotics if indicated.
- Place patient prone on two noncompressible bolsters with the lower bolster positioned at the break in the operating room (OR) table. The hips rest on the lower bolster. The lower ribcage rests on the upper bolster. The pannus should hang freely in between the bolsters to allow for the greatest amount of retroperitoneal working space. Place the operative side of the patient flush with that side of the table so that the table will not hinder the full range of motion of instruments, especially in the lateral-most port. If performing a bilateral adrenalectomy, the only patient repositioning necessary will be to shift the patient to the other edge of the bed (**FIG 1**).
- The lower back should be in a completely horizontal plane. This can be accomplished by lowering the leg portion of the OR table as much as possible to stretch the back and counter the natural convexity of the lower back.
- Raising the leg extension with the knees flexed and lower legs horizontal/parallel to the floor will help to prevent the patient from slipping further down on the bed.
- Flex arms at elbows, pad pressure points, and secure patient in place. Prep from midchest to just above buttocks.

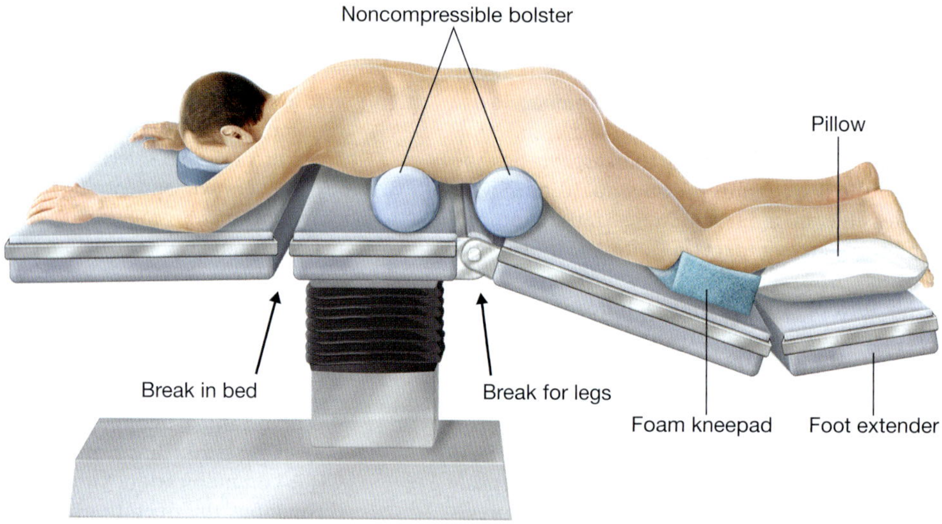

FIG 1 • Patient positioning for a laparoscopic retroperitoneal adrenalectomy.

PORT PLACEMENT

- Three ports (lateral, middle, and medial) (**FIG 2**)
  - Medial: 5-mm "pediatric" or short port. Place this just lateral to paraspinous muscle and a few centimeters inferior to the costal margin.
  - Middle: 10-mm port with a "donut" balloon. Place this halfway in between the medial and lateral ports.
  - Lateral: 5-mm pediatric or short port. Place this as laterally as possible.
- The middle port is placed first via a direct cutdown by making a transverse incision just large enough to admit a finger immediately inferior to the tip of 12th rib or the costal margin. The position of this port is determined as discussed earlier.
- Dissection proceeds through the subcutaneous tissue to the muscle just inferior to the costal margin by spreading with a Metzenbaum scissors. The retroperitoneal space is entered by blunt dissection with the Metzenbaum scissors through the fascia and muscle using a technique similar to placing a chest tube (except that the hole is made directly *inferior* to the costal margin). Feeling the smooth undersurface of the ribs provides confirmation that the correct space has been entered. Use blunt dissection with the finger both laterally and medially to develop space for the placement of the subsequent 5-mm ports

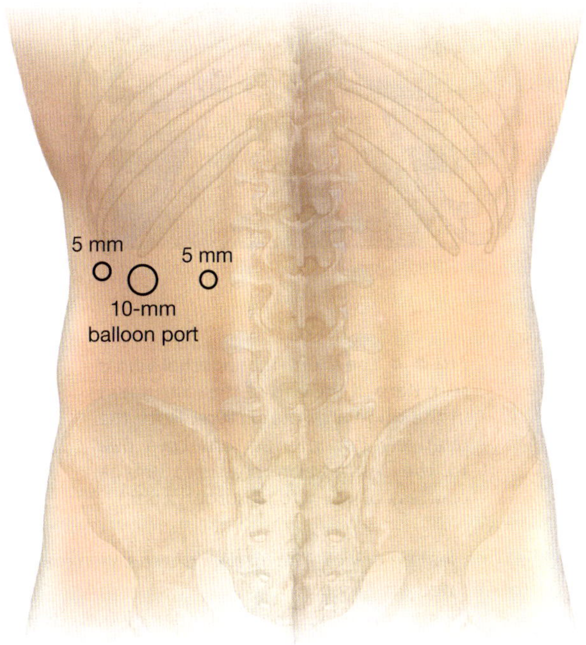

FIG 2 ● Right-sided port placement.

under direct palpation. Dissection should not be carried superiorly as this can make entering Gerota's fascia more challenging.

- Place the medial port 3 to 4 cm inferior to the costal margin just lateral to the paraspinous muscle entering the retroperitoneal space on a bias/angle cephalad of approximately 45 degrees such that the port enters the retroperitoneal space just inferior to the inferior margin of 12th rib. This angling of the port will improve visualization, obviating the need to torque the port.
- Place the lateral port just inferior to the costal margin as far laterally as possible.
- Place a balloon port in the middle port site to form a seal for the retroperitoneal insufflation.

DISSECTION OF THE RETROPERITONEAL SPACE

- Insufflate to 20 mmHg, liberally increasing as needed to maximum of 30 mmHg.
- Place camera into the middle port and a sealing device into the lateral port.

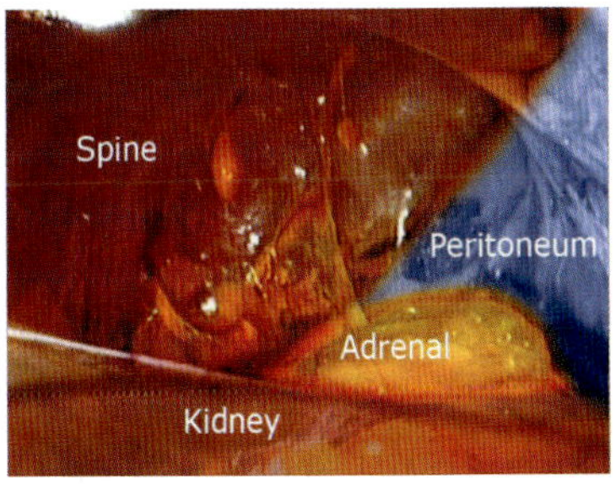

FIG 3 ● Retroperitoneoscopic view of the spatial relationships during initial dissection of a right adrenal gland. (Image courtesy of www.coachsurgery.com.)

- Enter Gerota's fascia bluntly and open it widely from left to right.
- Sweep the filmy posterior attachments of the periadrenal and perirenal fat anteriorly (i.e., toward the table). Continue this dissection to expose the peritoneum laterally, paraspinous muscle medially, and peritoneum superiorly.
- Switch camera to medial port and place a grasper into the middle port (FIG 3).
- Identify the superior border of the kidney. Starting laterally, divide the adrenal-renal connections using a combination of blunt and sharp dissection. Carry this dissection toward the paraspinous muscle following the superior contour of the kidney, which will allow the kidney to be retracted inferomedially.
- Carefully dissect the filmy plane between the adrenal gland and the paraspinous muscle medially to allow identification of the inferior vena cava during a right adrenalectomy or the inferior phrenic vein during a left adrenalectomy. The adrenal arteries will be in a plane that is posterior (i.e., away from the table) to the level of the adrenal vein. These arteries may be ligated with a sealing device.

IDENTIFICATION OF THE ADRENAL VEIN

- Right adrenal vein (FIG 4). Once the inferior vena cava is identified, follow the cava superiorly. The adrenal vein can typically be found entering the adrenal gland at the junction of the middle and superior third of the adrenal gland. The adrenal vein enters the adrenal gland anteriorly (i.e., toward the table). Divide the vein with clips or a sealing device.
- Left adrenal vein (FIG 5). Identify the adrenal vein either by tracing the inferior phrenic vein from superiorly to inferiorly or by dissecting the inferior border of the adrenal gland from lateral to medial until the confluence

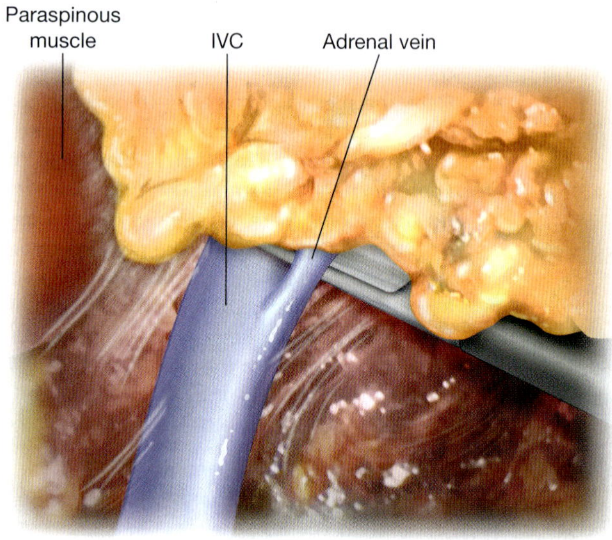

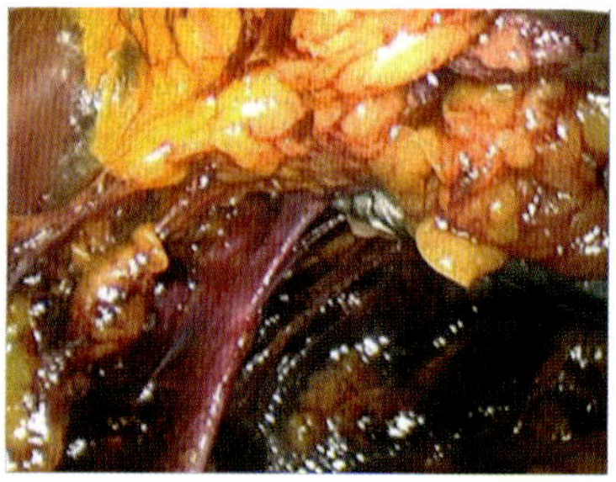

FIG 4 ● The short right adrenal vein is seen here at the end of the instrument in the middle of the picture. Note the relatively flat inferior vena cava due to the insufflation pressure. (Image courtesy of www.coachsurgery.com.)

of the adrenal vein and inferior phrenic vein is encountered. Ensure that the inferior-medial border of the adrenal gland is fully dissected from the surrounding tissue, as there is often a tongue of adrenal tissue extending toward the renal hilum. Divide the left adrenal vein with clips or a sealing device. The inferior phrenic vein may be either ligated or spared.

- Once the vein is divided, the remainder of the adrenal gland can be dissected with mostly blunt dissection and a minimum of sharp dissection.

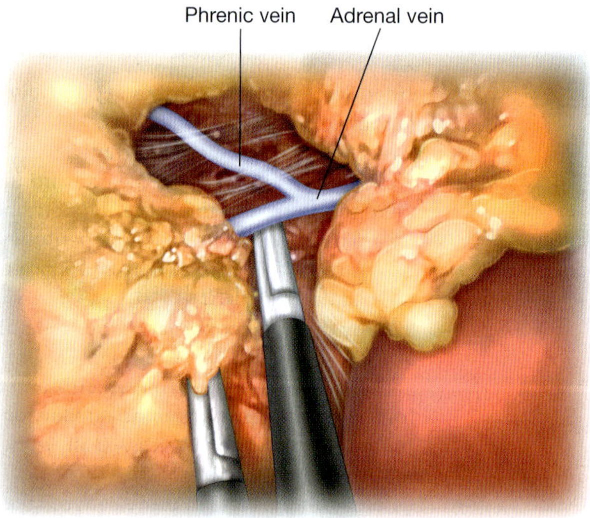

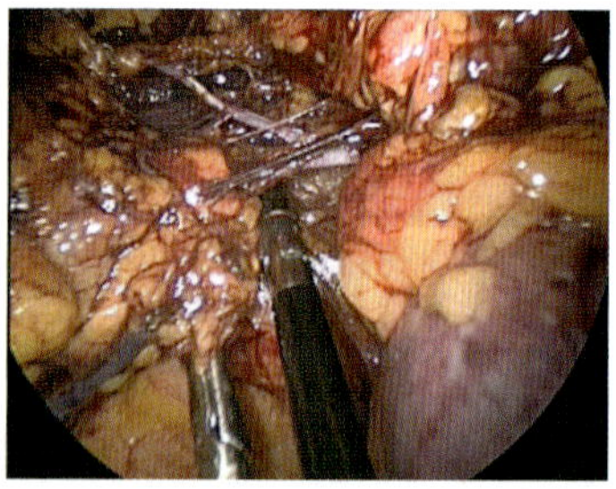

FIG 5 ● The left adrenal gland (notable for its distinct color that differentiates it from surrounding retroperitoneal fat) seen here at the end of the left adrenal vein (directly above the instrument in the middle of the picture). The left phrenic vein joins at an angle from above and can often be spared. The red-toned structure in the right foreground is the paraspinous muscle. (Image courtesy of www.coachsurgery.com.)

SPECIMEN EXTRACTION

- The adrenal gland can be placed in a specimen bag and removed through the middle port site, usually without the need to enlarge this site.
- Replace the middle port and inspect for hemostasis. Decrease insufflation to 5 to 7 mmHg to assist in identification of bleeding.
- A closed suction drain is not normally necessary.
- Remove the ports and close the middle port site fascia with a single absorbable figure-of-eight stitch, taking care to avoid the subcostal nerve.
- Close the skin with subcuticular stitches.

PEARLS AND PITFALLS

Patient positioning	■ Proper patient positioning is critical. ■ Make sure the rib cage and hips rest on the bolsters with the pannus hanging freely. ■ Place the operative side flush with the side of the table. ■ Lower the leg portion of the OR table to stretch the back so it is completely horizontal. Then raise the leg extension with the knees flexed to prevent the patient slipping down the bed.
Port placement and insufflation	■ The middle port is placed just inferior to the tip of 12th rib. Use blunt dissection with Metzenbaum scissors and fingers to enter the correct plane and allow the other two ports under direct palpation. ■ Make liberal use of increased insufflation pressures (20 to 30 mmHg) to improve visualization and hemostasis.
Dissection	■ Because of the nontraditional view of the anatomy, there is a longer learning curve associated with this approach. ■ Dissecting the superior pole of the kidney from lateral to medial and then retracting the kidney inferomedially allows for the best exposure to the adrenal gland and adrenal vein.

POSTOPERATIVE MANAGEMENT

- Remove the urinary catheter 4 to 6 hours postoperatively.
- Patients may ambulate and eat a regular diet on the day of surgery.
- Aldosteronoma. Draw potassium, aldosterone, and renin levels the morning after surgery. Stop potassium supplements and aldosterone antagonists. Implementation of the antihypertensive regimen differs from patient to patient. Some clinicians will choose to stop all antihypertensives and add them back as needed, whereas others will cut the patient's typical doses in half and add them back as needed. Typically, beta-blockers are continued postoperatively.
- Pheochromocytoma. Monitor hemodynamics closely and treat as indicated until stabilized. Stop all α-blockade. After removal of a pheochromocytoma, the major hemodynamic change to watch for is hypotension.
- Cortisol-producing tumor. Begin steroid taper. Consider keeping patients in-house for a day or two to begin the steroid taper under observed conditions.

COMPLICATIONS

- Bleeding. Significant bleeding occurs in less than 1% of cases. Increasing insufflation pressures as high as 30 mmHg often tamponades small bleeding sites. Even with a significant caval injury, increasing the insufflation pressure can cause tamponade that allows time either to repair the injury laparoscopically or to convert to an open procedure.
- Significant intraoperative hypertension occurs in 1% to 2% of cases.
- Conversion to an open operation occurs in approximately 1% of cases. Emergent conversion (such as for significant bleeding) should be done through a posterior approach, obviating the need for patient repositioning and minimizing the dissection needed to get to the affected area. Resection of the 12th rib improves exposure to the retroperitoneal space significantly. If conversion is not emergent, conversion to a laparoscopic transabdominal adrenalectomy or an open lateral approach should be considered.
- Incisional hernia, pneumothorax, and wound infection occur in less than 1% of cases.
- Hyperesthesia and abdominal wall laxity occur in approximately 5% to 8% of cases but are usually temporary.

RESULTS

- Walz et al. reported in 2006 a prospective study of 560 laparoscopic retroperitoneal adrenalectomies on 520 patients, demonstrating a 2% conversion rate, a median operating time of 55 minutes that decreased throughout the study, and a median intraoperative blood loss of 10 mL.
- More recently, Dickson et al. reported a prospective series of 118 laparoscopic retroperitoneal adrenalectomies on 109 patients. A conversion rate of 6.6% was reported, mainly due to a failure to maintain an adequate working space with CO_2 insufflation, not due to uncontrolled bleeding.

SUGGESTED READINGS

1. Dickson PV, Jimenez C, Chisholm GB, et al. Posterior retroperitoneoscopic adrenalectomy: a contemporary American experience. *J Am Coll Surg*. 2011;212:659–667.
2. Perrier ND, Kennamer DL, Bao R, et al. Posterior retroperitoneoscopic adrenalectomy: preferred technique for removal of benign tumors and isolated metastasis. *Ann Surg*. 2008;248:666–674.
3. Silberfein E, Perrier ND. Management of pheochromocytomas. In: Cameron JL, ed. *Current Surgical Therapy*. 10th ed. Philadelphia, PA: Elsevier; 2011:579–584.
4. Walz MK, Alesina PF, Wenger FA, et al. Posterior retroperitoneoscopic adrenalectomy—results of 560 procedures in 520 patients. *Surgery*. 2006;140:943–950.
5. Walz MK, Alesina PF, Wenger FA, et al. Laparoscopic and retroperitoneoscopic treatment of pheochromocytomas and retroperitoneal paragangliomas: results of 161 tumors in 126 patients. *World J Surg*. 2006;30(5):847–853.
6. Walz MK, Gwosdz R, Levin SL, et al. Retroperitoneoscopic adrenalectomy in Conn's syndrome caused by adrenal adenomas or nodular hyperplasia. *World J Surg*. 2008;32(5):847–853.

7. Giebler RM, Walz MK, Peitgen K, et al. Hemodynamic changes after retroperitoneal CO2 insufflation for posterior retroperitoneoscopic adrenalectomy. *Anesth Analg*. 1996;82(4):827–831.

Disclaimer: The views expressed in this presentation are those of the author and do not necessarily reflect the official policy or position of the Department of the Navy, Department of Defense, or the United States government.

Chapter 50 Laparoscopic Adrenalectomy—Lateral Approach

Geoffrey B. Thompson Anna Kundel

DEFINITION

- Lateral laparoscopic adrenalectomy is defined as a minimally invasive procedure to remove all or part of an adrenal gland via a lateral transperitoneal approach with the patient in a nearly full decubitus position.

ANATOMY

- The adrenal glands lie partially anterior, medial, and superior to the upper pole of the kidneys. The caudal limb of the left adrenal gland often lies in close proximity to the left renal hilum.
- The left adrenal vein frequently joins with the medially located inferior phrenic vein to form a common channel entering the left renal vein. This anatomic configuration, resulting in hormonal dilution within the common channel, is very important in understanding and interpreting the results of adrenal venous sampling (**FIG 1**).
- The right adrenal vein is short, often wide, and empties directly into the posterolateral aspect of the inferior vena cava. On occasion, additional right adrenal veins may drain directly into the inferior vena cava or the right hepatic vein. Arterial inflow to the adrenals is less predictable but generally arises as small arteries originating from the renal artery (inferior adrenal artery), the aorta (middle adrenal artery), and the inferior phrenic artery (superior adrenal artery).
- Paired small veins may accompany these arteries. It is these anatomic findings that allow for cortical-sparing adrenalectomy in familial pheochromocytoma syndromes, such as von Hippel-Lindau (vHL), neurofibromatosis type 1 (NF1), and multiple endocrine neoplasia type 2 (MEN-2) (**FIG 2**).
- Rarely, small rests of adrenocortical tissue may be found at sites near the adrenal bed or within the gonads. This has particular importance when treating corticotropin-dependent hyperadrenocorticism.

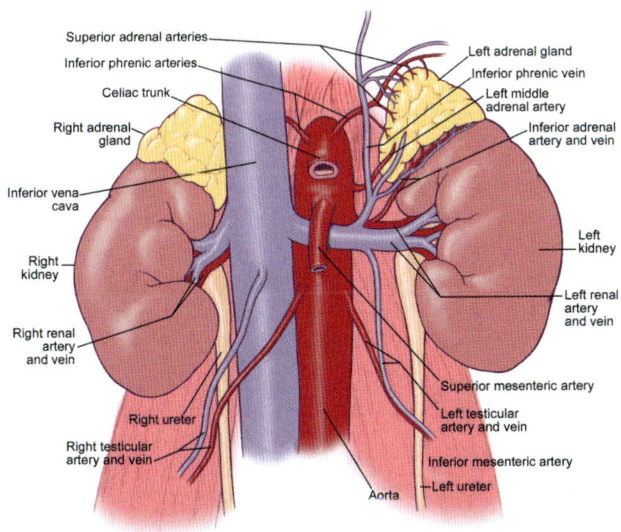

FIG 1 • Vascular anatomy of the adrenal glands.

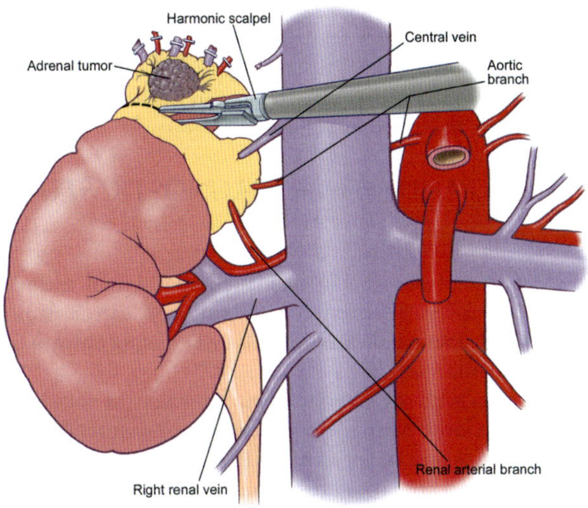

FIG 2 • Cortical-sparing adrenalectomy.

PATHOGENESIS

- Pheochromocytomas, aldosteronomas, and cortisol-secreting tumors produce catecholamines and hormones in an uncontrolled fashion, resulting in potentially life-threatening hormonal sequelae. Some of these tumors are seen in familial cases (MEN, vHL, NF1); most occur sporadically.

NATURAL HISTORY

- Untreated functional tumors can lead to death and disability. Undiagnosed adrenocortical carcinomas are most often fatal.

PATIENT HISTORY AND PHYSICAL FINDINGS

- Laparoscopic adrenalectomy is used for small functional and nonfunctional adrenal tumors, the latter being removed because of suspicion of underlying malignancy (either primary or metastatic).
- Adrenal incidentalomas are incidentally discovered (asymptomatic) adrenal masses, typically picked up on cross-sectional imaging studies performed for some other reason. For example, a patient comes to the emergency room with renal colic and a computed tomography (CT) with stone protocol is performed, revealing a ureteral calculus and an incidentally discovered 4-cm right adrenal mass.
- Indications for removal an adrenal incidentaloma include (1) a functional lesion because of the risk associated with excess hormonal sequelae; (2) a growing lesion or a lesion greater than 4 cm in diameter because of the risk of adrenocortical malignancy; or (3) an abnormal radiographic phenotype, which can be an indicator of an underlying malignancy.

Table 1: Absolute Contraindications to the Laparoscopic Approach

Obvious, large adrenocortical carcinomas
Pheochromocytomas >8 cm or clearly malignant pheochromocytomas associated with direct invasion, nodal metastases, or distant metastases
Extensive upper abdominal surgery in which the surgeon should consider a posterior endoscopic approach (see Chapter 49)

- Absolute contraindications to the lateral laparoscopic approach are described in Table 1.

IMAGING AND OTHER DIAGNOSTIC STUDIES

Diagnostic Studies

- Evaluation of an adrenal incidentaloma should include a 24-hour urine collection for fractionated catecholamines and total metanephrines or plasma metanephrines and normetanephrines.
- In patients who are hypertensive, regardless of their serum potassium level, plasma aldosterone concentration (PAC) divided by plasma renin activity (PRA) should be calculated to screen for primary aldosteronism. In the case of a high PAC:PRA ratio, confirmation of primary aldosteronism is obtained by salt loading and demonstration of a failure to suppress urinary aldosterone in a 24-hour sample. Autonomous cortisol secretion should be ruled out with an overnight 1 mg or 8 mg dexamethasone suppression test. The demonstration of autonomous cortisol secretion is confirmed by a two-day low-dose dexamethasone suppression test.
- Other studies available include a 24-hour urinary free cortisol level or demonstration of loss of diurnal variation between a.m. and p.m. plasma cortisol levels.
- Midnight salivary cortisol levels are also being used with increasing frequency for case detection of cortisol hypersecretion.
- Studies for estrogen and androgen excess are obtained when clinically indicated but are not routinely done.

Imaging

- Imaging of pheochromocytomas (**FIG 3**), aldosteronomas, cortisol-secreting tumors, and adrenocortical carcinomas is best performed with CT or magnetic resonance imaging (MRI). Tumors that are round, homogeneous, and low in Hounsfield units on CT scan with rapid washout of intravenous contrast are thought to represent lipid-rich cortical adenomas (**FIG 4**).

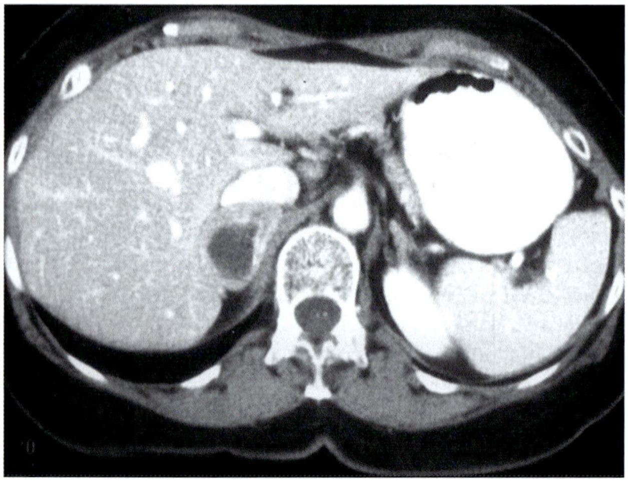

FIG 3 • CT scan of pheochromocytoma.

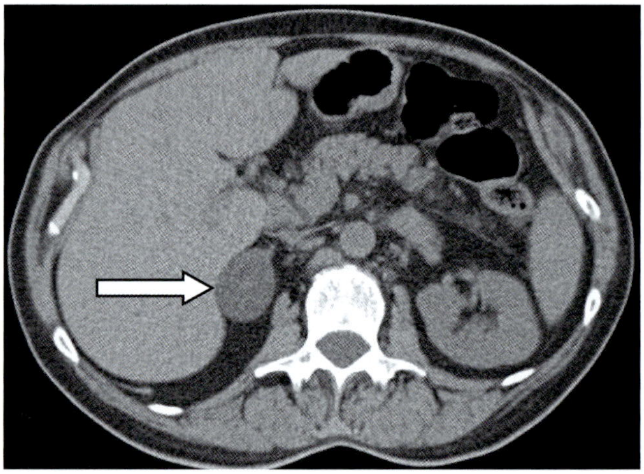

FIG 4 • CT scan of benign cortical adenoma.

- Malignancies tend to be large and heterogeneous, with areas of hemorrhage or necrosis associated with high Hounsfield units on CT and delayed washout of intravenous contrast (**FIG 5**). These lesions appear bright on T2 weighted MRI images.
- Approximately 25% of lesions 6 cm and greater are likely to be malignant, whereas 6% of lesions between 4 and 6 cm turn out to be primary malignancies. It is for this reason that the 4-cm cutoff is used. This avoids taking out an excessive amount of nonfunctional cortical adenomas while missing very few adrenocortical carcinomas.
- CT imaging is also valuable in picking up small aldosteronomas, but because of the high incidence of nonfunctional incidentalomas in patients older than 50 years of age, adrenal venous sampling has become the localizing procedure of choice for determining lateralization of an aldosterone-producing adenoma or hyperplasia.
- Metaiodobenzylguanidine (MIBG) scanning is useful for detecting occult pheochromocytomas, paragangliomas, metastatic disease, and multiple tumors in familial cases.

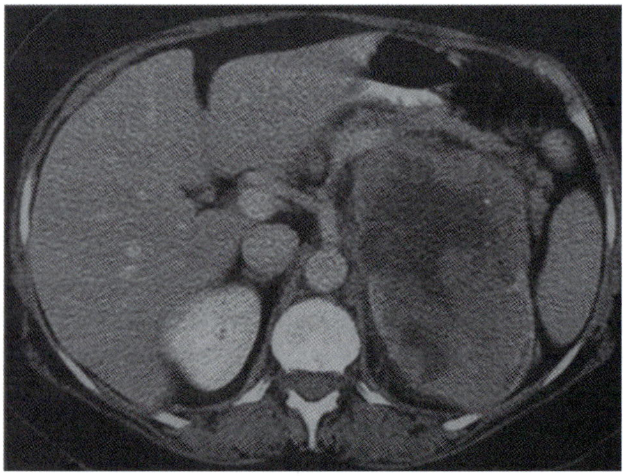

FIG 5 • CT scan of left adrenocortical carcinoma.

NONOPERATIVE MANAGEMENT

- Pheochromocytomas can be managed, albeit less effectively, with medical blockade (α-blockers). Aldosteronomas can be treated with mineralocorticoid receptor blockers, but this is not an ideal choice for younger patients.

SURGICAL MANAGEMENT

Preoperative Considerations

- Laparoscopic adrenalectomy via a lateral approach is indicated in the following circumstances:
  - All benign, functional adrenal masses less than 6 cm in maximal diameter (aldosteronomas, cortisol-secreting tumors) and pheochromocytomas less than 8 cm in diameter
  - All nonfunctional adrenocortical tumors greater than 4 cm but less than 6 cm in diameter
  - All nonfunctional tumors less than 4 cm in diameter demonstrating interval growth by cross-sectional imaging (CT or MRI)
  - All tumors regardless of size with a worrisome radiographic phenotype (high Hounsfield units on noncontrast CT, poor washout of intravenous contrast on CT, bright image on T2 weighted MRI)

Preoperative Preparation

- For pheochromocytomas, pharmacologic blockade (α-blockade for 7 to 10 days, then β-blockade for 24 to 48 hours preoperatively for atrial tachyarrhythmias and calcium channel blockers) is instituted. Effective circulating volume is restored using salt loading and increased fluid intake over a period of 10 to 14 days. α-Methyl-para-tyrosine, Demser® (Valeant Pharmaceuticals International, Inc, Montreal, Quebec, Canada), can be added in refractory cases.
- When treating aldosteronomas, optimal blood pressure control must be achieved and hypokalemia should be corrected. Mineralocorticoid receptor blockade is often instituted.
- The patient with Cushing's syndrome undergoes perioperative steroid preparation as well as prophylaxis for deep venous thrombosis, stress ulcer, and opportunistic infection.

Table 2: Equipment Typically Recommended to Perform a Lateral Laparoscopic Adrenalectomy

Four 10-mm trocars
An OptiView port
10-mm scopes, both straight and 30 degrees (occasionally 45-degree scopes are necessary)
Insufflator, light source, and camera
Two monitors: InsideView (LSI Solutions, Victor, NY)
5-mm Harmonic scalpel
L cautery tip
10-mm clip applier
Suction/irrigation apparatus

Surgical Equipment

- The equipment typically used to perform a lateral laparoscopic adrenalectomy in my practice is shown in Table 2.

Preoperative Steps

- In addition to one or two large-bore peripheral intravenous lines, a radial artery line should also be placed preoperatively. A central line should be used in the elderly, the infirmed, and select pheochromocytoma patients.
- General endotracheal anesthesia is used. Antibiotics and deep venous prophylaxis are administered.
- Nitroprusside, labetalol, nicardipine, and intravenous pressors should be readily available for pheochromocytoma patients.
- An orogastric tube is placed.

Positioning and Port Placement

- The patient is placed in (near-complete) lateral decubitus position with the side of the tumor facing.
- Three to four ports are placed on the left; the fourth port is used for a fan retractor in obese patients and the most medial port is used for a liver retractor for right-sided tumors. The ports should be spread out between the midaxillary line and the midabdomen, approximately two to three fingerbreadths below the costal margin.
- The OptiView® (Ethicon Endo-Surgery, Cincinnati, OH) system and a straight scope are used for introduction of the first trocar, typically along the anterior axillary line.
- Patient pressure is maintained between 14 and 18 mmHg.

LEFT ADRENALECTOMY

- The splenic flexure is mobilized using the L cautery with caudal displacement of the large bowel (FIG 6).
- The lateral splenic attachments are divided with medial rotation of the spleen and body and tail of the pancreas, exposing Gerota's fascia and the adrenal gland.
- The surgeon opens the avascular plane between the posterior aspect of the pancreas and the adrenal gland, much like opening a book. The adrenal vein often can be found directly across the "valley" from the splenic vein.
- The adrenal vein, inferior phrenic vein, and common channel are exposed.

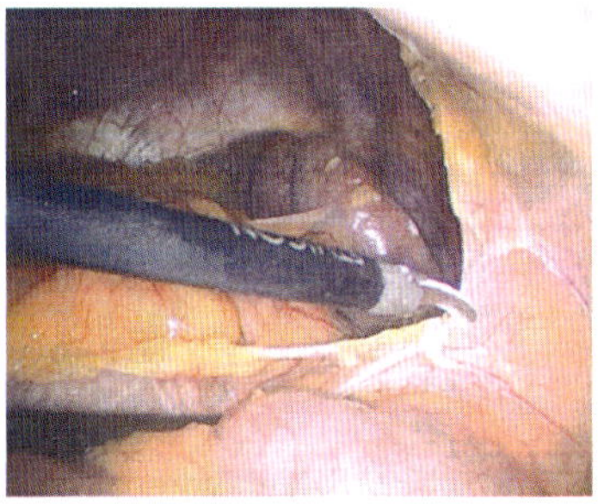

FIG 6 • Mobilization of splenic flexure.

- No attempts should be made to dissect out the renal artery and vein.
- The surgeon doubly clips the veins and divides them (**FIG 7**).
- The caudal tip of the adrenal gland is elevated away from the area of the renal hilum; very often, renal artery pulsation is visible.
- The surgeon dissects up along the medial aspect of the gland using the Harmonic scalpel. If the inferior phrenic vein does not fall away from the dissection, it may require further division between clips at this level.
- Arterial tributaries from the aorta can be divided using the Harmonic scalpel as can the inferior phrenic artery tributaries, as dissection is carried around the superior aspect of the gland (**FIG 8**).
- The plane between the adrenal gland and the kidney is dissected using the Harmonic scalpel. This can be performed just outside the edge of the adrenal gland or, when thin, just inside Gerota's fascia.
- The gland is then elevated anteriorly and a small arterial branch from the renal artery, often present, is divided with the Harmonic scalpel.
- Any remaining areolar attachments are divided and the gland is removed using a commercially available retrieval device (**FIG 9**).
- The adrenal bed is irrigated and aspirated completely, and hemostasis is ensured. A sheet of a topical hemostatic agent can be left within the adrenal bed for added hemostasis.

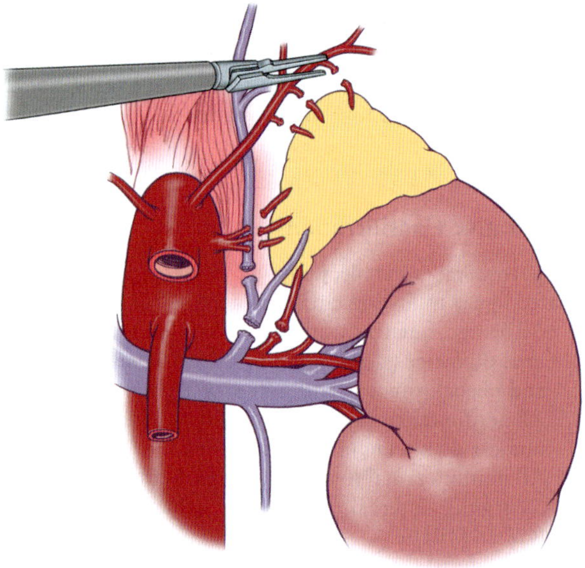

FIG 8 ● Division of arterial tributaries.

- If bladeless ports are used and dilation was not necessary for specimen retrieval, no deep fascial sutures are placed.
- Dilated port sites undergo fascial closure with interrupted suture, using a fascial closure device.
- Skin incisions are closed in a subcuticular fashion with an absorbable suture and are covered with Steri-Strips.
- Sterile dressings are applied.

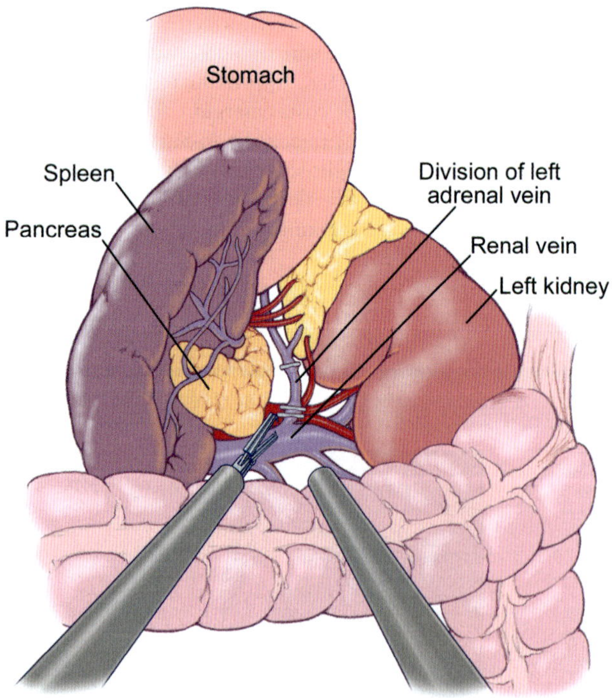

FIG 7 ● Division of left adrenal vein.

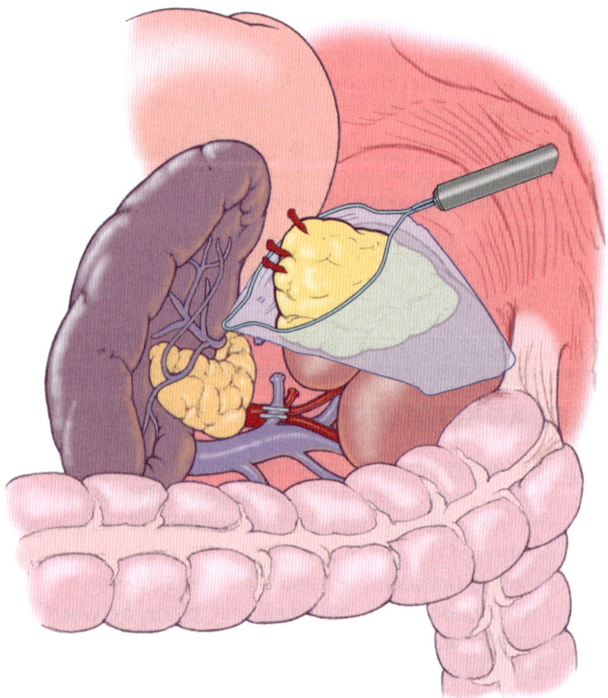

FIG 9 ● Retrieval of resected adrenal gland.

RIGHT ADRENALECTOMY

- Attachments to the right lobe of the liver are divided using the Harmonic scalpel so as to allow the liver to be fully retraced medially. This brings the adrenal gland and inferior vena cava into view (**FIG 10**).
- The peritoneum overlying the lateral border of the inferior vena cava is incised using the L cautery on a low setting.
- If possible, the right renal vein is exposed to define the lower limit of the dissection.
- A blunt-ended instrument is used to gently retract the adrenal gland away from the inferior vena cava (**FIG 11**).
- Using the L cautery or Harmonic scalpel, the areolar tissue posterior and lateral to the inferior vena cava is divided. This may contain arterial tributaries directly from the aorta.
- The dissection is carefully carried out along the lateral border of the inferior vena cava up to the level of the adrenal vein (**FIG 12**).
- If the adrenal vein is easily exposed at this stage, it can be doubly clipped and divided; otherwise, it can be done later when visualization is optimal (**FIGS 13, 14**).
- In a larger pheochromocytoma, the adrenal vein really should be divided after the gland has been mobilized to avoid venous congestion and bleeding.
- The superior pole, including its inferior phrenic artery branches, is mobilized using the Harmonic scalpel to free the gland from the diaphragm posteriorly. Care must be taken to control additional veins at the junction of the medial and superior portions of the gland.
- Using the distal right renal vein as a landmark, the caudal aspect of the gland is exposed, dissected, and elevated, often revealing a renal artery branch to the adrenal, which is divided using the Harmonic scalpel.
- Final step in the dissection is freeing the lateral aspect of the gland from the kidney using cautery or Harmonic scalpel.

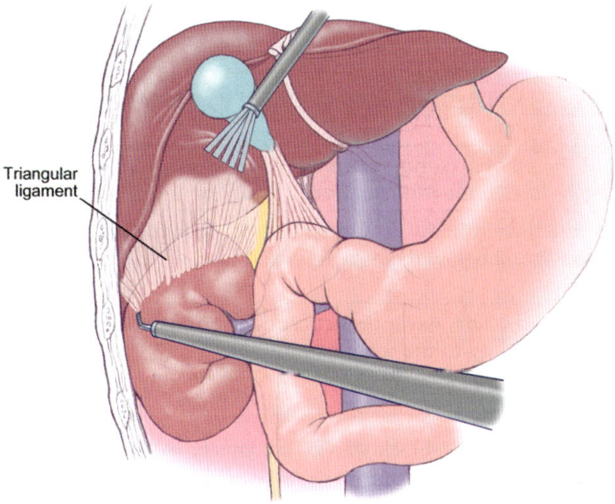

FIG 10 ● Liver retractor placement and division of triangular ligament.

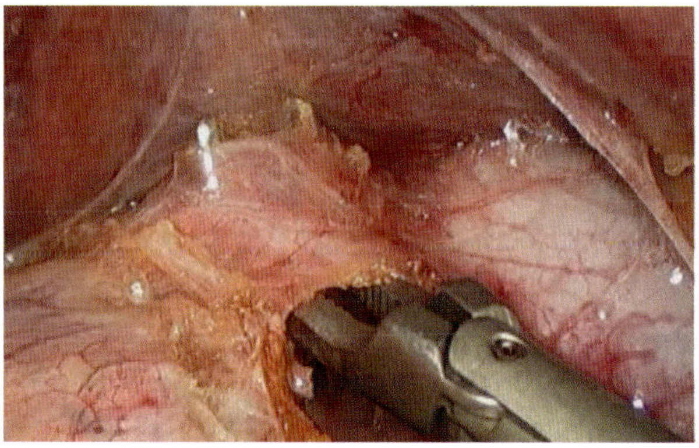

FIG 12 ● The right adrenal vein is encircled.

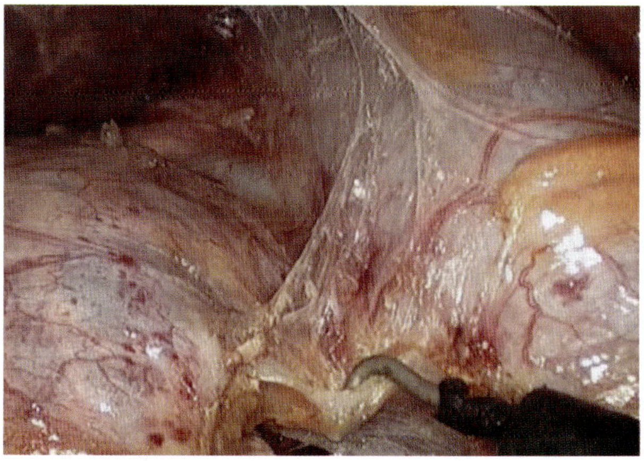

FIG 11 ● A right-sided pheochromocytoma is separated from the inferior vena cava.

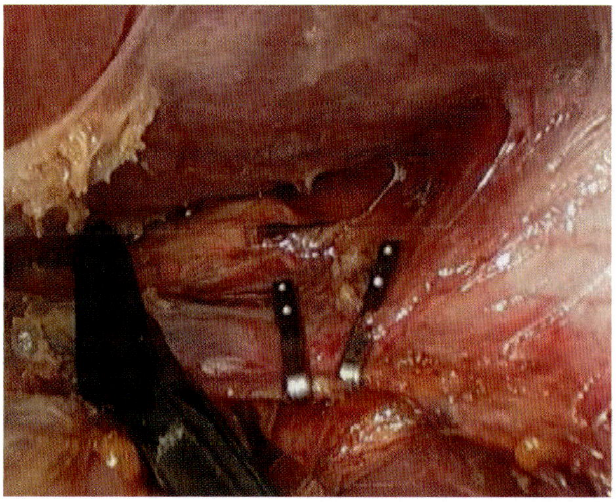

FIG 13 ● The right adrenal vein is doubly clipped and divided.

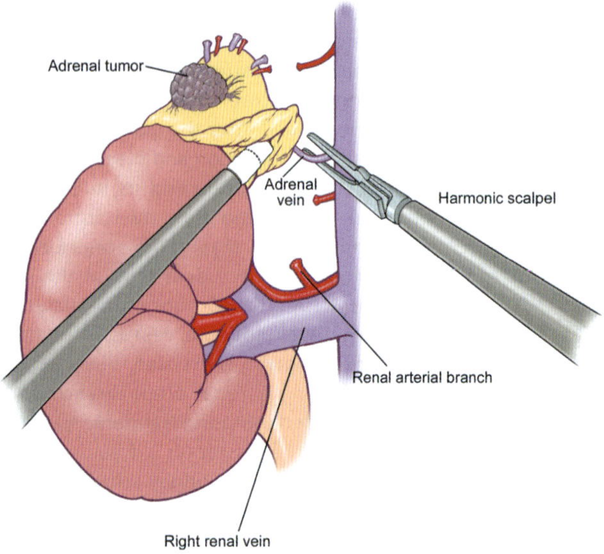

FIG 14 ● Division of right adrenal vein.

PEARLS AND PITFALLS

Adrenal vein	■ The adrenal vein does not have to be ligated as a first step in adrenalectomy; do it when it is safe and easy, even in patients with pheochromocytoma.
Accessory renal arteries	■ When dissecting on the posterior aspect of the adrenal gland, watch out for accessory renal arteries. If a large vessel is present, follow its course before considering ligation.
Low pressure bleeding	■ If bleeding occurs, remember that most of the time, it is low pressure bleeding. Pack the area with a sheetlike hemostatic agent. Work above and below the area, in which case, oftentimes, the bleeding site will become clear and manageable.
Renal hilum	■ Once the adrenal vein has been divided on the left side, never dissect caudally or posterior to the plane of the adrenal vein stump. This will avoid injury to the renal hilum.

POSTOPERATIVE CARE

Pheochromocytoma

- Pheochromocytoma (**FIG 15**) patients will often be mildly hypotensive, with systolic blood pressures in the 90s for 8 to 12 hours postoperatively. Greater or more prolonged falls in blood pressure accompanied by oliguria or tachycardia should prompt investigation for bleeding.
- All blood pressure medications should be stopped after the morning preoperative doses have been administered; the exception being β-blockers used long-term for ischemic heart disease. Rarely, pressors may be required, although volume replacement may be all that is necessary for a short period of time.
- Plasma metanephrines and normetanephrines are drawn prior to dismissal.

Primary Aldosteronism

- Patients with primary aldosteronism (**FIG 16**) may require decreasing antihypertensive agents for weeks and will need careful monitoring.

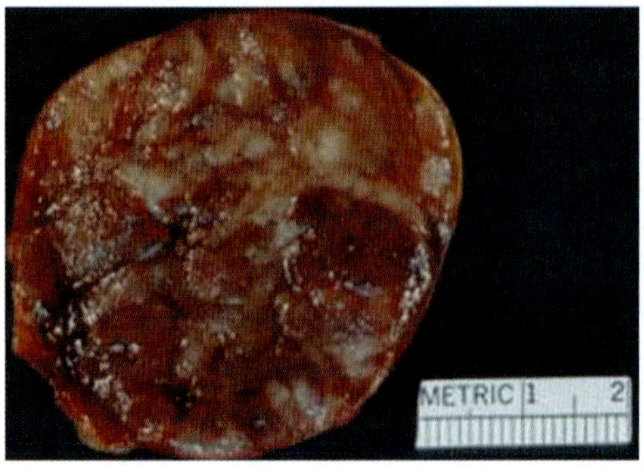

FIG 15 ● Pheochromocytoma.

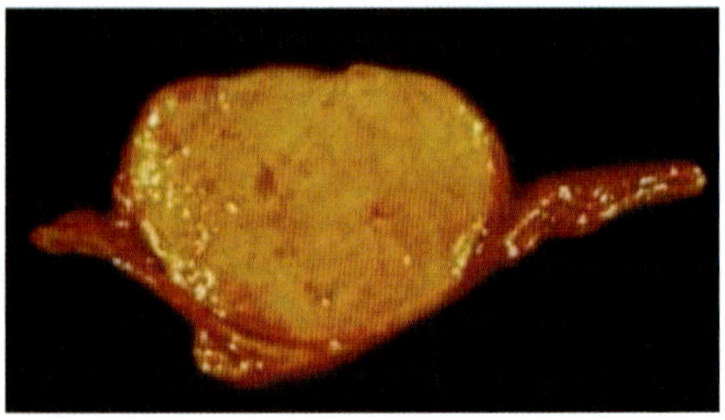

FIG 16 ● Aldosteronoma.

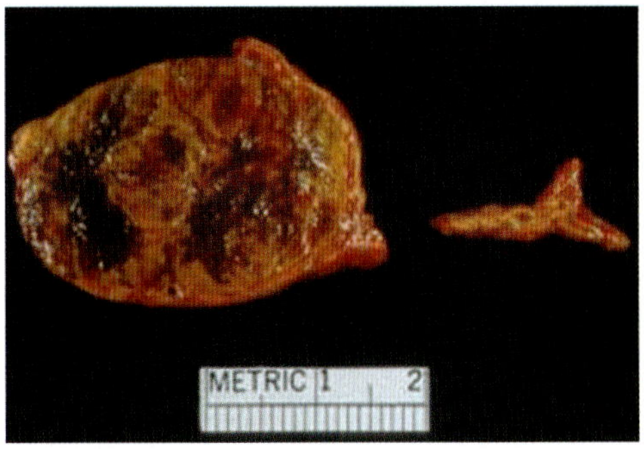

FIG 17 • Cortical-secreting tumor.

- Potassium supplements should be withheld and only given on an as-needed basis because severe hyperkalemia may otherwise ensue with ongoing supplementation.
- PAC is collected prior to dismissal, and serum potassium levels are checked weekly for the first month.

Cushing's Syndrome

- Patients with Cushing's syndrome (**FIG 17**) are released on a tapering steroid dose to be monitored and adjusted by their endocrinologist.
- Resumption of oral intake is rapid.
- Dismissal usually occurs within 24 to 48 hours after surgery.
- Hemoglobin, electrolytes, and creatinine are checked the day after surgery, along with a serum amylase in left adrenal gland patients to rule out pancreatic injury.
- Patients undergoing bilateral adrenalectomy for adrenocorticotropic hormone (ACTH)–dependent Cushing's syndrome require lifelong replacement of glucocorticoids and mineralocorticoids, with increased doses during times of stress (illness, trauma, surgery).

OUTCOMES

- Outcomes for laparoscopic adrenalectomy are no different than open procedures with regard to cure rates. Morbidity is certainly less (pain, return to work, paresthesias, hypesthesias, and bulging flank muscles).

COMPLICATIONS

- Bleeding
- Spleen, pancreatic, renal, colon, and gastric injury (rare)
- Diaphragmatic injury (pneumothorax)

SUGGESTED READINGS

1. Taskin HE, Siperstein A, Mercan S, et al. Laparoscopic posterior retroperitoneal adrenalectomy. *J Surg Oncol*. 2012;106(5):619–621.
2. Porpiglia F. Miller BS, Manfredi M, et al. A debate on laparoscopic versus open adrenalectomy for adrenocortical carcinoma. *Horm Cancer*. 2011;2:372–377.
3. Carnaille B. Adrenocortical carcinoma: which surgical approach? *Langenbeck Arch Surg*. 2012;397:195–199.
4. Nehs MA, Ruan DT. Minimally invasive adrenal surgery: an update. *Curr Opin Endocrinol Diabetes Obes*. 2011;18:193–197.
5. Brunt ML. Laparoscopic adrenalectomy. In: Eubanks WS, Swanstrom LL, Soper NJ, eds. *Mastery of Endoscopic and Laparoscopic Surgery*. Philadelphia, PA: Lippincott Williams & Wilkins; 2000:320–329.
6. Gagner M, Lacroix A, Bolte E. Laparoscopic adrenalectomy in Cushing's syndrome and pheochromocytoma. *N Engl J Med*. 1992; 327:1033.
7. Thompson GB, Grant CS, van Heerden JA, et al. Laparoscopic versus open posterior adrenalectomy: a case-control study of 100 patients. *Surgery*. 1997;122:1132–1136.

Chapter 51 Insulinomas

Douglas L. Fraker

DEFINITION

- Insulinomas are neoplasms arising from the beta cells of the pancreas. The vast majority are benign, sporadic, and unifocal.[1,2] These neoplasms release insulin in a dysregulated manner and therefore cause decreased blood sugar, resulting in neuroglycopenic symptoms. Surgical excision uniformly provides long-term cure for the majority of benign insulinomas and corrects all of the associated symptoms.

ANATOMY

- The beta cells of the pancreas are distributed amongst the pancreatic islets uniformly throughout the pancreas. For this reason, insulinomas can occur in all areas of the pancreas. Virtually all large series of insulinomas demonstrate that there is a uniform distribution related to the volume of pancreatic tissue.[3–5] Half of insulinomas occur in the pancreatic head, neck, and uncinate process and the other half are distributed across the body and tail of the pancreas. Most series report insulinomas only occurring within the parenchyma of the pancreas. They can be exophytic and extend off the surface and these exophytic lesions may not be appreciated by standard cross-sectional imaging. There are reports of less than 2% of insulinomas being located outside of the pancreas parenchyma.[1] Virtually all of these lesions are found in the wall of the duodenum and presumably, they occur within embryologic pancreatic rest tissue that is physically separate from the pancreatic parenchyma, such that the insulinoma occurs within the duodenal wall with a similar appearance to duodenal gastrinomas.
- In most surgical series, insulinomas are small, measuring under 2 cm in cross-sectional diameter. Because symptomatology is caused by release of hormone and not by direct effects of tumor mass, lesions as small as 5 to 6 mm may present with significant clinical symptoms. In most series, 90% to 97% of insulinomas are benign. The average size of malignant insulinomas is over 6 cm and the majority of those present with concurrent regional lymph node or hepatic metastases.[1,2]

NATURAL HISTORY

- Insulinomas cause virtually all of their symptoms due to excess circulation of insulin and the subsequent hypoglycemic effects. The first clinical case of insulinoma was described in 1927 when a patient who had severe hypoglycemic episodes had an abdominal operation with a large tumor of the pancreas and lymph node and liver metastases.[2] Extracts of this tumor actually were injected into animals and caused hypoglycemia. Allen Whipple described the triad carrying his name that is known to define the symptoms of insulinoma in 1938. *Whipple's triad* consists of hypoglycemia, documentation of hypoglycemia during periods of fasting, and relief of symptoms with administration of glucose. On analysis, this constellation of signs and symptoms is not truly a distinct triad but rather makes a single point of symptoms related to low blood sugar.[6]
- The majority of symptoms experienced by patients relate to lack of blood glucose to the central nervous system. These are called *neuroglycopenic symptoms* and can range from mild confusion to coma. Patients may experience visual disturbances and there are numerous reports in the literature of insulinoma being misdiagnosed as an epileptic seizure. A second set of symptoms relate to the sympathetic nervous system release of adrenaline due to the effects of the hypoglycemia. This catecholamine release leads to palpitations, diaphoresis, and tremors. In most series, the onset of symptoms initially noted by the patient may be years before the specific time of diagnosis of the insulinoma. The average interval from onset of symptoms to diagnosis is between 2 to 3 years but sometimes may exist for over 10 years. Patients adapt and know that when they experience their symptoms, intake of food, particularly carbohydrates, provide rapid relief; however, this practice of glucose intake may not be elicited when taking a clinical history. Although the majority of patients exhibit weight gain in the anabolic state of hyperinsulinemia, some patients maintain a normal weight.
- The vast majority of patients with insulinoma have sporadic tumors with no family history. A small proportion is associated with multiple endocrine neoplasia type 1 (MEN-1).[5] The most common functional neuroendocrine tumor in MEN-1 is gastrinoma; outnumbering insulinoma by three- or fourfold. Insulinoma is the second most common pancreatic tumor in this syndrome. Because patients with MEN-1 may have multifocal nonfunctional neuroendocrine tumors throughout the pancreas, it may be difficult to distinguish the lesion making insulin versus other tumors. Typically, the dominant neuroendocrine tumor is the insulinoma but occasionally, patients will have multiple large lesions. Intraoperative measurement of insulin from direct tumor aspiration has been reported as an adjunct to insulinoma identification in this unusual situation.

LABORATORY DIAGNOSIS

- The key to diagnosis of insulinoma is not with imaging but rather with biochemical testing. The cornerstone of diagnosing hypoglycemia is detecting glucose levels typically below 40 mg/dL. Additional blood tests that should be obtained are insulin levels, proinsulin levels, and C-peptide levels.[7] Virtually all patients will have a plasma insulin concentration greater than 5 μU/mL at the time of low blood glucose. The vast majority of patients have insulin levels greater than 10 μU/mL. The insulin to glucose ratio can define hypoglycemia due to insulinoma as opposed to other causes with high specificity and sensitivity.[8] The measurements of proinsulin levels and C peptide are helpful in eliminating the diagnosis of surreptitious insulin abuse. The majority of patients have a proinsulin to insulin ratio greater than 25% and a C-peptide concentration greater than 1.7 ng/mL.

- The gold standard for confirming the diagnosis of an insulinoma is a monitored 48-hour or 72-hour fast.[9,10] Patients are typically in the inpatient setting given intravenous normal saline without glucose or allowed to drink noncaloric compounds while monitored for clinical symptoms and sequential blood analysis. The vast majority of patients who truly have an insulinoma causing hypoglycemia become symptomatic within the first 24 hours of the fast and virtually 100% of patients will become symptomatic by 72 hours. As time progresses, patients' symptoms include decreased mental acuity, confusion, or other neuroglycopenic symptoms, which are documented by the nursing staff and physicians during the monitored fast. When symptoms reach a significant level, blood is drawn for glucose, insulin, and proinsulin before administering glucose to relieve the neurologic symptoms.

DIFFERENTIAL DIAGNOSIS

- The differential diagnosis of hypoglycemia includes surreptitious use of either insulin or oral hypoglycemic agents and noninsulinoma pancreatogenous hypoglycemia syndrome (NIPHS).[7,11] In general, blood tests for proinsulin, C peptide, as well as specific tests for sulfonylureas can eliminate the use of surreptitious agents. NIPHS is distinguished from insulinoma by the timing of hypoglycemia. These patients often do not become symptomatic during a 72-hour monitored fast but will become profoundly hypoglycemic after ingesting glucose orally.[7] Pathology often shows significant beta cell hypertrophy but does not show a mass on imaging.

IMAGING

- The vast majority of insulinomas are small and are located within the substance of the pancreatic parenchyma. The three choices of imaging that have been highly specific for identifying the insulinoma are contrast-enhanced computed tomography (CT) scan, magnetic resonance imaging (MRI) scan, or endoscopic ultrasound.[12,13] Insulinomas are hypervascular with very well-defined margins and have a classic appearance on enhanced CT and MRI scans (**FIGS 1** and **2**). They are oval-shaped, well-marginated, and show a characteristic vascular blush.[12] The limitations of imaging relate to the size of the lesions. Again, insulinomas may cause symptoms that mandate surgical resection for correction with sizes smaller than 5 to 6 mm. Small insulinomas are ones that would be potentially missed on cross-sectional imaging studies. Also, exophytic lesions which may not be surrounded by pancreatic parenchyma may be a challenge to identify on CT or MRI, particularly if they are small. Insulinomas located near the tip of the pancreatic tail are the most common location for false-negative imaging; insulinomas may be incorrectly identified as lymph nodes, accessory spleens, and splenic vessels.

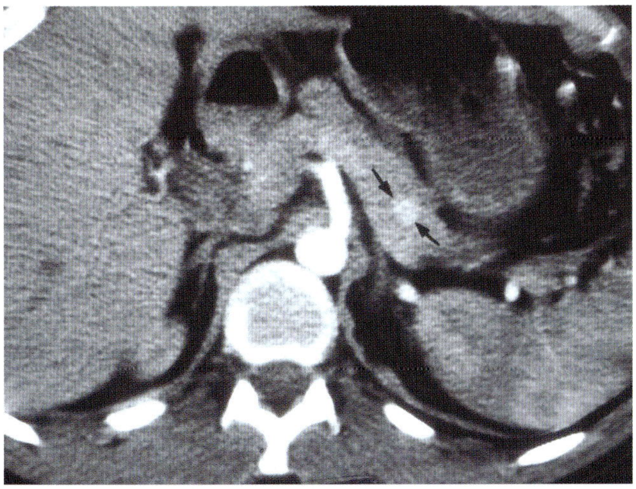

FIG 1 • Axial cut of MRI scan demonstrating an insulinoma in the body tail junction of the pancreas (marked by *arrows*). The insulinoma is small, oval shaped, and hypervascular compared to the surrounding pancreas.

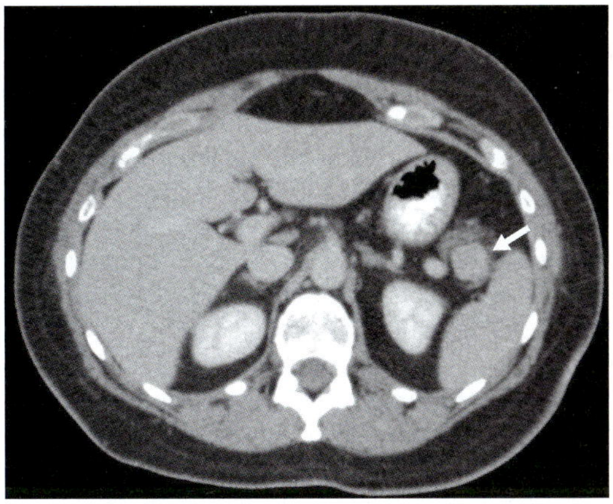

FIG 2 • Axial cut of a CT scan demonstrating a 2-cm insulinoma in the tail of the pancreas (marked by *arrow*). This scan, an MRI scan, and an endoscopic ultrasound all reported this lesion to be an accessory spleen as it was exophytic off the pancreas tail and had identical imaging characteristics as the spleen on all three imaging modalities.

- Since the early 1990s, a variety of institutions with large experience in insulinoma have used endoscopic ultrasound as the primary imaging technique.[12,13] Endoscopic ultrasound allows for direct imaging in three dimensions with very close field ultrasonography of the head, neck, and uncinate process. The pancreatic body is less well imaged as it can only be seen from the placement of the ultrasound probe within the stomach and depending on the patient's body habitus, the tail may be a blind zone for endoscopic ultrasound. The ultrasound appearance of insulinoma is an oval hypoechoic mass with well-defined margins (**FIG 3**). Endoscopic ultrasound also allows a relatively straightforward fine needle

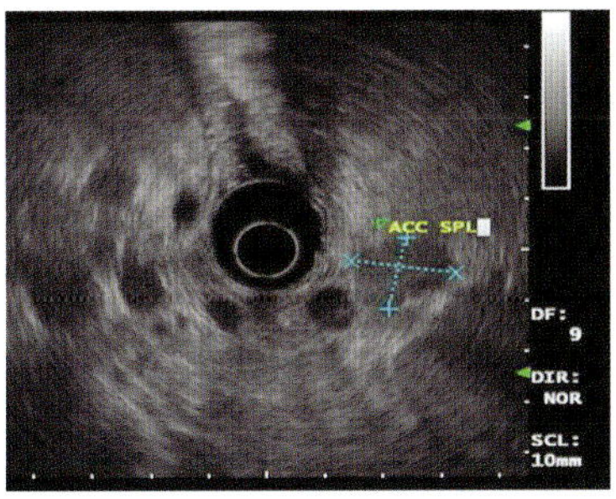

FIG 3 • Endoscopic ultrasound image of the same patient in **FIG 2**. The insulinoma is oval shaped and hypoechoic. The gastroenterologist has incorrectly labeled the insulinoma as accessory spleen.

aspiration biopsy, which would produce neuroendocrine cells on cytology to confirm the diagnosis. Positive imaging may occur with identification of peripancreatic lymph nodes that are often embedded on the surface of the pancreas or accessory spleen, which can be found on the surface or actually within the parenchyma of the pancreas primarily in the tail region. Standard fluorodeoxyglucose-positron emission tomography (FDG-PET) scans have been shown to be of limited value in insulinomas as these may not be particularly hypermetabolic lesions.[14] A recent report showed a specific targeting agent of indium-labeled glucagonlike peptide-1 receptor that was sensitive for insulinomas and also could allow the use of a handheld intraoperative probe to detect these lesions.[15] This technique is being developed in Switzerland and has not been widely adapted elsewhere.

- Despite the high sensitivity of cross-sectional imaging and endoscopic ultrasound, a portion of patients with well-documented biochemical insulinoma may have no lesions imaged.[16,17] Historically, an interventional radiology invasive procedure called portal venous sampling was used in which a transhepatic portal vein cannulation was performed and blood was drawn from various regions and tributaries from the portal vein and assayed for insulin.[18,19] Portal venous sampling has now been replaced by intraarterial calcium stimulation with hepatic vein sampling. In this technique, two catheters are placed: one in the right hepatic vein and a second standard arterial angiogram catheter advanced into arterial branches feeding the pancreas. Calcium is injected into branches of the splenic artery supplying the body or tail or branches of the superior pancreaticoduodenal artery off the gastroduodenal artery or the inferior pancreaticoduodenal artery off the superior mesenteric artery. Blood is drawn from the right hepatic vein at 0 second, 30 seconds, and 60 seconds after calcium infusion and an increased gradient of greater than twofold in the hepatic vein insulin levels is significant.[18] This procedure does not image insulinoma but rather identifies the region of production of insulin. It is a highly specific test and may be helpful in focusing efforts in the operating room to one area or the other. It may justify performance of a blind distal pancreatectomy for patients without imaged lesions that have gradient in the body and tail, but a blind pancreaticoduodenectomy is virtually never indicated.

NONOPERATIVE MANAGEMENT

- The choices for nonoperative management include diet modification or hypoglycemic agents. One approach for management of hypoglycemic symptoms is small frequent meals, particularly of slowly absorbed carbohydrates to provide more of a steady level particularly while patients are sleeping.[2,5] Diazoxide is a benzothiazide analog with antihypertensive effects but also with potent hyperglycemic effects. It inhibits insulin release from the beta cells and enhances glycogenolysis to also contribute to elevation of blood sugar. Side effects include sodium retention causing edema and some patients have nausea. A second agent that has been used for control of hypoglycemic symptoms in insulinoma is somatostatin analogs. However, due to relatively low expression of somatostatin receptors on most well-differentiated insulinomas, these have not been markedly effective.

PREOPERATIVE PLANNING

- The cornerstone to performing an insulinoma resection is being absolutely certain the patient has the disease proven by definitive biochemical workup. In patients who have imaged lesions, particularly if they are biopsied as neuroendocrine tumors or have classic appearance on CT or MRI, this provides very good evidence that the patient has the disease. In patients who have no definitive imaging of the site of the lesion, the surgeon has to review in detail the preoperative blood chemistries. This analysis includes reviewing the data related to a 72-hour fast, looking at concurrent glucose, insulin, and proinsulin levels as described earlier.
- It is very important for patients to either be the first case of the day or to be admitted to the hospital and have dextrose solution running so that they do not suffer from severe hypoglycemia while they are nil per os (NPO) prior to general anesthesia. In general, for abdominal procedures, anesthesiologists do not administer glucose-containing fluids as they are infused at a relatively rapid rate and patients are catabolic. When operating on patients with insulinoma, it is very important to communicate to the anesthesia team that dextrose needs to be administered often and frequent analysis of glucose levels need to be performed.

SURGICAL APPROACH AND PATIENT POSITIONING

- Over the past few decades, the majority of patients in most surgical series have been treated with an open surgical technique. There have been many recent reports of laparoscopic excision of insulinomas, particularly in the body and tail, with high success rate. We will describe primarily identification and resection of insulinomas using an open technique and also provide information on laparoscopic approaches.
- The approach for the open resection of an insulinoma is performed with the patient lying supine with either an upper midline incision or a bilateral subcostal incision. The vast majority of the substance of the pancreas can be assessed with an upper midline incision with the exception of the far distal tail, which may be somewhat difficult particularly in obese patients. For patients with a well-localized insulinoma in the head and neck, uncinate process, or proximal body, a midline incision is preferred if the patient's body habitus is appropriate. Any patient can be approached with a bilateral subcostal incision.

EXPOSURE OF THE PANCREAS

- The initial steps of an insulinoma resection is to briefly assess the liver, although insulinoma is a benign disease in the vast majority of patients, and if liver metastases existed, they should have been identified on preoperative imaging. The next step is exposure of the pancreas parenchyma. Exposure of the head and neck of the pancreas as well as uncinate process can be achieved with a Kocher maneuver (**FIG 4**). The duodenum and head of the pancreas are brought up from the retroperitoneal location to allow bimanual palpation for mass lesions as well as visual inspection of both the anterior and posterior surfaces of the pancreatic head. The greater omentum is taken off the transverse colon along its entire length using energy devices with the omentum reflected superiorly, pulling the stomach off the pancreas. There are avascular attachments of the posterior stomach to the anterior pancreas that can be divided sharply. There is always a bridge of vascular tissue from the right gastroepiploic to the middle colic vessels, which crosses anterior to the neck and proximal pancreatic body that needs to be controlled with either energy devices or suture ligation. By dissection along the inferior border of the pancreatic body and tail, the posterior surface can be exposed and the majority of the substance of the pancreatic body and tail can be palpated between two digits (**FIG 5**). By doing these maneuvers, 95% of the pancreatic parenchyma is accessible for palpation and virtually all of the anterior surface and most of the posterior surface of the body and proximal tail are accessible for visual inspection as well. The only inaccessible area is the very tip of the tail of the pancreas, which may be located completely behind the spleen and require dividing the lateral margins of the splenic ligaments to reflect the spleen medially and expose that area of the very tip of the pancreatic tail.
- Insulinomas are identified by a combination of visual inspection, palpation, and intraoperative ultrasound. Insulinomas are uniformly red-brown in color against the yellow-gray background of the pancreas and lesions near the surface or exophytic lesions can be easily identified by visual inspection (**FIG 6**). Neuroendocrine tumors have

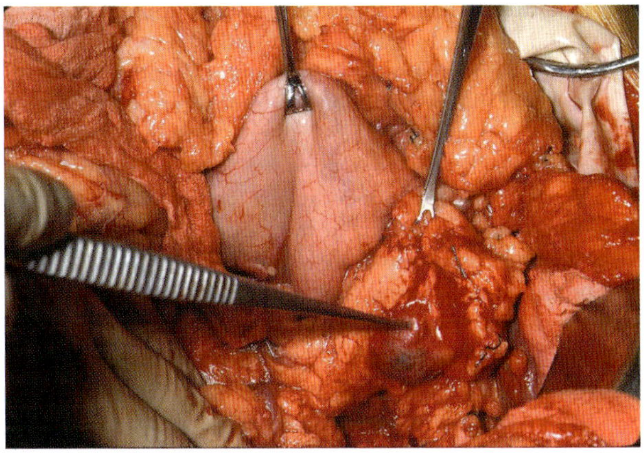

FIG 5 • The lesser sac is exposed by reflecting the stomach and omentum superiorly and the transverse colon inferiorly. By dividing the retroperitoneum at the inferior edge of the pancreatic body and tail, the posterior surface of the pancreas is visualized as well. A large posterior body insulinoma is seen pointed at by the forceps.

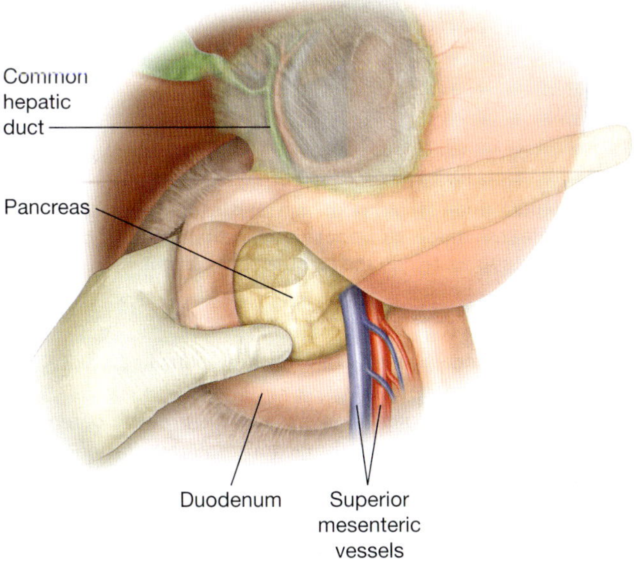

FIG 4 • The lateral retroperitoneal attachments of the duodenum are divided along the entire length of the duodenum from the pylorus to the superior mesenteric vessel. By doing the Kocher maneuver, the entire head and uncinate process can be palpated between two fingers. By clearing the surface, all of the anterior head and uncinate process and most of the posterior surface can be visually inspected.

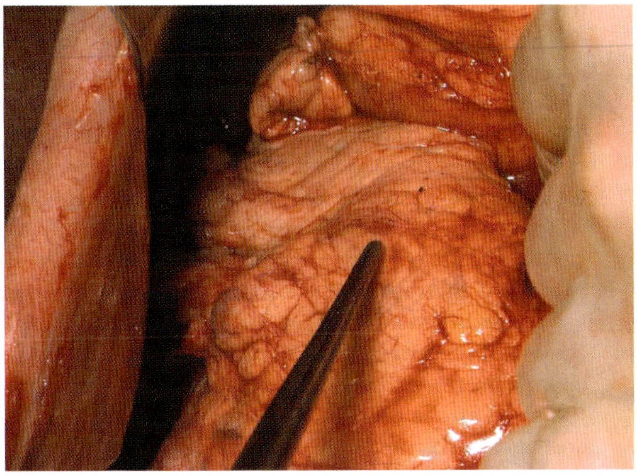

FIG 6 • The anterior surface of the body and tail of the pancreas is skeletonized and exposed by retracting the stomach superiorly (posterior stomach on the left side of the picture) and the transverse colon inferiorly (retracted by the hand on the right side of the picture). The forceps is pointing at a red-brown insulinoma near the surface of the body of the pancreas.

a classic ultrasound appearance and intraoperative ultrasound is a key to management (**FIG 7**). Even in patients with lesions of the head and uncinate process of the pancreas that are well seen by preoperative endoscopic ultrasound, it is mandatory to have intraoperative ultrasound available. The reason for having intraoperative ultrasound available is because if the small lesion is deep within the parenchyma of the pancreas, it is essential to know exactly where the insulinoma is located so an appropriate enucleation can be performed. It is impossible to use preoperative imaging alone to know where to cut into the pancreas in the same way breast surgeons need intraoperative localizing techniques to remove nonpalpable breast tumors.

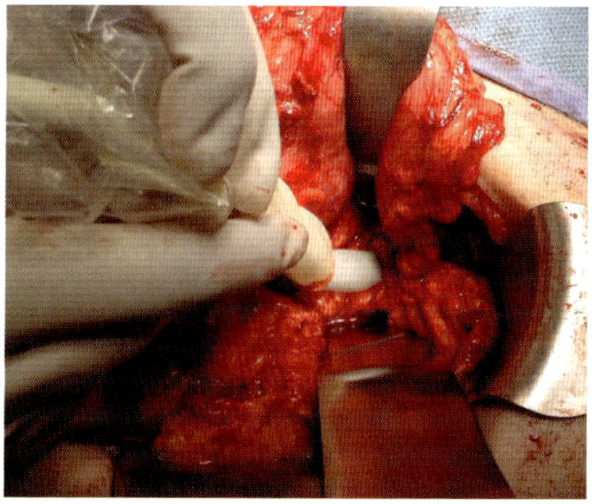

FIG 7 • The head, neck, body, tail, and uncinate process of the pancreas are exposed and the intraoperative ultrasound probe is placed directly on the pancreatic surface. Ultrasound not only identifies the insulinoma but can also demonstrate precise relationships to the pancreatic duct and main vessels.

EXCISION OF THE INSULINOMA

- After exposure and identification of the insulinoma, the choices for excision of the lesion are enucleation versus a segmental pancreatic resection. In most surgical series, the majority of insulinomas are removed by enucleation, with one-third or more removed by distal pancreatectomy with or without splenic preservation and a very small fraction removed with pancreaticoduodenectomy or a Whipple procedure. The ability to enucleate an insulinoma relates to how close the insulinoma is located to the pancreatic duct. For patients who have their lesion identified by preoperative imaging, the proximity of the insulinoma to the main pancreatic duct is known prior to surgery. The pancreatic duct generally runs along the length of the midline of the pancreas slightly superior and slightly toward the dorsal or deep side of the pancreas. The duct can virtually always be identified on intraoperative ultrasound as a tubular structure with no vascular flow within on color Doppler. Even in the case of insulinomas that are well localized on the pancreatic surface, routine use of intraoperative ultrasound is helpful, partly to look for additional lesions and mostly to identify the proximity of the insulinoma to the duct.
- For lesions that are on the surface or visible from the surface, enucleation is relatively straightforward (**FIG 8**). The reddish brown color of the insulinoma is easily differentiated from the glandular tissue of the pancreas. The plane on the capsule of the insulinoma is quite distinct and easily separated from the parenchyma with gentle traction. The attachment of the insulinoma to the pancreatic tissue can be controlled with ties, clips, or use of energy device such as a Harmonic scalpel. The large bleeding vessels could be treated with a suture ligature. Even lesions as large as 4 to 5 cm when they are exophytic off the surface can be enucleated as long as they are not near the main pancreatic duct such that all exocrine pancreas duct branches are controlled to prevent postoperative fistula.

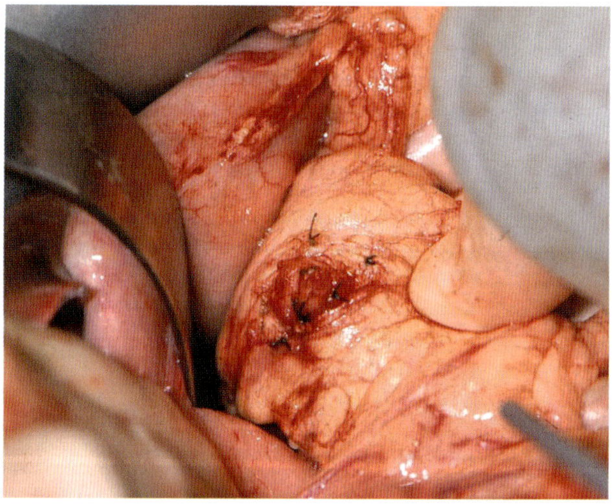

FIG 8 • Enucleation of the insulinoma seen in **FIG 6**. Ultrasound confirms the lesion does not abut the pancreatic duct and the insulinoma is enucleated on the capsule of the tumor.

- Enucleation of an insulinoma that is deep in the parenchyma and not seen by inspection requires continuous use of intraoperative ultrasound. Generally, insulinomas are softer in terms of their substance compared to the tissue density of the normal pancreas and therefore, unless lesions are quite large, they cannot be felt by manual palpation with a finger behind and a finger in front of the pancreas. Ultrasound is used to mark the precise location of the lesion and the distance from the pancreatic surface to the closest margin of the insulinoma can be accurately measured to know exactly how deep to go for an enucleation (**FIG 9**). In general, a cruciate incision centered

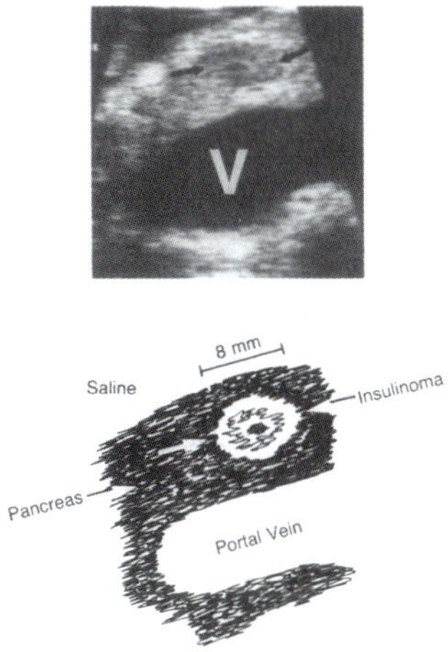

FIG 9 ● The *top panel* shows an image from an intraoperative ultrasound demonstrating the hypoechoic insulinoma indicated by the *black arrows*. The drawing on the *lower panel* shows the 8-mm insulinoma and the precise distance between the tumor and the underlying portal vein.

right over the mass is made using an energy device such as a Harmonic scalpel. Any sizable vessels are controlled with small hemoclips or ties as needed. Ultrasound is continuously used to monitor the progress of the enucleation to make certain the defect in the pancreas is aimed toward the tumor until the capsule of the insulinoma is seen. Once a small surface area of the tumor is definitely visualized, ultrasound becomes unnecessary as the tumor enucleation is completed, staying right on the capsule of the lesion just as for lesions located on the surface (**FIG 10**). Again, specific knowledge of the main pancreatic duct anatomy is crucial as an injury to the main duct by either making a defect in it or transecting it may lead

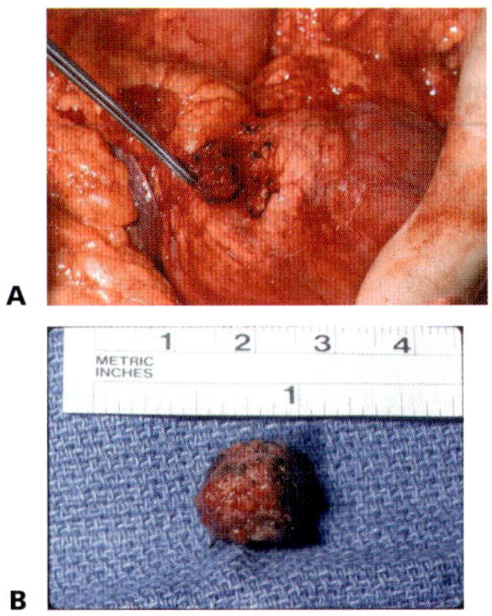

FIG 10 ● **A.** Enucleation of an insulinoma from the deep tissue of the head of the pancreas. Once the capsule of the insulinoma is seen, intraoperative ultrasound is no longer needed to guide the dissection. **B.** Intact pancreatic head insulinoma after enucleation. Small amounts of pancreatic parenchyma are attached to the lesion.

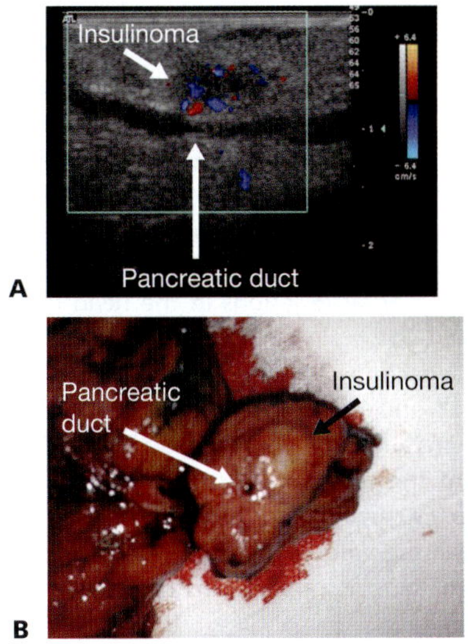

FIG 11 ● The patient had a small midbody insulinoma seen by CT scan. Intraoperative ultrasound **(A)** shows the insulinoma clearly but it indents the main pancreatic duct. Color Doppler ultrasound identifies the duct as there is no blood flow and the insulinoma is hypervascular. Due to the proximity of the main pancreatic duct to the insulinoma, a distal pancreatectomy was performed. **B** shows the insulinoma bordering a mildly dilated pancreatic duct. If the insulinoma was enucleated, there would be a high likelihood of a significant pancreatic leak.

to a significant pancreatic or cutaneous fistula that may require reoperation.

- For larger lesions or lesions that abut or distort the main pancreatic duct located in the body and tail of the pancreas, there is no question that the appropriate operation is a distal pancreatectomy (**FIG 11**). Again, intraoperative ultrasound is used to map the transection of the pancreas to the right of the lesion to get a margin. This resection can be either spleen preserving or a distal pancreatectomy plus splenectomy, depending on the preference of the operating surgeon. There are some minor advantages of preserving the spleen in adult patients but the incidence of postsplenectomy sepsis is exceedingly rare. Again, the location of the lesion is mapped out or if it is not visible on the surface, mapped using ultrasound. Distal pancreatectomy is generally done by dissecting the short gastric vessels along the greater curvature of the stomach using an energy device. At this point, when doing a distal pancreatectomy plus splenectomy, a large silk tie is placed around the splenic artery at the site of pancreatic transection to control blood inflow to the spleen. The lateral margins of the spleen are divided and the spleen and tail of the pancreas are reflected medially. The spleen and tail and body of the pancreas are reflected up and to the right off the left adrenal gland to the point of the targeted pancreatic transection line. The artery is then double ligated and divided, and the splenic vein is either stapled separately with vascular staples or stapled with the stapling device used to transect the pancreas.

A gas-powered stapler in which pressure can slowly be applied over 30 to 60 seconds to close the jaws of the stapling device minimizes fracturing the pancreatic parenchyma before firing the stapler load. Always inspect the margin and ensure complete excision of the insulinoma either by cutting into the pancreas on the back table or by having the pathologist do a gross evaluation of the specimen.

- Only for very large lesions in the head of the pancreas that abut the main pancreatic duct would a pancreaticoduodenectomy be performed for a benign insulinoma (**FIGS 11** and **12**). A Whipple procedure for insulinoma is a generally relatively straightforward procedure in terms of the resection portion as major vascular structures are virtually never invaded and can be done with pylorus-preserving technique. It may be somewhat more challenging to do the reconstruction as these patients typically have normal-sized pancreatic duct and bile duct, as even large insulinomas do not cause ductal obstruction, as well as a soft normal pancreas increasing the incidence of pancreatic leak.
- The most challenging situation for a surgeon is to be in the operating room and to be unable to identify the insulinoma.[17] Understanding the correct interpretation of the biochemical diagnosis of insulinoma should avoid the pitfall of operating on a patient who does not have the disease, which is a procedure obviously destined for failure. Historically, performance of a stepwise blind distal pancreatectomy with interval checks of blood glucose was advocated by some. In the era of high-resolution ultrasound, this blind resection of tissue should never be done. The key to success in this situation is the use of intraoperative ultrasound and evaluating areas where small insulinomas may be difficult to identify. Specifically, the very tip of the pancreatic tail lateral to the spleen, the uncinate process adjacent to the superior mesenteric vein, and the neck of the pancreas under the vascular bridge between the right gastroepiploic middle colic vessels should be closely examined.
- In the unusual or rare case of a malignant insulinoma, tumor debulking may be very beneficial in terms of controlling hypoglycemic symptoms. In general, this would require either a pancreaticoduodenectomy or distal pancreatectomy to remove the primary lesion and lymph node metastases. If there is limited number of liver metastasis, simultaneous liver resection or ablation may be performed. Chemoembolization also has benefit in controlling the hormone output from these hypervascular lesions and benefits the patients in terms of hypoglycemic control.

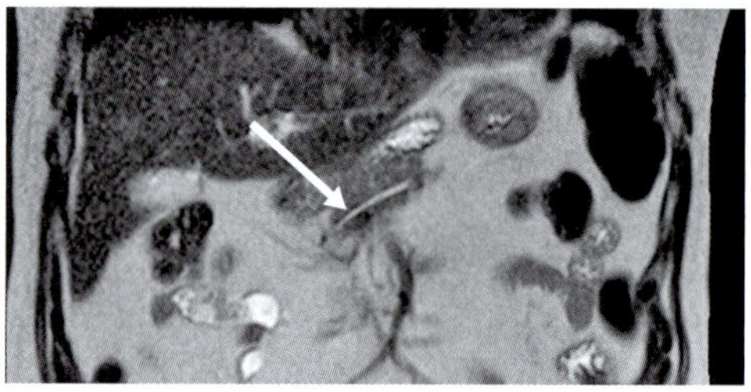

FIG 12 ● A coronal MRI scan shows a 2-cm insulinoma in close proximity to the main pancreatic duct in the head of the pancreas *(white arrow)*. After confirmation of the duct by intraoperative ultrasound, a pylorus-preserving pancreaticoduodenectomy was performed.

LAPAROSCOPIC RESECTION OF INSULINOMAS

- Although the majority of insulinomas are excised using standard open techniques described earlier, several surgeons have reported successful excision of insulinomas using laparoscopic techniques over the past two decades.[19–21] The precise location of the insulinoma and the success of preoperative localization studies are the keys to patient selection for laparoscopic excision.
- Insulinomas located in the body and proximal tail are the ones that are best approached by laparoscopy. Patients are positioned supine and a 30-degree scope is used in a central periumbilical port. The gastrocolic ligament is divided and the omentum and stomach are retracted superiorly to expose the pancreas at the base of the lesser sac. Laparoscopic ultrasound is used in an identical manner to intraoperative ultrasound in open procedures both to identify the insulinoma and the main pancreatic duct. Either enucleation or distal pancreatectomy is chosen based on tumor location again with the same decision-making process as in open procedures.
- Several studies, including a meta-analysis, have confirmed that laparoscopic removal of insulinomas is safe and has advantages over open excision. In institutional comparative studies, there was no difference in operative time, overall cure rate (which is uniformly 100%), and the incidence of pancreatic fistula. Length of hospital stay and blood loss generally favors laparoscopic excision. For surgeons who have experience in managing insulinomas and who have advanced laparoscopic skills, selected patients should have their insulinomas resected laparoscopically. However, as opposed to adrenalectomy in which video-assisted techniques are absolutely the standard of care, insulinoma procedures are much less common and the majority of procedures are still done with an open technique.

PEARLS AND PITFALLS

Indications	▪ Confirm definitive biochemical diagnosis by review of primary laboratory reports including glucose levels with simultaneous insulin, proinsulin, and C-peptide levels. ▪ Insist on a 72-hour monitored fast with appropriate documentation of symptoms and biochemical disease in patients with equivocal diagnosis and negative imaging.
Imaging	▪ Obtain cross-sectional imaging with either contrast-enhanced CT scan or MRI scan to look for hypervascular lesion. ▪ For image-negative patients, have endoscopic ultrasound performed by skilled invasive gastroenterologist. ▪ If definitive diagnosis and negative imaging by CT and endoscopic ultrasound (EUS), consider calcium-stimulated angiogram with hepatic vein sampling.
Exposure of pancreas	▪ Expose head and uncinate process by doing a complete Kocher maneuver all the way to the fourth portion of the duodenum. ▪ Expose body and tail by dividing gastrocolic ligament and reflecting omentum and stomach superiorly and colon inferiorly. ▪ Expose tip of pancreatic tail by dividing lateral attachments of the spleen.
Resection	▪ Be certain to have intraoperative ultrasound available to evaluate the insulinoma and the proximity of the main pancreatic duct. ▪ Decide between enucleation versus segmental pancreatectomy based on tumor size and relationship to the pancreatic duct.
Enucleation techniques	▪ For surface lesions, stay right on the capsule of the insulinoma using energy device or clips to divide and seal tissue. ▪ For deep lesions, continuously monitor progress with intraoperative ultrasound as pancreatic parenchyma is divided.

POSTOPERATIVE MANAGEMENT AFTER INSULINOMA RESECTION

- After excision of the entire insulinoma, patients recover almost instantaneously in terms of their glucose metabolism. Typically, blood sugars may rise to between 150 and 200 mg/dL or higher in the recovery room and for the first 24 to 48 hours, patients should be placed on appropriate sliding scale of insulin. It is certainly possible and has been reported that resection of an insulinoma may unmask a patient who has developed diabetes but the majority of these patients correct and normalize their glucose metabolism within 2 to 3 days.[22,23]
- The major postoperative complication from either a distal pancreatectomy or enucleation, either laparoscopic or open, is a pancreatic fistula.[24] The standard practice is to leave a closed suction drain adjacent to the enucleation site or the staple line and to leave that in until the patient is eating at least a low-fat diet. The color and character of the drain fluid can be monitored. If it is a serosanguineous color, it is likely to have a low pancreatic amylase content. Pancreatic fistulas normally present with a dishwater-gray discoloration and can be confirmed by measuring drain content amylase levels. Standard maneuvers to decrease pancreas secretion including nonfat diets or even using total parenteral nutrition should decrease pancreatic fistula outputs.

OUTCOMES AND ALTERNATIVES TREATMENT TO SURGERY FOR TREATMENT OF INSULINOMA

- In virtually all of the surgical series resecting insulinoma, there is uniformly a 100% long-term cure rate after excision of these small benign lesions.[3,4,25] The only exception would be inability to identify an occult insulinoma resulting in immediate operative failure. Because the vast majority of patients are cured by surgery, there has been no impetus to use nonsurgical treatments. Two percutaneous or endoscopic techniques have been reported.
- Ethanol injection to ablate insulinomas[26] and radiofrequency ablation[27] of lesions may provide nonsurgical resolution of hypoglycemic symptoms. Only for very selected patients who are poor surgical candidates should these ablative techniques be offered.

REFERENCES

1. Okabayashi T, Shima Y, Sumiyoshi T, et al. Diagnosis and management of insulinoma. *World J Gastroenterol*. 2013;19(6):829–837.
2. Mathur A, Gorden P, Libutti SK. Insulinoma. *Surg Clin North Am*. 2009;89:1105–1121.
3. Zhao YP, Zhan HX, Zhang TP, et al. Surgical management of patients with insulinomas: result of 292 cases in a single institution. *J Surg Oncol*. 2011;103:169–174.
4. Nikfarjam M, Warshaw AL, Axelrod L, et al. Improved contemporary surgical management of insulinomas. A 25 year experience of the Massachusetts General Hospital. *Ann Surg*. 1008;247:165–172.
5. Krampitz GW, Norton JA. Pancreatic neuroendocrine tumors. *Curr Prob Surg*. 2013;50:509–545.
6. Van Heerden JA, Edis AJ, Service FJ. The surgical aspects of insulinomas. *Ann Surg*. 1979;189(6):677–682.
7. Service FJ. Diagnostic approach to adults with hypoglycemic disorders. *Endocrinol Metab Clin North Am*. 1999;28(3):519–532.
8. Nauck MA, Meler JJ. Diagnostic accuracy of an "amended" insulin-glucose ratio for the biochemical diagnosis of insulinoma. *Ann Int Med*. 2012;157:767–775.
9. Van Bon A, Benhadi N, Endert E, et al. Evaluation of endocrine tests. D: the prolonged fasting test for insulinoma. *Neth J Med*. 2009;67(7):274–278.

10. Hirshberg B, Livi A, Bartlett DL, et al. Forty-eight hour fast: the diagnostic test for insulinoma. *J Clin Endocrinol Metab*. 2000;85(9):3222–3226.
11. Thompson GB, Service FJ, Andrews JC, et al. Noninsulinoma pancreatogenous hypoglycemia syndrome: an update in 10 surgically treated patients. *Surgery*. 2000;128:937–945.
12. McAuley G, Delaney H, Colville J, et al. Multimodality preoperative imaging of pancreatic insulinomas. *Clin Radiol*. 2005;60:1039–1050.
13. Atiq M, Bhutani MS, Bektas M, et al. EUS-FNA for pancreatic neuroendocrine tumors: a tertiary cancer center experience. *Dig Dis Sci*. 2012;57:791–800.
14. Tessonnier L, Sebag F, Ghander C, et al. Limited value of 18F-F-DOPA PET to localize pancreatic insulin-secreting tumors in adults with hyperinsulinemic hypoglycemia. *Endocrinol Metab*. 2010;95:303–307.
15. Christ E, Wild D, Forrer F, et al. Glucagon-like peptide-1 receptor imaging for localization of insulinomas. *J Clin Endocrinol Metab*. 2009;94:3298–4405.
16. Abboud B, Boujaoude J. Occult sporadic insulinoma: localization and surgical strategy. *World J Gastroenterol*. 2008;15(5):657–665.
17. Rostambeigi N, Thompson GB. What should be done in an operating room when an insulinoma cannot be found? *Clin Endocrinol*. 2009;70:512–515.
18. Guettier JM, Kam A, Chang R, et al. Localization of insulinomas to regions of the pancreas by intraarterial calcium stimulation: the NIH experience. *J Clin Endocrinol Metab*. 2009;94:1074–1080.
19. Hu M, Zhao G, Luo Y, et al. Laparoscopic versus open treatment for benign pancreatic insulinomas: an analysis of 89 cases. *Surg Endosc*. 2011;25:3831–3837.
20. Richards ML, Thompson GB, Farley DR, et al. Setting the bar for laparoscopic resection of sporadic insulinoma. *World J Surg*. 2011;35:785–789.
21. Su AP, Ke NW, Zhang Y, et al. Is laparoscopic approach for pancreatic insulinomas safe? Results of a systematic review and meta-analysis. *J Surg Res*. 2014;186:126–134.
22. Crippa S, Zerbi A, Boninsegna L, et al. Surgical management of insulinomas. Short- and long-term outcomes after enucleations and pancreatic resections. *Arch Surg*. 2012;147(1):261–266.
23. Roland CL, Lo CY, Miller BS, et al. Surgical approach and perioperative complications determine short-term outcomes in patients with insulinoma: results of a bi-institutional study. *Ann Surg Oncol*. 2008;15(12):3532–3527.
24. Zhao YP, Zhan HX, Cong L, et al. Risk factors for postoperative pancreatic fistula in patients with insulinomas: analysis of 292 consecutive cases. *Hepatobiliary Pancreat Dis Int*. 2012;11:102–106.
25. Placzkowski KA, Vella A, Thompson GB, et al. Secular trends in the presentation and management of functioning insulinoma at the Mayo Clinic, 1987-2007. *J Clin Endocrinol Metab*. 2009;94(4):1069–1073.
26. Levy MJ, Thompson GB, Topazian MD, et al. US-guided ethanol ablation of insulinomas: a new treatment option. *Gastrointest Endosc*. 2012;75(1):200–206.
27. Procházka V, Hlavsa J, Andrašina T, et al. Laparoscopic radiofrequency ablation of functioning pancreatic insulinoma: video case report. *Surg Laparosc Endosc Percutan Tech*. 2012;22(5):312–215.

Chapter 52 Surgery for Glucagonoma

Richard A. Prinz Catherine A. Madorin

DEFINITION

- Glucagonomas are pancreatic neuroendocrine tumors (PNETs) that arise from the glucagon-secreting alpha islet cells of the pancreas. They are very rare with an estimated incidence of 1/20,000,000 individuals.[1] Most are sporadic but 10% are associated with multiple endocrine neoplasia type 1 (MEN-1) syndrome.[2] Most glucagonomas are large (>5 cm) at diagnosis, with 70% to 90% of patients presenting with metastatic disease.[3] Operative treatment of a glucagonoma involves resection of the primary tumor as well as metastatic disease for cure when possible or to palliate hormonal or local symptoms.

PATIENT HISTORY AND PHYSICAL FINDINGS

- Glucagonoma is classically associated with the 4 "Ds": dermatitis, diabetes, depression, and deep vein thrombosis.
- The skin lesions associated with a glucagonoma are termed necrolytic migratory erythema and are pathognomonic for glucagonoma. It is a pruritic rash that occurs in the lower abdomen, lower extremities, perineum, perioral area, and feet (**FIGS 1** and **2**). It is seen in approximately 70% of patients and may be the initial presentation of the tumor.[4]
- Glucose intolerance is often mild and insulin administration usually is not required.
- Weight loss is often out of proportion to the amount of tumor burden and is due to the catabolic effect of excess glucagon.
- Stomatitis, glossitis, and diarrhea are other frequent findings.
- Psychiatric manifestations may include depression, anxiety, and psychoses.
- Glucagonoma creates a hypercoagulable state, and 30% of patients will experience a thromboembolic event.[5]
- A thorough personal and family history should be taken, with particular interest in other endocrinopathies because glucagonomas may be associated with MEN-1. Glucagonomas may also secrete secondary hormones, which may lead to Zollinger-Ellison syndrome in up to 10% of patients. Less commonly, they may secrete vasoactive intestinal polypeptide (VIP), pancreatic polypeptide, somatostatin, or adrenocorticotropic hormone (ACTH).[6]

DIAGNOSIS

- Diagnosis is confirmed by high levels of fasting serum glucagon (>1,000 pg/mL; normal, <150 pg/mL). Other conditions that cause hyperglucagonemia include hepatic insufficiency, stress, sepsis, and starvation, but levels rarely reach beyond 500 pg/mL.

IMAGING

- Glucagonomas are typically greater than 5 cm at time of diagnosis and are easier to localize preoperatively than most PNETs. Most glucagonomas are located in the body or tail of the pancreas. Rarely, they may be located outside the pancreas in the duodenal wall, accessory pancreatic tissue, or the kidney.
- Triple-phase computed tomography (CT) scan is the first-line localization study. Somatostatin receptor scintigraphy (SRS) can also be used and can identify extraabdominal spread to lymph nodes and liver.
- Endoscopic ultrasound (EUS), visceral angiography, and portal venous sampling may be required for glucagonomas that are difficult to identify, but this is very unusual.

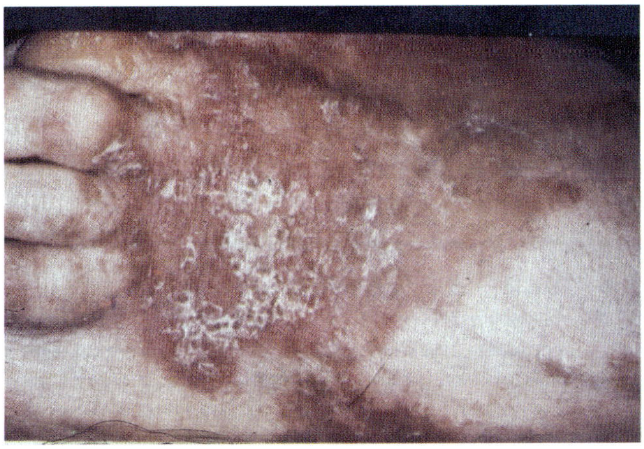

FIG 1 • Necrolytic migratory erythema of the lower extremity.

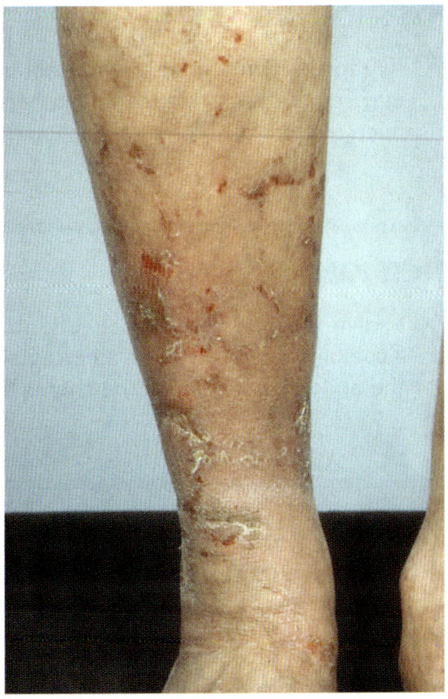

FIG 2 • Necrolytic migratory erythema of the lower extremity.

SURGICAL MANAGEMENT

- The goal of operative management of glucagonoma is an R0 resection including the primary tumor and all metastases. Patients who cannot undergo R0 resection benefit from tumor debulking because it can palliate symptoms due to excess glucagon by decreasing the levels of circulating hormone.
- If the tumor is limited to the pancreas, surgical resection can completely reverse all clinical manifestations of a glucagonoma. This demands a formal pancreatic resection due to the large size of the tumors, usually a distal pancreatectomy with or without splenectomy. Pancreaticoduodenectomy is required for tumors in the head of the gland. Resection should include peripancreatic lymph node dissection. Although smaller tumors may be technically amenable to enucleation, the high malignant potential of these tumors suggests caution with this approach (**FIG 3**).
- All nodal and hepatic metastases that can be safely removed should be excised. Hepatic metastases may be managed by either wedge resection or formal hepatic resection.
- Tumor debulking leads to a dramatic improvement in symptoms and the hormonal manifestations of glucagonoma may be diminished for years. Repeat debulking of recurrent disease may also prolong survival.
- In patients with MEN-1, consideration must be given to the presence of other functional and nonfunctional PNETs. If hyperparathyroidism is present as a component of the MEN-1 syndrome, it should be treated before addressing the pancreatic tumor to avoid problems with postoperative hypercalcemia.

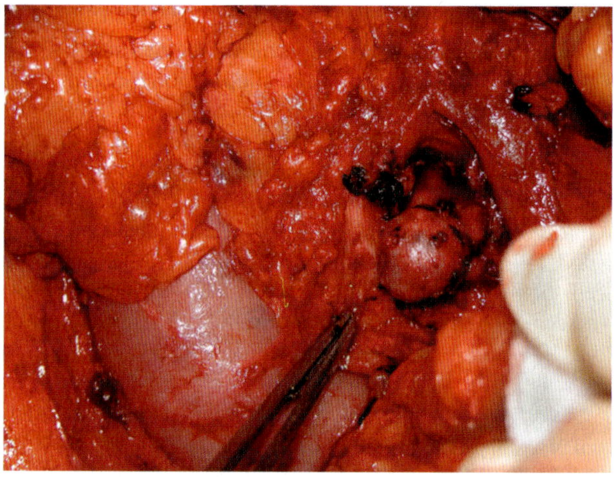

FIG 3 • Small glucagonomas (<2 cm) with no malignant features can be enucleated from the pancreas using cautery or an energy device to control bleeding. Intraoperative ultrasound should be used to avoid injury to the pancreatic duct.

Preoperative Planning

- Preoperative management is focused on treating the metabolic effects of excess glucagon and preventing or treating venous thromboembolism.
- Somatostatin analogue therapy with octreotide is titrated to symptomatic improvement. Total parenteral nutrition (TPN) may be needed if marked cachexia is present and may also help ameliorate necrolytic migratory erythema.
- Hyperglycemia and diabetes, when present, should be controlled.
- Patients should receive anticoagulation with Coumadin or low-molecular-weight heparin at the time of diagnosis. Preoperative placement of an inferior vena cava (IVC) filter may be necessary in patients with a history of thrombosis.

TECHNIQUES

POSITIONING

- As most patients present with metastatic disease and may require both pancreatic and hepatic resection, an open approach is preferred. For tumors confined to the pancreas, a laparoscopic approach may be possible. The open approach will be first described here.
- The patient is placed supine with arms either extended laterally or tucked according to surgeon preference.

INCISION

- Midline laparotomy, extended left subcostal, chevron, or a combination of these are all acceptable approaches to the abdomen and should be chosen based on surgeon preference and experience, the body habitus of the patient, and the possible need for hepatic or other organ resection.

DISTAL PANCREATECTOMY WITHOUT SPLENECTOMY

- After the abdomen has been explored, the lesser sac is entered by separating the greater omentum from the transverse colon. The short gastric vessels must be preserved to provide blood flow to the spleen.
- Mobilize the posterior wall of the stomach off the anterior surface of the pancreas and retract the stomach cephalad. The stomach may be held in place with retractors or stay sutures. The anterior body and tail of the pancreas should now be fully exposed (**FIG 4**).
- Incise the peritoneum along the inferior border of the pancreas along the length of the body and tail.

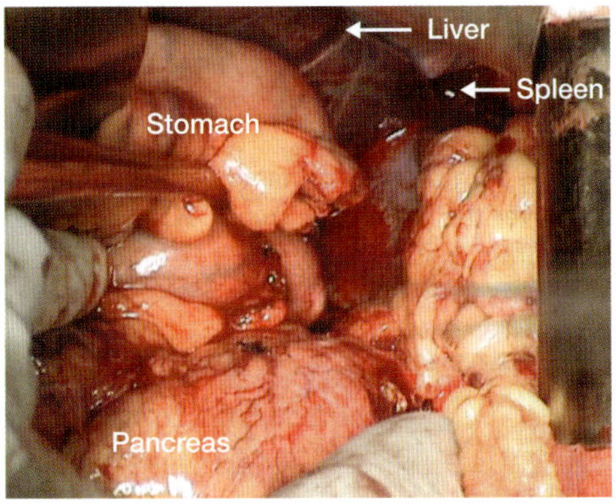

FIG 4 ● The anterior surface of the body and tail of the pancreas is exposed by entering the lesser sac thru the gastrocolic omentum and retracting the stomach cephalad.

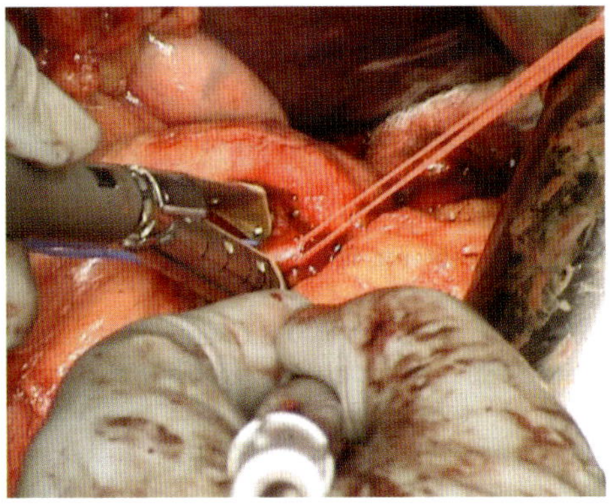

FIG 6 ● The splenic artery and vein are ligated with a vascular stapler as shown. Ligatures or suture ligatures may also be used according to surgeon preference.

Gently elevate the pancreas off the retroperitoneum using blunt dissection along the avascular plane.

- The splenic artery and vein, which run along the superior border of the pancreas (the vein runs posterior to the artery), will be elevated along with the rest of the pancreas.
- Determine the point of transection for the pancreas. This should be just to the left of the superior mesenteric vein in the pancreatic neck.
- Bluntly develop a plane between the splenic vessels and the pancreas at the point of transection. Place vessel loops around the splenic vessels to facilitate retraction and provide vascular control (FIG 5).
- Ligate the splenic artery and vein individually—ligatures, suture ligatures, or a vascular stapler (as shown) can be used according to surgeon preference (FIG 6).
- Divide the pancreas using a stapler with a vascular load. Multiple firings may be required (FIG 7). If there is bleeding from the staple line, place 2-0 sutures in a figure-of-eight pattern at the superior and inferior borders of the pancreas to secure the gastropancreatic arteries.
- Ligate, clip, or use an energy device to control the numerous small, short vessels connecting the splenic vessels to the pancreas along the entire body and tail. Control any bleeding that occurs on the splenic artery or vein with fine Prolene sutures.
- As the splenic vessels approach the hilum, they will branch into multiple tributaries. Care must be taken to avoid injury to these branches along the tail of the pancreas. The hilum of the spleen may be directly abutting or within 1 cm of the tail of the pancreas. Once fully dissected off the vessels, the specimen may be removed.
- Check the surgical bed for hemostasis. Omentum may be placed over the pancreatic stump. Placement of a closed suction drain is our preference.

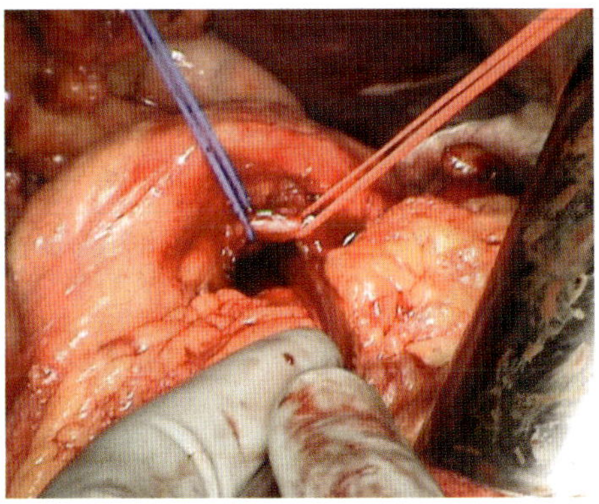

FIG 5 ● A plane is developed between the superior border of the pancreas and the splenic flexure at the point of transaction. Vessel loops are placed around the splenic vessels for retraction and vascular control.

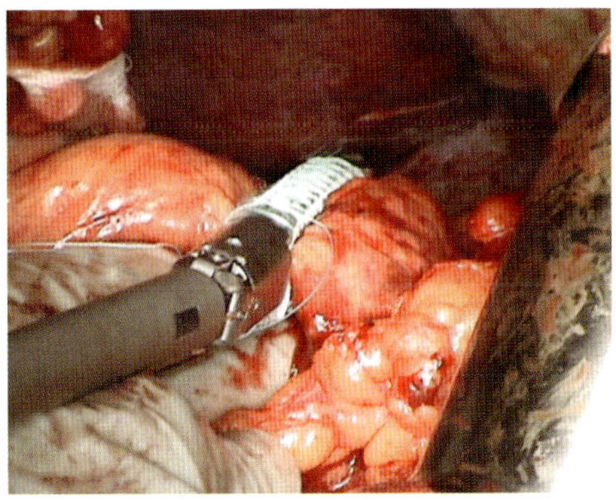

FIG 7 ● The pancreas is divided using a stapler with a vascular load.

DISTAL PANCREATECTOMY WITH SPLENECTOMY

- The exposure and mobilization of the pancreas proceed as described earlier.
- Divide the short gastric vessels.
- Mobilize the splenic flexure of the colon and retract it inferiorly.
- Divide the splenophrenic and splenocolic ligaments, and reflect the spleen and pancreatic body and tail up from the retroperitoneum.
- Once the point of transection of the pancreas has been determined, carefully isolate the splenic artery and vein and ligate them individually.
- Mobilize the splenic vessels along with the superior border of the pancreas.
- Divide the pancreas using a stapler with a vascular load. Multiple firings may be required. If there is bleeding from the staple line, place 2-0 sutures in a figure-of-eight pattern at the superior and inferior borders of the pancreas to secure the gastropancreatic arteries.
- The pancreas and spleen are then removed as specimen (**FIG 8**).
- Check the surgical bed for hemostasis. Omentum may be placed over the pancreatic stump. Placement of a closed suction drain is our preference.

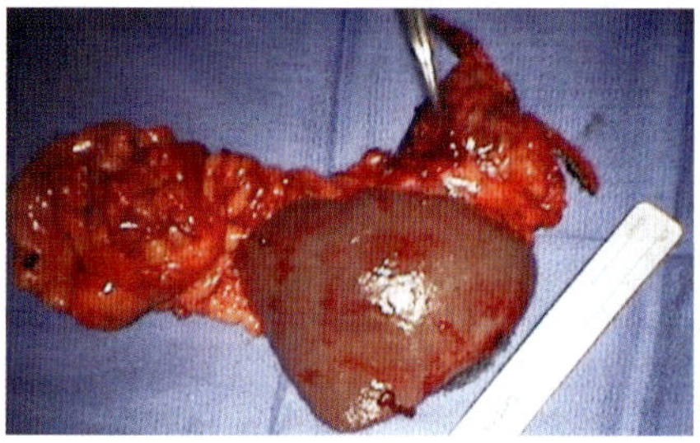

FIG 8 ● The body and tail of the pancreas have been removed en bloc. The instrument points to the tumor.

LAPAROSCOPIC DISTAL PANCREATECTOMY

Positioning and Port Placement

- Laparoscopic distal pancreatectomy is a suitable approach for patients with localized disease confined to the pancreas.
- The patient is placed supine.
- A 5- to 12-mm port is placed infraumbilically.
- A diagnostic laparoscopy is performed and so is a laparoscopic ultrasound of the liver.
- Any suspicious lesions are biopsied and sent for frozen section analysis. If metastatic disease or invasion into surrounding organs is identified, conversion to an open operation should be considered.
- Additional trocars are as shown in the figure (**FIG 9**).
- The anterior wall of the stomach is elevated and the lesser sac is entered through the gastrocolic ligament using an energy device.

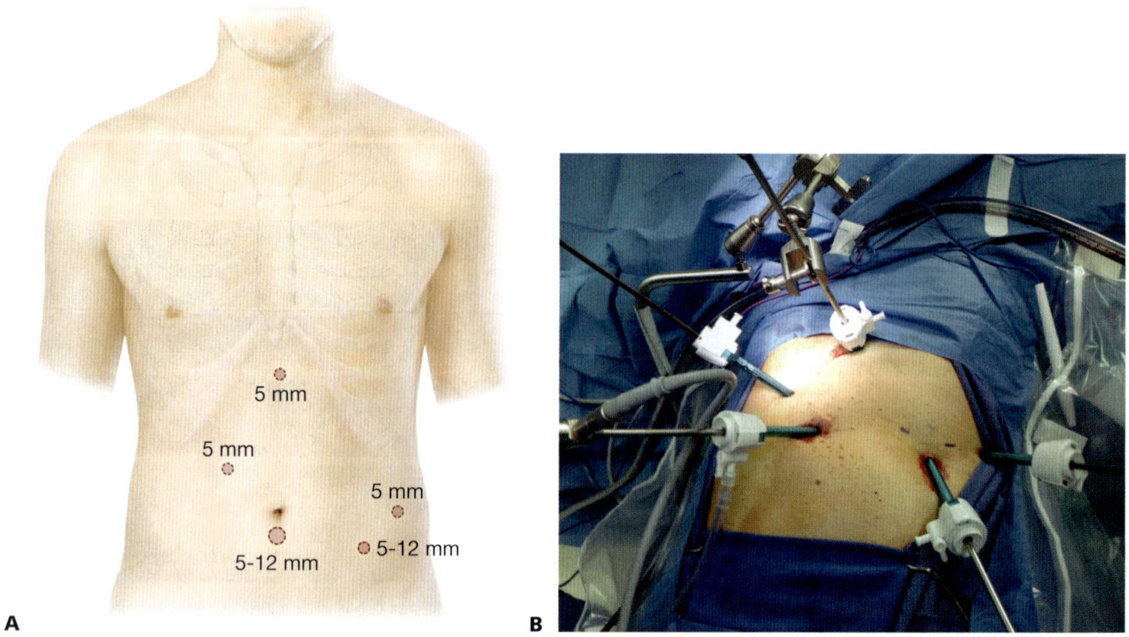

FIG 9 ● **A,B.** The position of the trocars for laparoscopic distal pancreatectomy is shown. A 5- to 12-mm trocar is placed at the umbilicus. A 5-mm trocar is placed subxiphoid for retraction. An optional assistant working port (5 mm) is placed in the right upper quadrant. Two working trocars, a 5- to 12-mm and another 5-mm, are placed in the left abdomen as shown. Trocar placement may be individualized for the patient.

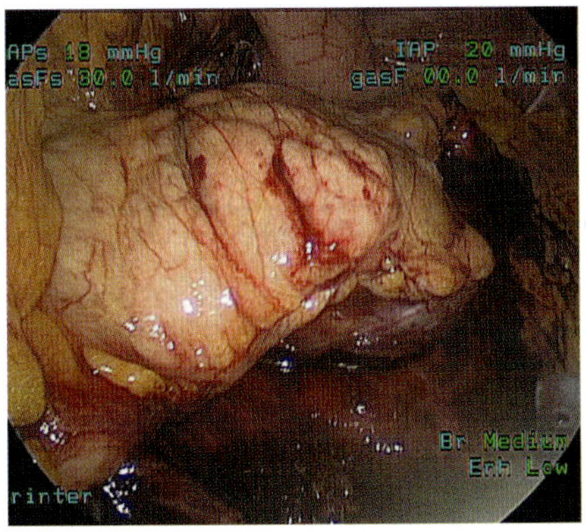

FIG 10 ● After entering the lesser sac through the gastrocolic ligament, the stomach is retracted superiorly and the transverse colon is mobilized inferiorly to expose the anterior surface of the pancreas.

- The splenic flexure of the colon is mobilized inferiorly and the transverse mesocolon is dissected away from the inferior border of the pancreas, allowing visualization of the anterior surface of the pancreas and the splenic artery (**FIG 10**).
- Laparoscopic ultrasound is used to delineate the extent of the tumor and the proximal position for transecting the pancreas. In the medial to lateral technique, the splenic vessels are isolated and circumferentially dissected at the proposed transaction site.
- The splenic artery and splenic vein are individually divided using an endoscopic stapler with a 2- to 2.5-mm cartridge as determined by the vessel size. The splenic vein may need to be transected with the pancreatic parenchyma.
- The peritoneum on the inferior edge of the pancreas is incised and dorsal dissection of the pancreas is done to create a window for placement of the stapler.
- The pancreas is then divided with a linear stapler cutter with a vascular cartridge sized to the thickness of the pancreas (**FIG 11**). The pancreas and spleen are then mobilized in a retrograde fashion from left to right.
- The specimen is placed in a plastic retrieval bag and the umbilical port incision is extended to allow its removal (**FIG 12**).
- This incision is closed and the abdominal cavity is reinsufflated and irrigated and hemostasis confirmed.
- A closed suction drain is placed through the most lateral port in the left upper quadrant down to the pancreatic sump and fixed to the skin with sutures.
- The trocars are removed under direct vision and all port sites are closed with absorbable sutures.

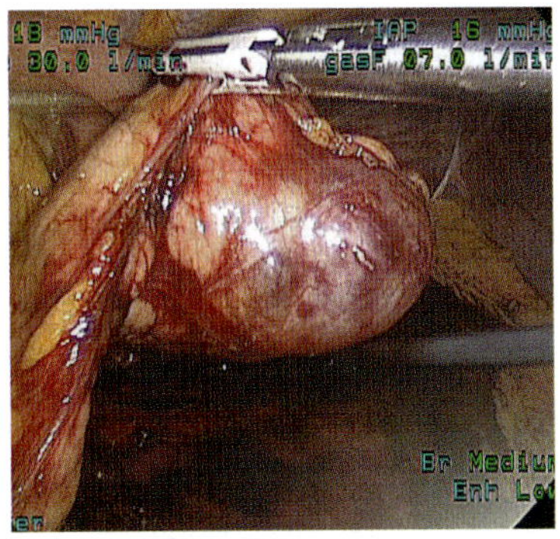

FIG 12 ● When the specimen has been completely dissected free, it is elevated and placed in a plastic retrieval bag.

Management of Hepatic Metastases

- Both curative intent resection and palliative intent resection are recommended for malignant glucagonoma (**FIG 13**). Other treatment options include hepatic artery occlusion or embolization, radiofrequency ablation, and cryoablation.
- Regional lymphadenectomy should be done because lymph node metastases are common.

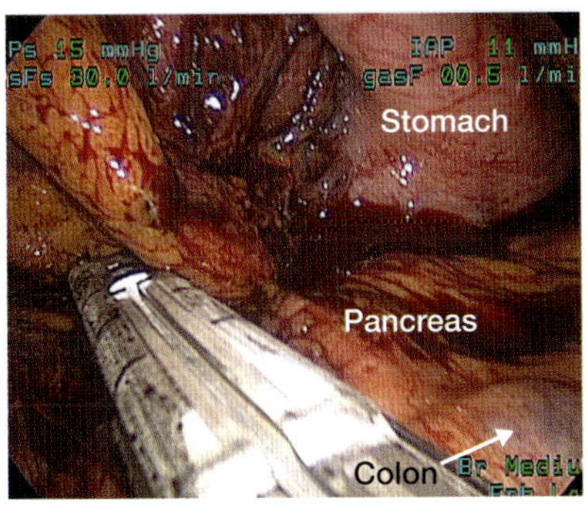

FIG 11 ● The pancreas is then divided with a linear stapler cutter with a vascular cartridge sized to the thickness of the pancreas. If the splenic vein could not be separated from the pancreas and individually ligated, it can be included with the pancreas transection.

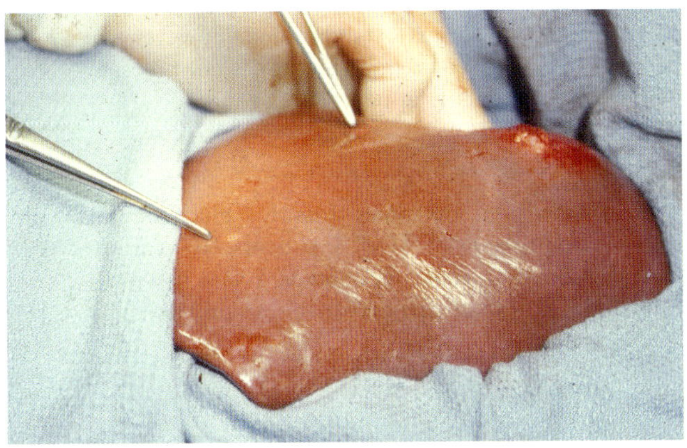

FIG 13 ● Glucagonoma metastases to the liver.

PEARLS AND PITFALLS

- MEN-1 patients with glucagonomas should have hyperparathyroidism addressed before surgical treatment for glucagonoma. Failure to do so may lead to uncontrolled hypercalcemia postoperatively.
- Although some tumors may be amenable to enucleation, formal pancreatic resection is preferred due to the high malignant potential of glucagonomas.
- Glucagonomas are associated with hypercoagulability and 30% of patients will have a deep vein thrombosis (DVT). Anticoagulation is recommended and serious consideration should be given to IVC filter placement preoperatively.
- Even if an R0 resection is not possible, patients may benefit tremendously from extensive debulking for palliation of symptoms.
- When performing a spleen-preserving distal pancreatectomy, care must be taken to avoid trauma to branches off the splenic vessels as you approach the tail of the pancreas. Remember, if extensive bleeding is encountered, the procedure can be changed to a distal pancreatectomy with splenectomy.
- Large tumors in the body of the pancreas may involve the splenic vein. In this situation, it may be helpful to divide the pancreatic neck early to better visualize the splenoportal confluence. If necessary, the splenic vein may be ligated flush with the superior mesenteric vein (SMV).
- The left adrenal may be located more superiorly than expected and may be injured by excessive medial retraction of the pancreas and spleen.
- Laparoscopic pancreatectomy without laparoscopic ultrasound is not recommended. Failure to use a laparoscopic ultrasound may result in a specimen that lacks part or all of the tumor.
- Pancreatic stump leak/fistula is one of the most common postoperative complications and may occur in up to 30% of patients. Consider octreotide for patients who do not respond to closed suction drainage or have high-output fistula. However, routine use of perioperative octreotide will not reduce the rate of fistula.

POSTOPERATIVE CARE

- Admission to the intensive care unit (ICU) is not mandatory and should be decided on a patient-by-patient basis. Management of pain, nasogastric intubation, and diet is similar to most major abdominal resections.
- Closed suction drain output should be tested for amylase and lipase before removal.
- Streptozocin is somewhat effective chemotherapy for both malignant tumors that are incompletely removed and their biochemical effects. Tumor regression is seen in 50% of patients and reduction in serum glucagon levels in over 60% of patients. Dacarbazine (DTIC) has also been used with some efficacy.
- Continued symptoms of excess glucagon after the operation should be treated with a somatostatin analog. However, routine perioperative use of octreotide therapy is not necessary and will not reduce the rate of pancreatic fistula.

OUTCOMES

- There is a paucity of outcomes data for glucagonoma. According to one study of MEN-1 patients, 10-year survival is approximately 50%.[7] In another, 5-year survival is approximately 50% following operative resection and adjuvant chemotherapy.[8]

COMPLICATIONS

- Patients may experience any postoperative complication associated with laparotomy such as superficial or deep wound infection, urinary tract infection, pneumonia, and cardiac dysrhythmia or ischemia.
- The risk of venous thromboembolism is elevated in patients with glucagonoma and the physician should remain vigilant about detection and treatment of thromboembolic events.
- Pancreatic leakage and fistula occur in up to 30% of patients undergoing distal pancreatectomy. This is managed by continued closed suction drainage in the stable patient. In a patient showing signs of infection, a CT scan should be obtained to look for abscess or inadequately controlled fistula. This can usually be treated with an additional percutaneous drain placed with image guidance. Consider octreotide therapy for persistent high-output fistulas. Operative drainage, endoscopic sphincterotomy, or stent placement may be necessary in patients not responding to percutaneous drainage.

REFERENCES

1. Franston S, Bloom SR. Glucagonomas. *Baillieres Clin Gastroenterol.* 1996;10:697–705.
2. Stacpoole PW, Jaspan J, Kasselberg AG, et al. A familial glucagonoma syndrome. Genetic, clinical, and biochemical features. *Am J Med.* 1981;70:1017–1026.
3. Economopoulos P, Christopoulos C. Glaucagonoma. *Ann Gastroenterol.* 2001;14(2):99–108.
4. Wermers RA, Fatourechi V, Wynne AG, et al. The glucagonoma syndrome. Clinical and pathologic features in 21 patients. *Medicine (Baltimore).* 1996;75:53.
5. Stacpole PW. The glucagonoma syndrome: clinical features, diagnosis, and treatment. *Endocr Rev.* 1981;2:347.
6. Wynick D, Williams SJ, Blooms SR. Symptomatic secondary hormone syndromes in patients with established malignant pancreatic endocrine tumors. *N Engl J Med.* 1998;319:605–607.

7. Levy-Bohbot N, Merle C, Goudet P, et al. Prevalence, characteristics, and prognosis of MEN 1-associated glucagonomas, VIPomas, and somatostatinomas: study from the GTE (Group de Tumeurs Endocrines) registry. *Gastroenterol Clin Biol.* 2004;28(11):1075–1081.
8. Lepage C, Ciccolallo L, DeAngelis R, et al. European disparities in malignant digestive endocrine tunmours survival. *Int J Cancer.* 2010; 126(12):2928–2934.

SUGGESTED READINGS

1. Chastain MA. The glucagonoma syndrome: a review of its features and discussion of new perspectives. *Am J Med Sci.* 2001;321(5):306–320.
2. Doherty GM, Jayarajan S. Rare functioning pancreatic endocrine tumors. In: Hubbard JG, Inabnet WB, Lo CY, eds. *Endocrine Surgery: Principles and Practice.* New York, NY: Springer; 2009: 523–532.
3. Doherty GM, Cheng SP. Rare neuroendocrine tumors of the pancreas. In: Sturgeon C, ed. *Endocrine Neoplasia.* New York, NY: Springer; 2010:253–270.
4. Jensen RT, Norton JA. Endocrine tumors of the pancreas and gastrointestinal tract. In: Feldman M, Friedman LS, Brandt LJ, eds. *Sleisenger and Fordtran's Gastrointestinal and Liver Disease.* 9th ed. New York, NY: Elsevier; 2010:505–508.

Index

Page numbers followed by *f* and *t* indicated figures and tables, respectively.

C

D

R

S